FIFTH EDITION

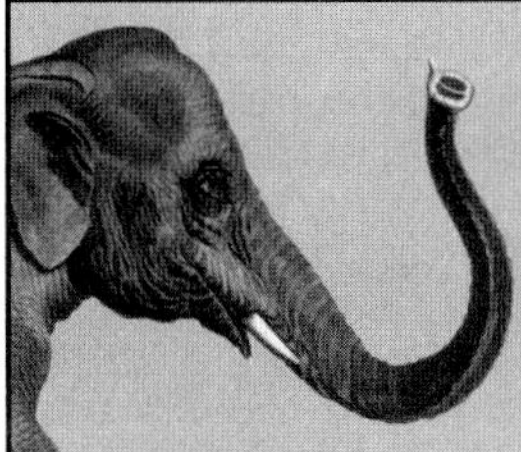

LANGE Q&A™

USMLE STEP 2

Carlyle H. Chan, MD, FAPA
Department of Psychiatry & Behavioral Medicine
Medical College of Wisconsin
Milwaukee, Wisconsin

McGraw-Hill
Medical Publishing Division

New York Chicago San Francisco Lisbon London Madrid Mexico City Milan
New Delhi San Juan Seoul Singapore Sydney Toronto

Lange Q&A™: USMLE Step 2, Fifth Edition

1 2 3 4 5 6 7 8 9 0 QPD/QPD 0 9 8 7 6 5

ISBN: 0-07-144770-9

Notice

Medicine is an ever-changing science. As new research and clinical experience broaden our knowledge, changes in treatment and drug therapy are required. The authors and the publisher of this work have checked with sources believed to be reliable in their efforts to provide information that is complete and generally in accord with the standards accepted at the time of publication. However, in view of the possibility of human error or changes in medical sciences, neither the authors nor the publisher nor any other party who has been involved in the preparation or publication of this work warrants that the information contained herein is in every respect accurate or complete, and they disclaim all responsibility for any errors or omissions or for the results obtained from use of the information contained in this work. Readers are encouraged to confirm the information contained herein with other sources. For example and in particular, readers are advised to check the product information sheet included in the package of each drug they plan to administer to be certain that the information contained in this work is accurate and that changes have not been made in the recommended dose or in the contraindications for administration. This recommendation is of particular importance in connection with new or infrequently used drugs.

This book was set in Palatino by International Typesetting and Composition.
The editor was Catherine A. Johnson.
The production supervisor was Richard Ruzycka.
Project management was provided by International Typesetting and Composition.
Quebecor World Dubuque was printer and binder.

This book is printed on acid-free paper.

Library of Congress Cataloging-in-Publication Data

Lange Q & A. USMLE, step 2 / [edited by] Carlyle H. Chan.
p. ; cm.
Includes bibliographical references and index.
ISBN 0-07-144770-9
1. Clinical medicine—Examinations, questions, etc. 2. Physicians—Licenses—United States—Examinations—Study guides. I. Title: Q & A. II. Title: USMLE, step 2. III. Chan, Carlyle H.
[DNLM: 1. Clinical Medicine—Examination Questions.]
RC58.L355 2005
616'.0076—dc22

2004065626

Contents

Color insert appears between pages 340 and 341.

Contributors

E. James Aiman, MD
Professor of Obstetrics and Gynecology
Medical College of Wisconsin
Froedtert Hospital
Milwaukee, Wisconsin

Ruric C. Anderson, MD
E. Stephen Kurtides Chair of Medical Education
Program Director in the Department of Medicine
Evanston Northwestern Healthcare
Evanston, Illinois

Rainer G. Gedeit, MD
Associate Professor of Pediatrics
Medical College of Wisconsin
Children's Hospital of Wisconsin
Milwaukee, Wisconsin

Seira Kurian, MD, MS, MPH
Assistant Professor
Health Policy Institute
Medical College of Wisconsin
Milwaukee, Wisconsin

Jon A. Lehrmann, MD
Assistant Professor of Psychiatry
Medical College of Wisconsin
Zablocki Veterans Administration Medical Center
Milwaukee, Wisconsin

Leslie F. Martin, MD, MPH
Assistant Professor of Preventive Medicine
Director, Office of International Affairs
Medical College of Wisconsin
Milwaukee, Wisconsin

Philip N. Redlich, MD, PhD
Associate Professor of Surgery
Associate Dean for Curriculum
Medical College of Wisconsin
Milwaukee, Wisconsin

Andrea L. Winthrop, MD
Associate Professor of Surgery
Medical College of Wisconsin
Children's Hospital of Wisconsin
Milwaukee, Wisconsin

Preface

Taking licensing examinations is a stressful but necessary endeavor. Extensive clinical exposure and comprehensive study, including rehearsing the examination process through a review book such as this one, can aid in the preparation. Such reviews can help you identify areas of content weakness as well as provide you an opportunity to familiarize yourself with the test format.

The questions in this book were constructed according to the parameters set forth in the USMLE Step 2 Bulletin. All of the subjects, types of questions, and techniques that will be encountered on the USMLE Step 2 have been updated and presented in this review. In addition to the questions in the six clinical disciplines, we have provided two practice tests covering all areas at the end.

The contributors are experienced educators and clinicians, several of whom have been either clerkship directors or medical student education directors for their respective specialties.

We believe this book will provide you with a valuable tool to assess your readiness to take the exam. We hope you will find the questions, explanations, and format to be of assistance to you in your review. Good luck!

Carlyle H. Chan, MD, FAPA

Review Preparation Guide

This book is designed for those preparing for the United States Medical Licensing Examination (USMLE) Step 2. It provides a comprehensive review, with more than 1000 clinical science multiple-choice questions and referenced, paragraph-length explanations of each answer. The last section of the book consists of two integrated practice tests for self-assessment purposes.

This introduction provides information on question types, question-answering strategies, specifics on the USMLE Step 2, and various ways to use this review.

The United States Medical Licensing Examination Step 2

The USMLE Step 2 is currently a 1-day (8-hours) computerized examination consisting of approximately 400 multiple-choice questions testing your knowledge in the clinical sciences.

Organization of this Book

This book is organized to cover sequentially each of the clinical science areas specified by the National Board of Medical Examiners (NBME). There are six sections, one for each of the clinical sciences, and an integrated practice test section at the end of the review. The sections are as follows:

1. Obstetrics and Gynecology (including biology of reproduction; fetus, placenta, and new-born; primary care of the OB/GYN patient; normal and abnormal clinical obstetrics; clinical gynecology)
2. Pediatrics (focusing on pediatric content and tasks and competencies)
3. Internal Medicine (including infectious disease, immunology, and allergy; diseases of the respiratory, cardiovascular, hematopoietic, gastrointestinal, renal, musculoskeletal, nervous, and integumentary systems; nutritional, metabolic, endocrine, oncologic, and fluid and electrolyte disorders; clinical pharmacology; legal medicine)
4. Surgery (including the general topics of physiology, anesthesiology, wounds, neoplasms, and forensic medicine; specific surgical treatment of the various body systems)
5. Psychiatry (including theories; social, community, and family relationships; assessment techniques; psychopathology; interventions; ethical and legal aspects of psychiatry)
6. Preventive Medicine (including biostatistics, epidemiology, disease control, provision of health services, and ethical and legal aspects of medicine)

7/8. Practice Tests (includes 275 questions from all six clinical sciences presented in an integrated format)

Each section is authored by an experienced teacher in the discipline. However, you will find that the author covers material of a general nature appropriate for Step 2. As a result, the basic concepts of clinical pathophysiology are covered. As in the examination itself, topics that might be classified as general or internal medicine are included in each section.

Each of the eight chapters is organized in the following order:

1. Questions
2. Answers and Explanations
3. References

The Practice tests in Chapters 7 and 8 also include subject lists.

These sections and how you might use them are discussed below.

Question Format

The style and presentation of the questions have been fully revised to conform with the USMLE. This will enable readers to familiarize themselves with the types of questions to be expected and practice answering questions in each format. Following the answer to each question, a reference refers the reader to a particular and easily available text for further reference and reading.

Each chapter contains multiple-choice questions (or *items*). Most of these are one best answer–single-item questions, some are one best answer–matching sets, and some are comparison–matching set questions. In some cases, a group of two or three questions may be related to one situation. In addition, some questions have illustrations (graphs, x-rays, tables, or line drawings) that require understanding and interpretation. Because the USMLE seems to prefer questions requiring judgment and critical thinking in the context of clinical situations, we have attempted to emphasize these questions.

One Best Answer–Single-Item Question. Most of the questions are posed in the A-type, or "one best answer–single-item" format. This is the most popular question format in most exams. It generally consists of a brief statement, followed by five options of which only ONE is entirely correct. The options on the USMLE are lettered A, B, C, D, and E. Although the format for this question type is straightforward, these questions can be difficult, because some of the distractors may be partially right. The instructions you will see for this type of question will generally appear as below:

DIRECTIONS: Each of the numbered items or incomplete statements in this section is followed by answers or by completions of the statement. Select the ONE lettered answer or completion that is BEST in each case.

The following is an example of this question type:

1. An obese 21-year-old woman complains of increased growth of coarse hair on her upper lip, chin, chest, and abdomen. She also notes menstrual irregularity with periods of amenorrhea. The most likely cause is

(A) polycystic ovary disease
(B) ovarian tumor
(C) adrenal tumor
(D) Cushing disease
(E) familial hirsutism

In the question above, the key word is "most." Although ovarian tumors, adrenal tumors, and Cushing disease are causes of hirsutism (described in the stem of the question), polycystic ovary disease is a much more common cause. Familial hirsutism is not associated with the menstrual irregularities mentioned. Thus, the most likely cause of the manifestations described can only be "(A) polycystic ovary disease."

Strategies for Answering One Best Answer–Single-Item Questions

1. Remember that only one choice can be the correct answer.
2. Read the question carefully to be sure that you understand what is being asked.
3. Quickly read each choice for familiarity. (This important step is often not done by test takers.)
4. Go back and consider each choice individually.
5. If a choice is partially correct, tentatively consider it to be incorrect. (This step will help you eliminate choices and increase your odds of choosing the correct answer.)
6. Consider the remaining choices and select the one you think is the answer. At this point, you may want to scan the item quickly to ensure you understand the question and your answer.
7. If you do not know the answer, make an educated guess. Your score is based on the number of correct answers, not the number you get incorrect. **Do not leave any blanks.**
8. The actual examination is timed for an average of 1.2 minutes per question. It is important to be thorough to understand the questions, but it is equally important for you to keep moving.

One Best Answer–Matching Set Questions. This format presents lettered options followed by several items related to a common topic. The directions you will generally see for this type of question are as follows:

DIRECTIONS (Questions 2 through 4): Each set of matching questions in this section consists of a list of lettered options followed by several numbered items. For each item, select the ONE best lettered option that is most closely associated with it. Each lettered option may be selected once, more than once, or not at all.

Below is an example of this type of question.

For each adverse drug reaction listed below, select the antibiotic with which it is most closely associated.

(A) tetracycline
(B) chloramphenicol
(C) clindamycin
(D) gentamicin

1. Bone marrow suppression

2. Pseudomembranous enterocolitis

3. Acute fatty necrosis of liver

Note that unlike the single-item questions, the choices in the matching sets *precede* the actual questions. However, as with the single-item questions, only one choice can be correct for a given question.

Strategies for Answering One Best Answer–Matching Set Questions

1. Remember that the lettered choices are followed by the numbered questions.
2. As with single-item questions, only one answer is correct for each item.
3. Quickly read each choice for familiarity.
4. Read the question carefully to be sure you understand what is being asked.
5. Go back and consider each choice individually.
6. If a choice is partially correct for a particular item, tentatively consider it to be incorrect. (This step will help you eliminate choices and increase your odds of choosing the correct answer.)
7. Consider the remaining choices, and select the one you think is correct.
8. If you do not know the answer, make an educated guess. Your score is based on the number of correct answers, not the number you get incorrect. **Do not leave any blanks.**
9. Again, the actual examination allows an average of 1.2 minutes per question.

Extended One Best Answer–Matching/Choosing Questions. The USMLE Step 2 uses a new type of matching question that is similar to the one above but can contain up to 26 lettered options followed by several items. The directions you will see for this type of question will generally read the same as those listed for the best answer–matching sets, because this is another version of the same question. An example of this type of question is:

(A) sarcoidosis
(B) tuberculosis
(C) histoplasmosis
(D) coccidioidomycosis
(E) amyloidosis
(F) bacterial pneumonia
(G) mesothelioma
(H) carcinoma
(I) fibrosing alveolitis
(J) silicosis

4. A right lower lobectomy specimen contains a solitary 1.2-cm-diameter solid nodule. The center of the nodule is fibrous. The periphery has granulomatous inflammation. With special stains, multiple 2- to 5-μm budding yeasts are evident within the nodule. Acid-fast stains are negative.

5. A left upper lobectomy specimen is received containing a 4.6-cm nodule with central cystic degeneration. Microscopically, the nodule is composed of anaplastic squamous cells. Similar abnormal cells are seen in a concomitant biopsy of a hilar lymph node.

6. After a long history of multiple myeloma, a 67-year-old male is noted to have abundant acellular eosinophilic deposits around the pulmonary microvasculature at autopsy. A Congo red special stain demonstrates apple green birefringence.

7. A large pleural-based lesion is found on chest x-ray of an asbestos worker. Electron microscopy of the biopsy shows abundant long microvilli.

Note that, as with other matching sets, the lettered options are listed first.

Strategies for Answering Extended One Best Answer–Matching/Choosing Questions

1. Read the lettered options through first.
2. Work with one item at a time.
3. Read the item through, then go back to the options and consider each choice individually.
4. As with the other question types, if the choice is partially correct, tentatively consider it to be incorrect.
5. Consider the remaining choices and select the answer.
6. Remember to make a selection for each item.
7. Again, the test allows for 1.2 minutes per item.

Answers, Explanations, and References

In each of the sections of this book, the question sections are followed by a section containing the answers, explanations, and references to the questions. This section: (1) tells you the answer to each question; (2) gives you an explanation/review of why the answer is correct, background information on the subject matter, and why the other answers are incorrect; and (3) tells you where you can find more in-depth information on the subject matter in other books and/or journals. We encourage you to use this section as a basis for further study and understanding.

If you choose the correct answer to a question, you can then read the explanation: (1) for reinforcement; and (2) to add to your knowledge about the subject matter (remember that the explanations usually tell not only why the answer is correct, but also why the other choices are incorrect). **If you choose the wrong answer** to a question, you can read the explanation for a learning/reviewing discussion of the material in the question. Furthermore, you can note the reference cited (e.g., *Last, pp. 478–484*), look up the full source in the References at the end of the section (e.g., Last JM, Wallace RB, Barrett-Connor E. *Maxcy-Rosenau-Last Public Health and Preventive Medicine*, 13th ed. Norwalk, CT: Appleton & Lange, 1992.), and refer to the pages cited for a more in-depth discussion.

Subject Lists

At the end of the practice tests of this book is a subject list for each subject area. These subject lists will help point out your areas of relative weakness, and thus help you focus your review.

For example, by checking off your incorrect answers on, say, the preventive medicine list, you may find that a pattern develops in that you are incorrect on most or all of the biostatistics questions. In this case, you could note the references (in the explanation section) for your incorrect answers and read those sources. You might also want to purchase a biostatistics text or review book to do a much more in-depth review. We think that you will find these subject lists very helpful, and we urge you to use them.

Practice Tests

The 275-question practice tests at the end of the book consist of questions from each of the six clinical sciences. The questions are grouped according to question type (one best answer–single-item, one best answer–matching sets, and comparison/matching sets, with the subject areas integrated. This format mimics the actual exam and enables you to test your skill at answering questions in all of the clinical sciences under simulated examination conditions.

The practice test section is organized in the following format: questions, answers and explanations, references, and subject lists (which, here, will also list the major subject heading).

How to Use this Book

There are two logical ways to get the most value from this book. We call them *Plan A* and *Plan B*.

In *Plan A*, you go straight to the practice tests and complete them. After taking the practice tests, you check your answers and then tick off those you got wrong on the subject lists on pages 309–310 and 365–366. The *number* of questions you got wrong will be a good indicator of your initial knowledge state, and the *types* of questions you got wrong will help point you in the right direction for further preparation and review. At this point, you can use the first six sections of the book, with the lists and discussions, to help you improve your areas of relative weakness.

In *Plan B*, you go through the clinical science sections (from OB/GYN to preventive medicine), checking off your answers, and then compare your choices with the answers and discussions in the book. Once you've completed this process, you can take the practice tests, check your answers as described above, and see how well prepared you are at this point. If you still have a major weakness, it should be apparent in time for you to take remedial action.

In *Plan A*, by taking the practice tests first, you get quick feedback regarding your initial areas of strength and weakness. You may find that you know all of the material very well, indicating that perhaps only a cursory review of the six clinical science sections is necessary. This, of course, would be good to know early on in your exam preparation. On the other hand, you may find that you have many areas of weakness (say, for example, in all of pediatrics and psychiatry and in some of the subspecialties of preventive medicine). In this case, you could then focus on these areas in your review—not just with this book, but also with textbooks of pediatrics and psychiatry.

It is, however, unlikely that you will not do some studying before taking the USMLE Step 2 (especially because you have this book). Therefore, it may be more realistic to take the practice tests *after* you have reviewed the six clinical science sections (as in *Plan B*). This, of course, will probably give you a more realistic test-type situation, because few of us can sit for an exam without study. In this case, you will have done some reviewing (from superficial to in-depth), and your practice tests will reflect this studying time. If, after reviewing the six clinical science sections and taking the practice tests, your scores still indicate some weaknesses, you can then go back into the clinical science sections and supplement your review with your texts.

Specific Information on the Step 2 Examination

The official source of all information with respect to the United States Medical Licensing Examination Step 2 is the National Board of Medical Examiners (NBME), 3930 Chestnut Street, Philadelphia, PA 19104. Established in 1915, the NBME is a voluntary, nonprofit, independent organization whose sole function is the design, implementation, distribution, and processing of a vast bank of question items, certifying examinations, and evaluative services in the professional medical field. Contact the NBME for information on registration requirements for the USMLE Step 2.

Standard Abbreviations

ACTH: adrenocorticotropic hormone
ADH: antidiuretic hormone
ADP: adenosine diphosphate
AFP: α-fetoprotein
AMP: adenosine monophosphate
ATP: adenosine triphosphate
ATPase: adenosine triphosphatase
bid: two times a day
BP: blood pressure
BUN: blood urea nitrogen
CT: computed tomography
CBC: complete blood count
CCU: coronary care unit
CNS: central nervous system
CPK: creatine phosphokinase
CSF: cerebrospinal fluid
DNA: deoxyribonucleic acid
DNase: deoxyribonuclease
ECG: electrocardiogram
EDTA: ethylenediaminetetraacetate
EEG: electroencephalogram
ER: emergency room
FSH: follicle-stimulating hormone
GI: gastrointestinal
GU: genitourinary
Hb: hemoglobin
HCG: human chorionic gonadotropin
Hct: hematocrit
IgA, etc.: immunoglobulin A, etc.
IM: intramuscular(ly)
IQ: intelligence quotient
IU: international unit
IV: intravenous(ly)
KUB: kidney, ureter, and bladder
LDH: lactic dehydrogenase
LH: luteinizing hormone
LSD: lysergic acid diethylamide
mRNA: messenger RNA
PO: oral(ly)
PRN: as needed
RBC: red blood cell
RNA: ribonucleic acid
RNase: ribonuclease
rRNA: ribosomal RNA
SC: subcutaneous(ly)
SGOT: serum glutamic oxaloacetic transaminase
SGPT: serum glutamic pyruvic transaminase
TB: tuberculosis
tRNA: transfer RNA
TSH: thyroid-stimulating hormone
WBC: white blood cell

CHAPTER 1

Internal Medicine

Ruric (Andy) Anderson, MD

Questions

DIRECTIONS (Questions 1 through 63): Each of the numbered items or incomplete statements in this section is followed by answers or completions of the statement. Select the ONE lettered answer or completion that is BEST in each case.

Questions 1 through 3

1. You evaluate a 70-year-old man who complains of muscle weakness. His appearance is remarkable for a periorbital heliotrope rash with edema and erythema on his upper chest, neck, and face (Fig. 1-1). Which of the following is the most likely diagnosis?

   (A) polymyositis
   (B) dermatomyositis
   (C) spinocerebellar degeneration
   (D) vasculitis
   (E) rheumatoid arthritis

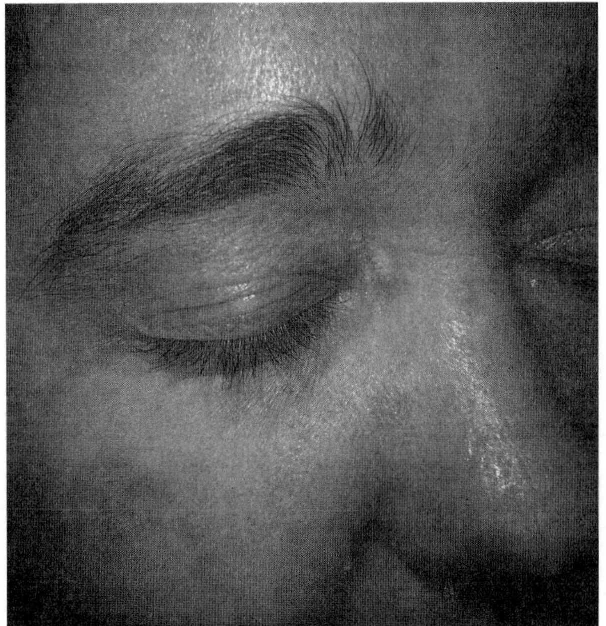

FIG. 1-1 *(Reprinted with permission from Hurwitz RM.* Pathology of the Skin. *Stamford, CT: Appleton & Lange, 1998.)*

2. Which of the following examination findings would this patient most likely have?

   (A) proximal muscle weakness
   (B) distal muscle weakness
   (C) ataxic gait
   (D) hyperactive deep tendon reflexes
   (E) inflamed small joints

3. Which of the following blood parameters is likely to be elevated?

   (A) serum creatinine
   (B) serum potassium
   (C) serum sodium
   (D) rheumatoid factor
   (E) creatinine phosphokinase

4. A 47-year-old man with diabetes and hypertension travels with his family to Mexico. The next morning after eating out at a local restaurant and despite drinking bottled water, he develops severe crampy abdominal pain and watery, frequent diarrhea. Which of the following is the best approach for his care?

   (A) ciprofloxacin × 3 days
   (B) penicillin × 5 days
   (C) tetracycline × 3 days
   (D) observation of symptoms
   (E) metronidazole × 10 days

5. Which of the following is the most likely diagnosis for the ulcerated lesion on the person's cheek shown in Fig. 1-2?

(A) squamous cell carcinoma
(B) malignant melanoma
(C) benign ulcerated nevus
(D) basal cell carcinoma
(E) hemangioma

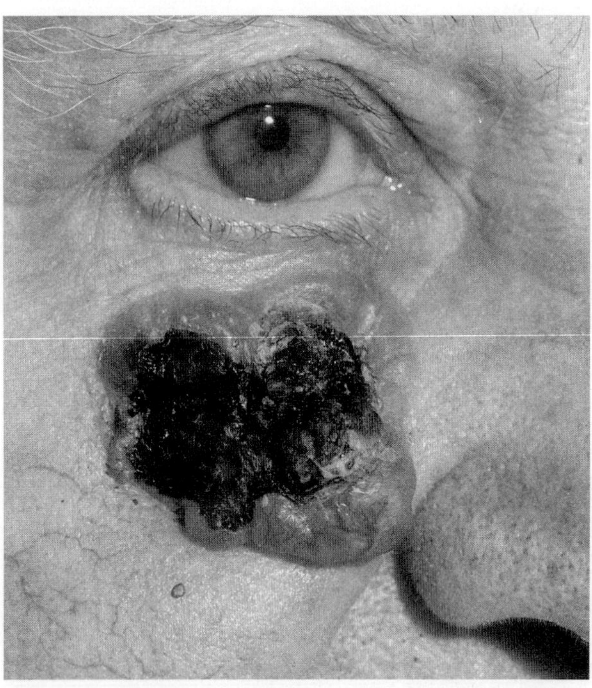

FIG. 1-2 *(Reprinted with permission from Fitzpatrick TB.* Color Atlas and Synopsis of Clinical Dermatology, *2nd ed. New York: McGraw-Hill, 1994.)*

Questions 6 through 8

A dentist asks you to evaluate a 42-year-old woman before tooth extraction.

6. Which of the following would prompt you to prescribe prophylactic antibiotics?

(A) midsystolic click at the left sternal border
(B) insulin-dependent diabetes
(C) a holosystolic, blowing murmur at the apex
(D) a history of congestive heart failure
(E) S_4 gallop

7. Which of the following is the prophylactic antibiotic of choice for dental procedures?

(A) amoxicillin
(B) vancomycin
(C) cephalexin
(D) penicillin
(E) clindamycin

8. In patients who are not intravenous (IV) drug users and who do not have prosthetic valves, which of the following organisms is the most common cause of bacterial endocarditis?

(A) *Enterococcus*
(B) *Streptococcus*
(C) gram-negative bacilli
(D) *Candida*
(E) *Pseudomonas*

9. A 36-year-old female complains of 5 days of fever, nasal congestion, sinus pressure, and postnasal drip. On examination, nasal discharge is yellow and the posterior pharynx is slightly erythematous. Tapping over the maxillary sinuses elicits mild pain. Which of the following is the most appropriate treatment for this patient?

(A) treatment of symptoms (analgesics, antipyretics, decongestants)
(B) a 7-day course of amoxicillin
(C) a 10-day course of amoxicillin-clavulanic acid
(D) a 14-day course of clarithromycin

Questions 10 through 12

You make the diagnosis of Marfan syndrome in a very tall 22-year-old man with long, thin extremities.

10. What other finding is associated with this disease?

(A) family history in 100% of the patients
(B) upward subluxation of the lenses
(C) mental retardation
(D) malar rash
(E) increased length of trunk compared with the limbs

11. The major cause of morbidity and mortality in Marfan patients is cardiac. Which of the following is a common complication?

    (A) pulmonary stenosis
    (B) ventricular septal defect (VSD)
    (C) pulmonary hypertension
    (D) aortic root dilatation
    (E) coronary artery disease (CAD)

12. Which of the following is the best way to monitor these patients for cardiovascular changes?

    (A) electrocardiogram (ECG)
    (B) chest x-ray (CXR)
    (C) angiography
    (D) pulmonary function tests
    (E) echocardiography

13. A 30-year-old woman is visiting you in your primary care office as a new patient. Overall, she is healthy. On taking a family history, you learn that her mother was diagnosed with colorectal cancer at the age of 50. When should this patient start being screened for colorectal cancer?

    (A) There is no proven benefit for colorectal cancer screening.
    (B) at age 40
    (C) at age 50
    (D) at age 60
    (E) at age 30

14. A 70-year-old man presents to urgent care complaining of a painful, swollen left knee. He previously has had no problems with this knee. Three days prior to onset, he went out dancing for 2–3 h but recalls no specific injury. Examination of the knee reveals a moderate-sized effusion and mild pain with any range of motion. Plain x-ray shows no fracture. Which of the following is the best next management?

    (A) MRI of knee
    (B) aspiration of effusion fluid
    (C) rest, ice, and leg elevation
    (D) physical therapy referral
    (E) arthroscopy

15. A 59-year-old woman complains of shortness of breath and aching left-sided chest pain that radiates to the left shoulder. Physical examination shows no abnormalities; her CXRs are shown in Fig. 1-3. Which of the following statements is true concerning this disease?

    (A) This tumor frequently metastasizes to distant sites.
    (B) Direct exposure to asbestos is required.
    (C) Most cases are associated with recent, massive exposure to asbestos.
    (D) Diffuse forms may be cured by chemotherapy alone.
    (E) Localized forms may be cured by surgery alone.

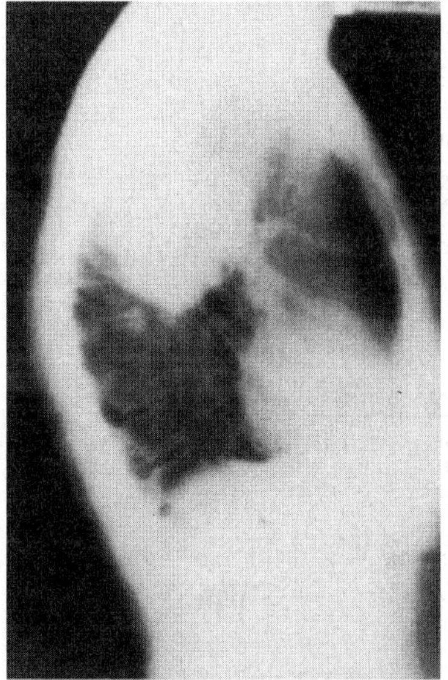

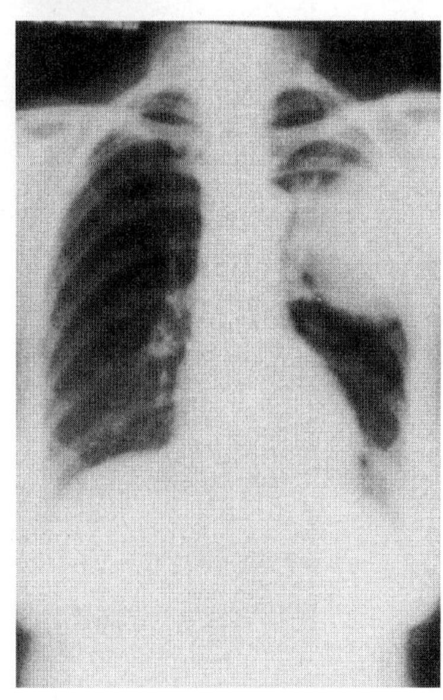

FIG. 1-3

16. A 23-year-old woman presents with "skipped heartbeats" and on cardiac examination is found to have a midsystolic click followed by a late systolic murmur. Echocardiogram shows prolapse of the mitral valve. Which of the following is true about this condition?

(A) Mitral valve prolapse is present in up to 10% of the population.
(B) Mitral valve prolapse is more common in men.
(C) Prophylaxis against bacterial endocarditis is never recommended.
(D) Risk of pulmonary embolism is high.
(E) Ventricular arrhythmias do not occur.

17. A 57-year-old man complains of worsening headache, nausea, and vomiting for 2 months. On examination, he is lethargic, confused, and has right-sided weakness. While waiting for a computed tomography (CT) scan, he develops status epilepticus, suffers cardiorespiratory arrest, and dies. His brain at autopsy is shown in Fig. 1-4. Which of the following is the most likely diagnosis?

(A) glioma
(B) meningioma
(C) craniopharyngioma
(D) pituitary adenoma
(E) acoustic neuroma

18. A 19-year-old high school senior complains of feeling "fat and ugly" despite being extremely thin. She takes small amounts of food at meals and occasionally gags herself to induce vomiting after meals. Which of the following is commonly associated with this disorder?

(A) menorrhagia
(B) metrorrhagia
(C) loss of body hair
(D) bradycardia
(E) thrombocytopenia

Questions 19 and 20

A 59-year-old woman had a left modified radical mastectomy for intraductal carcinoma 2 years previously. She presents with confusion, lethargy, and thigh pain. X-rays reveal a lytic lesion in the shaft of the femur.

19. Which of the following blood abnormalities is most likely?

(A) high glucose
(B) low calcium
(C) high potassium
(D) high calcium
(E) low magnesium

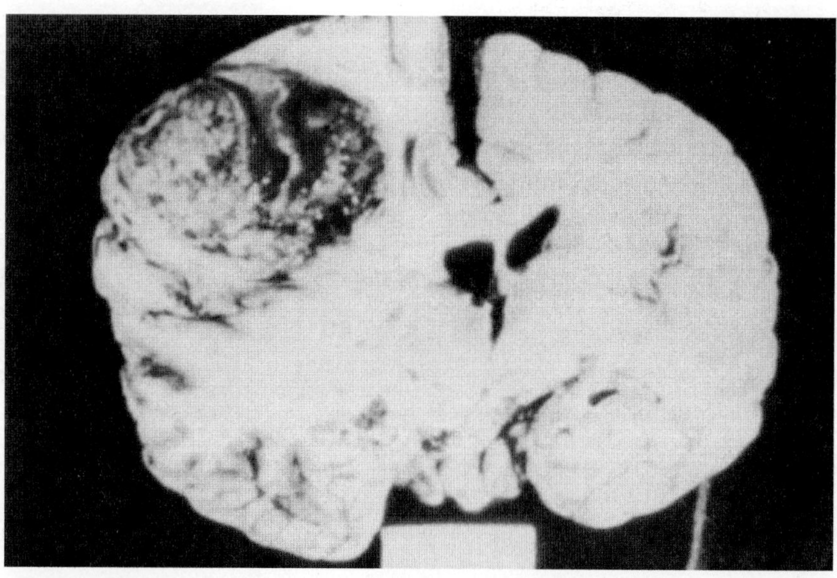

FIG. 1-4

20. Which of the following is the most appropriate initial therapy?

(A) radiotherapy to the femur
(B) vigorous saline infusion
(C) tamoxifen
(D) chemotherapy
(E) glucocorticoids

21. A 55-year-old retired policeman has had hypertension for about 15 years for which he takes hydralazine. He has a 35 pack-year tobacco history and continues to smoke one pack a day. On his visit, he complains about the appearance of his nose (Fig. 1-5) and asks if something can be done to decrease the redness. Which of the following statements is correct?

(A) Hydralazine does not play a role in his nasal erythema.
(B) Smoking probably aggravates the dilatation of the blood vessels on his nose.
(C) He should avoid alcohol and spicy foods.
(D) There is no effective topical therapy.
(E) Laser therapy will worsen the erythema.

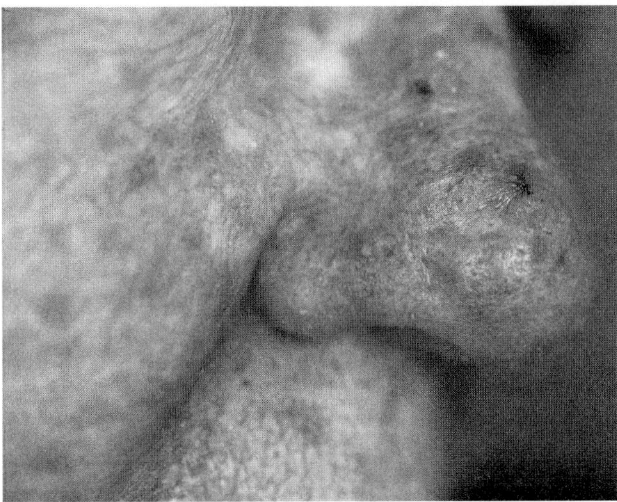

FIG. 1-5 *(Reprinted with permission from Hurwitz RM.* Pathology of the Skin. *Stamford, CT: Appleton & Lange, 1998.)*

22. A 46-year-old attorney is noted to have normal cholesterol levels but a very high fasting triglyceride level of 1600. He is otherwise healthy and has no risk factors for CAD. Which of the following statements is correct?

(A) Hypertriglyceridemia is a strong independent risk factor for premature CAD.
(B) Dietary modification is usually sufficient.
(C) High triglyceride levels are associated with elevated high-density lipoprotein (HDL) levels.
(D) Hypertriglyceridemia is usually associated with skin lesions.
(E) Control of triglyceride levels can prevent attacks of acute pancreatitis in patients with extreme hypertriglyceridemia.

23. A 60-year-old patient with long-standing diabetes has a creatinine of 3.6, which has been stable for several years. Which of the following antibiotics requires the most dosage modification in chronic renal failure?

(A) tetracycline
(B) gentamicin
(C) erythromycin
(D) nafcillin
(E) chloramphenicol

24. A 57-year-old man is on maintenance hemodialysis for chronic renal failure. Which of the following metabolic derangements can be anticipated?

(A) hypercalcemia
(B) hypophosphatemia
(C) osteomalacia
(D) vitamin D excess
(E) hypoparathyroidism

25. Which of the following is a degenerative disease of the central nervous system (CNS) caused by infectious proteins called prions?

(A) Creutzfeldt–Jakob disease (CJD)
(B) Alzheimer disease
(C) Parkinson disease
(D) Cushing disease
(E) Guillain–Barré syndrome

26. A 25-year-old man was admitted to the intensive care unit with a severe head injury, with fracture of the base of the skull. Approximately 18 h after the injury, he developed polyuria. Urine osmolality was 150 mOsm/L and serum osmolality was 350 mOsm/L. IV fluids were stopped, and 3 h later, urine output and urine osmolality remained unchanged. Five units of vasopressin were intravenously administered. Urine osmolality increased to 300 mOsm/L. Which of the following is the most likely diagnosis?

(A) central diabetes insipidus
(B) nephrogenic diabetes insipidus
(C) water intoxication
(D) solute overload
(E) syndrome of inappropriate antidiuretic hormone secretion (SIADH)

27. A 70-year-old man with a 60 pack-year smoking history presents with cough and weight loss. He describes recent diffuse darkening of his skin and his CXR shows a mass suspicious for lung cancer in the left hilum. His labs reveal hypokalemia. Which of the following is the most likely histology of his lung cancer?

(A) adenocarcinoma
(B) small cell
(C) squamous cell
(D) mesothelioma
(E) glioblastoma

28. A 47-year-old man is postoperative day number 2 after an open cholecystectomy. He becomes short of breath and a medicine consult is called to evaluate. Vital signs include a temperature of 100°F, pulse rate of 110/min, blood pressure (BP) of 110/60 mmHg, and respiratory rate of 24/min. Blood gas shows a pH of 7.52, carbon dioxide of 28, Po_2 of 58, and calculated bicarbonate of 20. What is the primary acid-base disorder in this patient?

(A) metabolic acidosis
(B) respiratory acidosis
(C) metabolic alkalosis
(D) respiratory alkalosis
(E) metabolic and respiratory acidosis

29. A 20-year-old female presents to the office complaining that her right eye has been itchy and watery. The patient reports that the onset was abrupt. The patient is noted to be afebrile with normal vital signs. Examination discloses a red eye with watery discharge. Minimal preauricular adenopathy is also found on examination. Tonometry is normal. Profuse tearing is noted (Fig. 1-6). Which of the following is the most likely diagnosis?

(A) viral conjunctivitis
(B) bacterial conjunctivitis
(C) foreign body reaction
(D) allergic conjunctivitis
(E) acute open-angle glaucoma

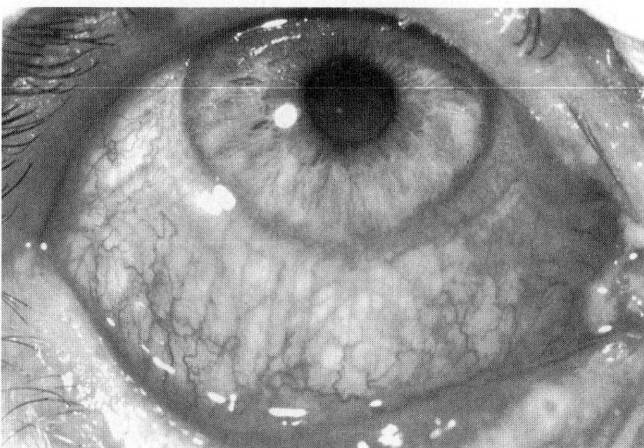

FIG. 1-6 *(Reprinted with permission from 1994 Managing the Red Eye: A Slide Script Program, San Francisco, American Academy of Ophthalmology, from Jenson HB, Baltimore RS.* Pediatric Infectious Diseases. *Stamford, CT: Appleton & Lange, 1995.)*

30. A 22-year-old man complains of low back pain and stiffness that is worse on arising and improves with exercise. On examination, he is found to have limited mobility of the sacroiliac joints and lumbar spine. A serum test for histocompatibility antigen HLA-B27 is positive. What is the most common extraskeletal manifestation of this disease?

(A) premature cataracts
(B) splenomegaly
(C) acute iritis
(D) aortic insufficiency
(E) pulmonary fibrosis

Questions 31 and 32

A 54-year-old man presents to the emergency department complaining of epigastric discomfort, which began while he was walking his dog after dinner about one-half hour earlier. He has not received medical care for several years. On examination, he is moderately obese and in obvious discomfort and seems restless. His BP is 160/98 mmHg, and his examination is otherwise unremarkable. His ECG is seen in Fig. 1-7.

31. Which of the following is the most likely diagnosis?

(A) gastroesophageal reflux
(B) costochondritis
(C) gastroenteritis
(D) inferior wall myocardial infarction
(E) anterolateral myocardial infarction

32. Which of the following is the most appropriate next step in management?

(A) trial of antacid immediately
(B) reassurance and arrange outpatient follow-up
(C) arrange for cardiac intensive care bed
(D) begin thrombolytic therapy in the emergency department
(E) arrange for cardiac catheterization

33. A 59-year-old woman who lives independently and has been doing well is hospitalized for pneumonia. She is started on ceftriaxone and azithromycin but continues to deteriorate and have high fever 4 days after admission. Which of the following factors is a poor prognostic sign in community-acquired pneumonia?

(A) age less than 60
(B) systolic BP = 160 mmHg
(C) leukocytosis = 15,000
(D) altered mental status
(E) mycoplasma pneumonia infected

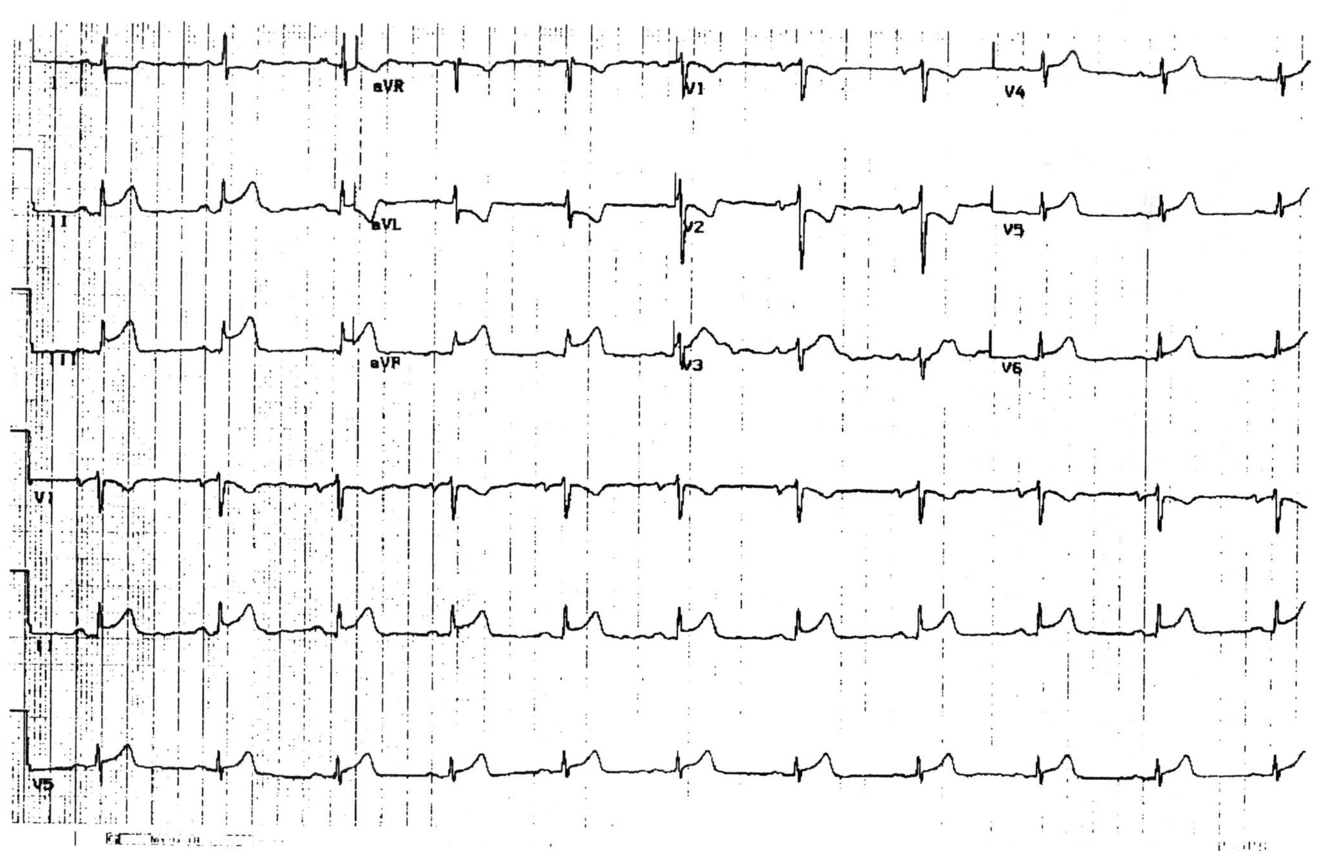

FIG. 1-7

34. A 32-year-old woman is referred to you by her dermatologist for further evaluation. She developed these changes gradually in the last year. Her hands are seen in Fig. 1-8. What other associated disease is most likely?

(A) acquired immune deficiency syndrome (AIDS)
(B) Addison disease
(C) lymphoma
(D) primary biliary cirrhosis
(E) Hashimoto's thyroiditis

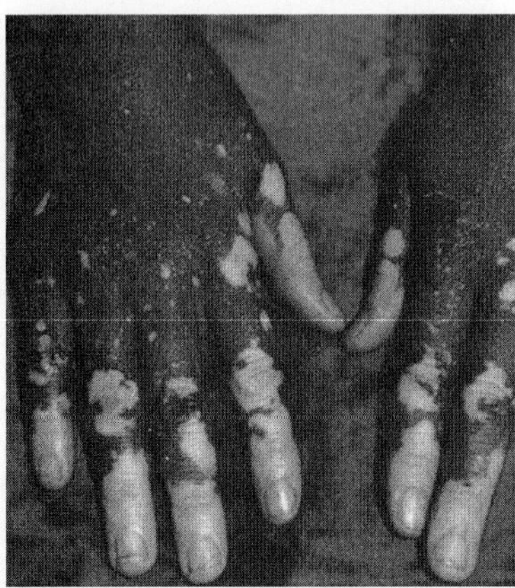

FIG. 1-8 *(Reprinted with permission from Bondi.* Dermatology Diagnosis & Therapy. *Stamford, CT: Appleton & Lange, 1991.)*

35. A 75-year-old man who developed diabetes within the last 6 months was found to be jaundiced. He has remained asymptomatic, except for weight loss of about 10 lbs in 6 months. On physical examination, he is found to have a nontender, globular, right upper quadrant mass that moves with respiration. A CT scan shows enlargement of the head of the pancreas, with no filling defects in the liver. What is the most likely cause of his painless jaundice?

(A) malignant biliary structure
(B) carcinoma of the head of the pancreas
(C) choledocholithiasis
(D) cirrhosis of the liver
(E) pancreatitis

36. Which of the following is a useful clue to the diagnosis of *Legionella* pneumonia?

(A) diarrhea
(B) rash
(C) pedal edema
(D) elevated serum glucose
(E) photophobia

37. A 60-year-old previously healthy man presents with massive rectal bleeding. Which of the following is the most likely diagnosis?

(A) diverticulosis of the colon
(B) ulcerative colitis
(C) external hemorrhoid
(D) ischemic colitis
(E) carcinoma of the colon

38. A 24-year-old man runs a marathon on an unusually hot and muggy day. Several hours later he becomes ill with fever, weakness, and painful swollen legs and passes dark brown urine. Which of the following is a common finding with this disorder?

(A) Urine orthotoluidine (Hematest) reaction will be negative.
(B) Serum will be pink.
(C) Serum creatine phosphokinase levels will be elevated.
(D) Serum haptoglobin levels will be elevated.
(E) Serum potassium levels will be below.

39. While examining a 46-year-old woman, you hear a diastolic murmur that is increased when the patient is in the left lateral decubitus position. You ask her to run in place for 3 min, and the murmur is found to be accentuated as well by exercise. What is the most likely valvular defect?

(A) aortic regurgitation
(B) mitral stenosis
(C) tricuspid stenosis
(D) pulmonic regurgitation
(E) VSD

Questions 40 and 41

A 70-year-old man presents with shuffling gait, tremor, masked facies, and rigidity which have progressed over the last 9 months. Parkinson disease is diagnosed.

40. In this patient, which neurotransmitter deficiency primarily is responsible for his symptoms?

(A) acetylcholine
(B) epinephrine
(C) norepinephrine
(D) dopamine
(E) cortisol

41. Which of the following is true about Parkinson disease?

(A) Over 10 million people in North America have Parkinson disease.
(B) Mortality is no higher in patients with Parkinson disease when compared to age-matched controls.
(C) The classic triad of major signs of Parkinson disease is memory loss, rigidity, and akinesia.
(D) The tremor in Parkinson disease is typically an intention tremor.
(E) Over 90% of patients with Parkinson disease have a good initial response to levodopa.

42. A 73-year-old man has been experiencing increasing drowsiness and incoherence. He has a history of arrhythmias and has fallen twice in the past 2 weeks. There are no focal deficits on neurologic examination. A contrast CT scan of the head is shown in Fig. 1-9. Which of the following is the treatment of choice?

(A) parenteral antibiotics
(B) antifungal therapy
(C) neurosurgical evacuation of the clot
(D) observation and a repeat CT scan in 1 month
(E) fibrinolytic therapy

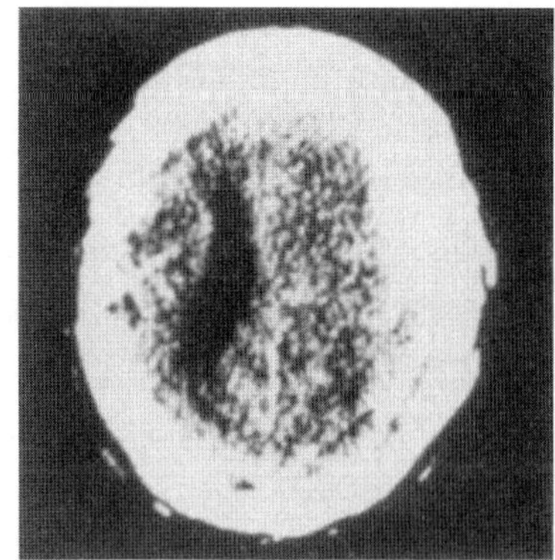

FIG. 1-9

43. A 63-year-old man complains of sudden onset of right-sided headache while at work. He rapidly becomes confused and lethargic. On examination, he is hemiparetic and has bilateral Babinski's signs. A CT scan of the head is shown in Fig. 1-10. What is the patient most likely to have?

(A) an arteriovenous malformation
(B) a carotid occlusion
(C) hypertension
(D) an underlying malignancy
(E) abnormal clotting studies

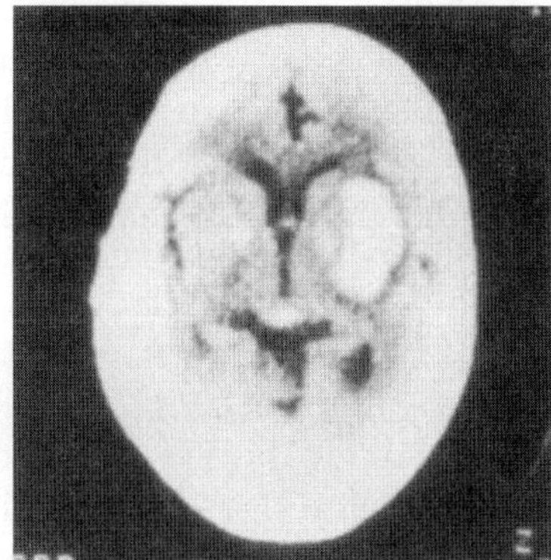

FIG. 1-10

44. A 54-year-old woman with diabetes is noted to have BP in the range of 140/90 mmHg on several occasions. Which of the following is the best next step in management?

    (A) initiate antihypertensive therapy
    (B) advise weight loss and recheck BP in 3 months
    (C) advise regular exercise and recheck BP in 3 months
    (D) no further intervention is necessary
    (E) follow-up in 6 months for recheck of BP

45. A 44-year-old man undergoes evaluation for worsening headaches. His posteroanterior and lateral arteriograms are shown in Fig. 1-11. Which of the following is the patient most likely to develop?

    (A) hypopituitarism
    (B) subarachnoid hemorrhage
    (C) hypercalcemia
    (D) tentorial herniation
    (E) chronic meningitis

Questions 46 through 48

A 35-year-old pharmacist complains of "hurting all over." Her pain is particularly bad in her upper back and shoulders, and she notes morning stiffness. On examination, her joints are not inflamed, but she has symmetric "tender points" in the posterior neck, anterior chest, lateral buttocks, medial knees, and lateral elbows. You make a preliminary diagnosis of fibromyalgia.

46. Which of the following is another characteristic symptom associated with this syndrome?

    (A) sleep disturbance
    (B) fever
    (C) rash on the extremities
    (D) muscle weakness
    (E) migratory joint inflammation

47. Which one of the following diagnostic tests should you order?

    (A) Lyme titers
    (B) electromyelography
    (C) sedimentation rate
    (D) spine radiographs
    (E) screening test for depression

48. Which of the following is the most appropriate therapeutic recommendation?

    (A) avoid most physical activity
    (B) trial of amoxicillin
    (C) benzodiazepine in low doses for sleep
    (D) low-dose steroid
    (E) low-dose antidepressant

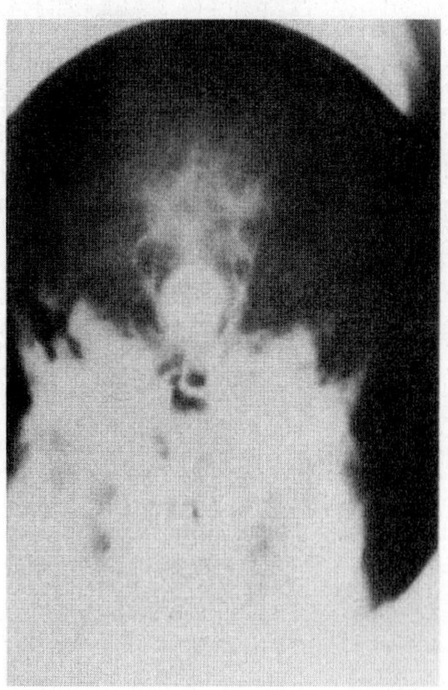

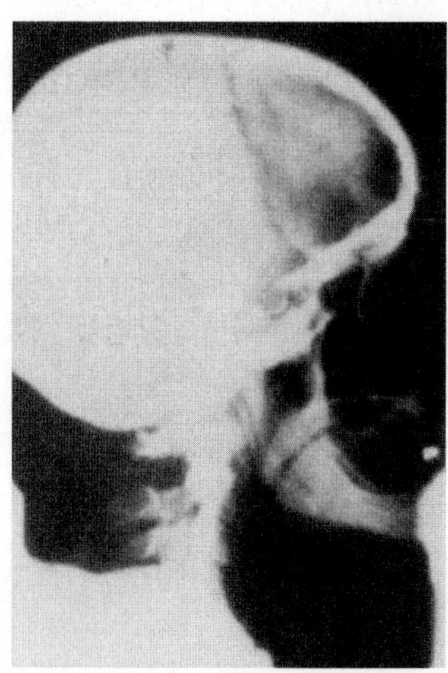

FIG. 1-11

49. A 62-year-old man is undergoing neurologic evaluation. His arteriogram demonstrates the lesion shown in Fig. 1-12. Which of the following deficits is compatible with this lesion?

(A) diplopia
(B) transient monocular blindness
(C) ataxia
(D) vertigo
(E) dysarthria

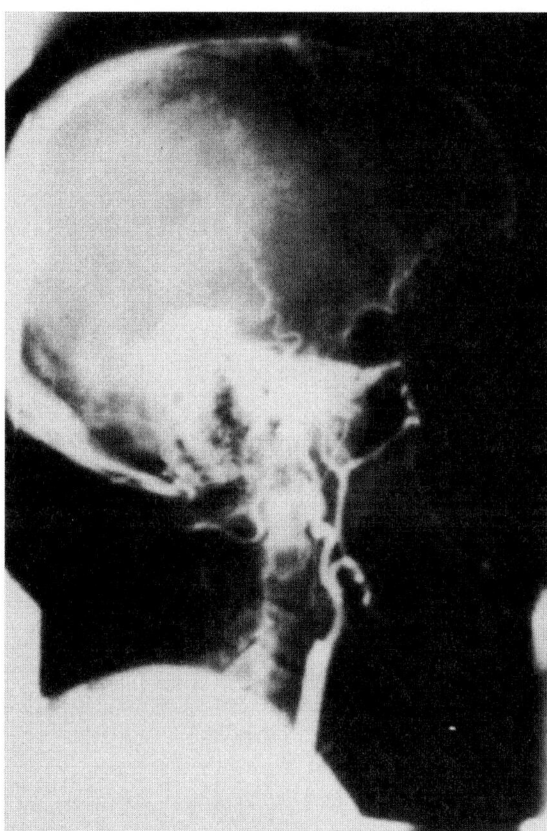

FIG. 1-12

Questions 50 and 51

A 30-year-old woman who has been human immunodeficiency virus (HIV) positive for 4 years was recently diagnosed with AIDS.

50. Which of the following meets the criteria for the case definition?

(A) oral thrush
(B) herpes zoster
(C) persistent lymphadenopathy
(D) peripheral neuropathy
(E) pulmonary tuberculosis

51. Which of the following immunologic abnormalities would be expected?

(A) increased numbers of $CD4^+$ (helper) T cells
(B) decreased number of $CD8^+$ (suppressor) T cells
(C) cutaneous anergy to usual skin test antigens
(D) normal B-cell function
(E) increased natural killer cell function

52. When you examine the back of an elderly gentleman, you note multiple brown papules and nodules having a "stuck on" appearance. These are shown in Fig. 1-13. The patient tells you they have been there for years. Which of the following is the most likely diagnosis?

(A) melanocytic nevi
(B) actinic keratoses
(C) seborrheic keratoses
(D) seborrheic dermatitis
(E) malignant melanoma

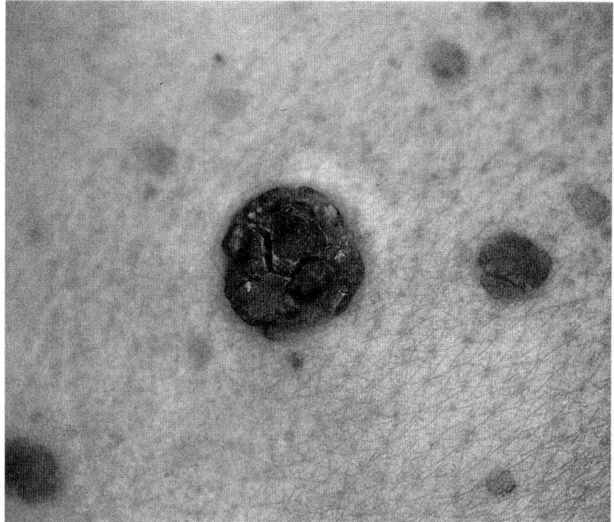

FIG. 1-13 *(Reprinted with permission from Hurwitz RM. Pathology of the Skin. Stamford, CT: Appleton & Lange, 1998.)*

Questions 53 and 54

A 58-year-old man is establishing care with you because his insurance changed. His old records have not yet arrived, but he is complaining of palpitations and lightheadedness, so you order the ECG shown in Fig. 1-14.

53. What is the underlying abnormality?

(A) right bundle branch block (RBBB)
(B) left bundle branch block (LBBB)
(C) accelerated junctional rhythm
(D) left anterior fascicular block
(E) intraventricular conduction delay

54. Which of the following is the most likely problem associated with this pattern?

(A) congenital heart disease
(B) severe aortic valve disease
(C) hypokalemia
(D) atrial septal defect (ASD)
(E) VSD

55. In a patient infected with HIV, which of the following laboratory parameters provides the most useful information about the current immunologic status of the patient?

(A) HIV RNA level
(B) white blood cell (WBC) count
(C) $CD4^+$ T-cell count
(D) $CD8^+$ T-cell count
(E) p24 antigen level

56. During a routine checkup, a 45-year-old executive is found to have hypercalcemia. Subsequent workup reveals elevated parathormone, decreased phosphorus, elevated chloride, and normal blood urea nitrogen (BUN), and creatinine in serum. Urinary calcium is above normal levels. What is the most likely etiology?

(A) multiple myeloma
(B) primary hyperparathyroidism
(C) hypervitaminosis D
(D) sarcoidosis
(E) milk alkali syndrome

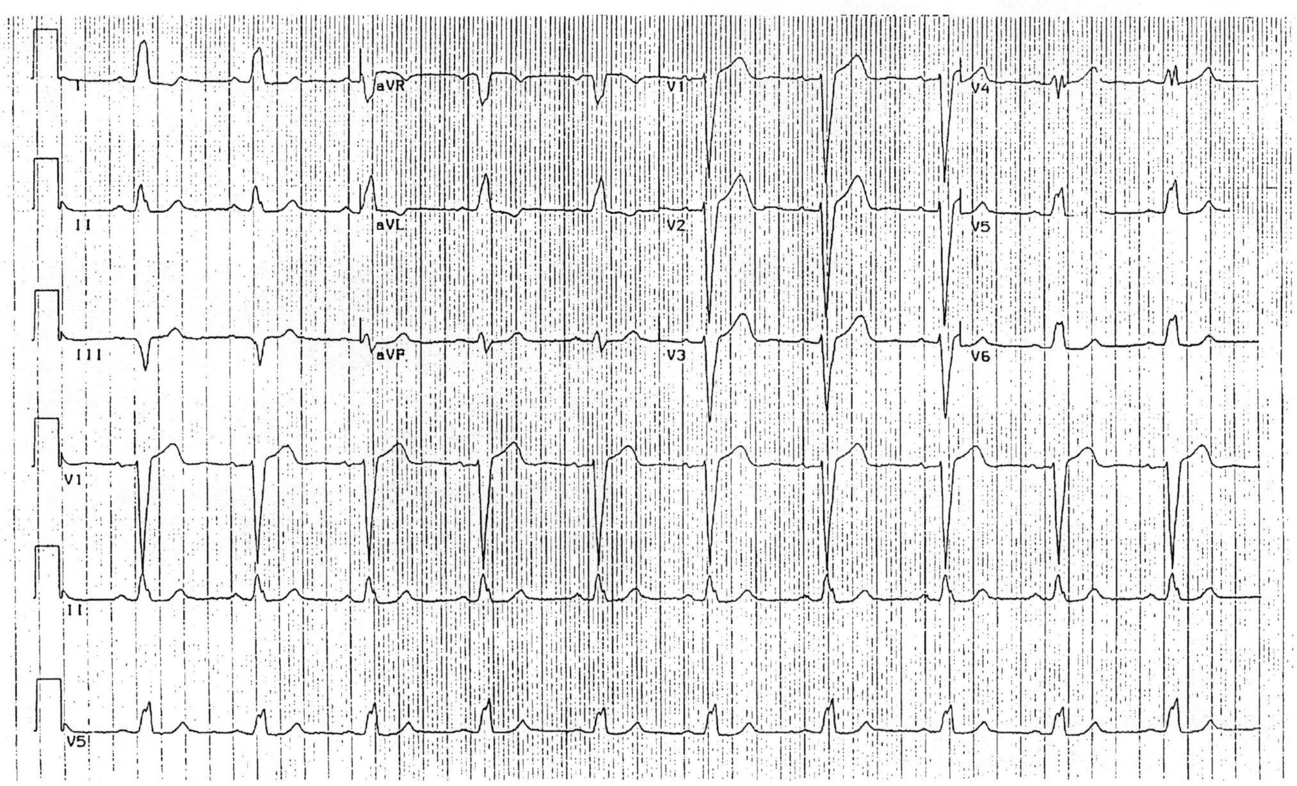

FIG. 1-14

57. A 62-year-old woman with a long-standing history of diabetes and hypertension presents for evaluation of hyperkalemia. Her room air arterial blood gas (ABG) and electrolytes are the following:

pH 7.38/Pco_2 34/Po_2 89
Na 140 Cl 106 BUN 51
K 5.9 CO_2 20 Cr 2.8

Which of the following is the underlying renal abnormality?

(A) renal tubular acidosis (RTA), type 2
(B) focal segmental glomerulonephritis
(C) interstitial nephritis
(D) RTA, type 4
(E) Barter syndrome

Questions 58 and 59

A 72-year-old man has the sudden onset of suprapubic pain and oliguria. His temperature is 38.0°C (100.4°F), pulse is 100/min, respiration rate is 12/min, and BP is 110/72 mmHg. Abdominal examination is remarkable only for a tender, distended urinary bladder.

58. Which of the following is the most appropriate immediate management of this patient?

(A) plain x-ray of the abdomen
(B) abdominal ultrasonography
(C) urethral catheter
(D) IV furosemide
(E) intravenous pyelogram (IVP)

59. Which of the following is the most likely cause of this condition?

(A) urinary tract infection
(B) prostatic hypertrophy
(C) posterior urethral valves
(D) renal carcinoma
(E) renal arterial occlusion

60. A 42-year-old woman is noted to have a multinodular goiter on examination. She has no symptoms and is clinically euthyroid. Which of the following statements about Hashimoto's thyroiditis is true?

(A) The condition is associated with prior radioactive exposure.
(B) Patients diagnosed with this disorder have an increased incidence of thyroid cancer.
(C) Corticosteroids are helpful in controlling the progression of the disease.
(D) Antinuclear antibodies are pathognomonic for this disease.
(E) Hashimoto's thyroiditis is an autoimmune disease.

61. A 55-year-old man complains of severe headaches over the past few weeks. Similar episodes have occurred in past years. Which of the following supports the diagnosis of cluster headaches?

(A) Pain-free intervals can last for days and then recur.
(B) Attacks of daily pain last for 4–8 weeks.
(C) The most common location of pain is occipital.
(D) Women are affected twice as commonly as men.
(E) Caffeine is the most effective treatment for an acute attack.

62. On the 2nd day after an appendectomy, a 33-year-old man complains of chest pain. Vital signs are: temperature 102°F, BP 130/70 mmHg, pulse rate 100/min, and respiration rate 22/min. Room air ABG reveals a pH of 7.50, Pco_2 of 29, and Po_2 of 49. His WBC count is elevated and CXR shows a right lower lobe infiltrate. Which of the following is the most likely diagnosis?

(A) pulmonary embolism
(B) myocardial infarction
(C) pneumonia
(D) asthma
(E) congestive heart failure

63. A 46-year-old woman presents with a 4-h history of left flank pain with fever and chills. On examination, her temperature is 103°F, pulse rate is 120/min, respiratory rate is 40/min, and supine BP is 80/40 mmHg. She has marked tenderness over the left flank and left upper quadrant of the abdomen without rebound. Urinalysis shows multiple red blood cells (RBCs), multiple WBCs, and WBC casts. Which of the following is the most likely diagnosis?

(A) appendicitis
(B) pyelonephritis
(C) cholelithiasis
(D) diverticulitis
(E) pelvic inflammatory disease

DIRECTIONS (Questions 64 through 78): Each set of matching questions in this section consists of a list of lettered options followed by several numbered items. For each item, select the ONE best lettered option that is most closely associated with it. Each lettered option may be selected once, more than once, or not at all.

Questions 64 through 66

For each patient with hepatitis, select the most likely type of viral hepatitis.

(A) hepatitis A
(B) hepatitis B
(C) hepatitis C

64. A 45-year-old woman presents with fever, anorexia, nausea, and diarrhea. Other patients in the community have presented similarly and have a common exposure at a local restaurant.

65. A 55-year-old male who is a former IV drug user presents with jaundice, ascites, and leg edema. A CT scan of the abdomen reveals a malignant-appearing mass in the liver.

66. A 43-year-old prison cook becomes ill with jaundice, malaise, and fever. Shortly thereafter, multiple prison inmates develop similar symptoms.

Questions 67 through 73

For each item, select the ONE best lettered option that is most closely associated with it. Each lettered heading may be selected once, more than once, or not at all.

(A) Cushing syndrome
(B) Addison disease
(C) Klinefelter syndrome
(D) hyperparathyroidism
(E) hypothyroidism
(F) pheochromocytoma
(G) acromegaly
(H) diabetes insipidus
(I) diabetes mellitus
(J) polycystic ovarian disease

67. A 42-year-old obese woman complains of hirsutism, amenorrhea, and difficulty becoming pregnant.

68. A 47-year-old man complains of fatigue and dizziness. On laboratory evaluation, he is noted to have significant hyponatremia and hyperkalemia.

69. A 55-year-old woman is having episodic palpitations, headaches, and sweating. On examination, her BP is elevated.

70. A 48-year-old man is being evaluated for diabetes and hypertension. On examination, he has mandibular enlargement and large hands.

71. A 35-year-old woman complains of constipation, hair loss, and dry skin.

72. A 45-year-old woman has noticed changes in the fat distribution on her body with excess fat over the posterior neck and upper back. On examination, she has high BP and abdominal striae. Laboratory evaluation shows a high glucose.

73. A 55-year-old man complains of abdominal pain and is found to have a kidney stone. Laboratory evaluation reveals hypercalcemia.

Questions 74 and 75

For each clinical setting described below, select the set of ABG determinations with which it is most likely to be associated.

	pH	Pa_{O_2}	Pa_{CO_2}
(A)	7.23	64	80
(B)	7.39	88	40
(C)	7.22	74	33
(D)	7.54	75	24
(E)	7.37	67	52

74. a 60-year-old man with morbid obesity

75. a 30-year-old woman with salicylate intoxication

Questions 76 through 78

For each antihypertensive agent listed below, select the set of undesirable side effects with which it is most commonly associated.

(A) cough, hyperkalemia, renal failure
(B) positive Coombs' test, hemolytic anemia, hepatitis
(C) hypokalemia, hyperuricemia, hyperglycemia
(D) sodium retention, heart failure, increased body hair
(E) increased angina, tachycardia, systemic lupus erythematosus (SLE)

76. hydrochlorothiazide

77. hydralazine

78. captropril

DIRECTIONS (Questions 79 through 113): Each of the numbered items or incomplete statements in this section is followed by answers or completions of the statement. Select the ONE lettered answer or completion that is BEST in each case.

79. A 34-year-old male presents to your clinic with acute bronchitis. This patient is immunocompetent and has no underlying heart or lung disease. Which of the following is the most appropriate treatment?

(A) 7 days of a macrolide antibiotic
(B) 7 days of a quinolone antibiotic
(C) 5 days of a macrolide antibiotic
(D) 5 days of a quinolone antibiotic
(E) rest and fluids

80. A 40-year-old patient of yours is planning to climb Mt. Everest. Which of the following is considered an important risk factor for high-altitude pulmonary edema?

(A) warm temperature
(B) history of asthma
(C) rate of ascent
(D) tall stature
(E) rate of descent

Questions 81 and 82

81. A previously healthy 19-year-old woman has the sudden onset of headache, profound myalgias, profuse vomiting, and diarrhea. The woman is near the end of her menstrual period and is using tampons. She appears to be suffering from toxic shock syndrome (TSS). Which of the following is the most likely skin finding?

(A) papular rash on the trunk
(B) scaly rash on the face
(C) pustular rash on the extremities
(D) macular erythroderma
(E) heliotrope facial rash

82. Which of the following is another common finding in TSS and is part of the case definition?

(A) hypertension: systolic BP 160 mmHg
(B) hyperreflexia
(C) fever with temperature 102°F
(D) elevated platelet count 400,000
(E) hypercalcemia

83. A 45-year-old man with HIV is being evaluated in clinic. His HIV diagnosis was made 6 months ago and he wants to know more about medication treatment options. Which of the following is an indication to initiate HIV medication treatment?

(A) CD4 count less than 700
(B) HIV viral load less than 55,000
(C) CD4 count greater than 700
(D) history of hepatitis A
(E) HIV viral load greater than 55,000

84. A 24-year-old female is infected with HIV from an unprotected sexual exposure. What is the median time for this patient to develop clinical disease if she is not treated?

(A) 6 months
(B) 1 year
(C) 5 years
(D) 10 years
(E) 15 years

85. A 52-year-old woman has had diabetes mellitus since childhood. She has controlled her glucose well and kept her glycohemoglobin (HgbA1C) below 7% (normal, 4–7%). For which of the following complications is she still at risk, despite excellent glucose control?

(A) autonomic dysfunction
(B) coronary heart disease
(C) blindness
(D) peripheral neuropathy
(E) peripheral vascular disease

86. A middle-aged White male presents to your office complaining of arthralgias, diarrhea, abdominal pain, and weight loss. On examination, you note generalized increased skin pigmentation. Which of the following is true regarding Whipple disease?

(A) Acute renal failure is a common complication.
(B) This disease usually strikes young adults before the third decade.
(C) It is predominantly a disease of women.
(D) Microscopic examination of the small intestine shows infiltration by large macrophages with periodic acid Schiff (PAS)-positive inclusions.
(E) It is associated with a gram-positive cocci.

Questions 87 and 88

87. A 42-year-old patient suffering from alcoholism has advanced liver disease with ascites. He is hospitalized for agitation and bizarre behavior. Which of the following findings is most helpful in making the diagnosis of hepatic encephalopathy?

(A) jaundice
(B) asterixis of the hands
(C) spider angiomas on the face and chest
(D) heme-positive stool
(E) positive fluid wave on abdominal examination

88. In the patient above, his blood ammonia level is twice his baseline. Which of the following is a likely precipitating factor?

(A) bleeding esophageal varices
(B) noncompliance with diuretic therapy
(C) excessive lactulose therapy
(D) insufficient protein ingestion
(E) recent alcohol ingestion

89. A 78-year-old woman comes to your primary care office practice with her son who is concerned about changes in her mood. She is less interested in going out to dinner and does not want to visit family or friends. Her language skills seem to have deteriorated over the last few years and her memory is not as sharp. Her gait and motor strength are normal. Which of the following is the most likely diagnosis?

(A) Parkinson disease
(B) anxiety disorder
(C) meningioma
(D) Alzheimer disease
(E) dysthymia

90. A 67-year-old man has a long history of constipation and recurrent, brief episodes of gripping lower abdominal pain. He is currently asymptomatic; his barium enema x-ray is shown in Fig. 1-15. Which of the following is the most appropriate therapy?

(A) surgical resection
(B) colonoscopy with biopsy
(C) histamine receptor antagonist
(D) corticosteroid rectal enema
(E) bulk-producing colloid, such as bran or psyllium

Questions 91 through 93

91. A 44-year-old secretary presents with a fever of 103°F, headache, and stiff neck. You entertain a diagnosis of bacterial meningitis and begin antibiotics immediately. With bacterial meningitis, which of the following is a likely finding in the cerebrospinal fluid (CSF)?

(A) leukocytes between 100 and 500/mm
(B) CSF pressure between 100 and 120 mm H_2O
(C) negative Gram stain
(D) glucose >120 mg/dL
(E) protein levels >45 mg/dL

92. In this otherwise healthy adult woman, what is the most likely infecting organism?

(A) group B *Streptococcus*
(B) *Staphylococcus aureus*
(C) *Hemophilus influenzae*
(D) *Streptococcus pneumoniae*
(E) *Listeria monocytogenes*

93. In the adult neutropenic patient, which of the following is the most likely organism to cause bacterial meningitis?

(A) group B *Streptococcus*
(B) *Staphylococcus aureus*
(C) *Hemophilus influenzae*
(D) *Streptococcus pneumoniae*
(E) *Listeria monocytogenes*

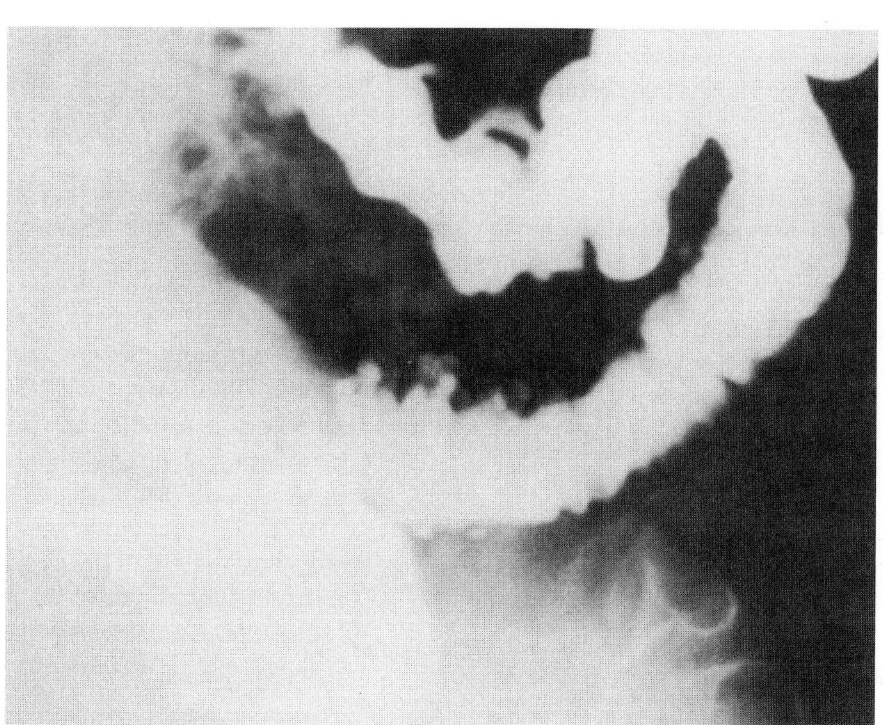

FIG. 1-15

94. A 50-year-old woman complains of worsening dyspnea of 1-month duration, but is otherwise asymptomatic. Lung examination is normal; her CXR is shown in Fig. 1-16. Which of the following is the most likely diagnosis?

(A) pulmonary tuberculosis
(B) lung metastases
(C) sarcoidosis
(D) mycoplasma pneumonia
(E) silicosis

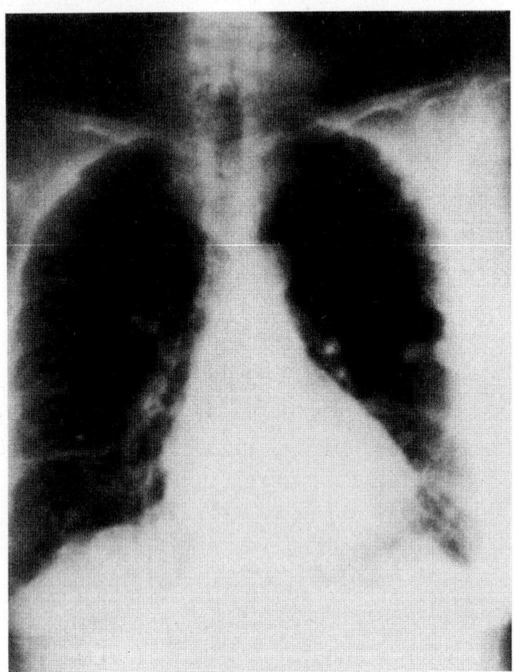

FIG. 1-16

95. A 63-year-old man complains of a new cough and of breathlessness after walking up a flight of stairs. Chest examination reveals late inspiratory crackles but no wheezes. There is a mild clubbing of the fingers. His CXR is shown in Fig. 1-17. Which of the following would be found on pulmonary function testing?

(A) increased arterial carbon dioxide pressure ($Paco_2$)
(B) normal compliance
(C) decreased carbon monoxide diffusing capacity (DLco)
(D) increased vital capacity
(E) increased oxygen saturation with exercise

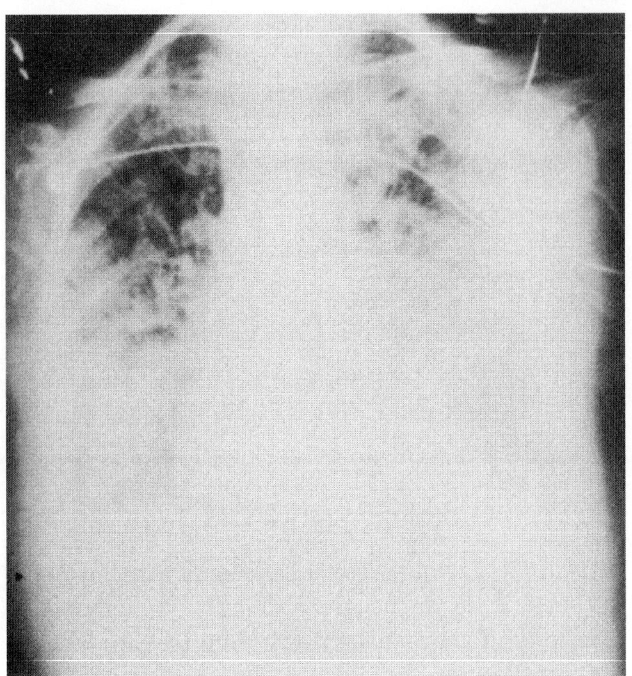

FIG. 1-17

96. A 23-year-old man presents complaining of severe crampy abdominal pain and blood in his stool over the past 2 days. A similar episode occurred a few months ago and spontaneously resolved. No history of travel. Abdominal x-ray shows mild colonic dilatation. Which of the following is the most likely diagnosis?

(A) ulcerative colitis
(B) Crohn disease
(C) irritable bowel syndrome
(D) celiac sprue
(E) Whipple disease

97. A 60-year-old man presents with a nonproductive cough for a week and generalized malaise. He also has noted some abdominal pain associated with diarrhea for the past few days. His temperature is 101.5°F and clinical examination is unremarkable. A CXR shows a left lower lobe infiltrate. His urinalysis shows 50 RBCs, and his BUN (30) and creatinine (1.6) are both mildly elevated. In light of the extrapulmonary symptoms and signs, which of the following is the most likely cause of his pneumonia?

(A) *Pseudomonas aeruginosa*
(B) *Staphylococcus aureus*

(C) *Hemophilus influenzae*
(D) *Streptococcus pneumoniae*
(E) *Legionella*

98. A 63-year-old man with chronic bronchitis presents to the emergency department with worsening shortness of breath. He is dyspneic, his respiratory rate is 32/min, and he has peripheral cyanosis. A chest examination reveals increased anteroposterior diameter and scattered rhonchi, but no wheezes or evidence of consolidation. His ABG determinations on room air are pH of 7.36, arterial oxygen pressure (Pao_2) of 40 mmHg, and $Paco_2$ of 47 mmHg. He is given oxygen by face mask while awaiting a CXR. His respiratory rate falls to 12/min, but his ABGs on oxygen are now pH of 7.31, Pao_2 of 62 mmHg, and $Paco_2$ of 58 mmHg. Which of the following is the most appropriate next step in the management of this patient?

(A) repeat the ABG
(B) initiate mechanical ventilation
(C) obtain a CXR
(D) check the oxygen delivery system
(E) decrease the fraction of inspired oxygen (Fio_2)

Questions 99 through 101

99. A 26-year-old man presents with a hard, painless testicular mass. At operation, frozen section reveals testicular cancer. Which of the following is a risk factor?

(A) family history of testicular cancer
(B) masturbation
(C) prior history of radiation exposure
(D) cryptorchidism
(E) maternal diethylstilbestrol (DES) during pregnancy

100. What is the most common cell type in testicular cancer?

(A) choriocarcinoma
(B) embryonal cell
(C) seminoma
(D) teratocarcinoma
(E) endodermal sinus

101. What serum marker can be used to monitor therapy?

(A) carcinoembryonic antigen (CEA)
(B) human chorionic gonadotropin (hCG)
(C) sedimentation rate
(D) lactic dehydrogenase (LDH)
(E) prostate-specific antigen (PSA)

102. A 55-year-old man with a 50 pack-year history of smoking presents with hemoptysis. CXR shows a left upper lobe mass and laboratory evaluation reveals hypercalcemia. Which of the following is the most likely diagnosis?

(A) small cell lung cancer
(B) tuberculosis
(C) squamous cell lung cancer
(D) adenocarcinoma of the lung
(E) metastatic testicular cancer

103. A 25-year-old man has the sudden onset of chest pain on the right side and dyspnea. On CXR, his trachea is deviated to the left. Which of the following should be anticipated on examination?

(A) rales on the left
(B) rales on the right
(C) hyperresonance on the left
(D) distant breath sounds on the right
(E) pleural friction rub on the left

104. A 65-year-old woman with a long history of uncontrolled hypertension and valvular heart disease presents for evaluation. She is fatigued and complains of swelling in her legs and shortness of breath. Which of the following is the distinguishing feature of left ventricular failure?

(A) elevated liver enzymes
(B) pulmonary edema
(C) ascites
(D) peripheral edema
(E) jugular venous distention

105. A 42-year-old man admitted with a high fever and leukocytosis is transferred to the intensive care unit in shock. Which of the following is a common finding in the early stages of septic shock?

(A) reduced cardiac output
(B) bradycardia
(C) decreased systemic vascular resistance (SVR)
(D) hypertension
(E) metabolic alkalosis

106. A 35-year-old man presents with acute low back pain after lifting a couch in his home. Pain is in the lumbosacral area and increases with walking and bending. Examination reveals paraspinal muscle spasm and tenderness and negative straight leg raise bilaterally. Which of the following is the best next step in managing this patient?

(A) bed rest for 1 week
(B) referral to an orthopedic specialist
(C) x-ray of lumbosacral spine
(D) treatment with anti-inflammatory medication and gradual return to normal activity
(E) referral to a pain clinic

107. A 54-year-old woman is brought to the ER with palpitations and dizziness. She has a history of arrhythmia. Adenosine is given and the patient converts to a sinus rhythm. Which of the following rhythms did this patient most likely present to the ER with?

(A) ventricular tachycardia
(B) atrial fibrillation
(C) atrial flutter
(D) paroxysmal supraventricular tachycardia
(E) ventricular fibrillation

108. A 48-year-old man complains of fatigue and shortness of breath. His hematocrit is 32% and hemoglobin is 10.3 g/100 mL. Peripheral blood smear reveals macrocytosis. His serum vitamin B_{12} level is 90 pg/mL (normal, 170–940); serum folate level is 6 ng/mL (normal, 2–14). Which of the following is the most likely cause of this patient's symptoms?

(A) poor dietary habits
(B) colonic diverticulosis
(C) regional enteritis
(D) chronic constipation
(E) vagotomy

109. A 62-year-old man presents with weakness and aching in his hips and shoulders which has progressed over the last few months. He reports generalized fatigue and malaise. Work-up includes a normal complete blood count, kidney and liver tests, and a sedimentation rate of 98. Which of the following is the most likely diagnosis?

(A) SLE
(B) diabetes
(C) Wegener's granulomatosis
(D) polymyalgia rheumatica
(E) Graves disease

110. A 33-year-old woman complains of generalized, throbbing headache that is worse in the morning and with coughing. She occasionally feels dizzy and nauseated. Examination is significant only for obesity and bilateral papilledema. A CT scan of the head is normal. At lumbar puncture, the opening pressure is 220 mm H_2O; CSF is clear, with protein of 12 mg/100 mL (normal, 15–45), glucose of 68 mg/100 mL (normal, 45–80), and no cells are seen. Which of the following is the most likely diagnosis?

(A) migraine headache
(B) multiple sclerosis
(C) malignant carcinomatosis
(D) pseudotumor cerebri
(E) glaucoma

111. A 55-year-old man is being evaluated for gradually increasing shortness of breath. He does not smoke and does not have any significant environmental exposures. Cardiac work-up is unremarkable and pulmonary function tests reveal decreased lung volumes and decreased total lung capacity and vital capacity. Which of the following is the most likely diagnosis?

(A) chronic pulmonary emboli
(B) obstructive lung disease
(C) adult-onset asthma
(D) tuberculosis
(E) interstitial lung disease

112. A 24-year-old man is found to be seropositive for HIV on a military induction screening test. Which of the following opportunistic infections is most likely to develop in this patient?

(A) *Pneumocystis carinii* pneumonia
(B) *Candida albicans* fungemia
(C) disseminated *Mycobacterium avium-intracellulare* infection
(D) cryptococcal meningitis
(E) cytomegalovirus retinitis

113. A 56-year-old man complains of fatigue, dyspnea on exertion, and palpitations. He has had a murmur since childhood. Examination reveals a lift at the left sternal border, split S_1, and fixed splitting of S_2. There is a grade 3/6 midsystolic pulmonic murmur and a 1/6 mid-diastolic tricuspid murmur at the lower left sternal border. CXR shows right ventricular enlargement and prominent pulmonary arteries. An ECG demonstrates atrial fibrillation with a RBBB. Which of the following is the most likely diagnosis?

(A) coarctation of the aorta
(B) ASD
(C) patent ductus arteriosus
(D) tetralogy of Fallot
(E) VSD

DIRECTIONS (Questions 114 through 119): For each item, select the ONE best lettered option that is most closely associated with it. Each lettered option may be selected once, more than once, or not at all.

(A) rheumatoid arthritis
(B) SLE
(C) Wegener's granulomatosus
(D) polyarteritis nodosa
(E) Goodpasture syndrome
(F) fibromyalgia
(G) osteoarthritis (OA)
(H) temporal arteritis
(I) sarcoidosis

114. A 70-year-old female with headaches and fevers notices visual changes. Her erythrocyte sedimentation rate (ESR) is 125.

115. A 40-year-old male with purulent, bloody sinus drainage, hemoptysis, and rising creatinine.

116. A 32-year-old White female with anemia, arthralgia, alopecia, and red blood cell casts on urinalysis.

117. A 38-year-old Black female with shortness of breath and bilateral hilar adenopathy on CXR.

118. A 45-year-old female with pain and visible swelling in her metacarpal-phalangeal joints bilaterally. Her distal interphalangeal joints appear normal.

119. A 60-year-old obese male with Heberden's nodes on his hands and chronic, severe left-sided knee pain.

DIRECTIONS (Questions 120 through 144): Each of the numbered items or incomplete statements in this section is followed by answers or completions of the statement. Select the ONE lettered answer or completion that is BEST in each case.

120. A 92-year-old man is referred from his nursing home for evaluation of lethargy. Examination is unrevealing, but laboratory results are significant for a serum sodium level of 118 meq/L (normal, 135–148). Serum osmolality is 260, urine osmolality is 450, and urine sodium is 80. Which of the following is the most likely cause of this patient's lethargy?

(A) hyperglycemia
(B) hyperlipidemia
(C) hyperproteinemia
(D) SIADH
(E) diabetes insipidus

121. Which of the following is the most common cause of nephrotic syndrome?

(A) diabetes mellitus
(B) Hodgkin's lymphoma
(C) heroin abuse
(D) malignant hypertension
(E) renal failure

Questions 122 and 123

122. A 33-year-old woman experiences visions of flashing lights followed by throbbing left-sided temporal pain and nausea. Which of the following is the most likely diagnosis?

(A) tension headache
(B) transient ischemic attack (TIA)
(C) temporal arteritis
(D) migraine headache
(E) cluster headache

123. This patient is most likely to benefit from acute treatment with which of the following substances?

(A) propranolol
(B) prednisone
(C) sumatriptan
(D) heparin
(E) oxygen

Questions 124 and 125

A 27-year-old female complains of dysuria and urinary frequency. Urinalysis reveals 10–20 WBCs per high-power field and numerous gram-negative bacteria. She denies fevers, chills, and has no flank pain or tenderness.

124. Which of the following statements concerning urinary tract infections is true?

(A) A single dose of an antibiotic may be sufficient treatment.
(B) Pregnant women with bacteriuria should not be treated if asymptomatic.
(C) Patients with flank pain or fever should be hospitalized.
(D) Hematuria indicates renal involvement.
(E) Urologic investigation is indicated after the treatment course is completed.

125. Which of the following bacteria is most likely responsible for this patient's urinary tract infection?

(A) *Klebsiella*
(B) *Chlamydia*
(C) *Escherichia coli*
(D) *Pseudomonas*
(E) *Candida*

126. A 49-year-old woman with a history of migraine headaches reports 6 days of persistent headache, nausea, and recurrent vomiting. On examination, the patient is orthostatic. Electrolytes show a bicarbonate of 42 and a blood gas is obtained revealing a pH of 7.53, carbon dioxide of 53, and Po_2 of 85. What is the underlying acid-base abnormality?

(A) metabolic acidosis
(B) metabolic alkalosis
(C) respiratory acidosis
(D) respiratory alkalosis
(E) respiratory alkalosis and metabolic acidosis

Questions 127 and 128

127. A 28-year-old man has the acute onset of colicky pain in the left costovertebral angle radiating into the groin, as well as gross hematuria. Abdominal x-ray discloses a stone in the left ureter. Which of the following is true concerning this disease?

(A) The majority of renal stones are radiolucent.
(B) Radiolucent stones are usually composed of uric acid.
(C) Staghorn calculi are associated with acid urine.
(D) Radiopaque stones usually contain cystine.
(E) Urate stones are associated with alkaline urine.

128. The patient spontaneously passes the stone, which is found to contain calcium oxalate. Which of the following is the most likely cause of this stone?

(A) chronic urinary tract infection
(B) vitamin D excess
(C) primary hyperparathyroidism
(D) idiopathic hypercalciuria
(E) RTA

129. A 30-year-old woman comes to your office for evaluation of fatigue and shortness of breath on exertion. Past medical history is unremarkable. Physical examination is remarkable only for mild pallor. Lung and cardiovascular examination are normal. Labs show a hematocrit of 28 with a mean corpuscular volume of 72. WBC count and platelet count are normal. On taking further history from the patient, which of the following patient questions would most likely confirm a diagnosis?

(A) What is your family history of colon cancer?
(B) What is your family history of heart disease?
(C) How much alcohol do you drink?
(D) Do you have attacks of pain in your joints?
(E) How heavy are your menstrual periods?

130. A 54-year-old man complains of cough, shortness of breath, and pleuritic left-sided chest pain. Examination and CXR are compatible with a large left-sided pleural effusion. At thoracentesis, the pleural fluid is straw colored and slightly turbid, with a WBC count of 53,000/mL, RBC count of 1200/mL, glucose of 42 mg/100 mL, total protein of 5 g/100 mL, LDH of 418 IU/L, and pH of 7.2. Simultaneous serum total protein is 8 g/100 mL (normal, 6–8 g/100 mL), and serum LDH level is 497 IU/L (normal, 52–149 IU/L). Gram stain is positive for gram-negative rods. Which of the following is the most likely cause of his pleural effusion?

(A) parapneumonic effusion
(B) congestive heart failure
(C) malignant effusion
(D) trauma
(E) nephrotic syndrome

131. A young woman with a history of seizures has a series of grand mal seizures in the emergency room. She is lethargic and has a nonfocal neurologic examination. Her blood gas reveals a pH of 7.12, carbon dioxide of 48, P_{O_2} of 86, and calculated bicarbonate of 16. How would you best characterize her underlying acid-base problem?

(A) respiratory acidosis
(B) metabolic and respiratory acidosis
(C) metabolic acidosis and respiratory alkalosis
(D) metabolic alkalosis and respiratory acidosis
(E) metabolic acidosis

132. A 43-year-old man with AIDS complains of shortness of breath and worsening diarrhea. His temperature is 98°F, respiration rate is 26/min, pulse rate is 100/min, and BP is 100/70 mmHg. His lung and heart examination are unremarkable. A room air ABG reveals: pH 7.10/P_{CO_2} 5/P_{O_2} 130/calculated bicarbonate 6. What is the primary acid-base disorder?

(A) respiratory acidosis
(B) respiratory alkalosis
(C) metabolic acidosis
(D) metabolic alkalosis

Questions 133 and 134

A 17-year-old girl notes an enlarging lump in her neck. On examination, her thyroid gland is twice the normal size, firm to rubbery, multilobular, nontender, and freely mobile. There is no adenopathy. Family history is positive for both hypo- and hyperthyroidism. Her serum triiodothyronine (T_3) and thyroxine (T_4) levels are low normal, and serum thyroid-stimulating hormone (TSH) is high normal. Technetium scan shows nonuniform uptake. Serum and antithyroglobulin titer is strongly positive.

133. What will thyroid biopsy of this patient most likely disclose?

- (A) giant cell granulomas and necrosis
- (B) polymorphonuclear cells and bacteria
- (C) diffuse fibrous replacement
- (D) lymphocytic infiltration
- (E) parafollicular cells

134. Which of the following is the most appropriate treatment for this patient?

- (A) corticosteroids
- (B) antibiotics
- (C) thyroid hormone
- (D) radioactive iodine
- (E) surgery

135. An obese 21-year-old woman complains of increased growth of coarse hair on her lip, chin, chest, and abdomen. She also notes menstrual irregularity with periods of amenorrhea. Which of the following is the most likely cause of this patient's symptoms?

- (A) polycystic ovary disease
- (B) an ovarian tumor
- (C) an adrenal tumor
- (D) Cushing disease
- (E) familial hirsutism

136. A 71-year-old woman is receiving parenteral methicillin for leg cellulitis. Over 2 days, she develops macroscopic hematuria, oliguria, and marked deterioration in renal functioning. Which of the following is suggestive of methicillin-induced acute interstitial nephritis?

- (A) protein in the urine
- (B) eosinophils in the urine
- (C) RBC casts in the urine
- (D) hyaline casts in the urine
- (E) myoglobin in the urine

137. A 52-year-old man is receiving a preoperative evaluation before elective surgery. He is asymptomatic and has a normal examination, but is noted to have a hemoglobin of 10.8, hematocrit of 33, with a mean corpuscular volume of 70 (normal, 82–92), and 6.1 million RBCs (normal, 4.5–5.0). Which of the following is the most likely diagnosis?

- (A) sickle cell anemia
- (B) iron-deficiency anemia
- (C) alpha-thalassemia major
- (D) beta-thalassemia minor
- (E) anemia of chronic disease

138. A 27-year-old woman presents with bloody stools. She is found to have multiple, irregular dark brown macules on her lips, buccal mucosa, hands, and feet. What is the most likely cause of her gastrointestinal (GI) bleeding?

- (A) esophageal carcinoma
- (B) jejunal hamartomas
- (C) gastric telangiectasia
- (D) intestinal neurofibromas
- (E) colonic hemangioma

Questions 139 and 140

A 42-year-old man camping in northern Wisconsin finds a tick embedded in his scalp. He presents to clinic a few days later after returning from his trip. He camps multiple times each summer and is fearful of Lyme disease.

139. Subsequent testing is positive for acute Lyme disease in this patient. Which of the following is a likely outcome in Lyme disease?

- (A) Thirty percent of patients have a slowly expanding skin lesion (erythema migrans) at the site of the tick bite.
- (B) Within weeks, 75% of untreated patients will develop neurologic manifestations.

(C) Fifty percent of untreated patients may develop chronic neuroborreliosis.
(D) Months after onset of illness, 60% of untreated patients will have intermittent attacks of joint swelling and pain.
(E) Joint involvement is primary in small joints (hands).

140. Which of the following persons is most in need of vaccination?

(A) a 20-year-old living in Chicago, IL
(B) an 85-year-old retiree living in Phoenix, AZ
(C) a 35-year-old living in the North Carolina mountains
(D) a 56-year-old who vacations in the Maine woods each summer
(E) a 45-year-old living in Boca Raton, FL

141. At a routine company physical examination, an asymptomatic 46-year-old man is found to have a BP of 150/110 mmHg, but no other abnormalities are present. Which of the following is the most appropriate next step in management?

(A) reassure the patient and repeat the physical examination in 12 months
(B) order an ECG
(C) initiate antihypertensive therapy
(D) obtain repeated BP recordings in your office and/or the patient's home or work site
(E) counsel the patient on dietary sodium reduction

142. A 58-year-old man carries the diagnosis of pseudogout (chondrocalcinosis). Which of the following is a common feature?

(A) uric acid deposits within joints
(B) episodic attacks of pain
(C) small joints affected more often than large joints
(D) predilection for women
(E) predilection for young people

143. A 25-year-old man presents with a large malignant melanoma on his back. There is no apparent lymphadenopathy (clinical stage 1). Which of the following is the most important prognostic factor?

(A) tumor thickness
(B) tumor diameter
(C) tumor location
(D) the patient's gender
(E) mitotic rate

144. What metabolic abnormality is the typical cause for the ECG changes seen in Fig. 1-18?

(A) hypokalemia
(B) hypercalcemia
(C) hypomagnesemia
(D) hyperkalemia
(E) hypocalcemia

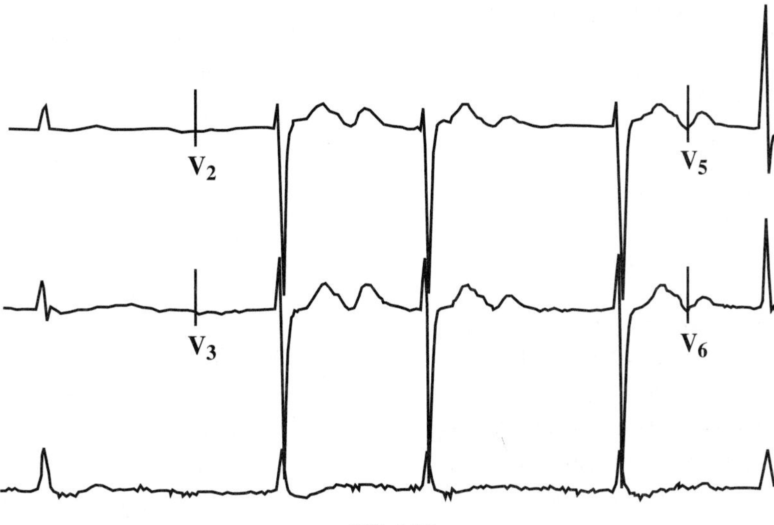

FIG. 1-18

Answers and Explanations

1. **(A)**

2. **(B)**

3. **(E)**

Explanations 1 through 3

The heliotrope, purple periorbital rash is seen with dermatomyositis and may even precede the muscle involvement. On examination, these patients will usually show proximal muscle weakness and may complain of difficulty getting up from a chair, climbing stairs, and raising the arms over the head. Ataxia may be present with cerebellar lesions. Deep tendon reflexes should be normal and there is no joint inflammation. Polymyalgia rheumatica generally occurs in older people but is not associated with muscle weakness. Spinocerebellar degeneration, vasculitis, and rheumatoid arthritis are not associated with this rash. Creatine phosphokinase is usually markedly elevated and muscle biopsy will confirm the diagnosis. Serum creatinine, sodium, and potassium should be normal, and rheumatoid factor should not be elevated. *(Kasper et al., pp. 2540–2544)*

4. **(A)** Ciprofloxacin is the drug of choice in a dose of 500 mg bid for 1–3 days because most cases of travelers' diarrhea are from *E. coli*. This patient's symptoms are moderate to severe and warrant antibiotic treatment which will decrease the frequency of bowel movements and duration of illness. Erythromycin and tetracycline are effective for *Vibrio* which is an uncommon cause of travelers' diarrhea. Metronidazole is used for *Clostridium difficile* enteritis. (*Kasper et al., pp. 727–728*)

5. **(D)** Basal cell carcinoma is the most common form of skin cancer and can present as an isolated papule or nodule or with ulceration. Although locally aggressive and destructive, they rarely metastasize. Fig. 1-2 shows a large ulcer with a rodent-like appearance with nodules at the border. Squamous cell carcinoma would be in the differential, but it does not ulcerate as often and is characterized by being hard nodules. Malignant melanomas are usually nodular and pigmented. It would be highly unusual for a benign nevus to ulcerate and have this appearance. A hemangioma is a red vascular lesion. (*Kasper et al., pp. 497–498*)

6. **(C)**

7. **(A)**

8. **(B)**

Explanations 6 through 8

Patients at high risk include those with previous endocarditis, prosthetic heart valves, valvular heart disease, and congenital heart lesions. Congestive heart failure, an S_4 gallop, and diabetes do not increase risk. Recommended antibiotic coverage for high-risk patients before dental procedures is amoxicillin 2 g po 1 h before the procedures. Penicillin-allergic patients can receive clarithromycin, cephalexin, cefadroxil, or clindamycin as prophylaxis. *Streptococci* and *Staphylococcus aureus* are responsible for the majority of community-acquired native valve endocarditis cases. In IV drug abusers, *S. aureus* is responsible for more than 50% of cases, and *Candida* and *Pseudomonas* for about 6% each. Patients with prior endocarditis are at high risk. Bacterial endocarditis carries a mortality rate of about 25%, and prevention is of paramount importance. In *S. aureus* endocarditis in injection drug users, mortality is only 10–15%. As many as 40% of cases occur without underlying heart disease. VSD, patent ductus arteriosus, and tetralogy of Fallot are most commonly associated; whereas, ASD is rarely a predisposing factor. (*Kasper et al., pp. 731–740*)

9. **(A)** The Clinical Practice Guidelines of the American College of Physicians (endorsed by CDC, American Academy of Family Physicians and the Infectious Disease Society of America) state that most cases of acute sinusitis in the ambulatory setting are due to viral infection and do not require antibiotic treatment or radiography. Therapy should be targeted toward symptoms and often include decongestants, antipyretics, and analgesics. Antibiotic treatment should be reserved for patients who have symptoms that persist or worsen (generally for more than 7 days). (*Piccirillo, pp. 902–910*)

10. **(B)**

11. **(D)**

12. **(E)**

Explanations 10 through 12

Marfan syndrome is an inherited disorder of connective tissue, but at least one-fourth of patients do not have an affected parent. Abnormal metabolism of collagen or elastin is suspected as the cause. Clinical features involve the eyes (upward subluxation of the lenses, myopia), cardiovascular system (aortic dilation, regurgitation, and aneurysms; mitral valve prolapse), and the skeleton (arachnodactyly, pectus deformity, joint laxity). Mental retardation and malar rash are not associated with Marfan. A frequent finding is increased length of the limbs as compared with the trunk. Aortic root dilatation is a serious complication that can lead to aortic regurgitation, dissection, and even rupture. Mitral valve prolapse is also seen, but pulmonary stenosis, VSD, pulmonary hypertension, and CAD are not increased with Marfan syndrome. Echocardiography should be performed to follow the course of the heart. The other tests will not reveal aortic root dilatation or aneurysm formation. (*Kasper et al., pp. 2329–2330*)

13. **(B)** Screening should begin approximately 10 years before the age of diagnosis of colorectal cancer in a first degree (parent or sibling) relative. Given that this patient's mother was diagnosed at age 50, this patient should start screening at age 40. The natural history of a colon polyp to develop into cancer is thought to be 10 years. Colorectal cancer screening has proven mortality benefit. (*Smith et al., pp. 27–43*)

14. **(B)** The presence of effusion generally signifies significant disease. Aspiration of the effusion will help in evaluation for hemarthrosis, septic arthritis, and inflammatory crystal disease. Each of these is important to identify and treat early. An MRI and/or arthroscopy would be later considerations. Orthopedic referral likely would be necessary. (*Ferrari and Bach, pp. 52–63*)

15. **(E)** The x-ray in Fig. 1-3 shows a large, pleural-based tumor in the left upper chest; this is most likely a mesothelioma. The tumor is locally invasive, so there are no signs of extrathoracic disease. Direct exposure or contact with asbestos is not required—tumors have occurred in families of asbestos workers. The exposure may be brief and mild, and there is typically a long latent period before appearance of the tumor, about 20–40 years. Surgery is curative in local cases. Diffuse malignant mesothelioma responds poorly to all treatments (surgery, radiotherapy, and chemotherapy). (*Kasper et al., pp. 1523, 1567*)

16. **(A)** Mitral valve prolapse can be diagnosed by auscultation and echocardiogram in as much as 10% of the population. They may be asymptomatic or complain of atypical chest pain, palpitation, shortness of breath, or weakness. An increasing number of complications are being recognized. Although they occur infrequently, they may be life threatening and demand careful evaluation of individuals at risk. Both supraventricular and ventricular arrhythmias occur, as may sudden death. Mitral insufficiency, if present, is usually insignificant but may progress and require valve replacement. There is an increased risk of infective endocarditis. Intraatrial thrombus formation may occur, predisposing to cerebral and peripheral embolism. Because the clot originates in the left atrium, however, pulmonary embolism does not occur more frequently in these patients. (*Kasper et al., pp. 1395–1396*)

17. **(A)** The autopsy specimen illustrated in Fig. 1-4 contains a large, multicolored, irregular tumor

invading the left hemisphere. There is hemorrhage, necrosis, and surrounding edema. The clinical and pathologic findings are most compatible with a diagnosis of malignant glioma (astrocytoma). Glioma is a highly malignant tumor of astrocytic cells and is the most common primary brain tumor. It infiltrates widely, often involving multiple lobes, as well as the opposite hemisphere via the corpus callosum. Prognosis is poor, with an average survival time of 6 months after diagnosis. Meningiomas are benign primary brain tumors that are usually slow growing and occur outside of the hemispheres, where they are well encapsulated and compress but do not invade brain tissue. Craniopharyngiomas arise from remnants of Rathke's pouch (the craniopharyngeal anlage). They are usually benign, well encapsulated, and found in or near the sella turcica. Acoustic neuromas arise from the root of the eighth cranial nerve in the cerebellopontine angle. Like meningiomas, they are encapsulated and compress rather than invade brain substance. (*Kasper et al., pp. 2452–2457*)

18. **(D)** The history of severe, self-induced weight loss with an abnormal attitude toward food, weight, and body image in an adolescent female strongly suggests anorexia nervosa. Common symptoms are amenorrhea, not menorrhagia or metrorrhagia, constipation, and cold intolerance. Examination frequently reveals cachexia, hypothermia, bradycardia, hypotension, hypercarotenemic skin, and increased lanugo-like body hair. Decreased thyroid and pituitary function are evident on laboratory tests, but thrombocytopenia and anemia are not common. (*Kasper et al., pp. 430–432*)

19. **(D)**

20. **(B)**

Explanations 19 and 20

Hypercalcemia is a common complication of malignancy. Mechanisms include bone metastases, humoral secretion (e.g., osteoclast-activating factor), prostaglandin, or ectopic parathormone production and immobilization. Hypercalcemia is often manifested by confusion and lethargy. The other metabolic abnormalities usually are not associated with confusion. Therapy is directed at increasing renal calcium clearance and inhibiting further bone resorption. Saline infusion raises the glomerular filtration rate and decreases calcium reabsorption in the proximal tubule. Under life-threatening circumstances, the infusion may need to be aggressive, as much as 6 L of saline daily plus furosemide. Radiotherapy will do nothing for the calcium. Tamoxifen is an antiestrogen used in the treatment of breast carcinoma and other malignancies. When used in the presence of bone metastases, it may contribute to hypercalcemia. Chemotherapy will not decrease the calcium levels. Glucocorticoids have an antitumor effect and reduce tumor production of humoral mediators, but act slowly. (*Kasper et al., pp. 2257–2261*)

21. **(C)** He should avoid alcohol and spicy foods because these along with the heat, emotional stress, and hot temperature foods can aggravate rosacea. Hydralazine is a vasodilator and could worsen his nasal erythema. Smoking vasoconstricts rather than dilates blood vessels. Metronidazole gel is an effective topical therapy. Laser therapy is usually done after the other interventions have been tried. (*Kasper et al., p. 295*)

22. **(E)** Increased risk for CAD from high triglyceride levels has not been established. Severely elevated triglycerides (1000 mg/100 mL) are a recognized risk factor for attacks of acute pancreatitis, and control of the triglycerides can prevent these attacks. Diet alone is usually not sufficient at these high levels. A National Institutes of Health Consensus Conference has recommended that treatment be initiated in all patients with triglycerides greater than 500 mg/100 mL to prevent acute pancreatitis. Skin lesions are not present with hypertriglyceridemia. (*Kasper et al., pp. 1430–1432*)

23. **(B)** Many drugs require dosage modifications in chronic renal insufficiency. Bioavailability, distribution, action, and elimination of drugs all may be altered. The aminoglycosides, vancomycin,

ampicillin, most cephalosporins, methicillin, penicillin G, sulfonamides, and trimethoprim all should be given in reduced dosage to patients with chronic renal failure. The small group of antibiotics not needing dosage modification includes chloramphenicol, erythromycin, and the isoxazolyl penicillins (nafcillin and oxacillin). (*Kasper et al., p. 1662, 19*)

24. **(C)** Chronic renal failure treated with hemodialysis results in predictable metabolic abnormalities. The kidneys fail to excrete phosphate, leading to hyperphosphatemia, and fail to synthesize $1,25(OH)_2D_3$. Vitamin D deficiency causes impaired intestinal calcium absorption. Phosphate retention, defective intestinal absorption, and skeletal resistance to parathyroid hormone (PTH) all result in hypocalcemia. Hypocalcemia causes secondary hyperparathyroidism, and the excess PTH production worsens the hyperphosphatemia by increasing phosphorus release from bone. These derangements impair collagen synthesis and maturation, resulting in skeletal abnormalities collectively referred to as renal osteodystrophy. Osteomalacia, osteosclerosis, and osteitis fibrosa cystica may all be seen. (*Kasper et al., pp. 1656–1657*)

25. **(A)** CJD is caused by an infectious protein called a prion. Patients typically are between 50 and 75 years of age and present with dementia and clonus. The disease is progressive and death occurs generally within a year of symptom onset. CJD is found throughout the world, and no consistent etiologic agent has been identified. (*Kasper et al., pp. 2495–2500*)

26. **(A)** Diabetes insipidus, a deficiency of pituitary antidiuretic hormone (ADH) (arginine vasopressin), causes water loss because of failure to facilitate reabsorption of water in the distal tubules and collecting ducts of the kidneys. In central diabetes insipidus, there is impaired production of vasopressin, and in nephrogenic diabetes insipidus, the distal renal tubules are refractory to vasopressin. In central diabetes insipidus, urine osmolality remains unchanged. If water intoxication were present, stopping IV fluids should have increased urine osmolality. With solute overload, serum osmolality would have been higher. In SIADH, urine osmolality is usually higher than serum osmolality. (*Kasper et al., pp. 251–258, 2098–2100*)

27. **(B)** Endocrine syndromes are seen in 12% of patients with lung cancer. Squamous cell carcinoma is associated with PTH-related peptide. Adrenocorticotrophic hormone (ACTH) and ADH secretion can be associated with small cell lung carcinoma. ACTH-secreting tumors are associated with darkening of the skin and hypokalemia. (*Kasper et al., pp. 508–509*)

28. **(D)** This patient has an elevated pH (normal is 7.40) indicating alkalosis. A low carbon dioxide level is consistent with a respiratory etiology of the alkalosis. This occurs when alveolar ventilation is increased relative to CO_2 production. Causes may include fever, anxiety, pain, pulmonary, and/or neurologic conditions. In a metabolic alkalosis, a high bicarbonate is seen (a bicarbonate of 20 is low normal). (*Paulson, pp. 103–109*)

29. **(A)** Viral (follicular) conjunctivitis most often presents with minimal discharge and itching as compared to the moderate-to-profuse discharge of bacterial conjunctivitis. While mild pain and photophobia may be noted in viral, bacterial, fungal, and allergic conjunctivitis, preauricular adenopathy is common in viral and fungal conjunctivitis only. Allergic conjunctivitis presents with minimal discharge and marked itching. The patient's young age and normal eye pressure (tonometry) helps to rule out glaucoma. (*Kasper et al., p. 166*)

30. **(C)** The clinical features of the patient described in the question are most compatible with ankylosing spondylitis, an inflammatory arthritis that occurs most often in young men. Early findings of low back pain and stiffness may progress to involve the entire spine with straightening (poker spine). The most common extraskeletal manifestation is acute anterior iridocyclitis, occurring in 25–30% of patients. Additional manifestations, which occur rarely, include heart block, aortitis with aortic insufficiency, and upper-lobe pulmonary fibrosis. Splenomegaly is associated with rheumatoid arthritis (Felty syndrome) but is not a feature of ankylosing spondylitis, nor are cataracts. (*Kasper et al., pp. 1993–1995*)

31. **(D)**

32. **(D)**

Explanations 31 and 32

This ECG reveals ST segment elevation in II, III, and AVF, indicating acute injury of the inferior wall of the myocardium. Inferior wall ischemia can be perceived as pain in the epigastric area. Anterolateral myocardial infarction would show loss of R-wave progression in V_4 through V_6. Although his symptoms could suggest gastroesophageal reflux or gastroenteritis, this ECG shows this a cardiac event. Costochondritis is not present by examination. When ST segment elevation is present, a patient should be considered a candidate for reperfusion therapy. If no contraindications are present, thrombolytic therapy should ideally be initiated within 30 min, right in the emergency department. The goal of thrombolysis is prompt restoration of coronary arterial patency. Thrombolytic therapy can reduce the risk of in-hospital death by up to 50% when administered within the first hour of symptoms, so time is of the essence. Arranging for a bed may waste time for limiting infarct size. Catheterization can be performed later when the patient is stable. The ECG would obviously preclude the other two options: immediate trial of antacid or reassurance and arranging outpatient follow-up. (*Kasper et al., pp. 1316–1318, 1444–1449*)

33. **(D)** Altered mental status is a poor prognostic sign in community-acquired pneumonia. Other patient factors include age greater than 65 years, systolic BP less than 90 mmHg or diastolic pressure less than 60 mmHg, temperature greater than 38.3°C, and leukocytosis greater than 30,000/mm or less than 4000/mm. *Streptococcus pneumoniae*, *Legionella*, and *Staphylococcus aureus* are the pathogens associated with poor prognosis, not *Mycoplasma*. (*Bartlett et al., pp. 811–838*)

34. **(E)** Up to 30% of cases of acquired vitiligo are associated with thyroid disease, especially Hashimoto's thyroiditis. It also may occur with pernicious anemia, diabetes, and other autoimmune disorders. Vitiligo has not been reported with AIDS. Addison disease, lymphoma, and biliary cirrhosis can be associated with hyperpigmentation. (*Kasper et al., pp. 285–301*)

35. **(B)** Adenocarcinoma of the pancreas arises from ductal epithelium. Because of fibrous tissue formation, the terminal bile duct occludes, causing jaundice. Typically, in the early stages, the patient is free of pain. With invasion of retroperitoneal structures, the patient may sometimes have severe and constant pain. Often, patients have a history of weight loss and present with unexplained diabetes. Because of gradual obstruction, the gallbladder distends, unless it has lost its distensibility because of previous scarring. Malignant biliary stricture, choledocholithiasis, and cirrhosis of the liver are ruled out by the appearance of the CT. Pancreatitis is rarely associated with jaundice and would be painful. (*Kasper et al., pp. 537–538*)

36. **(A)** The spectrum of infection with *Legionella* organisms ranges from asymptomatic seroconversion to Pontiac fever (a flu-like illness) to full-blown pneumonia. Cough is usually nonproductive initially. Malaise, myalgia, and headache are common. The diagnosis of *Legionella* infection is suggested by extrapulmonary signs and symptoms, including diarrhea, abdominal pain, azotemia, and hematuria. (*Kasper et al., pp. 870–874*)

37. **(A)** The causes of lower GI bleeding include hemorrhoids and anal fissure diverticulosis, carcinoma, vascular ectasia, colitis, and polyps. Carcinoma of the colon usually causes chronic GI bleeding, resulting in anemia. Diverticulosis and vascular ectasia are common causes of massive GI bleeding in the elderly patient. Inflammatory bowel disease can also cause massive GI bleeding but is more frequent in younger age group patients. Most patients with ischemic colitis will be quite sick and will have had symptoms before the onset of bleeding. (*Kasper et al., pp. 235–238*)

38. **(C)** The clinical features of the patient described in the question are characteristic of

rhabdomyolysis with myoglobinuria. Skeletal muscle injury releases large amounts of myoglobin into the circulation, and myoglobinuria produces a positive orthotoluidine reaction. Because myoglobin is quickly cleared from serum by the kidneys, the serum does not turn pink, as it does with hemoglobinemia. Muscle damage leads to elevated creatine phosphokinase levels and hyperkalemia. Myoglobin does not bind to haptoglobin as does hemoglobin, so serum haptoglobin levels are normal. The major complication of rhabdomyolysis is acute renal failure. (*Kasper et al., p. 744*)

39. (B) Heart sounds and murmurs can often be accentuated by various physiologic and pharmacologic maneuvers. These maneuvers aid in the differentiation of multiple valvular and other organic lesions from ordinary sounds. Mitral stenosis is a diastolic murmur that grows louder with increased flow across the stenotic valve, as in exercise. A VSD may be small; its murmur will fade with maneuvers favoring forward flow, such as vasodilatation with amyl nitrate. The murmur of aortic stenosis will grow louder with increased flow across the valve, as with amyl nitrate; it will diminish with maneuvers that decrease flow across the valve, as in stage two of the Valsalva maneuver. (*Kasper et al., pp. 1307–1311*)

40. (D)

41. ~~**(D)**~~ E

Explanations 40 and 41

Deficiency of dopamine primarily is responsible for the signs and symptoms of Parkison disease. Specifically, the loss of dopamine from the substantia nigra is thought to be primarily responsible for the akinesia and rigidity. Tremor, akinesia, and rigidity are the classic triad of signs seen in Parkison disease. The tremor typically is a resting tremor; often a "pill rolling" tremor is seen in the hand. Well over 90% of patients with Parkinson disease do have a good initial response to levodopa. (*Lang, pp. 1130–1143*)

42. (C) The CT scan shown in Fig. 1-9 demonstrates a smooth, biconvex lens-shaped mass in the periphery of the right temporoparietal region. This picture is characteristic of a subdural hematoma that is a result of laceration of veins bridging the subdural space. Unlike an epidural hematoma, which expands quickly and progresses rapidly to coma, a subdural hematoma is initially limited in size by increased intracranial pressure and expands slowly. Symptoms may follow the inciting trauma by several weeks. Altered mental status is often more prominent than focal signs and may progress from confusion to stupor to coma. Treatment consists of evacuation of the clot via burr holes. Antibiotics and antifungal agents have no role, and fibrinolytic therapy or delay in treatment could be harmful. (*Kasper et al., pp. 2449–2450*)

43. (C) The history and physical examination of the patient described in the question suggest either an intracerebral hemorrhage or a completed ischemic stroke. The CT scan that accompanies the question demonstrates a large hemorrhage in the region of the right basal ganglia with a surrounding zone of edema and narrowing of the ventricle. Patients with intracerebral hemorrhage often have a preceding history of hypertension. Carotid occlusion, malignancy, arteriovenous malformation, and coagulopathy all are much less likely causes of this disorder. In general, only cerebellar hemorrhages and cerebral hemorrhages that are easily reached are surgically evacuated. Most intracerebral hemorrhages are managed with general supportive care. (*Kasper et al., pp. 257, 2372*)

44. (A) The Hypertension Optimal Treatment Study and the U.K. Prospective Diabetes Study both showed benefit in targeting BP to the normal range in patients with diabetes (i.e., 130/85 mmHg). This patient has multiple readings of 140/90 mmHg and should be treated with antihypertensive medication. (*Kasper et al., pp. 1470–1480*)

45. (B) The arteriograms in Fig. 1-11 demonstrate a large aneurysm arising from the basilar artery. Intracranial aneurysms occasionally present with new onset or worsening of headaches or may be asymptomatic and found coincidentally during evaluation of an unrelated disorder. Frequently, they leak or rupture, resulting in a subarachnoid hemorrhage with sudden onset of severe headache and meningeal symptoms and signs (e.g., nuchal rigidity, photophobia). Rapid progression to stroke, coma, or death may follow. Intracranial aneurysms are not usually associated with hypercalcemia, hypopituitarism, or chronic meningitis and rarely cause tentorial herniation without rupturing. Surgical approaches to intracranial aneurysms include excision and ligation. (*Kasper et al., p. 1481, 86*)

46. (A)

47. (C)

48. (E)

Explanations 46 through 48

Sleep disturbance is a characteristic symptom associated with fibromyalgia. Patients awaken feeling tired. The examination, other than tenderness in 14 specific, symmetrical points, is usually normal. Fever, rash on the extremities, muscle weakness, and migratory joint inflammation point to Lyme disease or other rheumatologic disorders. A sedimentation rate should be normal. If elevated, it may point to another diagnosis. Lyme titers are not indicated unless the patient has symptoms or history suggestive of the disease. Electromyelography and spine radiographs are typically normal and unnecessary for help in establishing the diagnosis. Depression can be associated with pain, but screening for it early on does not make sense and might offend the patient. Low-dose antidepressants often help to correct the sleep pattern and result in relief of pain. Nonsteroidal anti-inflammatory agents can also be used as needed; low-dose steroid is not indicated. Exercise is also helpful, and patients should be encouraged to stay physically active. Amoxicillin is not used for fibromyalgia. Benzodiazepines have addictive potential and lose their effectiveness for sleep after a few weeks. (*Kasper et al., pp. 2055–2057*)

49. (B) The cerebral arteriogram shown in Fig. 1-12 reveals severe stenosis of the common carotid artery proximal to its bifurcation, as well as small lesions in the more distal vessels. Common manifestations are transient monocular blindness (amaurosis fugax), hemiparesis, hemisensory loss, aphasia, and homonymous visual field defects. Ataxia would be an unusual feature of carotid disease and, if present, would suggest involvement of the vertebrobasilar arteries, which results in dysarthria, diplopia, and vertigo. (*Kasper et al., pp. 2383–2384*)

50. (E)

51. (C)

Explanations 50 and 51

The new case definition for AIDS in 1993 added pulmonary tuberculosis, invasive cervical cancer, and recurrent pneumonia. This Centers for Disease Control and Prevention (CDC) classification system is divided into three categories: category A is symptomatic infection with HIV and includes acute illness and persistent lymphadenopathy; category B includes conditions attributed to HIV infection, such as oral thrush, herpes zoster, and peripheral neuropathy; category C is the AIDS surveillance cases. Anergy to common skin test antigens is a common finding with HIV infection. There **is** a decline in CD4 cell numbers, a relative increase in the number of T_8 cells, which results in a decreased T_4:T_8 ratio of less than 1. Functional abnormalities occur in both B cells and natural killer cells, which accounts for the increase in certain bacterial infections seen in advanced HIV disease. Elevation of beta$_2$ submicroglobulin, a serologic finding reflecting immunologic dysfunction, is a fairly reliable marker of progressive immunologic decline and the subsequent development of AIDS. (*Kasper et al., pp. 1071–1122*)

52. (C) This man has multiple seborrheic keratoses, which are very common, benign pigmented tumors that occur after age 30, especially on the trunk and face. Melanocytic nevi are usually small, circumscribed, pigmented macules or papules, rather than large "stuck-on" nodules. Actinic keratoses are red, scaly (not dark) lesions on the face and arms that are from sun-induced damage. Seborrheic dermatitis is a red, scaly rash along the scalp, eyebrows, and nasolabial folds. Malignant melanoma would be in the differential if it were a single lesion. (*Kasper et al., pp. 285, 497–503*)

53. **(B)**

54. **(B)**

Explanations 53 and 54

The wide notched R waves in V_5 and V_6 are characteristic for LBBB. In RBBB, there is an rSR′ complex in V_1 and QRS pattern in V_6. Accelerated junctional rhythm would not have P waves. Partial blocks, such as left anterior fascicular block, generally do not prolong the QRS duration substantially, but are associated with shifts in the frontal plane QRS axis (left axis deviation). With intraventricular conduction delay, the QRS is between 100 and 120 ms. LBBB is a marker of one of four conditions: severe aortic valve disease, ischemic heart disease, long-standing hypertension, and cardiomyopathy. RBBB is seen more commonly than LBBB in patients without structural heart disease, although RBBB also occurs with congenital heart disease and ASD or valvular heart disease. Hyper- but not hypokalemia may cause intraventricular conduction delay. Myocarditis does not usually lead to LBBB. (*Kasper et al., pp. 1315–1316*)

55. **(C)** The $CD4^+$ T-cell count provides information on the current immunologic status of a patient infected with HIV. HIV RNA level measures viral load and predicts what will happen to the $CD4^+$ count in the near future. WBC count is a nonspecific marker for infection. The p24 antigen assay is used for direct detection of HIV. $CD8^+$ count typically is not as important in monitoring immunologic status though the $CD4^+/CD8^+$ ratio sometimes is used. (*Kasper et al., pp. 1071–1122*)

56. **(B)** Primary hyperparathyroidism is characterized by hypercalcemia, hypophosphatemia, hyperchloremia, increased urinary calcium excretion, and an increase in serum parathormone level. Multiple myeloma is associated with hypercalcemia when there are many lytic lesions. Chronic ingestion of 50–100 times the normal requirement of vitamin D is required to produce hypercalcemia in normal people, so hypervitaminosis D is rare and parathormone levels would be suppressed. With milk alkali syndrome, which is caused by excess ingestion of calcium and absorbable antacids, parathormone levels would also be suppressed. In sarcoidosis, about 10% of patients have hypercalcemia attributable to increased intestinal absorption of calcium and increased production of 1,25(OH)2D. (*Kasper et al., pp. 2252–2263*)

57. **(D)** In type 4 RTA associated with diabetes and hypertension, damage to the juxtaglomerular apparatus in the glomeruli leds to decreased renin production. This results in a state of hypoaldosteronism, causing hyperkalemia and a nongap metabolic acidosis. (*Kasper et al., pp. 1699–1700*)

58. **(C)**

59. **(B)**

Explanations 58 and 59

Acute oliguria is a medical emergency requiring the immediate identification of any correctable cause. Distention of the urinary bladder indicates bladder outlet obstruction. Immediate management should be the passage of a urethral catheter to relieve the obstruction and provide urine for examination. An abdominal flat plate, ultrasonography, or IVP may yield a diagnosis but delay the relief of obstruction. Furosemide may be harmful if given while the bladder is obstructed. Bladder outlet obstruction may be caused by prostatic hypertrophy or prostatitis, stones, clots, malignancy, or urethral stricture; it may also be neurogenic. Posterior urethral valves are a congenital defect that could cause obstruction in children but rarely in adults. Renal carcinoma would not cause outlet obstruction. Renal arterial occlusion can cause acute renal failure but not obstructive uropathy. If urethral catheterization fails to relieve the obstruction, further evaluation, including radiographic or ultrasound studies, is in order. Suprapubic cystostomy may be necessary to empty the bladder. (*Kasper et al., pp. 1644–1652*)

60. **(E)** Hashimoto's thyroiditis, an autoimmune condition, is the leading cause of multinodular goiter in the United States. Although not unique to this condition, antimicrosomal antibodies are found in 70–95% of patients. Antinuclear antibodies are associated with SLE. Although an autoimmune process, steroids are of no benefit in this condition. One-third of patients experience progressive loss of glandular function, and eventually become hypothyroid, but there is no increased incidence of thyroid cancer. (*Kasper et al., pp. 2109–2113*)

61. **(D)** Men are affected by cluster headaches seven to eight times more often than women. Attacks are typically periorbital and may involve the temporal area. Cluster headaches typically occur daily over a 4- to 8-week period followed by pain-free intervals averaging 1 year. The periodicity of the attacks is often striking, with daily recurrences of pain often at the same hour. Pathogenesis is thought to be due to abnormal serotonergic neurotransmission. One hundred percent oxygen inhalation is most effective acutely. Drugs used to prevent cluster attacks include lithium, ergotamine, sodium valproate, and prednisone. (*Kasper et al., pp. 85–94*)

62. **(D)** Asthma is characterized by bronchospasm and typically causes a prolonged expiratory phase and retention of carbon dioxide. This degree of hypoxia (Po_2 of 49) generally would not be seen with asthma. Pulmonary embolism, congestive heart failure, myocardial infarction, or pneumonia all could lead to this degree of hypoxia. The constellation of fever, elevated white count, and localized infiltrate on CXR is most characteristic of pneumonia. The most likely etiology is perioperative aspiration related to general anesthesia. (*Kasper et al., pp. 209–210, 1535–1538*)

63. **(B)** Detection of leukocyte casts is pathognomonic for pyelonephritis. Common symptoms include fever, shaking chills, nausea, vomiting, and diarrhea. Flank tenderness over the affected kidney is very common. (*Kasper et al., pp. 1717–1720*)

64. **(A)**

65. **(C)**

66. **(A)**

Explanations 64 through 66

Hepatitis A is transmitted almost exclusively by the fecal-oral route. Large outbreaks have been linked to contaminated food products. Intrafamily and intrainstitutional spread also is common. Clinical severity usually is mild, and hepatitis A does not progress to chronicity. Hepatitis C more commonly progresses to chronicity (50–70% develop chronic hepatitis and 80–90% of these patients have evidence for chronic infection). Hepatitis C can lead to cirrhosis and hepatocellular carcinoma. Chronicity occurs in only 1–10% of patients with hepatitis B. (*Kasper et al., pp. 1822–1845*)

67. **(J)** Polycystic ovarian syndrome is characterized by infertility, hirsutism, obesity, and amenorrhea or oligomenorrhea. These patients have chronic anovulation and experience withdrawal bleeding after progestogen administration. (*Kasper et al., pp. 2204–2205*)

68. **(B)** Addison disease, or primary adrenocortical deficiency, commonly results in a low serum Na^+, a low serum Cl^-, and a high serum K^+. Aldosterone deficiency causes loss of sodium in the urine and contributes to the hyperkalemia. The original description of Addison disease summarizes well the key clinical findings: general languor and debility, feebleness of the heart's action, irritability of the stomach, and a peculiar change of the color of the skin. The hyperpigmentation of the skin is often seen on the elbows and in the creases of the hands. (*Kasper et al., pp. 2141–2143*)

69. **(F)** Pheochromocytoma is a secondary cause of hypertension. Pheochromocytomas secrete catecholamines; 80% are unilateral, solitary tumors, most often located in the adrenal

gland. Patients present with episodes of headache, palpitations, sweats, and a sense of apprehension. (*Kasper et al., pp. 2148–2152*)

70. **(G)** Acromegaly is caused by oversecretion of growth hormone, usually from a pituitary adenoma. Clinical manifestations are indolent, often not diagnosed for 10 or more years. Acral bony overgrowth leads to frontal bossing, increased hand and foot size, and mandibular enlargement. Growth hormone excess also commonly affects the cardiovascular system. Upper airway obstruction with sleep apnea is present in up to 60% of patients. (*Kasper et al., pp. 2090–2092*)

71. **(E)** The most common symptoms seen in patients with hypothyroidism include tiredness, weakness, dry skin, feeling cold, hair loss, difficulty concentrating with poor memory, constipation, and weight gain. (*Kasper et al., pp. 2109–2111*)

72. **(A)** Cushing syndrome is caused by overproduction of cortisol by the adrenal gland. Centripetal obesity occurs in 97% of patients, increased body weight in 94%, fatigability and weakness in 87%, and hypertension in 82%. Impaired glucose tolerance is common and attributable to increased hepatic gluconeogenesis and insulin resistance. (*Kasper et al., pp. 2134–2137*)

73. **(D)** In primary hyperparathyroidism, increased levels of PTH lead to hypercalcemia and hypophosphatemia. Patient symptoms and signs on presentation include kidney stones, peptic ulcers, mental status changes and less commonly, extensive bony resorption. (*Kasper et al., pp. 2252–2256*)

74. **(E)**

75. **(D)**

Explanations 74 and 75

ABG determinations are essential in the diagnosis of respiratory and acid-base disturbances. Extremely obese patients suffer from increased work of breathing, as well as elevation of the diaphragm with decrease in lung volume. The resultant hypoventilation is characterized by carbon dioxide retention leading to chronic respiratory acidosis with metabolic compensation (ABG set E in the question). When associated with somnolence, excessive appetite, and polycythemia, this is known as the pickwickian syndrome. Modest weight loss can lead to dramatic improvement in respiratory functioning. The earliest derangement in salicylate poisoning is hyperventilation, resulting in decreased $Paco_2$ and increased arterial pH (ABG set D). Eventually, there is CNS depression with somnolence and hypoventilation resulting in respiratory acidosis. ABG set A reflects acute respiratory acidosis (hypoventilation) without metabolic compensation. ABG set B is normal. ABG set C suggests metabolic acidosis with modest respiratory compensation. (*Paulson, pp. 103–109*)

76. **(C)**

77. **(E)**

78. **(A)**

Explanations 76 through 78

All of the drugs used to treat hypertension can cause adverse reactions, ranging from trivial to life threatening. Thiazide diuretics are associated with hypokalemia, causing arrhythmias; hyperuricemia, causing gout; and hyperglycemia, causing clinical diabetes. The vasodilator hydralazine can cause tachycardia with increased angina, tachycardia, and a lupus-like syndrome. As many as 10% of patients on an angiotensin-converting enzyme (ACE) inhibitor develop an annoying dry cough. Because they block aldosterone, they can lead to hyperkalemia. Renal failure has been noted with underlying kidney disease, such as bilateral renal artery stenosis. Coombs'-positive hemolytic anemia and hepatitis are idiosyncratic reactions to the central adrenergic-stimulant methyldopa. (*Kasper et al., pp. 1470–1480*)

79. **(E)** Routine treatment of uncomplicated acute bronchitis with an antibiotic is not recommended. Evidence suggests that the quality of

patient-physician communication is most important for patient satisfaction. (*Gonzales et al., pp. 521–529*)

80. (C) Incidence of high-altitude pulmonary edema is related to the rate of ascent, altitude reached, and degree of exertion. Cold temperature increases pulmonary artery pressure through sympathetic stimulation and is an independent risk factor. Recurrence rate may be as high as 60% in persons with a previous history of high-altitude pulmonary edema. These individuals have reduced ventilatory response to hypoxia and an exaggerated pulmonary pressor response to exercise and hypoxia. (*Hackett, pp. 107–114*)

81. (D)

82. (D)

Explanations 81 and 82

Toxin-producing *S. aureus* organisms have been implicated in the pathogenesis of TSS and are frequently cultured from the vagina and cervix of affected women. There is no diagnostic laboratory test, and diagnosis is based on the typical clinical findings. Diffuse macular erythroderma (sunburn-like rash) occurs in the first few days of illness, followed by desquamation, usually of the palms and soles 1–2 weeks later. Fever, hypotension, and multiorgan-system involvement (GI, CNS, muscular, renal, hepatic, hematologic) are also part of the case definition. Platelet counts are usually reduced below 100,000. Disorientation may occur but without such focal neurologic signs as hyperreflexia. Complications include shock, arrhythmias, renal failure, respiratory failure, and coagulopathy. Hypercalcemia is not a part of the picture. (*Kasper et al., pp. 816–819*)

83. (E) Adherence to a drug regimen is critical to prevent resistance. Treatment usually should be offered to patients who are symptomatic from their HIV infection. Asymptomatic patients should have antiretroviral therapy offered if their CD4 counts are less than 350 or plasma HIV viral load is greater than 55,000 copies. Counseling about risks and benefits of treatment is critical. (*Department of Health and Human Services, p. 97*)

84. (D) The median time from initial infection with HIV to the development of clinical disease is 10 years. The rate of disease progression is highly variable and directly correlates with HIV RNA levels. With high levels of HIV RNA, the disease progresses faster. During the asymptomatic period of HIV infection, $CD4^+$ cells decline at an average rate of 50/μL per year. Some patients do not progress and show little if any decline in $CD4^+$ counts over time. (*Kasper et al., pp. 1093–1094*)

85. (B) Diabetes mellitus is associated with hyperglycemia, disease of the microvasculature (retinopathy, nephropathy, neuropathy), and large-vessel disease. Severe peripheral vascular disease is also common. The Diabetes Control and Complications Trial demonstrated that tight control can decrease complications of microvascular disease significantly, but does not seem to affect CAD. (*Kasper et al., pp. 2161–2169*)

86. (D) Whipple disease is a systemic illness characterized by arthralgias, diarrhea, abdominal pain, and weight loss. The usual patient is a middle-aged White male. Reported in 1907 by George Whipple, it has been associated with a bacillus, which has only recently been identified. The disease can affect nearly every organ system, although it usually involves the GI tract, heart, and CNS. Renal failure is not a common complication. (*Kasper et al., pp. 1770–1774*)

87. (B)

88. (A)

Explanations 87 and 88

Hepatic encephalopathy is a syndrome of declining intellectual function, altered state of consciousness, and neurologic abnormalities in the setting of advanced liver disease. Other findings include hyperactivity, delirium, agitation, and personality changes, progressing to confusion, somnolence, and coma. Asterixis (lapses of sustained muscle contraction) or "flapping tremor" is common. Jaundice, spider angiomas, and ascites can be present in alcoholic liver disease without the presence of encephalopathy. Precipitating factors must be looked for and reversed if possible. GI bleeding (due to esophageal varices, gastritis, ulcer, and so forth) increases the nitrogen load in the gut and reduces cerebral perfusion. Excessive diuresis with prerenal azotemia increases extrahepatic circulation of urea and ammonia production, so noncompliance with diuretics would decrease ammonia levels. Lactulose acidifies the stool, traps ammonia and other nitrogenous substances, and decreases their absorption from the gut so excessive lactulose would decrease ammonia levels. Excessive protein intake is a common precipitant. (*Kasper et al., pp. 1867–1869*)

89. **(D)** Classic features of Alzheimer syndrome include amnestic memory impairment, deterioration of language, and visuospatial deficits. Gait disturbances and motor and sensory changes are uncommon until late phases of the syndrome. Mood change and apathy are commonly seen in early stages of Alzheimer syndrome and typically continue for the duration of the disease. Psychotic features may be seen in middle and late phases of the syndrome. (*Cummings, pp. 56–67*)

90. **(E)** The barium enema x-ray shown in Fig. 1-15 reveals multiple sigmoid diverticuli. Most cases of colonic diverticular disease do not require surgery, even for active GI bleeding. Colonoscopy is not necessary unless the barium enema reveals additional lesions or the diagnosis is in doubt. Histamine H_2 receptor antagonists such as cimetidine and ranitidine are useful for treating peptic ulcer disease but not for diverticulosis. Rectal corticosteroid enemas have a role in inflammatory bowel disease, but not in diverticular disease. Appropriate management of the acute attack consists of bed rest, liquid diet, and perhaps anticholinergics. Thereafter, a high-fiber diet should be prescribed to help prevent further recurrences. Bran, raw vegetables, legumes, and hydrophilic colloids such as psyllium seed derivatives are all useful. (*Kasper et al., pp. 1795–1797*)

91. **(E)** The Gram stain is positive in three-fourths of bacterial meningitis cases. Leukocyte counts average between 5000 and 20,000; CSF pressure is consistently elevated usually above 180 mm H_2O; glucose levels are usually lower than 40 mg/dL, or less than 40% of blood glucose; and protein levels are higher than 45 mg/dL in 90% of cases. (*Kasper et al., pp. 2471–2475*)

92. **(D)** *S. pneumoniae* is the most common cause of adult meningitis in people over 30 and accounts for about 15% of cases. *H. influenzae* is the most common cause in children over 1 month old. Group B *Streptococcus* is an important cause of neonatal meningitis, but is very rare in adults. *Staphylococcus*, *E. coli*, and *Klebsiella* may be seen with penetrating head wounds or postneurosurgic procedures. (*Kasper et al., pp. 2471–2477*)

93. **(E)** Although *Listeria* still represents only a fraction of total cases (about 10%) of meningitis, it is seen in diabetes and cancer patients, alcoholic, elderly, and immunocompromised patients. (*Kasper et al., pp. 2471–2477*)

94. **(B)** The CXR shown in Fig. 1-16 contains multiple bilateral pulmonary parenchymal nodules varying in size and shape, most compatible with metastatic disease to the lungs. Other possibilities are bronchogenic carcinoma or fungal granulomas (e.g., histoplasmosis or coccidiosis). Sarcoidosis usually presents with bilateral hilar adenopathy and rarely with multiple pulmonary nodules. Tuberculosis presents with a cavitating lesion, pleural effusion, or miliary pattern. Typical findings in silicosis are diffuse nodular fibrosis and eggshell calcification of hilar or bronchopulmonary lymph nodes. The CXR of patients with mycoplasma pneumonia usually shows patchy infiltrates involving the lower lobes and spreading from the hila. The finding of metastatic nodules on CXR should prompt a search for the primary tumor. (*Kasper et al., p. 562, 1497, 1556*)

95. (C) The CXR shown in Fig. 1-17 shows a diffuse reticulonodular pattern consistent with interstitial lung disease. The hilar nodes are enlarged, suggesting lymphadenopathy. This is a nonspecific picture and may be caused by a large number of diseases. Occupational exposure to dust, gas, or fumes; sarcoidosis; idiopathic pulmonary fibrosis; and lung disease associated with the rheumatic diseases are the more common factors. Despite the diverse causes, there is a common pathogenesis: injury leads to alveolitis, which progresses to fibrosis. Abnormalities on pulmonary function testing are also similar: restrictive disease characterized by decreased lung volumes (vital capacity, total lung capacity) and decreased compliance. Loss of the alveolar capillary bed leads to decreased carbon monoxide diffusing capacity. Arterial oxygen pressure (PaO_2) may be normal at rest but is decreased with exercise. Arterial carbon dioxide pressure (PaCO_2) may be normal or decreased because of hyperventilation, but it is not usually elevated in pure interstitial lung disease. (*Kasper et al., pp. 1554–1556*)

96. (A) Ulcerative colitis typically presents between the ages of 15 and 25 years with symptoms of diarrhea with blood and abdominal pain. Involvement begins in the rectum and is limited to the colon. Crohn disease can occur anywhere in the GI tract and may present with obstructive symptoms. Both of these disorders can produce extraintestinal finding including erythema nodosum, arthritis, and uveitis. (*Toy et al., pp. 157–163*)

97. (E) The spectrum of infection with *Legionella* organisms ranges from asymptomatic seroconversion to Pontiac fever (a flu-like illness) to full-blown pneumonia. Cough is usually nonproductive initially. Malaise, myalgia, and headache are common. The diagnosis of *Legionella* infection is suggested by extrapulmonary signs and symptoms, including diarrhea, abdominal pain, azotemia, and hematuria. (*Kasper et al., pp. 870–874*)

98. (E) Patients with advanced chronic obstructive pulmonary disease (COPD) are at risk for development of acute respiratory failure. Common precipitants are infections, increased secretions, and superimposed bronchospasm. Oxygen therapy is effective in reversing the hypoxemia associated with respiratory failure. A risk of such therapy peculiar to patients with COPD is worsening hypercapnia. Affected patients are thought to have lost their respiratory center's sensitivity to hypercapnia, so that their primary stimulus to breathe is hypoxemia. When the hypoxemia is corrected, they may lose their stimulus to breathe and develop carbon dioxide narcosis with worsening acidosis, confusion, stupor, and eventually coma. Because of this, the usual approach is to begin with a low fraction of inspired oxygen (FIO_2) and increase gradually. Serial ABGs are obtained to ensure that as PaO_2 improves, PaCO_2 does not increase. In some cases, even the lowest FIO_2 causes carbon dioxide retention, and mechanical ventilation is required. In the case presented in the question, a lower FIO_2 should be used before mechanical ventilation is initiated. (*Kasper et al., pp. 1547–1553*)

99. (D)

100. (C)

101. (B)

Explanations 99 through 101

Testicular cancer is the most common cancer in men between the ages of 20 and 40. Predisposing factors include cryptorchidism, hernias, and testicular atrophy. Abdominal testes are at higher risk than inguinal cryptorchid testes. Family history of testicular or prostate cancer, radiation exposure, or maternal DES seems to play no role. Testicular cancers are divided into nonseminoma and seminoma subtypes. Seminoma represents about 50% of all tumors and generally follows a more indolent course. The primary tumor is treated by inguinal orchiectomy regardless of cell type. Pure seminomas do not require retroperitoneal lymph node dissection, because radiation is usually adequate therapy. Nonseminomatous testicular tumors (embryonal cell, teratocarcinoma, choriocarcinoma, endodermal sinus) are usually treated by retroperitoneal dissection. Serum alpha-fetoprotein (AFP) and hCG levels are markers that are important for diagnosis and as prognostic indicators and are used to monitor therapy. Serum LDH level is often elevated with bulky tumors but is not as specific as either AFP or hCG. CEA is a nonspecific marker elaborated by many adenocarcinomas. PSA is a marker associated with prostate cancer. (*Kasper et al., pp. 550–552*)

102. (C) Squamous cell lung cancers may be associated with hypercalcemia due to tumor secretion of PTH-like substances. Small cell cancers may secrete ACTH or ADH. These are examples of paraneoplastic syndromes. Other paraneoplastic manifestations may include peripheral neuropathy, endocrine syndromes such as thyrotoxicosis and hematologic conditions such as polycythemia and thrombocytopenic purpura. (*Toy et al., pp. 345–353*)

103. (D) In the patient described in the question, the movement of the trachea to the left suggests a difference between right and left pleural pressures, either a reduction in pressure on the left or a rise in pressure on the right. The acute onset of right-sided chest pain in an otherwise healthy young man suggests a pneumothorax. On the side of the pneumothorax, we would expect increased resonance and distant breath sounds because of the air trapped in the pleural space between the lung and chest wall. No rales or rhonchi would be expected. A pleural friction rub suggests an inflammatory process involving the left chest, a finding not likely on the basis of the patient's presentation. (*Kasper et al., pp. 1568, 77–79*)

104. (B) Congestion secondary to left ventricular failure may lead to pulmonary edema. Failure of the right side of the heart results in peripheral edema and jugular venous distention, and liver enzymes may be elevated secondary to liver congestion. (*Kasper et al., pp. 1370–1371*)

105. (C) The usual early hemodynamic response to sepsis is a hyperdynamic circulation. This includes tachycardia, elevated cardiac output, and decreased systemic resistance. Septic shock may then progress with intractable hypotension, metabolic acidosis, reduced cardiac output, and death. (*Kasper et al., pp. 1603–1607*)

106. (D) In younger patients, low back pain tends to be mild and self-limited, typically resolving in 4–6 weeks. Patients should be encouraged to remain active and symptom control can be achieved with pain medications. Two percent of adults each year miss work due to back pain. If pain symptoms persist, further investigation such as x-ray evaluation and orthopedic or pain clinic referral may be warranted. (*Toy et al., pp. 227–233*)

107. (D) The majority of paroxysmal supraventricular tachycardias respond to adenosine, because they involve a reentrant circuit including the atrioventricular node. Adenosine is ineffective in the termination of the majority of other atrial or ventricular tachycardias, although it may slow the ventricular response to an atrial tachycardia. (*Kasper et al., p. 17, 1349*)

108. (C) The most common causes of megaloblastic anemia are folate and vitamin B_{12} deficiencies. Vitamin B_{12} deficiency rarely results from inadequate intake, but has been associated with strict vegetarianism. Decreased absorption may be due to insufficient intrinsic factor (as in pernicious anemia and after gastrectomy), malabsorption of the intrinsic factor-vitamin B_{12} complex in the terminal ileum (as in regional enteritis, sprue, pancreatitis, and after ileectomy), or competition for vitamin B_{12} by gut bacteria (as in the blind loop syndrome and *Diphyllobothrium latum* infections). Because diverticulosis and constipation do not interfere with stomach or small-bowel functioning, they are not causes of vitamin B_{12} deficiency. (*Kasper et al., pp. 601–607*)

109. (D) Polymyalgia rheumatica is characterized by bilateral aching and stiffness of the proximal parts of the arms and thighs with associated weakness and generalized fatigue. The sedimentation rate typically is significantly elevated. This condition can coexist with the syndrome of temporal arteritis which is a chronic vasculitis of large- and medium-sized vessels, usually including cranial branches of the aortic arch arteries. Graves disease is an autoimmune thyroid disease and Wegner's granulomatosis typically involves the sinuses, lungs, and/or kidneys. (*Toy et al., pp. 447–453*)

110. **(D)** Pseudotumor cerebri is a disorder of increased intracranial pressure that has no obvious cause. The typical patient is an obese young woman who complains of headache and is found to have papilledema. Slight decrease in visual fields and enlargement of blind spots may also be observed. Neurologic examination is otherwise normal, and the patient appears to be healthy. CSF is under increased pressure and may have slightly low protein concentration, but is otherwise normal. CT scan, arteriogram, and other x-ray studies are usually normal. The most serious complication is severe visual loss, which occurs in about 10% of affected persons. Treatment with a carbonic anhydrase inhibitor decreases intracranial pressure by decreasing production of CSF. Weight loss is important but often unsuccessful. If the carbonic anhydrase inhibitor and weight loss fail, or if visual loss develops, lumboperitoneal shunting or optic nerve sheath fenestration are important maneuvers to prevent blindness. (*Kasper et al., pp. 169–170*)

111. **(E)** Interstitial lung disease is characterized by decreased lung volumes, decreased vital capacity, and decreased total lung capacity. Causes include pulmonary diseases such as interstitial fibrosis and extrapulmonary issues from poor breathing mechanics such as scoliosis or myasthenia gravis. Obstructive lung disease is characterized by decreased FEV1 and total lung capacity that is normal or increased. (*Toy et al., pp. 309–315*)

112. **(A)** Although thrush and esophagitis attributable to *C. albicans* are common manifestations of AIDS-related immunodeficiency, fungal dissemination and sepsis are extremely rare. Although not uncommon, opportunistic infections in these patients, disseminated *M. avium-intracellulare*, cryptococcal meningitis, and cytomegalovirus retinitis, are less common than *P. carinii* pneumonia, which is the presenting infection in 20% of HIV patients and develops in about 50% of all AIDS patients. (*Kasper et al., pp. 1105–1110*)

113. **(B)** ASD is the second most common form of congenital heart disease in adults, after a bicuspid aortic valve. The murmur heard in childhood is often considered innocent, and symptoms do not appear until adulthood. A left-to-right shunt of blood between the atria causes right ventricular overload and increased pulmonary circulation. These result in the classic findings of a pulmonic systolic ejection murmur, late pulmonic valve closure with wide splitting of S_2, and a tricuspid flow murmur. CXR has signs of cardiomegaly and pulmonary overcirculation. Characteristic ECG changes are atrial fibrillation and an incomplete or complete RBBB. In the more common ostium secundum type of ASD, there is often right axis deviation; whereas, the ostium primum type has a left axis deviation pattern. Coarctation of the aorta, patent ductus arteriosus, and VSDs are not associated with the findings of the patient described in the question, and tetralogy of Fallot would not present in adulthood. (*Kasper et al., p. 1385*)

114. **(H)** Temporal arteritis occurs almost exclusively in patients over 55 years of age. The classic clinical findings are fever, anemia, high ESR, and headache. Other manifestations may include malaise, fatigue, anorexia, weight loss, sweat, and arthralgias. Headache may be associated with a tender, thickened, or nodular temporal artery. Diagnosis often is made clinically and can be confirmed by a temporal artery biopsy. Patients respond well to glucocorticoid therapy. (*Kasper et al., pp. 2008–2009*)

115. **(C)** Wegener's granulomatosis affects males and females equally, can occur at any age, and is extremely rare in Blacks. Patients typically present with severe upper respiratory tract symptoms. Nasal perforation and saddle nose deformity may occur. Pulmonary involvement (cough, hemoptysis, or dyspnea are common presenting symptoms/signs) is present in 85–90% of patients, renal disease in 70–80% of patients, eye involvement in 50–55%, and skin lesions in 40–50%. Anti-neutrophil cytoplasmic antibodies (C-ANCA) is positive in 90% of patients. ESR typically is high. (*Kasper et al., pp. 2004–2006*)

116. (B) SLE is characterized by tissue and cell damage from pathogenic autoantibodies and immune complexes. 90 percent of patients are women in child-bearing years and the disease is more common in African Americans. Multiple organ system manifestations can occur, including musculoskeletal (arthralgias, myalgias), cutaneous (malar rash, photosensitivity, hair loss), renal (nephritis, nephritic syndrome), nervous (seizures, hadaches), cardiopulmonary (pericarditis, pleuritis), hematologic (anemia, leukopenia). (*Kasper et al., pp. 1960–1967*)

117. (I) Sarcoidosis is a relatively common disease. In the United States, most patients are Black (ratio ranges from 10:1 to 17:1). The disease is systemic, and the lung is almost always affected (primarily an interstitial lung disease). Seventy-five to ninety percent of patients have enlarged intrathoracic lymph nodes, usually the hilar nodes. (*Kasper et al., pp. 2017–2022*)

118. (A) Rheumatoid arthritis affects approximately 0.8% of the population. Women are affected three times more often than men. Synovial inflammation causes tenderness, swelling, and limitation of motion. Most often the arthritis is symmetric and characteristically involves certain joints such as the wrist and the proximal interphalangeal and metacarpophalangeal joints. (*Kasper et al., pp. 1968–1976*)

119. (G) Risk factors for OA include age, obesity, major trauma, and repetitive joint use. Bony enlargements of the DIP joint (Heberden's nodes) are the most common form of idiopathic OA. Obesity is a risk factor for knee OA. With severe OA of the knee in particular, obesity is thought to play a large role in pathogenesis. (*Kasper et al., pp. 2036–2040*)

120. (D) Hyponatremia is a common metabolic derangement. Facititious hyponatremia is seen with severe hyperlipidemia or hyperproteinemia (which lower plasma water content) and with hyperglycemia due to water movement out of cells. In the absence of these abnormalities, diagnosis is based on an estimation of circulating blood volume (CBV). Decreased CBV and hyponatremia are associated with diuretic use, dehydration, edematous states (congestive heart failure and cirrhosis of the liver), osmotic diuresis (e.g., glycosuria), or adrenal insufficiency. Hyponatremia with normal CBV can be due to the SIADH secretion in which urine osmolality and urine sodium are "inappropriately" high. Diabetes insipidus is a cause of hypernatremia. (*Kasper et al., pp. 2102–2104*)

121. (A) The nephrotic syndrome is characterized by proteinuria of greater than 3 g/day. Hypoalbuminemia, edema, and lipemia are other defining features. The nephrotic syndrome may result from a primary glomerular disease, such as focal glomerulosclerosis. It is associated with many other systemic diseases, such as lymphoma, and the use of drugs such as heroin. In North America, the most common cause is diabetes mellitus. (*Kasper et al., pp. 1684–1685*)

122. (D)

123. (C)

Explanations 122 and 123

The typical migraine attack consists of a visual aura with flashes, scintillating scotomata (field loss), or fortification spectra followed by a throbbing unilateral temporal headache. There may be associated vestibular, GI, or neurologic symptoms. Attacks are often precipitated by stress, fatigue, or foods that contain tyramine (e.g., cheese, yogurt, nuts) or phenylethylamine (wine, chocolate). Symptoms peak within an hour of onset and persist for hours to days. A positive family history is found in as many as 50% of cases. Tension headaches are more often bilateral and described as band like or vise like and are not usually associated with visual auras. TIAs more typically present as transient monocular blindness without aura or headache. Temporal arteritis may present as painless loss of vision without aura, but is usually in older people. Cluster headaches are much more common in men. Sumatriptan is a newer medication that stimulates the serotonin 5-HT receptors to produce cranial vasoconstriction and reduce vascular inflammation. It comes in oral, injectable, and nasal spray form. Ergotamine tartrate, antiemetics, and analgesics may also be used in the acute treatment of migraine headache. Prophylactic medications such as propranolol, dipyridamole, and methysergide are ineffective for acute attacks. Avoidance of known precipitants and control of stress are also important in prevention. (*Giammarco et al., pp. 71–85*)

124. (A)

125. (C)

Explanations 124 and 125

Urinary tract infections are extremely common in young women and in debilitated, bedridden patients. For simple infections uncomplicated by fever, chills, or flank pain, a single dose of an antibiotic may be curative. In the presence of symptoms suggesting renal parenchymal infection (i.e., pyelonephritis), treatment should continue for as long as 2 weeks, and parenteral antibiotics may be required (e.g., ampicillin plus an aminoglycoside). Bacteriuria in pregnant women should be treated regardless of symptoms; whereas, bacteriuria in patients with indwelling catheters should probably be treated only in the presence of symptoms. Chronic suppressive antibiotic therapy in the latter group has not been shown to be useful. Radiologic investigation for underlying anatomic abnormalities should be undertaken in girls up to age 6, in all males after their first infection, and in women of any age with recurrent urinary tract infections. The most common pathogen is *E. coli,* accounting for greater than 80% of infections. Other organisms frequently encountered include *Klebsiella, Proteus, and Enterobacter* species. (*Kasper et al., pp. 1715–1720*)

126. (B) The pH of 7.53 indicates alkalosis as the primary disorder (normal pH is 7.40). A high bicarbonate is consistent with a metabolic cause of the alkalosis. The high carbon dioxide of 53 (normal is 40) is compensating for the primary disorder (alkalosis) in attempt to bring the pH closer to normal. Metabolic alkalosis results from the kidney holding on to bicarbonate. Processes which maintain persistent high reclamation of bicarbonate include renal insufficiency, decreased volume, decreased chloride, hypokalemia, hypercapnea, mineralocorticoid excess. (*Paulson, pp. 103–109*)

127. (B)

128. (D)

Explanations 127 and 128

More than 90% of renal stones are visible on a plain abdominal x-ray, and the majority contain calcium oxalate. Staghorn calculi usually contain magnesium ammonium phosphate (triple phosphate or struvite) and are associated with alkaline urine. This is commonly encountered in chronic urinary tract infections with urea-splitting bacteria (especially *Proteus* species). Radiolucent stones often contain urea, which is associated with acidic urine. A small percentage (fewer than 10%) of renal stones contain cystine. The most common cause of calcium stone disease is idiopathic hypercalciuria. Almost half these patients will excrete more than 4 mg of calcium/kg body weight/24 h in the absence of hypercalcemia. Causes of hypercalciuria to be ruled out are sarcoidosis, hyperthyroidism, and Paget disease of bone. Idiopathic hypercalciuria is believed to result from either increased GI absorption of calcium, increased calcium resorption from bone, or excessive renal calcium leakage into the urine. (*Kasper et al., pp. 1710–1714*)

129. (E) Iron-deficiency anemia characteristically is a hypochromic, microcytic anemia. Causes of iron-deficiency anemia include menstrual loss, inadequate diet, malabsorption, chronic inflammation, and chronic blood loss. Colon cancer could lead to chronic blood loss and iron-deficiency anemia. This, however, would be very uncommon in a young patient without a family history of colon cancer. Alcohol causes a macrocytic anemia. (*Kasper et al., pp. 588–591*)

130. (A) Although the differential diagnosis of a pleural effusion is large, the diagnostic possibilities may be narrowed by classifying the fluid as transudative or exudative. Exudates are characterized by a pleural fluid-to-fluid serum protein ratio greater than 0.5, pleural fluid LDH greater than 200 IU/L, or pleural fluid-to-fluid serum LDH ratio greater than 0.6. Other common findings in exudative effusions are a WBC count greater than 1000/mL, glucose less than 60 mg/100 mL, and grossly hemorrhagic fluid. Causes of transudative effusions include CHF, nephrotic syndrome, cirrhosis with ascites, and myxedema. Causes of exudative fluid are parapneumonic effusion, neoplasm, pulmonary infarction, tuberculosis, viral disease, and fungal infection. A low pleural fluid pH (<7.30) limits the differential diagnosis to empyema, carcinoma, collagen vascular disease, esophageal rupture, tuberculosis, or hemothorax. Uncomplicated parapneumonic effusions have WBC counts under 40,000/mL, normal glucose levels, and a pH under 7.30; a positive Gram stain or culture constitutes a complicated parapneumonic effusion. These tend to loculate and form adhesions if not immediately and thoroughly drained by chest tube placement. (*Kasper et al., pp. 1565–1567*)

131. (B) The pH is 7.12, indicating acidosis as the primary disorder. A low bicarbonate is consistent with a metabolic cause of the acidosis and a high carbon dioxide is consistent with a respiratory cause of the acidosis. Therefore, both are contributing as primary problems. The metabolic source likely is lactic acidosis from muscle breakdown resulting from the seizures. The respiratory source likely is related to the patient's postictal state after the seizures. (*Paulson, pp. 103–109*)

132. (C) The pH is 7.10, which indicates the primary disorder to be an acidosis. The low bicarbonate and the low carbon dioxide both are indicative of a metabolic cause for the acidosis. For the primary cause of the acidosis to be respiratory, the carbon dioxide would need to be greater than 40. In this case, the patient is compensating for the metabolic acidosis by breathing down his carbon dioxide level. (*Paulson, pp. 103–109*)

133. (D)

134. (C)

Explanations 133 and 134

The patient described in the question most likely has Hashimoto's thyroiditis, also called autoimmune or chronic lymphocytic thyroiditis. It is the most common cause of thyroiditis in the United States and is encountered more frequently in women than in men. Patients note progressive thyromegaly but are usually euthyroid at the outset. Hypothyroidism may appear years later, often heralded by an elevated serum TSH level. Diagnosis is based on the history, examination, heterogeneous uptake on thyroid scan, and the presence of antithyroid and antithyroglobulin antibodies. If the diagnosis is still in doubt, needle biopsy will demonstrate lymphocyte infiltration, sometimes in sheets or forming germinal centers. Subacute (de Quervain's, granulomatous) thyroiditis will show polymorphonuclear cells, necrosis, and giant cells. Bacteria may not be present in acute suppurative thyroiditis. Thyroid infiltration and replacement by rock-hard, woody, fibrous tissue is typical of Riedel's struma. C-cell hyperplasia is associated with medullary thyroid carcinoma. Hashimoto's thyroiditis is treated with thyroid hormone. Lower doses (0.10–0.15 mg/day) of levothyroxine are used to treat hypothyroidism alone; whereas, higher doses (0.15–0.30 mg/day) suppress TSH release and diminish goiter size. Partial resection may result in enlargement of the remaining gland. Steroids, antibiotics, and radioiodine have no role in therapy. (*Kasper et al., pp. 2109–2113*)

135. (A) As many as 85% of women with hirsutism, obesity, and menstrual irregularities have polycystic ovary disease (Stein–Leventhal syndrome). Excessive luteinizing hormone (LH) response to gonadotropin-releasing hormone is thought by many to be the primary problem, resulting in ovarian theca-cell hyperplasia and hypersecretion of androgens. Others have found deficiencies of the ovarian enzymes involved in estrogen biosynthesis. Diagnosis is based on an elevated LH level, decreased follicle-stimulating hormone (FSH) level, and an LH/FSH ratio greater than 2:5. Combination estrogen-progestin therapy suppresses the androgen production. Less common causes of hirsutism are drug induced (e.g., testosterone, anabolic steroids), adrenal tumor or hyperplasia, Cushing disease, and ovarian tumors. Familial hirsutism is not associated with menstrual abnormalities or obesity. (*Kasper et al., pp. 275–277*)

136. **(B)** Drug-induced acute interstitial nephritis is a frequent cause of reversible renal failure. Methicillin, penicillin, diuretics, nonsteroidal anti-inflammatory drugs (NSAIDs), and allopurinol all have been implicated. An immune basis is postulated, and the acute azotemia may be associated with signs of an allergic reaction: fever, arthralgias, rash, and blood and urine eosinophilia. Discontinuing the offending agent may reverse the renal failure, so a high degree of suspicion and early diagnosis is vital. Steroids are commonly given and may further improve renal function. RBC casts in the urine are diagnostic of glomerulonephritis and are not associated with interstitial nephritis. (*Kasper et al., p. 248, 1705*)

137. **(D)** A low hematocrit can be seen with all of the anemias listed, but is usually much lower (low 20s) in sickle cell anemia. A low mean corpuscular volume (MCV) is associated with iron-deficiency anemia or beta-thalassemia, but a normal or high number of RBCs is characteristic of beta-thalassemia minor. In iron deficiency, the red cell count is usually below normal, and there is an elevated red cell distribution width. Cells are usually normocytic normochromic with anemia of chronic disease. Patients with alpha-thalassemia major have moderate-to-severe hemolytic anemia early in life. (*Kasper et al., pp. 330–334, 594–599*)

138. **(B)** Several familial skin disorders have associated GI manifestations. The patient described in the question most likely has Peutz–Jeghers syndrome, which is associated with hamartomatous polyps of the GI tract. These occur most frequently in the jejunum but may be found anywhere between the stomach and the rectum. Malignant transformation of the polyps occurs in 2–3% of cases. Tylosis (hyperkeratosis of palms and soles) is associated with esophageal carcinoma. Hereditary hemorrhagic telangiectasia (Rendu–Osler–Weber disease) often involves bleeding of the GI tract. The blue rubber bleb nevus syndrome also causes bleeding due to GI hemangiomas. Neurofibromatosis (von Recklinghausen disease) is characterized by café au lait spots with cutaneous and intestinal neurofibromas. (*Kasper et al., p. 198, 302*)

139. **(D)**

140. **(D)**

Explanations 139 and 140

Lyme disease primarily manifests in large joints, especially the knee. Eighty percent of patients have a slowly expanding skin lesion (erythema migrans) at the site of the tick bite. Within weeks, 15% of untreated patients will develop neurologic manifestations. Five percent of untreated patients may develop chronic neuroborreliosis. Other potential disease manifestations include neurologic (headaches, encephalitis, chronic axonal polyneuropathy), skin (erythema migrans), and cardiac (atrioventricular block, pericarditis). Lyme disease typically occurs in three distinct areas: the Northeast from Maine to Maryland, the Midwest in Wisconsin and Minnesota, and in the West in northern California and Oregon. The disease is transmitted by the ticks of the Ixodes ricinus complex. (*Steere, pp. 115–125*)

141. **(D)** Before any laboratory evaluation or therapy, the presence of hypertension must be carefully documented. When characteristic end-organ changes are not apparent on physical examination, the presence of hypertension can best be documented by demonstrating a persistent elevation of BP. Although a single observation of mildly elevated BP does not justify either an evaluation for secondary causes or initiation of treatment, it should not be ignored. The patient should be rescheduled for additional BP measurements on several occasions within the next few weeks. There is no need to obtain an ECG or begin counseling if this is not true hypertension. (*Kasper et al., pp. 1468–1471*)

142. **(B)** Pseudogout (chondrocalcinosis) is caused by crystalline deposition in the joints of calcium pyrophosphate dihydrate. It afflicts middle-aged and elderly persons, with males affected slightly more often. Asymptomatic periods punctuated by acute attacks are common. Large joints are affected more than the small ones, with the most frequently involved site being the knee. (*Kasper et al., pp. 2057–2058*)

143. **(A)** Among patients with clinical stage 1 primary melanoma, tumor thickness has been consistently shown to be the best indicator of prognosis. This is true even when regional lymph node metastases are subsequently discovered (clinical stage 1 but pathologic stage 2). Tumors less than 0.85 mm thick are associated with the most favorable prognosis, and those greater than 3.65 mm in thickness are associated with the least favorable. Tumor thickness is also related to the rate at which death occurs. Tumor location, mitotic rate, and the patient's gender are less powerful determinants of prognosis, and tumor diameter is relatively unimportant. (*Kasper et al., pp. 498–503*)

144. **(A)** Leads V_2 and V_3 show U waves. U waves are associated with prolonged ventricular repolarization and are seen in patients who are hypokalemic. (*Kasper et al., p. 260*)

REFERENCES

Bartlett JG, Breiman RF, Mandell LA, et al. Community-acquired pneumonia in adults: guidelines for management. *Clin Infect Dis* 1998;26: 811–838.

Kasper DL, Braunwald E, Fauci A, et al. *Harrison's Principles of Internal Medicine*, 16th ed. New York, NY: McGraw-Hill, 2005.

Byrne TN. Spinal cord compression from epidural metastases. *N Engl J Med* 1992;327:614–619.

Cummings JL. Alzheimer's disease. *N Engl J Med* 2004;351:56–67.

Department of Health and Human Services, Henry J. Kaiser Family Foundation. Guidelines for the use of antiretroviral agents in HIV-1-infected adults and adolescents. Bethesda, MD: Department of Health and Human Services, Henry J. Kaiser Family Foundation, 2004, March 23, p. 97 [355 references].

Ferrari JD, Bach BR. Knee pain in adults: when to manage, when to refer. *J Musculoskel Med* 1998;15(3):52–63.

Freedberg IM, Eisen AZ, Wolff K, et al. *Fitzpatrick's Dermatology in General Medicine*, 6th ed. New York, NY: McGraw-Hill, 2003.

Giammarco R, Edmeads J, Dodick D. *Critical Decisions in Headache Management*. Hamilton, Ont.: BC Decker, 1998.

Gonzales R, Bartlett J, Besser R, et al. Principles of appropriate antibiotic use for treatment of uncomplicated acute bronchitis: background. *Ann Intern Med* 2001;134:521–529.

Goroll AH, Lawrence AM, Mulley AG. *Primary Care Medicine*, 3rd ed. Philadelphia, PA: JB Lippincott, 1995.

Hackett PH, Roach RC. High-altitude illness. *N Engl J Med* 2001;345:107–114.

Hogan DE. The emergency department approach to diarrhea. *Emerg Clin North Am* 1996;14:673–692.

Hurst JW. *Medicine for the Practicing Physician*. Stamford, CT: Appleton & Lange, 1996.

Lang AE, Lozano AM. Parkinson's disease. First of two parts. [Review] *N Engl J Med* 1998;339(15): 1044–1053.

Lang AE, Lozano AM. Parkinson's disease. Second of two parts. [Review] *N Engl J Med* 1998;339(16): 1130–1143.

Light RW. Parapneumonic effusions and empyema: current management strategies. *J Crit Illn* 1995;10: 832–842.

Paulson WD. Identifying acid-base disorders: a systematic approach. *J Crit Illn* 1999;14(2):103–109.

Piccirillo JF. Acute bacterial sinusitis. *N Engl J Med* 2004;351:902–910.

Relman DA, Schmidt TM, MacDermott RP, et al. Identification of the uncultured bacillus of Whipple's disease. *N Engl J Med* 1992;327:293–301.

Smith RA, Cokkinides V, Eyre HJ. American Cancer Society guidelines for the early detection of cancer, 2003. *CA Cancer J Clin* 2003;53(1):27–43.

Steere AC. Lyme disease. *N Engl J Med* 2001;345: 115–125.

Toy EC, Patlan JT, Cruse SE, et al. *Case Files: Internal Medicine*. New York, NY: McGraw-Hill, 2004.

CHAPTER 2

Obstetrics and Gynecology

E. James Aiman, MD

Questions

DIRECTIONS (Questions 1 through 106): Each of the numbered items or incomplete statements in this section is followed by answers or completions of the statement. Select the ONE lettered answer or completion that is BEST in each case.

1. A 27-year-old woman has used oral contraceptives (OCs) without problems for 5 years. However, she just read an article about complications of OCs in a popular women's magazine and asks you about the risks and hazards of taking OCs. You correctly tell her which of the following?

(A) The risk of developing ovarian cancer is increased.
(B) The risk of developing pelvic inflammatory disease (PID) is increased.
(C) The risk of developing endometrial cancer is decreased.
(D) The risk of bearing a child with major congenital anomalies is increased if taken while pregnant.
(E) The risk of ectopic pregnancy is increased.

Questions 2 through 4

The mother of a 3-year-old girl brings her daughter to see you because the girl developed breasts 6 months ago. The girl has had no vaginal bleeding, and there is no pubic hair. She takes no medication.

2. Which of the following is the most appropriate next diagnostic step?

(A) an ultrasound of the pelvis
(B) a pelvic examination under general anesthesia
(C) computed tomography (CT) scan of her head
(D) a serum estradiol concentration
(E) a serum follicle-stimulating hormone (FSH) concentration

3. The tests you ordered are normal for a prepubertal girl. Which of the following is the most likely diagnosis?

(A) ingestion of the mother's OC pills
(B) a granulosa cell tumor
(C) 21-hydroxylase deficiency
(D) polycystic ovary syndrome
(E) premature thelarche

4. Which of the following is the most appropriate management of this girl?

(A) pituitary suppression with a gonadotropin-releasing hormone (GnRH) agonist
(B) laparoscopy
(C) assurance that the condition is benign and self-limiting
(D) corticosteroid suppression of adrenal function
(E) breast biopsy

5. After an appropriate diagnostic evaluation, a 59-year-old woman with postmenopausal bleeding had a total abdominal hysterectomy and bilateral salpingo-oophorectomy (TAH-BSO). The pathologic diagnosis is adenocarcinoma of the endometrium. An endometrial adenocarcinoma that is confined to the uterus and extends more than 50% through the myometrium is at which stage?

(A) IC
(B) IIA
(C) IIB
(D) IIIA
(E) IVA

6. A 39-year-old woman at 16 weeks' gestation complains of headaches, blurred vision, and epigastric pain. Her blood pressure is now 156/104 mmHg. Her uterine fundus is palpable 22 cm above her symphysis pubis. Fetal heart tones could not be heard with a handheld Doppler. She has 3+ proteinuria. Which of the following is the most likely diagnosis?

(A) anencephaly
(B) twin gestation
(C) maternal renal disease
(D) hydatidiform mole
(E) gestational diabetes mellitus

7. A 23-year-old woman develops painful vulvar vesicles that contain intranuclear inclusions on cytologic examination. She is 22 weeks pregnant. Which of the following statements about genital herpes is correct?

(A) Acyclovir should be prescribed from 36 gestational weeks until after delivery in women with primary herpes anytime during pregnancy.
(B) Herpes cultures from the cervix should be obtained weekly beginning at 36 weeks' gestation.
(C) An active genital herpetic lesion any time after 20 weeks' gestation requires a cesarean section.
(D) Intrauterine infection with herpes is common after 20 weeks in women with primary herpes.
(E) Pitocin induction of labor should be started within 4 h after ruptured amniotic membranes in a woman at term with active genital herpes.

8. A 63-year-old woman has a 3-cm pruritic lesion on her right labia majora that she has noted for approximately 9 months. She has been treated with various topical creams and ointments for vulvar candidiasis without resolution of her symptoms or lesion. When you examine this woman, the lesion is still present. Which of the following is the most appropriate intervention?

(A) Papanicolaou (Pap) smear of the lesion
(B) colposcopy of the lesion
(C) biopsy of the lesion
(D) wide local excision of the lesion
(E) vulvectomy

Questions 9 through 11

A 48-year-old woman had a biopsy of a friable, bleeding lesion on her cervix. She had not had a pelvic examination or Pap smear for about 12 years. The biopsy is reported as invasive squamous cell carcinoma of the cervix. On bimanual examination, there is induration to the side wall of her pelvis.

9. Which of the following is the stage of her cervical cancer?

(A) IA
(B) IB
(C) IIB
(D) IIIB
(E) IV

10. To complete the staging of her cancer according to International Federation of Gynecology and Obstetrics (FIGO) standards, she should have which of the following?

(A) lymphangiogram
(B) pelvic venogram
(C) cystoscopy

(D) magnetic resonance imaging (MRI) scan of her abdomen
(E) laparoscopy

11. Which of the following is the most important prognostic factor for 5-year survival after appropriate treatment of cervical cancer?

(A) presence of high-risk strains of human papilloma virus (HPV)
(B) stage of the cancer
(C) age of the patient
(D) histologic grade of the tumor
(E) presence of positive regional (pelvic) lymph nodes

12. A 35-year-old G3P3 woman has been experiencing bilateral breast pain for the past year. Breast examination and mammography are normal. Conservative measures have failed. Which of the following medications is most likely to bring relief?

(A) clomiphene
(B) tamoxifen
(C) danazol
(D) hydrochlorothiazide
(E) medroxyprogesterone

13. A 23-year-old married woman consults you because she and her husband have never consummated their marriage because she has severe pain with attempts at vaginal penetration. Her pelvic examination is normal except for involuntary tightening of her vaginal muscles when you attempt to insert a speculum. Which of the following conditions would best be treated with the use of vaginal dilators?

(A) primary dysmenorrhea
(B) vaginismus
(C) deep-thrust dyspareunia
(D) anorgasmia
(E) vulvar vestibulitis

14. At a follow-up routine prenatal visit, the uterine fundus of a healthy 23-year-old pregnant woman is palpated halfway between her symphysis pubis and umbilicus. Which of the following is the most appropriate test to order at this stage of her pregnancy?

(A) serum human immunodeficiency virus (HIV) titer
(B) glucose tolerance test
(C) amniocentesis
(D) maternal serum alpha-fetoprotein (MSAFP)
(E) cervical culture for group B *Streptococcus* (GBS)

15. A 58-year-old woman with stage II epithelial ovarian cancer undergoes successful surgical debulking followed by chemotherapy with carboplatin and radiation therapy. Subsequently, she develops nonpitting edema of both legs and pain and numbness in her legs. Which of the following is the most likely cause of her pain and numbness?

(A) nerve damage caused by the pelvic lymphadenectomy
(B) lymphedema
(C) carboplatin therapy
(D) radiation therapy
(E) recurrent ovarian cancer

16. A 13-year-old girl had growth of breast buds at 11 years, followed by the appearance of pubic hair between the ages of $11^1/_2$ and 12 years. Which pubertal event is most likely to occur next?

(A) beginning of accelerated growth
(B) menarche
(C) Tanner stage 5 breast development
(D) maximal growth rate
(E) Tanner stage 5 pubic hair

17. A 32-year-old G2P1 woman is now 13 weeks pregnant. Her first pregnancy was uncomplicated, and she delivered vaginally at 39 weeks' gestation 9 years ago. She has a history of rheumatic heart disease. She currently denies dyspnea, dizziness on standing, or syncope with exertion. Which of the following is most helpful in determining the functional capacity of this patient during pregnancy?

(A) an electrocardiogram
(B) elevated diaphragms and an enlarged cardiac silhouette on chest film
(C) pedal edema
(D) an S_3 heart sound
(E) the presence or absence of symptoms

18. Labor and vaginal delivery occur successfully in a 29-year-old woman after administration of oxytocin (Pitocin) for 9 h. Spontaneous onset of labor at term is the result of which of the following?

(A) cortisol production in the amniotic cavity
(B) prostaglandin release from the fetal membranes
(C) prolactin produced in the decidua
(D) fetal pituitary secretion of oxytocin from the neurohypophysis
(E) events that are currently uncertain

19. At 24 weeks' gestation, where are most fetal red blood cells produced?

(A) the yolk sac
(B) spleen
(C) bone marrow
(D) liver
(E) lymph nodes

Questions 20 and 21

A 27-year-old woman with amenorrhea of 6 months' duration relates a 4-month growth of thick, black hair on her face, chest, and abdomen. She takes no medications with androgenic effects. Her family history is negative for hirsutism. The hirsutism is confirmed by your examination. Her pelvic examination is normal other than a mild male pubic hair pattern.

20. Which of the following is the most appropriate next step in her evaluation?

(A) serum prolactin concentration
(B) 24-h urine for 17-ketosteroid excretion
(C) serum dehydroepiandrosterone sulfate (DHEAS) concentration
(D) CT scan of the pituitary sella
(E) pelvic ultrasound

21. Your evaluation of this hirsute, amenorrheic woman is normal except for a significantly increased serum DHEAS concentration. Additional history discloses that her menses have always been somewhat irregular since menarche at age 10 years. She has a 23-year-old sister with irregular menstrual intervals and hirsutism to a lesser degree. This patient has a blood pressure of 96/64 mmHg. Which of the following is the most likely diagnosis?

(A) polycystic ovary syndrome
(B) 21-hydroxylase deficiency
(C) 11-hydroxylase deficiency
(D) 17-hydroxylase deficiency
(E) Sertoli–Leydig cell tumor

22. A 31-year-old pregnant woman 6–7 weeks from her last menses comes to the emergency department of your hospital complaining of lower abdominal pain for 3 h. The pain is diffuse in the lower abdomen but worse on the right side. Her serum human chorionic gonadotropin (hCG) concentration is 9600 mIU/mL. Which of the following is the strongest evidence that she has a tubal ectopic pregnancy?

(A) absence of an extrauterine sac on ultrasonography
(B) absence of blood on culdocentesis
(C) absence of a mass on bimanual examination
(D) absence of an intrauterine sac on ultrasonography
(E) her hCG concentration

23. A 22-year-old primiparous woman is in premature labor at 30 weeks' gestation. Despite administration of tocolytic agents, it seems she will deliver soon. Pulmonary maturity might be enhanced by the administration of which of the following drugs?

(A) magnesium sulfate
(B) betamethasone
(C) hydroxyprogesterone
(D) chloroprocaine
(E) digitalis

24. A 28-year-old woman with 28-day menstrual cycle is attempting to conceive and is considering the use of a home ovulation predictor kit to time intercourse at ovulation. She asks you what day of her menstrual cycle her luteinizing hormone (LH) peak is most likely to occur. What should you tell her?

(A) day 12
(B) day 14
(C) day 18
(D) day 20
(E) day 27

25. A 48-year-old woman with five children complains of urinary incontinence with coughing and stair climbing. She likely has genuine stress urinary incontinence if loss of urine

(A) is secondary to involuntary bladder contractions
(B) is associated with a strong desire to void immediately
(C) occurs in relation to anxiety or depression
(D) occurs when intravesical pressure exceeds maximal urethral pressure
(E) is due to increased intravesical pressure associated with bladder distention

26. An 18-year-old nullipara has suddenly stopped menstruating. She recently lost 8.6 kg when she started long-distance running. The laboratory test most consistent with her cause of secondary amenorrhea is

(A) a serum prolactin level of 86 ng/mL (normal <20)
(B) a serum LH level of 48 mIU/mL (normal 6–35)
(C) a serum estradiol level of 128 pg/mL (normal 40–300)
(D) a serum FSH level of 3 mIU/mL (normal 5–18)
(E) a serum testosterone level of 156 ng/dL (normal 40–110)

27. A 22-year-old woman with cystic fibrosis is engaged to be married and asks you about childbearing. How should you advise her?

(A) An amniocentesis should be done to detect fetal cystic fibrosis.
(B) Pregnancy is contraindicated because maternal mortality is significantly increased.
(C) Her children have a 25% chance of having cystic fibrosis.
(D) Pregnancy and delivery are usually successful with special care and precautions.
(E) She should use nasal oxygen throughout pregnancy to minimize fetal hypoxemia.

28. On the first pelvic examination of an 18-year-old nulligravida, a soft, fluctuant mass is found in the superior aspect of the right labia majora. This is asymptomatic. She tells you it has been present for several years and seems to be enlarging slightly. There is no defect in the inguinal ring. Which of the following is the most likely diagnosis?

(A) vulvar varicosities
(B) inguinal hernia
(C) femoral hernia
(D) cyst of the canal of Nuck
(E) granuloma inguinale

29. Your patient has just had twins and wonders if there is any way to determine whether the twins are identical. You correctly tell her that

(A) close examination of the placenta can often provide this answer
(B) there is no way to tell unless one is a girl and one a boy
(C) only matching of human lymphocyte antigens could determine this with certainty
(D) identical twins occur only once in about 80 births of twins
(E) it is unlikely because the birth weights differed by more than 200 g

30. An 11-year-old girl has her first menses. Both ovaries contain approximately how many oocytes?

(A) 7 million
(B) 1 million
(C) 500,000
(D) 50,000
(E) 5000

31. A healthy 29-year-old gravida 2 woman at 39 weeks has been in labor for 3 h. She had a positive vaginal-anal culture for GBS at 37 weeks' gestation. Which one of the following statements is correct?

(A) Asymptomatic rectovaginal colonization is present in 60% of pregnant women.
(B) The transmission rate from mother to baby is approximately 25%.
(C) A rectovaginal culture should have been obtained at the first prenatal visit.
(D) Neonatal sepsis occurs in 1% of colonized mothers.
(E) Treatment with penicillin in labor is necessary only for heavy colonized mothers.

32. A 25-year-old women has vulvar condylomata. Which one of the following statements is correct?

(A) It is caused by herpes virus, type 2.
(B) It is sexually transmitted.
(C) A biopsy should be done to exclude verrucous carcinoma.
(D) The lesions usually regress and disappear spontaneously.
(E) Endometrial hyperplasia occurs more frequently.

33. A 24-year-old nullipara is being evaluated for infertility. On pelvic examination, she has a single cervix. A diagnostic laparoscopy shows a double uterine fundus. Which of the following is the most likely diagnosis of her uterine anomaly?

(A) septate uterus
(B) unicornuate uterus
(C) bicornuate uterus
(D) didelphic uterus
(E) a diethylstilbestrol (DES) exposed uterus

34. A 58-year-old G6P4Ab2 diabetic woman who weighs 122.6 kg (270 lb) has her first episode of vaginal bleeding in 5 years. Her physician performs an outpatient operative hysteroscopy and dilatation and curettage (D&C). Which of the following is an indication for the procedure and the most likely diagnosis?

(A) endometrial cancer because of her high parity
(B) endometrial cancer because of her obesity
(C) cervical cancer because of her age
(D) cervical cancer because of her diabetes
(E) ovarian cancer because of her obesity

35. A pregnant woman is being followed by a nephrologist for chronic glomerulonephritis. Which of the following findings is normal at 28 weeks' gestation?

(A) blood pressure of 132/86 mmHg
(B) blood urea nitrogen (BUN) of 21 mg/100 mL
(C) serum creatinine of 1.1 mg/100 mL
(D) glomerular filtration rate (GFR) of 130 mL/min
(E) glycosuria with a plasma glucose of 130 mg/100 mL

36. A 25-year-old woman has a positive cervical culture for *Neisseria gonorrhoeae*. She has had at least two positive cultures for gonorrhea treated in the past. She is afebrile and has no symptoms. The incidence of penicillin-resistant gonorrhea in some areas of the United States is currently as great as 10%. Because of this, the recommended treatment for gonorrhea includes which of the following?

(A) 125 mg intramuscular ceftriaxone as a single dose
(B) 1 g spectinomycin
(C) 2 g ampicillin orally as a single dose
(D) 2 g intramuscular cefoxitin
(E) 2 g metronidazole as a single dose

37. A 37-year-old pregnant woman with type 2 diabetes mellitus and chronic hypertension is 35 weeks pregnant. Which of the following is the best test to screen for fetal well-being?

(A) nonstress test (NSTs)
(B) oxytocin challenge test
(C) amniocentesis
(D) fetal movement counting
(E) fetal biophysical profile

38. A 31-year-old primigravida develops gestational diabetes mellitus and is managed appropriately during pregnancy. She asks you about the consequences of gestational diabetes to her and her fetus. Which one of the following statements is correct?

(A) The risk of fetal anomalies is increased.
(B) The risk of stillbirth is increased if her fasting blood sugars are elevated.
(C) The risk of a growth restricted newborn is increased.
(D) Insulin is the preferred treatment to maintain euglycemia.
(E) The risk of fetal macrosomia is not increased with gestational diabetes.

Questions 39 and 40

39. A 27-year-old woman develops spiking fevers to 104°F on her first postpartum day. She was placed on broad-spectrum antibiotics, including anaerobic coverage. However, she still has spiking fevers to 103°F on her third postpartum day. She had prolonged ruptured membranes and an 18-h labor before delivery with low forceps. She denies dysuria, increased frequency, and hematuria. On examination, her uterus is firm and appropriately involuted. Lochia is minimal. She has mild tenderness diffusely in her lower abdomen. Her white blood count is 18,000/mm^3. Which of the following is the most likely diagnosis?

(A) pyelonephritis
(B) infected episiotomy
(C) mastitis
(D) septic pelvic thrombophlebitis
(E) appendicitis

40. Which of the following is the most appropriate therapy for this woman?

(A) continue broad-spectrum antibiotics
(B) discontinue antibiotics and begin intravenous heparin
(C) continue the broad-spectrum antibiotics and add intravenous heparin
(D) perform a D&C
(E) TAH-BSO

41. A 27-year-old woman has carcinoma *in situ* of the cervix. By colposcopy, the squamocolumnar junction is completely visible, and the lesion does not extend into the endocervical canal. Which of the following is the most appropriate treatment for this woman?

(A) cryosurgery
(B) loop electroexcision procedure (LEEP)
(C) total hysterectomy
(D) radical hysterectomy
(E) local radiation therapy

42. A 16-year-old girl is brought to see you by a social worker. She has run away from home several times in the past 6 months. Her school grades have dropped noticeably. She has been arrested twice in the last month for shoplifting. She appears healthy and intelligent. Which of the following is the most plausible explanation for her behavior?

(A) boredom with school
(B) cocaine abuse
(C) incest
(D) depression
(E) peer pressure

Questions 43 and 44

You see a 23-year-old woman in the emergency department because she states that she was raped 3 h ago.

43. Which of the following history or physical findings are sufficient to document a diagnosis of rape on her record?

(A) bruises on her torso
(B) acid phosphatase from a pool of vaginal fluid
(C) nonmotile sperm in the vagina
(D) motile sperm in the cervical mucus
(E) none of the above permit a diagnosis of rape

44. Which of the following infections is most likely to occur in this woman as a result of her rape?

(A) HIV
(B) syphilis
(C) gonorrhea
(D) trichomonas
(E) hepatitis B

45. A 19-year-old primigravid woman at 39 weeks' gestation is in active labor, and her cervix is 4 cm dilated, 90% effaced. Her amniotic membranes have been ruptured for 4 h. Contractions are strong at 2- to 3-min intervals and of 60- to 70-s duration. For the past 30 min, repetitive variable decelerations of the fetal heart rate have occurred. They have lasted 60–90 s, and the fetal heart rate has dropped as low as 60 beats per minute (BPM). You explain that there is a risk that the baby will become hypoxic and recommend a cesarean section. She refuses. Which of the following is the most appropriate course of action?

(A) obtain permission for the cesarean section from her mother
(B) perform a cesarean section as an emergency
(C) obtain a court order permitting a cesarean section
(D) counsel her carefully about the fetal risks but accede to her wishes
(E) assign her care to another obstetrician

Questions 46 and 47

46. A 35-year-old primigravid woman with a history of cyclic menses at 28- to 30-day intervals began her last menses on August 18. A home pregnancy test was positive on September 20. At her first prenatal visit, she asks you what the duration of pregnancy is and what her due date is. You tell her that the average number of days from the onset of menses to delivery is

(A) 250
(B) 260
(C) 270
(D) 280
(E) 290

47. With reference to the above patient, you tell her that her expected delivery date (EDD) is

(A) May 18
(B) August 18
(C) May 11
(D) August 11
(E) May 25
(F) June 1

Questions 48 and 49

A 44-year-old woman had a normal Pap smear 3 years ago. Her menstrual periods occur monthly and last 5 days. She has had intermenstrual and postcoital spotting intermittently for the past 6 months. The pelvic examination is normal.

48. Which of the following is the most appropriate test to perform?

(A) an endometrial biopsy
(B) an endocervical curettage
(C) a conization of the cervix
(D) a Pap smear
(E) a hysteroscopy

49. All tests performed on the woman were normal. She returns 1 year later for her annual gynecologic examination. On speculum examination, she has a visible 7-mm lesion on her cervix that bleeds on contact. Which of the following is the most appropriate procedure to perform?

(A) colposcopy
(B) cervical biopsy
(C) Pap smear
(D) conization of the cervix
(E) vaginal hysterectomy

50. A 24-year-old woman lost her previous two pregnancies at approximately 20 weeks' gestation, without having noted any contractions. She is currently at 15 weeks' gestation and denies having uterine contractions. Her cervix is undilated and uneffaced. Which of the following is the most appropriate management of this patient?

(A) bed rest
(B) terbutaline
(C) hydroxyprogesterone
(D) DES
(E) a cervical cerclage

51. A 24-year-old woman has a MSAFP of 0.5 MOM (multiples of the median) at 17 weeks' gestation. Which of the following fetal abnormalities is most likely to occur with this MSAFP?

(A) spina bifida
(B) omphalocele
(C) gastroschisis
(D) bladder exstrophy
(E) trisomy 21

52. A 69-year-old woman with diabetes mellitus complains of urinary incontinence. Her diabetes is well controlled with oral hypoglycemic agents. She has no complaints other than the wetness. Which of the following tests is most likely to demonstrate the cause?

(A) urinalysis
(B) urine culture and sensitivity
(C) intravesical instillation of methylene blue
(D) the Q-tip test
(E) measurement of residual urine volume

53. A 48-year-old G5P5 woman has genuine stress incontinence (GSI). Kegel exercises have not helped, and her incontinence is gradually worsening. Her urethrovesical junction (UVJ) is prolapsed into the vagina, and her urethral closure pressure is normal. Which of the following procedures will most likely cure her incontinence?

(A) retropubic urethropexy
(B) anterior colporrhaphy
(C) suburethral sling procedure
(D) needle suspension of paraurethral tissue
(E) paraurethral collagen injections

54. On a routine annual examination, a 43-year-old woman is found to have a 2-cm mass in the lateral aspect of her right breast. Which of the following is the most appropriate next step in management?

(A) repeat the breast examination after her next menses
(B) mammography
(C) fine-needle aspiration
(D) open biopsy
(E) segmental resection

55. A 37-year-old pregnant woman has a genetic amniocentesis at 16 weeks' gestation. A concurrent ultrasound shows normal fetal anatomy. Her prenatal course has been unremarkable. Her prenatal labs include a B-negative blood type, a negative rubella antibody titer, a negative hepatitis B surface antigen, and a hematocrit of 31%. Which of the following is the most appropriate management for this woman?

(A) rubella immunization at the time of the amniocentesis
(B) a serologic test for the presence of hepatitis B surface antibody
(C) a follow-up ultrasound in 1 week to assess for intraamniotic bleeding
(D) administration of Rh immune globulin at the time of the amniocentesis
(E) chorionic villus biopsy at the time of the amniocentesis

Questions 56 through 58

A 23-year-old pregnant woman at 5 postmenstrual weeks took coumadin until about 3 days after her menses was due. She has monthly menses. A home pregnancy test was positive on the day she took coumadin. She takes coumadin because of a history of deep vein thrombosis and pulmonary embolism. She is concerned that the coumadin will cause birth defects.

56. You tell her that the conceptus is most susceptible to teratogenesis at what stage of pregnancy?

(A) between menses and ovulation
(B) from ovulation to implantation
(C) between implantation and the day of expected menses
(D) between the day of expected menses and 12 postmenstrual weeks
(E) during the second and third trimesters

57. You advise this woman to do which of the following?

(A) Abort the pregnancy because the fetus is likely to have birth defects.
(B) Have an ultrasound in 1–2 weeks to search for fetal anomalies.
(C) Have a genetic amniocentesis at 16 postmenstrual weeks.
(D) Begin prenatal care because the probability of birth defects is low.
(E) Take 10 mg vitamin K to reverse the effects of coumadin.

58. Which of the following is the treatment of choice during pregnancy for this woman?

(A) coumadin
(B) heparin
(C) aspirin
(D) tissue plasminogen activator (TPA)
(E) vena caval filter

59. A 19-year-old primigravida at term has been completely dilated for $2^1/_2$ h. The vertex is at 2 to 3 station, and the position is occiput posterior. She complains of exhaustion and is unable to push effectively to expel the fetus. She has an anthropoid pelvis. Which of the following is the most appropriate management to deliver the fetus?

(A) immediate low transverse cesarean section
(B) immediate classical cesarean section
(C) apply forceps and deliver the baby as an occiput posterior
(D) apply Kielland forceps to rotate the baby to occiput anterior
(E) cut a generous episiotomy to make her pushing more effective

Questions 60 and 61

A 22-year-old woman whose last pregnancy was terminated by salpingostomy for removal of a tubal pregnancy is attempting to conceive.

60. Which of the following is the average number of ovulatory cycles to achieve a pregnancy by normally fertile couples?

(A) 1
(B) 3
(C) 6
(D) 8
(E) 10

61. This woman is aware that her chances of another tubal pregnancy are increased. What is the earliest that a serum β-hCG will be positive?

(A) 4 days after fertilization
(B) during the week before the expected date of menses
(C) on the day of the expected menses
(D) 1 week after the missed menses
(E) 2 weeks after the missed menses

Questions 62 and 63

A 46-year-old G3P3 woman has had postcoital spotting for 6 months. On pelvic examination, she has a fungating, exophytic lesion arising from her cervix that is approximately 2 cm in diameter. Biopsy of this lesion is interpreted as invasive squamous cell carcinoma of the cervix. There is no evidence of extension of the cancer onto the vagina. The parametria are not indurated by bimanual examination. CT scan of her pelvis and abdomen discloses enlarged paraaortic lymph nodes and metastatic lesions in the parenchyma of her liver.

62. Which of the following is the FIGO stage of her cancer?

(A) IA
(B) IB
(C) IIA
(D) IIIB
(E) IVB

63. This woman's childbearing is complete. She is a healthy woman who is close to ideal body weight, exercises regularly, and does not smoke. Which of the following is the most appropriate treatment of this woman?

(A) TAH-BSO
(B) radical hysterectomy with pelvic and paraaortic lymph node dissection
(C) pelvic exenteration
(D) multiagent chemotherapy
(E) combined brachytherapy and external radiation therapy

64. A pregnant woman has been taking phenytoin (Dilantin) for a seizure disorder. She is concerned that the drug will cause fetal abnormalities. Which of the following defects is the most common anomaly associated with phenytoin?

(A) atrial septal defect
(B) ventricular septal defect
(C) cleft lip/palate
(D) spina bifida
(E) hydrocephalus

65. When counseling pregnant women about the dangers of drug use during pregnancy, they should be told that the rate of spontaneous major malformations in newborns is what?

(A) less than 1%
(B) 2–4%
(C) 6–8%
(D) 10–12%
(E) more than 12%

Questions 66 and 67

A 34-year-old woman just delivered a 4100-g boy after a 15-h labor, including a $2^1/_2$-h second stage. During the repair of a midline episiotomy, there is a marked increase in the amount of vaginal bleeding.

66. Which of the following is the most common cause of immediate postpartum hemorrhage?

(A) retained placental fragments
(B) uterine atony
(C) cervical laceration
(D) vaginal laceration
(E) disseminated intravascular coagulation

67. Which of the following is the best immediate management of the probable cause of this postpartum hemorrhage?

(A) massage and compression of the uterine fundus
(B) intravenous administration of 20 units of oxytocin
(C) intramuscular administration of 0.2 mg methylergonovine
(D) insertion of a gauze pack into the uterine cavity
(E) hypogastric artery ligation

Questions 68 through 72

A 55-year-old woman has a bloody discharge from her left breast. A mammogram discloses a cluster of microcalcifications 3 cm beneath her left nipple.

68. Which of the following is the best next step in her evaluation?

(A) cytologic evaluation of the nipple discharge
(B) fine-needle aspiration under radiologic guidance
(C) MRI of the breast and axillary nodes
(D) open biopsy of the left breast
(E) segmental mastectomy

69. Which of the following is the principal advantage of a fine-needle aspiration of a breast mass?

(A) It reassures the patient if it is negative.
(B) It reduces the number of open breast biopsies.
(C) It differentiates between noninvasive and invasive cancer.
(D) It replaces the need for subsequent mammography.
(E) It helps to determine the extent of *in situ* breast carcinoma.

70. Which of the following factors is associated with the greatest lifetime risk for developing breast cancer?

(A) obesity
(B) early menarche
(C) late menopause
(D) age
(E) having a mother with a history of breast cancer

71. Which of the following is the most common type of breast cancer?

(A) inflammatory carcinoma
(B) lobular carcinoma *in situ*
(C) lobular infiltrating carcinoma
(D) infiltrating ductal carcinoma
(E) ductal carcinoma *in situ*

72. Which of the following is the best predictor of survival after appropriate treatment of breast cancer?

(A) an initial tumor 1 cm or smaller in diameter
(B) the presence of estrogen receptors
(C) the presence of progesterone receptors
(D) a well-differentiated tumor
(E) axillary nodes negative for cancer

73. A 39-year-old woman known to have fibrocystic disease of the breast complains of persistent fullness and pain in both breasts. Which of the following drugs will be most effective in relieving her symptoms?

(A) tamoxifen
(B) bromocriptine
(C) medroxyprogesterone acetate
(D) danazol
(E) hydrochlorothiazide

74. A couple consults you because each has neurofibromatosis and wish to know what their reproductive possibilities are. You should tell them that

(A) the disease is lethal and results in spontaneous abortion of homozygous fetuses
(B) 25% of the females will be affected
(C) 50% of all offspring will be homozygous for the abnormal gene

(D) 75% or more of their offspring will have the disease
(E) 25% of their offspring will be unaffected

75. A 26-year-old woman complains of a vaginal discharge causing burning and itching of the perineum. The pH of the discharge is 4.5. Which of the following is the most likely cause of her discharge?

(A) monilial vaginitis
(B) trichomonas vaginitis
(C) chlamydial cervicitis
(D) gonococcal cervicitis
(E) bacterial vaginosis

Questions 76 and 77

76. A wet smear of a vaginal discharge is illustrated in Fig. 2-1. Which of the following is the most likely cause of the discharge?

(A) monilial vaginitis
(B) trichomonas vaginitis
(C) *Chlamydia trachomatis*
(D) *N. gonorrhoeae*
(E) bacterial vaginosis

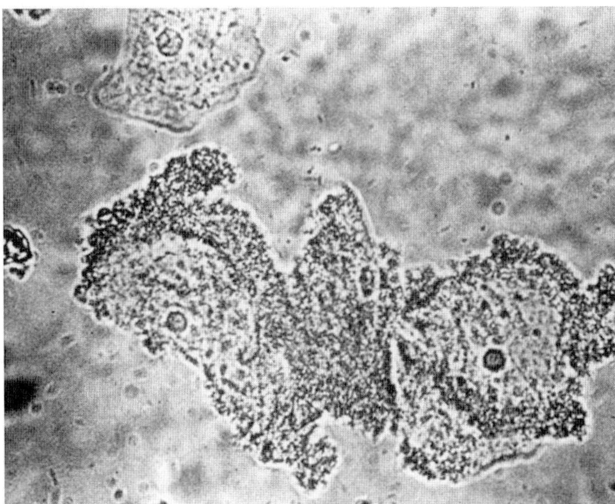

FIG. 2-1

77. Which of the following is the most appropriate treatment for the discharge illustrated in Fig. 2-1?

(A) clindamycin
(B) erythromycin
(C) metronidazole
(D) miconazole
(E) doxycycline

78. A 37-year-old man and his wife seek help for their 5-year history of primary infertility. Her infertility investigation is normal. However, the husband has an ejaculate volume of 0.4 mL, and there are no sperm in the ejaculate. A qualitative test for fructose in the semen is negative. Which of the following is the most likely diagnosis?

(A) germ cell aplasia
(B) bilateral occlusion of the vasa deferentia
(C) 17α-hydroxylase deficiency
(D) congenital absence of the vasa deferentia
(E) Klinefelter syndrome

Questions 79 and 80

79. A healthy 27-year-old male and his partner have been attempting to conceive for more than 1 year. As part of their evaluation he has a semen analysis. His ejaculate volume is 3.5 mL, sperm concentration is 8 million/mL, sperm motility is 65%, oval forms comprise 60% of the sperm, and fructose is present in the ejaculate. Which of these semen parameters is abnormal and suggests that this couple's infertility may be due to a male factor?

(A) ejaculate volume
(B) sperm concentration
(C) sperm motility
(D) sperm morphology
(E) presence of fructose

80. The man is treated with clomiphene for a presumptive diagnosis of male factor infertility. Though clomiphene is an unproven and unapproved therapy for male infertility, what is the earliest there should be an improvement in his semen parameters?

(A) 33 days
(B) 53 days
(C) 73 days
(D) 93 days
(E) 120 days

Questions 81 through 83

A 39-year-old pregnant woman with chronic hypertension and one prior pregnancy is now at 38 weeks' gestation. She comes to labor and delivery with profuse vaginal bleeding and abdominal pain of sudden onset.

81. Which of the following is the most likely diagnosis?

(A) bloody show
(B) vaginal laceration from coitus
(C) cervicitis
(D) placenta previa
(E) placental abruption

82. If the patient has a placental abruption, which of the following is the most likely risk factor?

(A) advanced maternal age
(B) low parity
(C) coitus immediately before the onset of bleeding
(D) hypertension
(E) a step aerobic class immediately before the onset of bleeding

83. This patient has an external fetal monitor placed. Uterine tone seems to be increased, and there are occasional variable decelerations of the fetal heart to 90 BPM. Which of the following is the most appropriate management?

(A) tocolysis with a β-receptor agonist
(B) Pitocin induction of labor
(C) continued monitoring of mother and baby
(D) amniotomy
(E) cesarean section

Questions 84 through 86

A 58-year-old woman with stage IIB squamous cell carcinoma of the cervix is receiving radiation therapy.

84. At which phase is a cell most sensitive to ionizing radiation?

(A) mitosis
(B) ribonucleic acid (RNA) synthesis
(C) deoxyribonucleic acid (DNA) synthesis
(D) protein synthesis
(E) the resting phase

85. This woman is to receive external radiation therapy. Which of the following is the usual dose to treat invasive cervical cancer?

(A) 500–1000 centigray (cGy)
(B) 1500–2000 cGy
(C) 4500–5000 cGy
(D) 7500–8000 cGy
(E) 9500 to 10,000 cGy

86. Which of the following is the earliest complication of radiation therapy?

(A) diarrhea
(B) hemorrhagic cystitis
(C) vaginal stenosis
(D) ureteral fibrosis
(E) rectovaginal fistula

87. A 45-year-old woman has bilateral breast pain that is most severe premenstrually. On palpation, there is excessive nodularity, tenderness, and cystic areas that diminish in size after menses. Which of the following is the most likely diagnosis?

(A) fibrocystic disease
(B) fibroadenomas
(C) intraductal papilloma
(D) breast cancer
(E) engorgement attributable to increased prolactin

88. Which feature of fibrocystic disease of the breast is associated with the greatest risk of developing breast cancer?

(A) number of nodules
(B) serous nipple discharge
(C) size of the dominant mass
(D) presence of epithelial hyperplasia
(E) presence of a palpable axillary node

89. A 35-year-old woman at 30 weeks' gestation discovers a lump in her left breast. Examination reveals a 2–3 cm, firm nodule in the upper outer quadrant. Which of the following is the most appropriate next step in the management of this patient?

(A) observation until after delivery
(B) thermography
(C) application of hot packs
(D) breast ultrasound
(E) fine-needle aspiration

90. A 1-cm carcinoma of the breast is diagnosed by an excisional biopsy in a 36-year-old woman at 14 weeks' gestation. The axillary nodes are negative. Which of the following is the best management of this patient?

(A) terminate the pregnancy immediately and treat the breast cancer
(B) monitor the mass throughout pregnancy with serial breast ultrasounds
(C) induce labor at 34 weeks' gestation, then give chemotherapy
(D) perform a cesarean delivery at 36 weeks and treat the breast cancer
(E) modified radical mastectomy at the time of diagnosis

Questions 91 through 94

A woman at 31 weeks' gestation complains of feeling dizzy and lightheaded when she lies on her back. She is Rh negative but denies vaginal bleeding, abdominal trauma, or abdominal pain. The diagnosis is probably the supine hypotensive syndrome.

91. This results in which of the following?

(A) a decreased fetal heart rate
(B) an increased frequency of uterine contractions
(C) a decreased tolerance to pain
(D) a decreased effect of epidural analgesia
(E) an increased risk of placental abruption

92. During this woman's labor, the nurse describes the presenting part as engaged when the woman is 6 cm dilated. Which of the following is the most accurate definition of engagement in a woman with a vertex presentation?

(A) The vertex has passed through the pelvic inlet.
(B) The vertex reaches the pelvic floor.
(C) The biparietal diameter has passed through the pelvic inlet.
(D) The biparietal diameter has reached the pelvic floor.
(E) The vertex is at 1 station.

93. In which of the following circumstances is the administration of anti-D immune globulin unnecessary?

(A) threatened abortion and first-trimester bleeding
(B) genetic amniocentesis at 16 weeks' gestation
(C) at 28 weeks
(D) at 40 weeks with the onset of labor
(E) after delivery of an Rh-positive fetus

94. She has an uncomplicated spontaneous vaginal delivery with an estimated blood loss of 450 mL. Her infant is Rh positive and she receives 300 μg of Rh immunoglobulin (one vial) within 72 h after delivery. This dose is sufficient to prevent Rh isoimmunization after what amount of fetal red cells enters the maternal circulation?

(A) 5 mL
(B) 30 mL
(C) 100 mL
(D) 200 mL
(E) 300 mL

Questions 95 through 97

A 19-year-old primigravida is at 39 weeks' gestation. Her prenatal course had been normal since her first visit at 9 weeks' gestation. Her blood pressure is now 144/96 mmHg. She has 2+ proteinuria. Her patellar reflexes are hyperactive.

95. Which of the following is the most likely diagnosis?

(A) acute glomerulonephritis
(B) essential hypertension
(C) pheochromocytoma
(D) preeclampsia
(E) polycystic kidneys

96. Which of the following is the most appropriate treatment of this patient?

(A) bed rest
(B) oral magnesium sulfate
(C) a thiazide diuretic
(D) propranolol
(E) induction of labor

97. Magnesium sulfate may be the preferred treatment in this patient if she is not at least at 37 weeks' gestation, and there is no evidence of fetal distress. What is the purpose of magnesium sulfate?

(A) tocolysis to prevent preterm labor
(B) decrease her blood pressure into the normal range
(C) reduce the risk of eclampsia
(D) increase uteroplacental blood flow
(E) prevent fetal hypertension

Questions 98 and 99

A 39-year-old multiparous woman has a retained placenta 60 min after the vaginal birth of a 3650-g healthy boy. There was no episiotomy and no lacerations of her perineum, vagina, or cervix. She now has profuse vaginal bleeding and her blood pressure is 80/50 mmHg with a pulse rate of 120/min. Her uterine fundus is firm.

98. Which of the following is the probable etiology of her postpartum hemorrhage?

(A) cervical laceration
(B) uterine atony
(C) Couvelaire uterus
(D) acute thrombocytopenia
(E) placenta accreta

99. Which of the following is the most appropriate treatment to control the hemorrhage?

(A) transfusion with whole blood
(B) uterine packing
(C) supracervical hysterectomy
(D) hypogastric artery ligation
(E) intravenous administration of methylergonovine

100. Ligation of the hypogastric (internal iliac) artery effectively controls intractable pelvic hemorrhage because

(A) there is no collateral circulation to the uterus
(B) uterine blood flow is stopped
(C) arterial pulse pressure to the uterus is reduced
(D) clotting in uterine capillaries is enhanced
(E) blood flow is shunted to the ovarian veins

Questions 101 through 103

A 53-year-old woman with five adult children complains of losing urine shortly after coughing or jumping. She occasionally loses urine while lying in bed if she happens to cough vigorously. She is unable to stop the urine once it has begun to flow.

101. Which of the following is the most likely diagnosis?

(A) GSI
(B) a vesicovaginal fistula
(C) a urethrovaginal fistula
(D) an atonic bladder
(E) detrusor dyssynergia

102. Which of the following would most likely confirm the cause of this woman's incontinence?

(A) a urine culture
(B) a Q-tip test
(C) urethroscopy
(D) urethrocystometry
(E) an intravenous pyelography (IVP)

103. Which of the following is the treatment of choice for this woman's urinary incontinence?

(A) a course of nitrofurantoin
(B) a selective serotonin reuptake inhibitor (SSRI)
(C) oxybutynin chloride (Ditropan)
(D) vaginal hysterectomy and anterior colporrhaphy
(E) a Marshall–Marchetti–Krantz urethropexy

Questions 104 through 106

A 14-year-old girl complains of monthly pelvic pain for the past 6 months. She has never menstruated. Breast development began at the age of $11^1/_2$ years, and pubic hair first appeared about the age of 12 years. Accelerated linear growth occurred about 1 year ago. On examination, there are no palpable abdominal masses, although the suprapubic region is tender to deep palpation. The external genitalia are normal, but there is no vaginal orifice. There is an outward bulge between the labia minora and a slight bluish tinge in this area. On rectal examination, there is a soft mass palpated anterior to the lower rectum. The uterus is palpated and feels somewhat enlarged and tender for a nulligravid adolescent.

104. Which of the following is the most likely diagnosis?

(A) vaginal agenesis
(B) androgen insensitivity
(C) labial adhesions
(D) imperforate hymen
(E) transverse vaginal septum

105. Which of the following is the most likely explanation for her enlarged, tender uterus?

(A) pregnancy
(B) uterine fibroids
(C) hematometra
(D) adenomyosis
(E) endometrial cancer

106. Which of the following is the treatment of choice for this patient?

(A) McIndoe vaginoplasty
(B) hysterectomy
(C) laparoscopy
(D) hymenotomy
(E) gonadectomy

DIRECTIONS (Questions 107 through 115): For each item select the ONE best lettered option that is the most likely diagnosis of vaginal bleeding in pregnancy. Each lettered option may be selected once, more than once, or not at all.

(A) threatened abortion
(B) gestational trophoblastic disease
(C) cervicitis
(D) placenta previa
(E) placental abruption
(F) uterine rupture
(G) placenta accreta
(H) uterine inversion
(I) uterine atony
(J) vaginal laceration
(K) tubal pregnancy

107. A 28-year-old pregnant woman at 32 weeks' gestation suddenly begins profuse, painless vaginal bleeding. Her prenatal care began at 7 weeks and had been uncomplicated. She last had sexual intercourse 7 days ago. She denies abdominal trauma. Her uterus is soft and nontender, and the fetal heart rate is 132 BPM.

108. A 23-year-old pregnant woman at 16 weeks' gestation begins to have light vaginal bleeding several hours after sexual intercourse. She has no abdominal discomfort. Her prenatal course has been uneventful and fetal heart tones were heard at 12 weeks. Her uterus is midway between her symphysis pubis and umbilicus, and is soft and nontender. Fetal heart tones are now 148 BPM. Her cervix is undilated.

109. A 15-year-old girl began her last menstrual period (LMP) 14 weeks ago. She had a positive pregnancy test 6 weeks ago. On examination, her uterine fundus is at the level of the umbilicus. Fetal heart tones are not heard and no fetus is seen by abdominal ultrasound.

110. A 39-year-old pregnant woman with chronic hypertension at 37 weeks' gestation presents with heavy vaginal bleeding and complains of lower abdominal pain. She also has noted diminished fetal movement since the bleeding began 3 h previously. On physical examination her uterus is firm (*rock hard*) and very tender. Fetal heart tones are in the range of 160–170 BPM.

111. A 32-year-old pregnant woman has a low forceps vaginal delivery after a 3-h second stage of labor. One hour later the nurse informs you she has excessive vaginal bleeding. On examination, her uterus is firm and nontender, and the uterine fundus is at the umbilicus.

112. A 21-year-old woman last menstruated 6 weeks ago. Her menses are usually every 28–30 days. She has a past history of chlamydia. One week ago she had a positive home pregnancy test. She complains of mild left lower quadrant pain. Quantitative serum chorionic gonadotropin (hCG) concentrations 2 days ago and today are 6850 and 7685 mIU/mL, respectively. No intrauterine pregnancy is identified by transvaginal ultrasound.

113. A 29-year-old pregnant woman at 38 weeks' gestation presents to your labor and delivery unit complaining of dizziness, heavy vaginal bleeding, and loss of fetal movement. She had been having uterine contractions for approximately 4 h, but these stopped when the bleeding began. Her previous pregnancy was delivered by classical cesarean section because of a transverse lie.

114. A 31-year-old woman has an uncomplicated labor and vaginal delivery of a healthy 3400-g male infant. However, her placenta has not yet delivered 2 h after the delivery of her child. Under appropriate anesthesia manual extraction of the placenta is attempted, but the placenta is removed in fragments. She continues to have excessive vaginal bleeding after manual removal of her placenta. Her first child was delivered by a low transverse cesarean section because of fetal distress.

115. A 34-year-old woman, gravida 5, has a 17-h first stage, a 3.5-h second stage ending with a spontaneous vaginal delivery of a 4400-g infant, and a 15-min third stage of labor. Immediately after the placenta delivers, she has profuse vaginal bleeding. On examination, her perineum is intact and there are no vaginal or cervical lacerations. Her uterus is soft and the uterine fundus is 4–5 cm above her umbilicus.

Answers and Explanations

1. **(C)** The incidence of ovarian cancer in OC users is 50% less than that found in nonusers. The incidence of PID is also decreased by 50% in OC users. The risk of endometrial cancer is decreased by 50% after 1 year of OC use, and the protective effect seems to persist after stopping the OC. In well-controlled studies, there is no increase in the risk of having a child with a major malformation, cardiac malformation, or limb abnormality. The risk of ectopic pregnancy is reduced by 90%, perhaps because the risk of any pregnancy approaches zero when the OC is taken correctly. (*Speroff and Fritz, pp. 894–895, 901–902, 904–905*)

2. **(D)** Breast development in an infant or young child is the consequence of increased estrogen secretion, exposure to exogenous estrogens, or increased response of breast tissue to normal, prepubertal amounts of estrogen. After excluding exposure to exogenous estrogens (e.g., OCs, estrogen creams), increased response to estrogen is more common than increased estrogen secretion from the ovaries or adrenal glands when breast development is the only sign of precocious puberty. The uterus and adnexa can be palpated abdominally in prepubertal girls if they are pathologically enlarged. For this reason, an estrogen-secreting ovarian tumor (granulosa cell is the most common type) is usually palpable, and an ultrasound examination is unnecessary. For the same reason, a pelvic examination under anesthesia is not necessary, especially if the serum estradiol concentration is normal. CT scan of the head and a serum FSH concentration are unnecessary if breast development is the only sign of precocious puberty, and the serum estradiol concentration is normal in the prepubertal range. (*Yen et al., pp. 396–398*)

3. **(E)** Premature thelarche is a disorder that probably occurs as a consequence of increased sensitivity of breast tissue to the low levels of circulating estradiol in prepubertal girls. The disorder occurs most commonly before the age of 3 years. The estradiol concentration may be normal in young girls ingesting estrogen if the serum estrogen concentration is not obtained at the time the estrogen is ingested. A negative medication history is helpful to exclude this possibility. The absence of a palpable lower abdominal mass and a prepubertal concentration of estradiol exclude a granulosa cell tumor. Adrenal 21-hydroxylase deficiency and polycystic ovary syndrome are function disorders that require the stimulation of adrenocorticotropic hormone (ACTH) and pituitary gonadotropins (FSH and LH), respectively, to become clinically apparent. Neither disorder appears until after the onset of puberty. Moreover, both are associated with androgen excess and masculinization, not estrogen excess and precocious breast development. (*Yen et al., p. 398*)

4. **(C)** Premature thelarche is a benign, self-limited disorder that does not progress. Breast development may actually regress, though the regression may not be complete. The girl and her parents should be assured that the events of puberty will be normal at a normal age. Examination of the girl should be repeated at 3- to 6-month intervals for about 1 year to be certain that additional pubertal events do not occur (such as growth of pubic hair, accelerated linear growth, and vaginal bleeding). Because pituitary and adrenal functions are normal for a prepubertal girl, therapy with a GnRH agonist (Lupron, Synarel, and so forth) or a corticosteroid is ineffective and inappropriate. Although breast cancer is a rare possibility in prepubertal girls, the presence of bilateral breast buds effectively excludes this diagnosis. A breast biopsy may destroy breast anlage, and these girls will not have breast development at puberty. (*Yen et al., p. 398*)

5. **(A)** In general, gynecologic cancers confined to the organ of origin are stage I. Thus, this patient has a stage I cancer. In 1988, FIGO revised the staging of endometrial cancer from a clinical staging to surgical staging. Cancer limited to the endometrium is stage IA. Myometrial invasion less than 50% is stage IB, and myometrial invasion more than 50%, but not involving the serosa, is stage IC. (*DiSaia and Creasman, p. 140; Hoskins et al., p. 924*)

6. **(D)** The onset of preeclampsia before the 20th week of pregnancy is clinically seen only with a hydatidiform mole. Advanced maternal age, uterine size greater than gestational weeks, and the absence of a fetal heartbeat are added features to suggest gestational trophoblastic disease. Hydramnios, which can be associated with anencephaly and other fetal developmental abnormalities, also predisposes to preeclampsia, but its onset does not occur before 24 weeks. Renal disease, diabetes mellitus, and chronic hypertension also increase the likelihood of preeclampsia, but not before 24 weeks of pregnancy. The incidence of preeclampsia is increased in twin gestation, but again, its onset is not before 24 weeks. (*Cunningham et al., pp. 835–847*)

7. **(A)** Acyclovir prescribed from 36 gestational weeks until after delivery reduces the probability of a cesarean section, although in one study of a small number of patients there were no cases of neonatal herpes in either the treatment or control group. Nonetheless, acyclovir (a class C drug) and newer antiviral drugs (valacyclovir, famciclovir, both class B) should be given to women with either a primary outbreak or a recurrence during pregnancy. Weekly cultures are unreliable to exclude active herpes lesions in pregnancy and are not recommended for basing a decision to perform a cesarean section. A cesarean section should be performed if a woman develops an active cervical or vaginal lesion at term. However, genital herpetic lesions before 36 weeks do not necessitate a cesarean section, because there is no evidence that vertical transmission to the fetus is increased until the pregnancy is within 2–4 weeks of delivery. Intrauterine infections via transplacental or transmembrane transmission of the herpesvirus are rare. Most infections of the infant occur after passage through an infected birth canal. A cesarean section should be performed at term if the amniotic membranes rupture in a woman with an active herpetic lesion in the genital area, regardless of the duration of membrane rupture. (*ACOG Practice Bulletin, Number 8, October 1999*)

8. **(C)** Vulvar carcinoma must be considered in any postmenopausal woman with pruritus, especially in the presence of a visible lesion. The appropriate management is to biopsy the lesion after disinfecting the area and infiltrating with 1% Xylocaine. A 3–4 mm dermal punch is useful to obtain the biopsy. Colposcopy alone is less reliable for vulvar lesions compared to cervical abnormalities because the technique requires the topical application of 3–5% acetic acid, which penetrates a keratinized squamous epithelium (the vulva) less than a nonkeratinized squamous epithelium (the cervix). Multiple biopsies should be obtained for a large, confluent lesion or a multifocal vulvar lesion. Wide local excision may be appropriate for small lesions, but is more difficult in an outpatient setting. Vulvectomy is reserved for women with biopsy-proven vulvar carcinoma. (*Hoskins et al., pp. 778–780*)

9. **(D)** Cancer of the cervix that has not invaded cervical stroma is stage 0 carcinoma *in situ*. Cancer that has invaded the cervical stroma but has not spread beyond the cervix is stage I. Involvement of the upper vagina or parametria (but not to the pelvic sidewall) is stage II. Stage III is involvement of the lower third of the vagina (IIIA) or parametria to the pelvic side wall (IIIB). Extension outside the reproductive tract is stage IV. (*Hoskins et al., p. 848*)

10. **(C)** The intent of staging is to judge the results of various treatments and to compare treatment results worldwide. Because advanced procedures such as venography, lymphangiography, MRI or CT scans, and laparoscopy are not universally available, staging of cervical cancer remains primarily clinical. Such tests

as cystoscopy, proctosigmoidoscopy, barium enema, IVP, and plain radiographs of the abdomen and chest are permitted. Evidence of mucosal cancer confirmed by biopsy at the time of cystoscopy changes her diagnosis to stage IV cervical cancer. (*Hoskins et al., pp. 846–849*)

11. **(B)** Stage of the cancer is the most important prognostic factor. Women with stage IA cervical cancer have a 95% 5-year survival. This decreases progressively to 80, 64, 38, and 14% for stages IB, II, III, and IV, respectively. The other choices are prognostic factors but relate to the stage of the cancer. Women with high-risk serotypes (strains) of HPV tend to develop cervical neoplasia at a younger age. More advanced stages of cervical cancer tend to have less differentiated tumors and a greater probability of pelvic and paraaortic lymph node metastasis. Pelvic lymph node metastasis will be found in 5% or fewer of women with stage I cervical cancer, with a progressive increase as the stage advances to 55% of women with stage IV cervical cancer. (*Hoskins et al., pp. 857–859*)

12. **(B)** Breast discomfort is a problem premenstrually for many women. Simple palliative measures include administration of vitamin E, 600 units daily, and limiting methylxanthines by eliminating coffee and other caffeine-containing substances, although the mechanism of action is not well understood. Danazol (Danocrine), in doses of 200–400 mg daily, is often effective in relieving breast pain. Clomiphene may have estrogenic side effects and worsen breast pain. Many women receiving progesterone note breast discomfort secondary to fluid retention. There is no evidence that diuretics such as hydrochlorothiazide relieve breast pain. In one comparison study, tamoxifen (a selective estrogen receptor modulator) was more effective than danazol. (*Speroff and Fritz, pp. 588–589*)

13. **(B)** Vaginismus is the painful, involuntary spasm of the musculature of the pelvis and lower third of the vagina. It may respond to properly administered dilator therapy, although there is a lack of conclusive evidence. Deep-thrust dyspareunia is often the result of pelvic pathology, such as fibroids, endometriosis, ovarian cysts, pelvic adhesions, and others. Anorgasmia is usually a psychologic disorder best dealt with by a psychologist or psychiatrist expert in sexual counseling and therapy. Sexual or physical abuse should be considered and the woman questioned about this possibility. Vulvar vestibulitis is an inflammatory condition of uncertain (perhaps multiple) etiology and is usually treated with topical glucocorticoids. Failure of medical therapy may require surgical excision of the affected area. (*McGuire and Hawton, pp. 1–24*)

14. **(D)** The fundal height corresponds to 16 gestational weeks. Between 15 and 20 weeks, screening for open neural tube defects should be offered. In addition to MSAFP, the American College of Obstetricians and Gynecologists recommends hCG and unconjugated estriol to screen for Down syndrome and trisomy 18 as well. This triad of tests is called a triple screen or triple marker screen. Reported sensitivity of the triple screen is between 57 and 67% and the false positive rate is 5%. An abnormal result must be evaluated further by ultrasonography to identify the presence or absence of open neural tube defects or abdominal wall defects (increased MSAFP) or trisomy disorder (decreased MSAFP and unconjugated estriol, increased hCG). In skilled hands, an ultrasound reduces the risk of such an anomaly by 95%. If the diagnosis is still uncertain, the woman should be offered amniocentesis for measurement of alpha-fetoprotein (AFP) and acetylcholinesterase activity (increased in neural tube defects) and karyotype of fetal skin cells. Although testing for HIV can be done any time, it is most appropriate at the first prenatal visit, because earlier onset of prophylaxis with acquired immune deficiency syndrome (AIDS) drugs reduces the risk of transmission to the fetus significantly. Routine culture for GBS is not recommended because of the high recurrence rate after treatment and the low attack rate to the fetus. Amniocentesis is not a screening procedure and is reserved for those women with a specific indication, such as elevated MSAFP, low MSAFP (risk of Down syndrome), advanced maternal age, and others. A glucose tolerance test may be appropriate if there is a

clinical indication for diabetes mellitus: previous macrosomic infant or stillbirth, strong family history of diabetes mellitus, persistent glycosuria, previous gestational diabetes, or elevated random serum glucose concentration. (*Cunningham et al., p. 984; Creasy et al., pp. 237–239*)

15. **(C)** The nonpitting edema of her legs is likely the result of lymphedema. This may cause discomfort or pain in her legs, but not hypesthesia. The most likely cause of the peripheral neuropathy is the carboplatin. Toxicity at doses higher than 100 mg/m^2 limit its use and also limit the ability to study various doses alone and in combination with other chemotherapeutic agents, such as paclitaxil (Taxol), which may also cause peripheral neuropathy. Nonetheless, the combination of tumor debulking, pelvic and paraaortic lymph node dissection, combination paclitaxil and carboplatin, and radiation offers the longest disease-free interval. (*Hoskins et al., pp. 1021–1024*)

16. **(D)** The mean age of onset of any pubertal event is approximately 11 years, beginning with the appearance of breast buds. Pubic hair appears approximately 6 months later, and this is followed by the peak height velocity (greatest rate of linear growth per unit time). Six to 12 months later, menstrual bleeding begins. Increased rate of growth begins early in the pubertal process. The sequence of pubertal events and the approximate age of appearance of each event is sufficiently predictable that significant variation in age of onset or sequence should lead to an evaluation of a cause of abnormal puberty. (*Speroff and Fritz, pp. 365–372*)

17. **(E)** There is no clinically applicable test for accurately measuring functional capacity of the heart. The most helpful guide to functional status is the mother's symptoms or the lack of symptoms. Enlargement of the heart and elevation of the diaphragm on a chest x-ray in pregnancy are normal findings. Pedal edema in mild degrees is also a very common finding. An S_3 in pregnancy is an abnormal finding and indicates cardiac disease but is not in and of itself predictive of functional status. (*Cunningham et al., pp. 1182–1184*)

18. **(E)** Although many mechanisms involving the fetal pituitary axis, placental membranes, decidual secretions, and fetal-placental interaction have been investigated, no mechanism has been established for the initiation of labor in humans. Cortisol mechanisms probably initiate labor in sheep, and sheep generally are the experimental animals used to study human parturition. It has, however, been shown that this mechanism does not incite labor in humans. Women who are pregnant with an anencephalic fetus often do not begin labor until after 42 weeks, but they do begin spontaneous labor even in the absence of a fetal pituitary gland. The most current thinking is that a fetal-placental-uterine interaction initiates labor. It is uncertain exactly how the pieces fit in this puzzle. (There is a comprehensive and complex review of the physiologic and biochemical processes of human parturition in Cunningham et al.) (*Cunningham et al., pp. 262–281; Scott et al., p. 35*)

19. **(D)** The first site of hematopoiesis in the fetus is the yolk sac. Between 12 and 24 weeks' gestation, the fetal liver makes the largest contribution. After 28 weeks, the fetal bone marrow is the most important site. (*Cunningham et al., pp. 145–147*)

20. **(C)** Hirsutism occurs when a woman is exposed to increased amounts of biologically active androgens, or when hair follicles are extrasensitive to normal amounts of androgens. Women with regular menstrual intervals usually have familial hirsutism, and it usually begins at or soon after puberty. Hirsutism associated with menstrual disturbances usually means exposure to increased amounts of androgens, either endogenous secretion from the ovaries or adrenal glands or ingestion of a drug with androgenic effects. The amenorrhea suggests increased androgen exposure, while the negative drug history suggests an endogenous source. Testosterone may arise from the ovaries, the adrenal glands, and from extraglandular formation. A serum testosterone

concentration is not helpful to distinguish which source of androgen is responsible for hirsutism. Furthermore, the serum testosterone level is often misleadingly low, because increased production rates of testosterone stimulate an increase in the rate of removal (the metabolic clearance rate) of testosterone from the circulation. The degree of hirsutism is the best gauge of the amount of excessive androgen production. Most virilizing ovarian tumors are palpable in young women, and a pelvic ultrasound is useful only when the bimanual examination is inadequate. Elevated prolactin levels may cause amenorrhea but do not cause hirsutism. There is no use for measurement of urinary androgen (17-ketosteroid or 17-ketogenic steroid) excretion in modern gynecology. The best next step is to measure a serum DHEAS concentration, because it is elevated in adrenal disorders and normal or only slightly elevated in ovarian causes of hirsutism. (*Speroff and Fritz, pp. 504–519*)

21. **(B)** A history of irregular menses from menarche suggests a functional disorder, such as polycystic ovary syndrome or attenuated adrenal hyperplasia attributable to an inherited enzyme deficiency. The absence of a unilateral ovarian mass on pelvic examination, the positive family history, and the early menarche favor a diagnosis of attenuated adrenal hyperplasia over that of a virilizing ovarian tumor. Women with 17-hydroxylase deficiency or 11-hydroxylase deficiency are hypertensive. Women with 17-hydroxylase deficiency are also sexually infantile, not hirsute, because they are unable to produce androgens or estrogens in normal amounts. Women with 21-hydroxylase deficiency may have salt wasting and hypotension if the enzyme deficiency is sufficiently severe. (*Speroff and Fritz, pp. 510–511*)

22. **(D)** At serum hCG concentrations above the discriminatory zone (usually about 4000 mIU/mL), transvaginal sonography should reveal an intrauterine pregnancy. The absence of such a finding suggests either an extrauterine pregnancy or a spontaneous abortion. Higher levels of hCG are necessary before an extrauterine gestational sac may be seen by sonography. At each week of gestation, hCG concentrations normally vary by a large amount. For this reason, a single measurement is not helpful, although serial measurements to determine whether the hCG fails to double in 48 h is helpful to suggest a failing pregnancy (ectopic or intrauterine). Nonclotting blood obtained from the cul-de-sac by a culdocentesis may be the result of a ruptured ectopic pregnancy or a ruptured ovarian cyst. An adnexal mass is palpated in only 50% of women with an ectopic pregnancy. (*Scott et al., pp. 92–94*)

23. **(B)** The only agents currently recognized to enhance production of fetal pulmonary surfactant are glucocorticoids. There is good evidence that pulmonary immaturity is reduced by 50% when corticosteroids are given to mothers at a gestational age less than 31 weeks. Also, there is evidence that neonatal death is decreased by about 50% with corticosteroid therapy, and other major infant morbidity is reduced as well (intraventricular hemorrhage, necrotizing enterocolitis). To achieve these benefits, delivery must be delayed 48 h. Of the agents listed, magnesium sulfate can prevent eclamptic seizures and may inhibit uterine contractions. The other agents have no role in the treatment of fetal lung immaturity. (*Creasy et al., pp. 456–460*)

24. **(B)** The LH surge classically triggers ovulation 14 days before the onset of the subsequent menstrual period. Subtract 14 days from the typical cycle length to estimate the cycle day of the LH surge and ovulation. It is pertinent to remind this woman that her probability of conceiving in each cycle is no higher than 15–20%, even with intercourse timed to the preovulatory LH surge. (*Speroff and Fritz, pp. 212–216*)

25. **(D)** GSI occurs when there is immediate involuntary loss of urine with increased intravesical pressure greater than maximal urethral pressure in the absence of detrusor contractions. These women can usually stop the flow of urine by voluntary contraction of the muscles that close the urethra. Loss of urine with a strong desire to void immediately suggests urge incontinence, often occurring as a result of detrusor contractions. Loss of urine associated with seemingly unrelated conditions should raise the suspicion of a drug-associated incontinence. Maximal bladder distention and greatly increased bladder capacity suggest a diagnosis of an atonic bladder with overflow incontinence. (*Scott et al., p. 846; Copeland, pp. 1061–1065*)

26. **(D)** Women with amenorrhea owing to weight loss and stress have decreased hypothalamic secretion of GnRH, and secondarily decreased serum levels of FSH and LH. As a consequence, serum estradiol levels will be low. While women with weight loss amenorrhea may have mild hirsutism, it is probably the result of a decreased estrogen secretion and decreased estrogen:androgen ratio, rather than an increase in serum testosterone levels. (*Speroff and Fritz, pp. 438–449*)

27. **(D)** With improved care, women with cystic fibrosis now survive into the reproductive age and are capable of carrying a pregnancy successfully. No special precautions such as prolonged hospitalization, oxygen supplementation, bed rest, or others are necessary. Likewise, there is no need for routine cesarean section or other labor modifications, except ensuring adequate hydration and normal serum electrolytes. An amniocentesis is unnecessary. There is no constituent of amniotic fluid that is diagnostic of cystic fibrosis. Also, the fetus is at risk for cystic fibrosis only if the father is a carrier. If not, the fetus will be a carrier only. Chorionic villus biopsy can be done to determine whether the fetus has cystic fibrosis if the father carries one of the 150+ alleles for cystic fibrosis or the couple had a previously affected child. It is becoming the standard of care to screen routinely pregnant women for the cystic fibrosis gene. Currently, routine screening will identify approximately 80% of carriers of the cystic fibrosis gene. (*Creasy et al., pp. 968–971*)

28. **(D)** The most likely diagnosis is a cyst of the canal of Nuck. These arise from inclusions of the peritoneum at the inferior insertion of the round ligament into the labia majora. They are analogous to a spermatic cord hydrocele and are typically found at the superior aspect of the labia majora. Vulvar varicosities usually involve most of the labia, occur in older and parous women, and have a classical "bag of worms" appearance. Given the physical findings, a hernia is unlikely. An ultrasound may be useful to distinguish a hernial sac from a cyst of the canal of Nuck. One-third of women with a cyst of the canal of Nuck may have a coexistent inguinal hernia. (*Scott et al., p. 622*)

29. **(C)** Different-sex twins must be dizygous. Prenatal ultrasound can detect monochorionic, monoamnionic twins, and these must be monozygous. For same-sex twins, careful examination of the amnionic membranes after birth can reveal monozygous twins if the placental membranes are monochorionic. Dichorionic membranes can occur with either monozygous or dizygous twins. Ultimately, assessment of DNA polymorphism is the best way to determine twin zygosity. (*Creasy et al., pp. 65–66*)

30. **(C)** The maximum number of oocytes is 6–7 million at approximately 20 gestational weeks. At birth, the number of oocytes has decreased to about 1 million, and the number at puberty is 300,000–500,000. Women at menopause still have a small number of oocytes, a number insufficient to produce an amount of estrogen to prevent vasomotor symptoms. By simple mathematics, women lose approximately 1000 oocytes per menstrual cycle: one by ovulation and the remainder by follicular atresia. (*Speroff and Fritz, pp. 106–107*)

31. **(D)** Approximately 20% of pregnant women have positive rectovaginal cultures. Vertical transmission rates from mother to baby is approximately 75%. A rectovaginal culture is not indicated at the first prenatal visit because the pregnant woman may subsequently convert from a negative to a positive culture. For this reason, all pregnant women should have a rectovaginal culture at 36–37 gestational weeks. If the woman goes into preterm labor before a culture is obtained, she should be treated with penicillin (gentamicin if she is penicillin allergic). The rate of neonatal sepsis is 1% of colonized mothers, a serious infection that may cause

pneumonia, meningitis, and death. (*Creasy et al., pp. 754–757*)

32. (D) Condyloma acuminata are caused by HPV, a sexually transmitted infection. A biopsy is unnecessary in young women, but should be done in older (age uncertain) to exclude verrucous carcinoma. The warts do not regress and are usually present for years without treatment. Without treatment they may enlarge, especially in women taking OCs or other forms of estrogen. Vulvar intraepithelial neoplasia and cervical dysplasia occur more frequently in women with condylomata, but not endometrial hyperplasia. (*Scott et al., pp. 616–617*)

33. (C) A single cavity uterus forms from fusion of paired Müllerian ducts followed by dissolution of the fused medial walls. Uterine anomalies can be divided into five distinct categories: (a) failure of formation of one or both Müllerian ducts (unicornuate uterus or absent uterus, respectively); (b) failure of fusion of the Müllerian ducts (didelphic uterus, with two cervixes and two vaginal canals separated by a longitudinal septum); (c) partial fusion of the Müllerian ducts (bicornuate uterus); (d) failure of dissolution of the fused medial walls of the Müllerian ducts (septate uterus); and (e) DES exposed uterus. A fetus exposed to DES (or any estrogen) in the first trimester will often develop a T-shaped uterine cavity. The pathophysiology of this abnormality is unknown. In this patient, a single cervix and a double uterine fundus indicate a bicornuate uterus. (*Speroff and Fritz, pp. 1079–1080*)

34. (B) Obesity, advanced age, and hepatic disease are associated with an increased risk of endometrial adenocarcinoma. While postmenopausal bleeding is most commonly caused by atrophic changes in the genital tract, cancer must be considered. Cervical cytology and examination of endometrial histology are absolutely indicated. The risk of endometrial cancer is increased approximately threefold in diabetic women, and obese women have a three- to fourfold increased risk. High parity is a risk factor for cervical cancer; low parity is a risk factor for ovarian and endometrial cancer. Postmenopausal bleeding is a sign of ovarian cancer only if the malignancy secretes estrogen to stimulate the endometrium. An office endometrial biopsy has a sensitivity of about 90%. If postmenopausal bleeding persists, a D&C with hysteroscopy should be done. A D&C alone samples about 50% of the endometrium. For this reason, many gynecologists are performing a hysteroscopy and directed endometrial biopsy in addition to a D&C. (*Hoskins et al., p. 920*)

35. (D) Blood pressure tends to drop slightly in normal pregnancy. This woman's blood pressure of 132/86 mmHg is definitely higher than would be expected and suggests the possibility of chronic hypertension. Because the GFR in pregnancy increases normally by as much as 50% to a peak of approximately 160 mL/min, serum creatinine and BUN should be less than 0.9 and 13 mg/100 mL, respectively. The observed values in this patient are elevated for pregnancy. The renal threshold for glucose normally decreases in pregnancy. Therefore, glycosuria does not always mean diabetes in pregnancy. Several plasma glucose measurements should be obtained in pregnant women with glycosuria to correlate urinary and plasma glucose levels. (*Creasy et al., pp. 111–118*)

36. (A) The current treatment guideline from the Centers for Disease Control and Prevention for uncomplicated gonococcal infections is ceftriaxone 125 mg IM one time. Cefixime 400 mg orally, ciprofloxacin 500 mg orally, or ofloxacin 400 mg orally are alternatives. Each is given as a single dose. To the chosen drug is added azithromycin, 1 g orally, or doxycycline, 100 mg orally twice daily for 7 days. The second drug is added to treat *C. trachomatis*, which is present in almost 50% of women with gonorrhea. Sexual partners should be treated at the same time. (*MMWR, pp. 36–37*)

37. (E) Of the choices listed, a biophysical profile is the best assessment of fetal well-being. This assesses multiple fetal variables: breathing movement, body or limb movements, tone and posture, fetal heart rate pattern, and amniotic fluid volume. A NSTs, oxytocin challenge test, and fetal movement counts assess only one determinant of fetal well-being. An amniocentesis has no value in assessing fetal well-being, but may be appropriate to determine fetal lung maturity if induction of labor before 40 gestational weeks is indicated because of her chronic illnesses. Fetal Doppler studies to assess systolic:diastolic (SD) ratio may be a better test of fetal well-being and a significant decrease or reversal of the ratio is an indication for delivery. (*Creasy et al., pp. 362–376*)

38. (B) Unlike women with overt or pregestational diabetes mellitus, the risk of fetal anomalies is not increased in women with gestational diabetes. Stillbirth rates are increased in women with gestational diabetes if their fasting plasma glucose concentrations are elevated, but not with elevated postprandial glucose concentrations only. The risk of a growth restricted infant is increased in women with long-standing diabetes and vascular disease, but not in women with gestational diabetes. There is a slight increase in the frequency of fetal macrosomia (birth weight over 4000 g), though shoulder dystocia and brachial plexus injury are infrequent. (*Cunningham et al., pp. 1363–1367*)

39. (D) The diagnosis of septic pelvic thrombophlebitis should be considered in women suspected of having a pelvic infection, but who fail to respond promptly to broad-spectrum antibiotics and continue to have spiking fevers after 3–4 days. Pyelonephritis is unlikely because of the location of her discomfort and the absence of urinary tract symptoms. A urinalysis and urine culture are, however, appropriate for this woman. An infected episiotomy is unlikely because these women complain of severe perineal pain. Postpartum mastitis usually does not occur until after the third to fourth postpartum day. Pregnant women with appendicitis typically have mid- to upper abdominal pain because of the displacement of the appendix by the enlarged uterus. (*Cunningham et al., pp. 681–682*)

40. (A) Septic pelvic thrombophlebitis is believed to occur in some women as a complication of bacterial endomyometritis. Blood cultures are positive in approximately 25% of cases. The range of organisms causing endomyometritis should be considered in the choice of antibiotics. Broad-spectrum and usually multiple antibiotics should be continued until she becomes afebrile. Intravenous heparin was considered standard therapy for septic pelvic thrombophlebitis until recent studies found that heparin alone or heparin with antibiotics did not shorten the febrile course compared with antibiotics alone. The absence of focal, severe tenderness of the uterus makes the diagnosis of endomyometritis and/or retained placenta unlikely. A D&C is appropriate only for retained placental tissue, which should be suspected in women with subinvolution of the uterus, marked uterine tenderness, and increased lochia. A hysterectomy is rarely indicated in postpartum women, especially when the diagnosis is septic pelvic thrombophlebitis. (*Cunningham et al., pp. 681–682*)

41. (B) Cryosurgery and electrocautery have the advantage of being office procedures and, therefore, treatments with relatively low cost. However, cryosurgery has at least two drawbacks: lack of tissue for histologic examination and the possibility that recurrences will not be detected by cytology or colposcopy. The latter problem occurs because the cryosurgery can cause the formation of a new squamocolumnar junction that grows over persistent or recurrent dysplastic cells. Any type of hysterectomy will effectively eradicate the lesion but is too much therapy for the problem. Local radiation is inappropriate for cervical cancer *in situ* but is usually the principal mode of therapy for stage II or greater invasive cervical cancer. The LEEP procedure has several advantages. A tissue specimen can be examined to be certain that the margins are disease free. The procedure can be done in the office with a paracervical anesthetic block. The procedure does not decrease the value of future cervical cytology or colposcopy. (*Hoskins et al., pp. 844–846.*)

42. (C) Incest should be suspected in a child or adolescent with behavioral changes, anger, guilt, lying, stealing, school failure, running away, and sleep disturbances. The physician should ask appropriate questions, such as, "Were you physically or sexually abused?" The question must be asked in a nonjudgmental manner. In many states, physicians have a legal requirement to report suspected abuse to Child Protective Services. The prevalence of child sexual abuse is conservatively estimated at 20%. The sexual abuse is committed by a family member in approximately 80% of instances. The other choices may describe some of her problems, but only incest encompasses all her problems. (*Copeland, pp. 486–497*)

43. **(E)** Each of the first four choices may be present in a woman who was raped. However, rape is a legal statement rather than a medical term. You should record your findings in the medical record and record a diagnosis of "alleged sexual assault." (*Copeland, pp. 487–497*)

44. **(D)** In one published study, trichomonas was the most likely infection to occur in sexually assaulted adult women. The risk of acquiring HIV with a single act of sexual intercourse is estimated to be less than 1%. Results from a study by the CDC show that the risk of acquiring syphilis or gonorrhea is 3 and 6–12%, respectively. The risk of acquiring hepatitis B is uncertain. Gonorrhea and chlamydia are the most common sexually transmitted infections in sexually abused children. (*ACOG Educational Bulletin, No. 242 November 1997*)

45. **(D)** In many states, a pregnant woman under the age of 21 years is considered an emancipated minor and is the only person who may make legal decisions pertaining to the pregnancy. Although an immediate cesarean section is indicated because of the severe fetal heart rate decelerations, to perform it without her permission violates the ethical principle of autonomy. This is a principle that states that human beings should have their wishes respected as autonomous persons if they are capable of self-determination. Obtaining a court order may fulfill the ethical principle of beneficence, a physician acting to do no harm and to help the patient. In this situation, the ethical (moral) decision is complicated by a conflict between beneficence and autonomy. However, proceeding with a cesarean section exposes the obstetrician to a legal charge of battery. Assigning her care to another physician is a standard and accepted solution when there is a moral conflict between patient and physician. However, this is not an acceptable option in an emergency situation. The obstetrician is at risk for abandonment. Although not a satisfying choice, the choice most ethically sound is to counsel her carefully, but eventually accede to her wishes. Placing her in the lateral position, giving her oxygen by mask, and providing adequate intravenous hydration should be instituted to minimize the risk of fetal hypoxia. (*Scott et al., pp. 1037–1042*)

46. **(D)** The mean duration of human pregnancy is 266 days from conception. To this is added 14 days for the interval between the onset of the last menses and the conception date. Thus, it is important to ascertain the range of days for each woman's menstrual cycles. The more variable a woman's menstrual cycles are, the less certain is the estimated due date calculated from the LMP. The standard deviation of pregnancy duration is ±17 days. Thus, 95% of human pregnancies will deliver between 263 and 297 days after the onset of the LMP. (*Cunningham et al., p. 226*)

47. **(E)** Calculation of the EDD is by using Naegele's rule. Seven days are added to the first day of the LMP, then 3 months are subtracted. Application of Naegele's rule is accurate only for women who have regular menstrual cycle intervals of 28–30 days. (*Cunningham et al., p. 226*)

48. **(D)** Postcoital spotting and intermenstrual spotting in a woman with cyclic menses is suggestive of a cervical abnormality, rather than an endometrial hormonal abnormality. In the absence of a visible lesion, a Pap smear that includes cells from both the ectocervix and endocervix is the preferred method of evaluation, especially when the woman has no history of cervical pathology or a normal Pap smear in the recent past. Endometrial biopsy and hysteroscopy assess the endometrium, not the

cervix. A conization of the cervix should be reserved for women with documented cervical neoplasia when determination of the extent of the lesion is necessary. An endocervical curettage is usually reserved for women with unsatisfactory Pap smears and persistent abnormal bleeding. (*Scott et al., p. 925*)

49. (B) Pap smear and colposcopy are screening tests appropriate when there is no visible cervical pathology. In the presence of a lesion, pathologic evaluation is necessary to make a diagnosis. An office cervical biopsy is the procedure of choice to establish the diagnosis. If the diagnosis from the biopsy is cancer, a conization of the cervix is indicated to determine the extent of the disease surface spread as well as depth of stromal invasion. As a general principle, cytology is a screening tool, not a diagnostic test, and any visible lesion (vulvar, vaginal, or cervical) should be biopsied for a definitive diagnosis. (*Scott et al., pp. 926–927*)

50. (E) The patient described in the question has a classic history of an incompetent cervix: expulsion of a fetus without labor. It is believed to be caused by previous cervical trauma, DES exposure, or, most commonly, a congenital defect in cervical stroma. In the absence of preterm labor, there is no indication for terbutaline or other tocolytic agents. DES is contraindicated in pregnancy, but was used in the past to treat repeated pregnancy loss. Hydroxyprogesterone is a progestational compound that is being used by some hospitals for patients in premature labor, but its use is controversial. Bed rest is occasionally encouraged by some practitioners for patients with a history of premature deliveries. The probability of a successful pregnancy after a cervical cerclage increases from 20% to approximately 80%. It is crucial to eliminate the possibility of preterm labor before placing a cerclage. (*Creasy et al., pp. 603–619*)

51. (E) Production of AFP begins in the yolk sac and then moves to the fetal liver and, to a lesser extent, the fetal gastrointestinal tract. Choices (A) through (D) result in an increased maternal serum AFP (MOM greater than 2.0) because all are open defects of the fetus that result in an increase in amniotic fluid concentrations and then maternal serum concentrations of AFP. Trisomy 21 (Down syndrome) is associated with a decreased MSAFP. In clinical practice, measurement of MSAFP is combined with serum chorionic gonadotropin (hCG) and unconjugated estriol (E3). These three tests are commonly called a triple screen or triple marker screen and together improve the sensitivity over each test alone. Approximately 60% of trisomy 21 fetuses in women under age 35 years, and more than 75% in women over 35 will be detected using a multiple marker screening test. Screening for these defects is most sensitive between 16 and 18 gestational weeks, but the test should be offered to all pregnant women between 15 and 22 gestational weeks. (*Cunningham et al., pp. 979–985*)

52. (E) The combination of aging and diabetes suggests the likelihood of a neurologic defect in the bladder, resulting in overflow incontinence. This occurs when the detrusor muscle becomes hypotonic or atonic. Such women complain of voiding small amounts but still having the feeling of a full bladder. In addition, these women are incontinent of small amounts of urine and are unable to stop the flow. This helps to distinguish those with overflow incontinence from those with GSI; the latter are able to voluntarily increase urethral pressure enough to stop urine flow. Cystitis commonly causes urgency and increased urinary frequency, but not incontinence. Urinalysis and urine culture are not likely to be revealing in this patient, but should be done routinely in all incontinent women. Instillation of methylene blue into the bladder after placement of a vaginal tampon should be done when a vesicovaginal fistula is suspected. This occurs most often following gynecologic surgery and should be suspected in women complaining of constant urine leakage. The Q-tip test is useful to demonstrate posterior urethral rotation found in women with GSI. (*Scott et al., pp. 849–856*)

53. (A) In a patient with GSI, a retropubic approach offers the best long-term cure of the incontinence. The Burch procedure and the Marshall–Marchetti–Krantz procedure are the most common retropubic procedures. With an anterior colporrhaphy, plication sutures are placed at the UVJ in an effort to support and elevate it. Long-term results are not as good as a retropubic urethropexy or a suburethral sling. A suburethral sling procedure is used when urethral closing pressure is low, less than 20 cm H_2O. A needle suspension procedure is most often done when there is associated genital prolapse with potential incontinence. Collagen injections at the UVJ have been attempted to obstruct the urethra partially. Incontinent patients who may benefit the most from collagen injections are those with intrinsic sphincter deficiency and a fixed bladder neck. (*Scott et al., pp. 856–866*)

54. (C) The presence of a dominant mass requires immediate evaluation. While all women with a dominant mass should have a mammogram, this is a screening test. A fine-needle aspiration is a diagnostic tool that will resolve whether the mass is cystic or solid. Any fluid or tissue obtained should be sent for cytologic evaluation to further aid in the diagnosis. If clear or cloudy fluid is aspirated, and the mass disappears, the woman should have a repeat breast examination in 1 month. If the mass remains after aspiration, if the fluid is bloody, or if there is a residual mass on a follow-up visit in 1 month, an open biopsy should be done. A segmental resection is a therapeutic option for a circumscribed carcinoma, but is not an appropriate diagnostic tool. (*Scott et al., pp. 895–898*)

55. (D) Rh immune globulin should always be administered to an Rh-negative pregnant woman who sustains any trauma or has any type of invasive procedure, such as an amniocentesis. Detectable fetomaternal hemorrhage occurs in 6% of women having an amniocentesis and 1% of Rh-negative women will develop Rh isoimmunization after amniocentesis (without Rh immune globulin). The immune globulin reduces the risk of subsequent Rh sensitization during the pregnancy, which could result in severe erythroblastosis fetalis. Although chorionic villus biopsy might be an alternative to amniocentesis, it is done earlier in pregnancy, and occasionally must be followed by an amniocentesis after 14 weeks' gestation because of the possibility that maternal decidua was analyzed. Rubella immunization should be given after delivery to avoid the theoretical risk of a congenital rubella syndrome from the administration of the live vaccine. The presence of hepatitis B surface antibody suggests immunity to hepatitis B but is unrelated to amniocentesis. Intraamniotic bleeding is a complication of amniocentesis but occurs at the time of the procedure. The amniotic fluid will appear bloody. (*Creasy et al., pp. 262–263*)

56. (D) The conceptus is remarkably resistant to the toxic and teratogenic effects of most drugs until about 2 postconceptual weeks (4 postmenstrual weeks). Although certain drugs may be toxic to oocytes, their effect will be to prevent conception or cause an early spontaneous abortion. The developing conceptus is not exposed to maternal toxins or teratogens until after implantation and establishment of a blood supply from mother to fetus. Even after implantation, the fetus is relatively resistant to teratogens for about 1 week. Organogenesis is complete by the end of the first trimester. Congenital abnormalities are, therefore, unlikely in the second and third trimesters. (*Cunningham et al., p. 1007*)

57. (D) From the information in Question 56, it is apparent that the fetus is relatively resistant to teratogenic effects of drugs until about 2 weeks after conception. A recommendation to abort the pregnancy cannot be made on medical probability, although the woman may choose this, because she does not wish to take any chance of having an affected child. Ultrasound is incapable of detecting anomalies until at least 12–14 postmenstrual weeks. The fetal warfarin syndrome does not cause chromosomal abnormalities, and a genetic amniocentesis is not indicated. Vitamin K reverses the anticoagulant effects of coumadin but does not alter the risk that the fetus will develop anomalies. (*Cunningham et al., pp. 1006–1007*)

58. (B) Heparin is the drug of choice for anticoagulation in pregnancy. Little of it crosses the placenta, and it is not associated with congenital birth defects. Experience with low molecular weight heparin in pregnancy is increasing and appears to be safe for mother and fetus. In full therapeutic doses, low molecular weight heparin offers the advantage of less or no monitoring of its anticoagulant effect. Coumadin readily crosses the placenta and is associated with birth defects in 15–25% of fetuses exposed throughout the first trimester. Aspirin is ineffective as an anticoagulant, although the risk of maternal or fetal bleeding (e.g., placental abruption, fetal intracranial bleeding) is increased. There is no clinical experience with TPA in pregnancy. Because pregnancy itself is a thrombogenic condition, anticoagulation throughout pregnancy is indicated. Vena caval filters offer no advantage over heparin and require an invasive procedure. (*Cunningham et al., pp. 1237–1239*)

59. **(C)** The station of the vertex indicates that the fetal head is on the perineum. A cesarean section, either low transverse or classical, is inappropriate unless an operative vaginal delivery is unsuccessful. In women with an anthropoid pelvis, the transverse, interspinous diameter of the bony pelvis is narrow, and the anteroposterior diameter of the pelvis is relatively long. In this circumstance, a forceps rotation should not be done and delivery should be in the occiput posterior. The indication for forceps is maternal exhaustion; women with an anthropoid pelvis usually have a spontaneous vaginal delivery. In women with a gynecoid pelvis, the transverse and anteroposterior diameters are more equal, and rotation of the fetal head to occiput anterior would be an acceptable choice. Soft-tissue resistance to delivery is not great enough that an episiotomy will permit slight expulsive efforts by the mother to deliver the fetal head. (*Cunningham et al., pp. 489–494*)

60. **(B)** Fecundability is the ability to achieve a pregnancy, and the rate per ovulation in couples with no impediment to fertility is approximately 25%. Fecundity is the ability to achieve a live birth within one ovulatory cycle. Fecundity is approximately 15% per cycle in normally fertile couples. Using the 25% fecundability rate, 25 of 100 couples will achieve a pregnancy in the first menstrual cycle of effort. In the second cycle, 25% of the remaining 75 couples will achieve a pregnancy, approximately 19 women. This is a cumulative pregnancy rate of 44%. Twenty-five percent of the remaining 56 women will conceive in the third cycle, approximately 14 women. The cumulative conception rate after three cycles is approximately 58%. However, nearly 50% of all conceptions do not progress to a live birth, ending as a very early unrecognized spontaneous abortion, a recognized first-trimester abortion, a second-trimester loss, or a third-trimester stillbirth. (*Speroff and Fritz, p. 1013*)

61. **(B)** Although messenger RNA for hCG is present in 6- to 8-cell embryos (preimplantation), hCG cannot be detected in the maternal circulation until soon after implantation, approximately 7 days after conception or 7 days before the expected date of menses. Although hCG cannot be detected in maternal blood as early as 4 days after fertilization, maternal serum estradiol and progesterone concentrations in the luteal phase are higher in conception cycles. This is suggestive that the embryo is capable of preimplantation signaling. Clinically, pregnancy should be detected as early as possible because of the increased risk of another tubal pregnancy. If a pregnancy test is not done until 1 week following the missed menses, a transvaginal ultrasound should be done soon thereafter to ascertain if there is an intrauterine gestational sac. The serum hCG concentration must be greater than approximately 1500 mIU/mL for transvaginal ultrasonography to be reliable. Waiting 2 weeks after the expected menses to obtain a pregnancy test is too late—the risk of a ruptured tubal pregnancy and intraperitoneal hemorrhage increases with advancing gestation. (*Speroff and Fritz, pp. 74–78*)

62. **(B)** Cervical cancer is currently the only female reproductive tract cancer staged clinically according to FIGO standards. FIGO also requires that the clinical staging be based on technologies generally available worldwide, including third world countries. For this reason, lymphangiography, angiography, CT or MRI scans, laparoscopy, or hysteroscopy are not permitted to stage cervical cancer. Stage I cancer is confined to the cervix. Stage IA is microscopic cancer without a visible lesion. Stage IB is macroscopic cancer visible to the eye. Stages II–IV have spread beyond the cervix. Because of the presence of abnormal paraaortic lymph nodes and hepatic changes consistent with metastases, she is actually a stage IVB. (*Hoskins et al., pp. 846–849*)

63. **(E)** Although this 46-year-old woman is staged as a IB, she should be treated as a stage IVB because of the findings on CT scan. Methods of staging that are similar allow institutions to compare results of treatment without having to account for different staging procedures and criteria. A simple TAH-BSO is appropriate therapy only for women with carcinoma *in situ* of the cervix (CIN III, stage 0). Women with stage I or IIA may be treated with radical hysterectomy or with radiation therapy. Beyond stage IIA, only radiation therapy is acceptable. A pelvic exenteration is indicated when there is a central recurrence after maximal dose radiation therapy. Platinum-based chemotherapy has been used for women with metastases or recurrence after radiation therapy. It is considered palliative. Recently, several have used chemotherapy as primary therapy for bulk disease. There are no randomized control trials to document that chemotherapy is superior to surgery or radiation. (*Hoskins et al., p. 861*)

64. **(C)** As many as 30% of fetuses exposed to phenytoin had minor craniofacial and digital anomalies. Cleft lip/palate, hypertelorism, broad nasal bridge, and epicanthal folds are the craniofacial anomalies observed. Hypoplasia of the distal phalanges and nails are the digital anomalies. In addition, these infants may have growth and cognitive deficiencies. Trimethadione, another anticonvulsant, causes similar anomalies. Spina bifida occurs in 1–2% of infants whose mothers took valproic acid during pregnancy. (*Cunningham et al., p. 1013; Creasy et al., p. 284; Scott et al., p. 238*)

65. **(B)** Approximately 3% of live born infants have a major congenital anomaly detected at birth. The incidence increases to 6–7% later in childhood. Chromosomal and single-gene defects account for 10–25% of human malformations. Fetal infections (3–5%), maternal disease (4%), and drugs and medications (<1%) account for the remaining recognized causes of human malformations. Sixty-five to 75% of malformations have an unknown or multifactorial etiology. (*Creasy et al., pp. 329–330, 1296*)

66. **(B)** The main mechanism by which hemostasis is achieved following delivery is contraction of the myometrium to compress the uterine vessels that had been supplying the placenta. Lack of effective myometrial contraction (i.e., uterine atony) is the major cause of postpartum hemorrhage. If the uterus is found to be firmly contracted, then other factors, such as cervical or vaginal lacerations or a coagulopathy, must be sought. (*Scott et al., pp. 48–49*)

67. **(A)** Immediate management is bimanual massage and compression of the uterine fundus by placing one fist into the anterior vaginal fornix and the other hand abdominally posterior to the uterus. The uterine massage is often enough to cause myometrial contractions and slowing of the bleeding. Oxytocin or an ergot alkaloid (e.g., methylergonovine) should then be administered if bimanual massage of the uterus is ineffective. Insertion of a gauze pack is never indicated because it is rarely effective. It may actually worsen the bleeding by preventing contraction of the myometrium. Persistent bleeding from the uterus despite these measures may indicate uterine rupture, retained placental fragments, or placenta accreta. If a careful curettage of the uterine lining fails to remove any placental fragments and decrease uterine bleeding, hypogastric artery ligation or a hysterectomy must be considered. (*Scott et al., pp. 48–49*)

68. **(D)** Both the bloody nipple discharge and the microcalcifications are indications for an open breast biopsy. Although there are benign-appearing radiographic calcifications, clusters of calcification are associated with a

25% chance of a cancer. An open biopsy is still preferred in most centers, because a fine-needle biopsy has about a 20% false negative rate. Cytology is a screening tool. In the presence of significant risk factors for cancer, a tissue diagnosis is mandatory. Imaging studies are also screening tools with a false negative and a false positive rate, making such studies inappropriate for diagnosis. (*Scott et al., pp. 893–898*)

69. **(B)** The advantages of a fine-needle aspiration of a breast mass are that it can distinguish between a cystic and solid lesion, and it reduces the number of open breast biopsies when it is positive for cancer. However, a negative needle biopsy is nondiagnostic (and nonreassuring), and an open biopsy is still necessary. A fine-needle biopsy does not differentiate between noninvasive and invasive cancer, nor does it delineate the extent of *in situ* disease. Most breast surgeons will not perform definitive surgery (e.g., mastectomy or lumpectomy with lymph node dissection) without histologic confirmation of cancer: core-needle biopsy, surgical biopsy, or frozen section at the time of lumpectomy or mastectomy. (*Scott et al., pp. 895–896*)

70. **(E)** The factor associated with the greatest lifetime risk for developing breast cancer is age of the woman. Hereditary breast cancers account for 5–10% of all breast cancers and give the woman a relative risk of approximately 2. The relative risk is 4 with two first-degree relatives. Increased lifetime estrogen exposure is a minor risk factor for breast cancer. Obesity, early menarche, late menopause, and low parity are associated with an increased lifetime estrogen exposure and are minor risk factors for breast cancer. Most epidemiologic studies have concluded that menopausal estrogen replacement does not increase the risk of breast cancer. However, several such studies have observed a statistically significant increased relative risk of breast cancer with postmenopausal hormone replacement, usually a relative risk of approximately 1.5. Estrogens are considered promoters of breast cancer rather than inducers or initiators. (*Scott et al., pp. 890–893*)

71. **(D)** Infiltrating ductal carcinoma accounts for approximately 80% of all breast carcinomas. Infiltrating lobular carcinoma accounts for approximately 9%, and the others 5% or less. (*National Comprehensive Cancer Network*)

72. **(E)** In women with a primary tumor of 1 cm or less, the recurrence risk is less than 10%. Women with positive sex-steroid receptors in the tumor also have a better prognosis for several reasons: the tumor tends to be more well differentiated, and 5-year therapy with tamoxifen significantly reduces recurrence. However, the strongest predictor of disease-free survival is axillary lymph nodes negative for metastasis. Survival decreases as the number of positive lymph nodes increases. (*Hoskins et al., pp. 1155–1159*)

73. **(D)** Danazol, in oral doses of 100, 200, or 400 mg daily for 4–6 months, relieves breast pain and reduces nodularity in 90% of women. The beneficial effects often last for several months after discontinuation of the drug. Tamoxifen is a synthetic antiestrogen that competes with estrogen receptors in the breast. Relief of symptoms has been achieved in approximately 70% of women in small studies, and seems to be more effective in women with cyclic rather than continuous pain. Bromocriptine inhibits prolactin secretion, not recognized as a cause of fibrocystic breast disease and mastodynia. Oral progestins (e.g., medroxyprogesterone acetate), depot medroxyprogesterone acetate (Depo-Provera), or OCs may provide symptomatic relief, but symptoms usually return after these are stopped. Hydrochlorothiazide provides unpredictable relief of symptoms. (*Copeland, pp. 1120–1122*)

74. **(D)** This is an autosomal-dominant disorder. Both parents are carriers of the abnormal gene (N), which is on chromosome 17. If each parent is a heterozygote (Nn, where n is the normal gene), 25% of their offspring will have a normal genotype, nn. Fifty percent of their offspring will be affected heterozygotes (Nn), and the remaining 25% will be homozygous affected (NN). If either parent or both are homozygous for the abnormal gene (NN), 100% of the offspring will be affected. As an autosomal disorder, there is no sex predilection; males and females are affected with equal frequency. Prenatal diagnosis is available. (*Creasy et al., p. 260*)

75. **(A)** The normal pH of the vagina is 3.8–4.2. In women with a vaginal discharge, a pH less than 5.0 suggests monilial vaginitis or a physiologic discharge of normal squamous cells desquamated from the vaginal epithelium. A pH greater than 5.0 suggests some type of bacterial infection, such as bacterial vaginosis or trichomonas vaginitis. The other possibility is an atrophic vaginal epithelium. Both chlamydia and gonorrhea infect the cervix and do not change the vaginal pH. (*Scott et al., pp. 585–589*)

76. **(E)** Clue cells are shown in Fig. 2-1. This indicates bacterial vaginosis. Clue cells are vaginal squamous cells with indistinct margins that are studded extensively with coccobacilli. Trichomonas infection is caused by a unicellular protozoon. The organism on wet smear with normal saline is fusiform, slightly larger than white blood cells, and has flagella at one end. The flagella cause the motion on wet smear that is diagnostic. Monilial vaginitis is best demonstrated by placing a small amount of the discharge in 10% potassium hydroxide (KOH) and observing for branching hyphae. *N. gonorrhoeae* and *C. trachomatis* cannot be seen on a wet smear. (*Scott et al., pp. 588–589*)

77. **(C)** The treatment of choice for bacterial vaginosis is metronidazole, also an effective treatment for trichomonas vaginitis. The dose is 375–500 mg orally twice daily for 1 week. A single daily dose of 750 mg was recently approved. Vaginal metronidazole gel or clindamycin cream are also approved forms of treatment. Concurrent therapy of the male partner is controversial. Treatment in pregnancy is recommended, because there is a potential association of bacterial vaginosis and preterm labor and delivery. (*Scott et al., pp. 588–589; Cunningham et al., p. 713*)

78. **(D)** The normal ejaculate volume is 2–5 mL, and the bulk of the ejaculate is from the seminal vesicles. The reduced ejaculate volume may be the result of an incomplete collection or may indicate absence of the seminal vesicles. Fructose is the reducing sugar produced by the seminal vesicles, and its absence establishes a diagnosis of congenital absence of the vasa deferentia and seminal vesicles. This explains the azoospermia (absence of sperm; aspermia is absence of an ejaculate). Men with germ cell aplasia have only Sertoli cells in their seminiferous tubules. Their ejaculate volumes are normal, and fructose is present. Likewise, men with occlusion of the vasa deferentia will be azoospermic but have a normal ejaculate volume containing fructose. Men with 17α-hydroxylase deficiency will have hypertension, be sexually infantile, and have azoospermia, because the enzyme deficiency prevents the secretion of normal amounts of cortisol, androgens, and estrogen, but an increased secretion of mineralocorticoids. Men with Klinefelter syndrome have patent vasa deferentia and seminal vesicles; their ejaculate volumes will be normal and contain fructose. (*Speroff and Fritz, pp. 1143–1146*)

79. **(B)** The WHO suggests a minimal sperm concentration of 20 million/mL for normal conception rates of 15–20% per ovulation. However, sperm motility (percentage and velocity; >50% with forward progression), sperm morphology (30% or more oval forms, using strict criteria), coital frequency, and others must be considered. Stated otherwise, a sperm concentration of 10 million/mL may be associated with normal fertility if the sperm motility and morphology are better than average and coital frequency is three to four times per week. (*Speroff and Fritz, p. 1144*)

80. **(D)** The cycle of spermatogenesis is 73 ± 5 days. This is the time required for maturation of spermatogonia to spermatozoa. The cycle is at different stages along the seminiferous tubules, necessary to ensure the presence of sperm in each ejaculate. Further, spermatozoa require approximately 3 weeks to traverse the ductal system and appear in the ejaculate. Knowing this has important implications, any therapy intended to stimulate spermatogenesis must be continued for at least the duration of one spermatogenic cycle to determine whether there is a beneficial effect. (*Speroff and Fritz, pp. 1135–1139*)

81. **(E)** Painful vaginal bleeding is most likely the result of placental abruption, premature separation of the placenta. Bloody show is a normal sign of impending or early labor. The bleeding is scant and intermingled with clear mucus. Bleeding from a vaginal laceration following coitus is not associated with abdominal pain. A history of coitus followed immediately by bleeding suggests this diagnosis. Bleeding from cervicitis is most often spotting and not associated with abdominal pain. Classically, bleeding with a placenta previa is painless. (*Creasy et al., pp. 371–378*)

82. **(D)** Maternal hypertension is the most common risk factor for a placental abruption. The relative risk is 3.8 for parous women and 1.6 for nulliparous women. In one published report, half of the women with an abruption severe enough to kill the fetus had hypertension, and half of these had evidence of chronic vascular disease. Advanced maternal age without confounding factors such as diabetes or hypertension is not a risk factor for placental abruption. High parity is associated with an increased risk of placental abruption. Vigorous coitus can cause a vaginal laceration, but not abdominal pain. While blunt abdominal trauma may cause a placental abruption, routine forms of exercise are not a risk factor for placental abruption. (*Creasy et al., pp. 371–378*)

83. **(E)** At term, a placental abruption severe enough to cause fetal distress warrants immediate delivery. If the pregnancy is remote from term, temporizing measures may be considered, such as observation. However, delivery should be achieved if the mother becomes hemodynamically unstable. Tocolysis is ineffective in relaxing the uterus and has the added disadvantage of causing vasodilation of an already under-filled vascular system. Amniotomy and Pitocin-induction will not cause delivery rapidly enough to prevent further deterioration of the fetus. Evidence of fetal distress makes continued monitoring unacceptable. (*Creasy et al., pp. 371–378*)

84. **(A)** Cells are most sensitive to radiation during mitosis. For this reason, rapidly dividing cells are the most radiosensitive. Fractionation of radiation doses provides effective tumor treatment without increasing the rate of complications to normal tissues. (*Hoskins et al., pp. 335–336*)

85. **(C)** The most common dose of radiation therapy for invasive cervical cancer is 4500–5000 cGy, or 45–50 Gy. Lower doses tend to result in treatment failures and higher doses are associated with greater complication rates. External beam radiation is combined with vaginal brachytherapy. (*Hoskins et al., pp. 866–870*)

86. **(A)** Each of the choices are potential complications of radiation therapy. Diarrhea and nausea may occur during the course of radiation treatment. The others are postradiation complications that usually do not occur sooner than 6 months after completing radiation. The likelihood of these complications is related to dosage, volume treated, and tissue sensitivity. Diseases that affect circulation (e.g., diabetes mellitus, hypertension) and prior abdominal surgery also increase the risk of complications. (*Scott et al., pp. 933–934*)

87. **(A)** The classic symptom of fibrocystic breast disease is cyclic bilateral breast pain. The pain and associated diffuse breast engorgement is most severe premenstrually. Cystic changes palpated premenstrually typically are smaller postmenstrually. Fibroadenomas are firm, rubbery, freely mobile, solid, and usually solitary masses. Intraductal papilloma does not cause diffuse breast symptoms. Spontaneous and intermittent nipple discharge is the classic sign of an intraductal papilloma. Intraductal carcinoma is more likely if there is a discharge from multiple ducts. Breast cancer should be suspected when a solitary firm nodule does not change throughout the menstrual cycle. A mammogram is helpful, but any suspicious mass should be biopsied. Hyperprolactinemia can cause breast engorgement, but the pain is usually mild, and cystic areas tend not to vary in size. (*Scott et al., p. 898*)

88. (D) Fibrocystic disease includes a variety of histologic findings. Typical is proliferation and hyperplasia of the lobular, ductal, and acinar epithelium. Histologic variants include variable-sized cysts, adenosis, fibrosis, duct ectasia, apocrine metaplasia, and others. Ductal epithelial hyperplasia and apocrine metaplasia with atypia are the findings associated with the greatest risk of subsequent breast cancer. The presence of histologic atypia increases the woman's chance of breast cancer fivefold. (*Scott et al., p. 898*)

89. (E) Breast cancer is rare in women younger than 35 years, and the approximate incidence of breast cancer in pregnancy is 1 in 3000 deliveries. Survival rates from breast cancer in pregnancy are less than in nonpregnant women of comparable age. However, this is due to delayed diagnosis, not a biological effect of pregnancy. Despite the pregnancy, the presence of a dominant mass requires histologic evaluation. Temporizing measures (choices A through D) are inappropriate in the presence of a dominant mass. Imaging studies of the breast during pregnancy are difficult to interpret because of the ductular and glandular hypertrophy of pregnancy. (*Hoskins et al., pp. 515–517*)

90. (E) Breast cancers in young women tend to be aggressive tumors and estrogen receptor negative, both of which worsen the prognosis. For this reason, the cancer should be treated surgically, usually a modified radical mastectomy to minimize the need for adjuvant radiation or chemotherapy with wide local excision or a lumpectomy. There is little convincing evidence that termination of pregnancy improves the prognosis. (*Cunningham et al., pp. 1233–1235; Hoskins et al., pp. 515–517*)

91. (A) In late pregnancy, the large uterus commonly compresses the inferior vena cava and impedes return of blood from the lower extremities to the heart. This may be sufficient to reduce cardiac output. In approximately 10% of women, arterial hypotension occurs, which can result in diminished uteroplacental blood flow and a decreased fetal heart rate. None of the other options occur as a result of this syndrome. Management is to have the woman roll onto her side or lean forward if she is sitting. Both these maneuvers cause the uterus to fall away from the inferior vena cava. (*Cunningham et al., p. 210*)

92. (C) The strict definition of the cardinal movement of labor, called engagement, is given as choice C. Among other things, this means that the presenting part is fixed in the true pelvis and a prolapsed umbilical cord is unlikely to occur. Often, the fetal head is considered to be engaged when the vertex is at 0 station, the level of the ischial spines. Although engagement is conclusive evidence of an adequate pelvic inlet, its absence is not always indicative of pelvic contraction. Nevertheless, the incidence of pelvic contraction is higher in primigravid women whose presenting part is not engaged. (*Cunningham et al., pp. 65–66*)

93. (D) Anti-D immune globulin should be given at the time of any vaginal bleeding, trauma, or invasive procedure (e.g., amniocentesis) during pregnancy. Although maternal isoimmunization usually occurs as a result of fetomaternal transfusion at the time of delivery, a small percentage of women become isoimmunized during pregnancy. Anti-D immune globulin is routinely given to unsensitized Rh negative women at 28 weeks' gestation to reduce this risk. Anti-D immune globulin must also be administered within 72 h after the birth of an Rh-positive infant. Administration at 40 weeks' gestation before the onset of labor is unnecessary if the infant is Rh negative and may be ineffective if the infant is Rh positive and there is a significant fetomaternal transfusion. (*Cunningham et al., pp. 986–987*)

94. (B) One vial of Rh immunoglobulin will prevent Rh isoimmunization if the amount of fetal whole blood entering the maternal circulation is 30 mL or less. If the woman has a condition where a greater amount of fetal blood may enter the maternal circulation, the amount of fetal blood should be estimated by submitting a maternal blood sample for a Kleihauer-Betke test. The dose of Rh immunoglobulin is then based on the results of this test. (*Scott et al., pp. 317–319*)

95. **(D)** In a previously healthy woman with an uncomplicated pregnancy, the appearance of hypertension and proteinuria in the third trimester is preeclampsia. The other disorders usually are present throughout the pregnancy, may develop earlier than the third trimester, and may present with hypertension or proteinuria, but not necessarily both. (*Cunningham et al., pp. 569–570*)

96. **(E)** The treatment of preeclampsia with a certain term pregnancy (>37 weeks' gestation) is delivery of the infant. Induction of labor with oxytocin (Pitocin) is the preferred method of delivery, provided the preeclampsia is not severe, the HELLP syndrome (hemolysis, elevated liver enzymes, low platelets) does not develop, or fetal distress does not occur. A cesarean section should be performed if any of these develop, and vaginal delivery is not imminent. (*Cunningham et al., pp. 591–595*)

97. **(C)** The only effect of magnesium sulfate is to reduce the risk of seizures with eclampsia. Although magnesium sulfate is commonly used as a tocolytic in idiopathic preterm labor, this is not its purpose in pregnant women with preeclampsia. Blood pressure is not reduced by magnesium sulfate; intravenous hydralazine or labetalol are safe antihypertensive agents when given in small, intermittent doses for diastolic blood pressures greater than 105–110 torr. Uteroplacental blood flow, decrease in preeclampsia, is unaffected by magnesium sulfate. Magnesium sulfate should be continued for 24 h after delivery because of the continued risk of eclamptic seizures. (*Cunningham et al., pp. 598–600*)

98. **(E)** A placenta accreta must be suspected if the placenta does not separate spontaneously by 30 min after delivery of the infant, especially if a plane of dissection cannot be identified with attempts to remove the placenta manually. The examination immediately after birth eliminates the possibility of a cervical laceration, although the lower genital tract should be reinspected to be certain that a laceration was not overlooked. With uterine atony, the fundus is boggy and larger than expected, unlike the firm uterus found in this woman. A Couvelaire uterus occurs as a complication of placental abruption with concealed hemorrhage. Blood intravasates between myometrial fibers and diminishes the capacity of the myometrium to contract. Although acute blood loss may lead to thrombocytopenia, the bleeding is the cause rather than the consequence of the low platelet count. (*Cunningham et al., pp. 640–643*)

99. **(D)** Hypogastric artery ligation, angiographically directed arterial embolization, and hysterectomy are acceptable treatment options. The choice depends on the experience of the obstetrician, the rapid availability of an interventional radiology team, and the hemodynamic status of the patient. If a hypogastric artery ligation is unsuccessful, then a hysterectomy is necessary. Blood should be transfused to maintain hemodynamic stability but is never the sole treatment with placenta accreta. In one study, one-fourth of the women died who had a uterine pack inserted after manual removal of the placenta. This was four times higher than in those who had an immediate hysterectomy. Administration of ergot alkaloids is a treatment option only when postpartum hemorrhage is attributable to uterine atony. (*Cunningham et al., p. 642*)

100. **(C)** Bilateral hypogastric artery ligation converts the arterial system into a venous system; thereby, reducing the pulse pressure by as much as 85%. Subsequent menstrual function and fertility are normal, in part because of the rich collateral circulation to the uterus. The procedure is successful in approximately 50% of cases. The procedure is not technically easy to perform, and an intimate knowledge of the local anatomy is essential to prevent injury to the hypogastric vein or ureter. (*Creasy et al., pp. 942–943*)

101. **(E)** Two clues to the diagnosis of detrusor dyssynergia are loss of urine in the recumbent position and inability to stop the urine loss once the stream has begun. Generally, large

volumes of urine are lost because of the inability to stop the flow of urine. With GSI, urine is lost only in the upright position when intraabdominal and intravesical pressure exceed urethral closing pressure, such as with coughing. Women with GSI are able to stop the flow of urine voluntarily and, therefore, the volume of urine lost is small. With GSI, urine loss with coughing is immediate. Women with a vesicovaginal or urethrovaginal fistula will complain of a watery vaginal discharge. Women with an atonic bladder typically void small amounts and complain that the bladder still feels full (which it is). This is a disorder seen in women with neurologic dysfunction of the bladder, such as multiple sclerosis and diabetic neuropathy. (*Scott et al., pp. 849–856*)

102. (D) Although a urine culture is a standard part of the evaluation of women with loss of urine, this woman's history is not consistent with acute cystitis. A Q-tip test is done to assess the angle the urethra makes with the horizontal in the relaxed and voiding circumstances. Though intended to differentiate GSI from other causes of incontinence, it has not proved to be sufficiently sensitive to make this distinction reliably. Urethroscopy is appropriate if a urethrovaginal fistula or urethral diverticulum is suspected. Urethrocystometry is one name for a test that measures the pressure-volume relationship in the bladder. It should be done in most women with incontinence as the most sensitive test to distinguish the various causes of incontinence. An IVP is of little value in determining the cause of incontinence. (*Scott et al., pp. 849–856*)

103. (C) Antibiotics are useful only when there is evidence of cystitis. SSRIs are antidepressants that have not been shown to improve incontinence with detrusor dyssynergia. Surgery is of no value and may actually worsen incontinence in women with detrusor dyssynergia. Bladder retraining, in which the patient embarks on a programmed progressive lengthening of the interval of voiding, forms the basis of therapy. While such retraining is occurring, the use of anticholinergic drugs, such as oxybutynin chloride (Ditropan), propantheline (Pro-Banthine), or flavoxate (Urispas), seems to improve the results over use of either alone. (*Scott et al., pp. 859–860*)

104. (D) The cyclic pain with bulging between normal labia is the classic history for an imperforate hymen. Ninety-five percent of women with vaginal agenesis also have agenesis or hypoplasia of the uterus and do not menstruate. The cyclic pain suggests that this girl has a uterus and is menstruating back through her fallopian tubes into her abdominal cavity. The presence of a uterus and normal pubic hair excludes androgen insensitivity. Normal appearing labia exclude the possibility of labial adhesions, an uncommon disorder that almost always occurs in prepubertal girls before estrogen production begins. Transverse vaginal septa are usually found higher in the vagina; bulging and discoloration of the hymen would not be found. (*Copeland, pp. 204–206*)

105. (C) The absence of a vaginal orifice effectively eliminates pregnancy as a diagnosis, although a urine pregnancy test in any amenorrheic women is reasonable. Both uterine fibroids and endometrial cancer are exceedingly rare in young women. Adenomyosis (endometriosis involving the myometrium) and endometriosis of other pelvic structures are later sequelae of imperforate hymen because of the retrograde menstruation. Hematometra is the most likely explanation. This is a condition whereby the endometrial cavity becomes distended with menstrual blood in any woman with obstruction to menstrual outflow. (*Copeland, pp. 204–206*)

106. (D) A hymenotomy is done by making three or four stellate incisions in the hymen and using fine suture only to secure hemostasis. This should be done once the diagnosis of imperforate hymen is made because endometriosis is a complication of retrograde menstruation. A McIndoe vaginoplasty is done when the diagnosis is vaginal agenesis, and the uterus is nonfunctioning or absent. After creating a space between the urethra and bladder anteriorly and the rectum posteriorly, a split-thickness skin graft from the buttocks is placed over a mold and inserted into this space. Within 5–7 days, the skin graft adheres to the walls of the created space. It is difficult to impossible to perform a McIndoe procedure and establish a permanently patent connection to a functioning uterus. For this reason, a hysterectomy is usually done in those women with vaginal agenesis who have a functioning uterus. The diagnosis in this girl is obvious enough that a laparoscopy adds nothing to the management. Girls with an imperforate hymen have a normal upper genital tract, normal ovaries, and a 46,XX karyotype. Thus, there is no indication for a gonadectomy. Urinary tract anomalies occur in as many as 30% of women with Müllerian duct anomalies (e.g., Müllerian agenesis, septate uterus, bicornuate uterus) and less often in women with isolated vaginal anomalies. (*Copeland, pp. 204–206; Speroff et al., pp. 420–421*)

107. **(D)** Painless vaginal bleeding in the third trimester is most often due to a placenta previa. The diagnosis is easily confirmed by abdominal ultrasound. No vaginal/cervical examination or vaginal ultrasound should be done because these may damage the placenta and cause further bleeding and fetal compromise. Delivery is by cesarean section. (*Cunningham et al., pp. 619–663*)

108. **(C)** Light vaginal bleeding following sexual intercourse is likely of cervical origin because of the increased blood flow to the pelvic organs in pregnancy and eversion of the endocervix that occurs as a result of the increased estrogen production. The absence of abdominal pain and tenderness, the appropriate size of the uterus and the spotting rather than overt bleeding tend to exclude threatened abortion as the cause of this woman's bleeding. (*Scott et al., pp. 643–648*)

109. **(B)** Gestational trophoblastic disease is more common in women at the extremes of reproductive age. Uterine size larger than her gestational age calculated from her last menses, the absence of fetal heart tones, and the absence of a fetus by ultrasound confirm the diagnosis. Treatment is evacuation of the uterus. (*Cunningham et al., pp. 619–663*)

110. **(E)** The features that make placental abruption the most likely diagnosis are the amount of bleeding, chronic hypertension, and an excessively firm (even titanic) uterus that is tender to palpation. Women with a placental abruption may have no bleeding if placental separation occurs only in the center of the placenta. The other signs of pain and tenderness will be present. (*Cunningham et al., pp. 619–663*)

111. **(J)** The use of forceps and the presence of a firm, nontender uterus of appropriate size suggest vaginal laceration as the cause of postpartum bleeding. The diagnosis is confirmed by a speculum examination. A cervical laceration should also be considered and the cervix carefully inspected at the time of the speculum examination. (*Cunningham et al., pp. 619–663*)

112. **(K)** Vaginal spotting accompanied by pelvic discomfort in a woman with a prior sexually transmitted infection suggest the diagnosis of an ectopic (tubal) pregnancy. Serum hCG concentrations should increase by at least 67% in 2 days during the first 6–8 weeks of pregnancy. The subnormal increase in this woman's serum hCG concentrations increases the probability of an ectopic pregnancy. However, approximately 15% of women with a normal intrauterine pregnancy will have a subnormal rise in hCG concentrations. Also, approximately 15% of women with an ectopic pregnancy will have a 48-h rise in serum hCG concentrations greater than 67%. At hCG concentrations over 5000 mIU/mL, the absence of an intrauterine pregnancy by transvaginal ultrasound provides additional evidence for the diagnosis of an ectopic pregnancy. (*Scott et al., pp. 89–103*)

113. **(F)** The clinical features that make uterine rupture the most likely diagnosis are profuse bleeding coincident with cessation of uterine contractions and labor in a woman with a prior classical cesarean section (vertical incision in the uterine fundus). Uterine rupture is uncommon in women with a prior low transverse cesarean section and rare in women with no scar on her uterus. The standard of care is that all women with a previous classical cesarean section be delivered by repeat cesarean section at term before the onset of labor. (*Cunningham et al., pp. 646–652*)

114. **(G)** Placenta accrete is suggested by the difficulty with manual removal of the placenta in a woman with a prior cesarean section. Placenta accrete is also more common over any previous uterine incision, such as a myomectomy. Placenta accrete is also more common in women with placenta previa and there is greater than an eightfold increase in women with an AFP higher than 2.5 MOM. The safest and most appropriate treatment is a hysterectomy. (*Cunningham et al., pp. 640–642*)

115. **(I)** Prolonged labor with delivery of a macrosomic fetus (greater than 4000 g) in a highly parous woman are the risk factors for uterine atony. The diagnosis is confirmed by a boggy, noncontracted uterus that is larger than expected after a normal delivery. Treatment is a combination of manual massage of the uterus, oxytocin, blood transfusion to maintain hemodynamic stability, and careful inspection of the vagina, cervix, and uterus to exclude a vaginal or cervical laceration or retained placental fragments. Ergot derivatives or prostaglandins should be administered if the above measures fail to cause the myometrium to contract. Uterine artery embolization is an unproven therapy. A hysterectomy is necessary if all measures fail to stop the postpartum hemorrhage. (*Cunningham et al., pp. 619–663*)

REFERENCES

ACOG Educational Bulletin. *Sexual Assault*. Number 242, November 1997.

ACOG Practice Bulletin. *Management of Herpes in Pregnancy*. Number 8, October 1999.

Copeland LJ. *Textbook of Gynecology*, 2nd ed. Philadelphia, PA: W.B. Saunders, 2000.

Creasy RK, Resnik R, Iams JD. *Maternal–Fetal Medicine: Principles and Practice*, 5th ed. Philadelphia, PA: W.B. Saunders, 2004.

Cunningham FG, Gant NF, Leveno KJ, et al. *Williams Obstetrics*, 21st ed. New York, NY: McGraw Hill, 2001.

DiSaia PJ, Creasman WT. *Clinical Gynecologic Oncology*, 5th ed. St. Louis, MO: Mosby, 1997.

Hoskins WJ, Perez CA, Young RC. *Principles and Practice of Gynecologic Oncology*, 3rd ed. Philadelphia, PA: Lippincott Williams & Wilkins, 2000.

McGuire H, Hawton K. Cochrane Database of Systematic Reviews. 2004;3:1–24.

Center for Disease Control and Prevention. MMWR Morbidity and Mortality Weekly Report. *Recommendations and Reports. Sexually Transmitted Diseases Guidelines*, Vol. 51, No. RR-6. May 10, 2002.

National Comprehensive Cancer Network. *Breast Cancer Treatment Guidelines.* Version 3, 2003. Updated recommendations for adjuvant hormonal therapy (BINV-D). Available at http://www. cancer. org/downloads/CRI/NCCN_Breast_Cancer_ 2002.pdf

Scott JR, Gibbs RS, Karlan BY, Haney AF (eds.). *Danforth's Obstetrics and Gynecology*, 9th ed. Philadelphia, PA: Lippincott Williams & Wilkins, 2003.

Speroff L, Fritz MA. *Clinical Gynecologic Endocrinology and Infertility*, 7th ed. Philadelphia, PA: Lippincott Williams & Wilkins, 2005.

Yen SSC, Jaffe RB, Barbieri RL. *Reproductive Endocrinology: Physiology, Pathophysiology and Clinical Management*, 4th ed. Philadelphia, PA: W.B. Saunders, 1999.

CHAPTER 3

Pediatrics

Rainer G. Gedeit, MD

Questions

DIRECTIONS (Questions 1 through 108): Each of the numbered items or incomplete statements in this section is followed by answers or completions of the statement. Select the ONE lettered answer or completion that is BEST in each case.

1. A 2-year-old child was recently adopted from India. She appears to be healthy, and there are no abnormal symptoms. Her weight and height are at 25th percentile for age. Her examination is normal. On screening, you find a positive TB skin test using purified protein derivative (PPD) with 20-mm induration. She has a history of receiving a BCG vaccination at birth. Your management plan is to

(A) obtain a chest x-ray and treat only if this is abnormal
(B) obtain a chest x-ray and initiate prophylactic treatment with isoniazid (INH)
(C) repeat the test in 3–6 months
(D) attribute the positive PPD to the BCG vaccination and do serial yearly x-rays
(E) obtain sputum cultures

2. A baby is born to a mother who is positive for hepatitis B surface antigen (HBsAg). Your plan is to

(A) give the infant a hepatitis B immunization
(B) give the infant hepatitis B immune globulin (HBIG)
(C) give the infant a hepatitis B immunization and HBIG
(D) obtain liver function tests and hepatitis serology of the infant
(E) give the HBIG only if the child is positive for HBsAg

3. In an adolescent presenting with pityriasis rosea, which of the following would be an appropriate blood test to order?

(A) Venereal Disease Research Laboratory (VDRL)
(B) complete blood count (CBC)
(C) hepatitis A immunoglobulin M (IgM)
(D) fluorescent antinuclear antibody (FANA)
(E) glucose

4. A parent brings in a 5-year-old boy being treated for acute lymphocytic leukemia (ALL). He states a friend who is staying with them at their home has just come down with chicken pox. Your patient has not had chicken pox or received immunization with varicella vaccine. What is the appropriate treatment?

(A) acyclovir given IV
(B) varicella vaccine
(C) varicella immune globulin (VZIG)
(D) varicella vaccine and VZIG
(E) acyclovir given IV for 7 days, varicella vaccine, and VZIG

5. A young mother claims that her 4-week-old child sleeps best on his stomach. You tell her that the safest sleep position for infants is which of the following?

(A) on the back
(B) on the stomach
(C) on the side
(D) on the back with the head elevated by a pillow
(E) in the parents' bed

6. You receive a call from a parent who says they have just received a letter from their daycare center that an employee has hepatitis A. Which of the following is the best treatment plan?

(A) Obtain hepatitis A serology and give hepatitis A immune globulin.
(B) Treat with hepatitis A immune globulin.
(C) Obtain hepatitis A serology and give hepatitis A vaccine.
(D) Give hepatitis A vaccine.
(E) No treatment is needed.

7. A 5-year-old child was hit in the right eye by a toy. He is rubbing at his eye, which is watering profusely. There is a small abrasion at the corner of the eye. He is mildly photophobic, but his pupils are equal, symmetric, and reactive to light and accommodation. His vision is normal. Which of the following is the most appropriate next step in the management of this patient?

(A) Perform a fluorescein dye stain of the cornea to determine if there is a corneal abrasion.
(B) Refer him immediately to an ophthalmologist.
(C) Irrigate the eye with sterile normal saline.
(D) Discharge him to home with antibiotic eye ointment.
(E) Apply a patch to the eye and follow up in a week.

8. A 9-month-old male is in for a well-child checkup. He is greater than 90th percentile for height, and he weighs 25 lb. He no longer fits in his infant car seat, which is only recommended for use by children under 20 lb. Which of the following is the safest car seat option for him?

(A) to remain in the rear-facing infant seat until he is 1 year old, in the rear seat of the car
(B) turn the infant seat to face forward, in the rear seat of the car
(C) a rear-facing car seat suitable for a larger child (20–40 lb), in the rear seat of the car
(D) a forward-facing car seat suitable for a larger child (20–40 lb), in the rear seat of the car
(E) a forward-facing car seat suitable for a larger child (20–40 lb), in the front seat of the car

9. A 2-month-old infant is brought to the emergency department with irritability and lethargy. The parents state that he was well until he rolled off the couch onto the floor yesterday. On examination, he is inconsolable and afebrile. The fontanels are full and tense. He has a generalized tonic-clonic seizure. Which of the following is the most important initial diagnostic study to order?

(A) serum calcium, phosphorus, and magnesium levels
(B) analysis of cerebrospinal fluid (CSF)
(C) cranial computed tomography (CT) scan
(D) serum ammonia level
(E) serum acetaminophen level

10. A 7-year-old girl presents with hives, which developed after a bee sting. She has no other symptoms. The hives resolve with diphenhydramine. Which of the following is the most appropriate management?

(A) Write a prescription for diphenhydramine in case she is bitten again.
(B) Provide an Epi-pen Jr (epinephrine auto injector) to be carried at all times, as well as a prescription for diphenhydramine.
(C) Admit to the hospital for observation for delayed hypersensitivity symptoms.

(D) Refer her to an allergist for desensitization.
(E) Order a skin-prick test with hymenoptera venom.

11. A 2-year-old boy has had a purulent drainage from the right nostril for a week. He is afebrile and has had no associated symptoms, such as cough. Which of the following is the most likely diagnosis?

(A) sinusitis
(B) nasal polyps
(C) an upper respiratory infection
(D) a foreign body in the right nostril
(E) allergic rhinitis

Questions 12 and 13

12. A 5-year-old boy has a history of bed-wetting about four to five times a week. He has recently begun to attend kindergarten. He was toilet trained (dry during the day) by age 3 but has never been consistently dry at night. He denies any dysuria or frequency. There is no history of increased thirst or frequent urination. The urinalysis is negative for blood, protein, glucose, or ketones; there are no white cells or bacteria; the specific gravity is 1.020. Which of the following is the most likely diagnosis?

(A) a urinary tract infection
(B) primary nocturnal enuresis
(C) secondary enuresis caused by stress of the new school
(D) diabetes mellitus
(E) diabetes insipidus

13. The parents request some treatment for this condition. Which of the following is the most appropriate treatment for a child of this age?

(A) bladder stretching exercises
(B) intranasal DDAVP (desmopressin acetate)
(C) imipramine
(D) conditioning therapy with a bed-wetting alarm
(E) reassurance of the parents and restriction of fluids before bedtime

14. A 14-year-old boy complains of breast enlargement on the left side. He denies pain, discharge, or any drug use. He is on no medications and is otherwise healthy. On physical examination, his sexual maturity rating (Tanner) is stage II for both genitalia and pubic hair growth. Initial management should include which of the following?

(A) magnetic resonance imaging of the head
(B) urine drug screen for marijuana
(C) chromosome analysis
(D) reassurance that this is a normal condition
(E) ultrasound imaging of the abdomen and testes

15. A mother brings in her 3-year-old girl because she felt a smooth mass on the left side of her belly when she was giving her a bath. Which of the following is the most likely diagnosis?

(A) Wilms' tumor
(B) neuroblastoma
(C) acute lymphoblastic leukemia
(D) Hodgkin disease
(E) hepatoblastoma

Questions 16 through 19

An 11-month-old girl presents to your office with a fever of 39°C she has had for 2 days. She has also vomited frequently and had decreased fluid intake. She looked tired and ill but on examination, had no apparent source of infection. She appeared to be 5–10% dehydrated.

16. You decide to obtain a urine specimen for analysis and culture. Which of the following is the best method?

(A) Collect a midstream "clean catch" specimen.
(B) Collect a catheterized specimen.
(C) Place an adhesive bag to collect urine.
(D) Obtain urine from a diaper.
(E) Collect urine after she urinates in a potty chair.

17. Her urinalysis shows a urine specific gravity of 1.030, trace blood, and protein. Nitrite and leukocyte esterase are both positive. Microscopic examination of unspun urine shows >100 white blood cells (WBCs) and 0–5 red blood cells (RBCs)/high-power field, as well as many bacteria. A urine culture is sent. Which of the following is the most appropriate management plan?

(A) Treat only if the culture is positive.
(B) Admit for intravenous (IV) hydration and IV antibiotics.
(C) Treat with intramuscular ceftriaxone and have her follow-up in the office the following day.
(D) Treat with trimethoprim-sulfamethoxazole, and have her follow-up in the office the following day.
(E) Prescribe amoxicillin and start oral hydration.

18. Her urine culture is positive at 24 h. Which of the following is the most likely organism?

(A) *Klebsiella*
(B) *Escherichia coli*
(C) *Staphylococcus saprophyticus*
(D) *Proteus*
(E) *Enterococcus*

19. After the infection has been treated, which one of the following tests should be considered?

(A) no tests are needed
(B) renal ultrasound
(C) voiding cystourethrogram (VCUG)
(D) renal ultrasound and a VCUG
(E) radionucleotide renal scan

20. A 3-month-old infant is brought to your office in the winter with a history of 1 day of vomiting, followed by 3 days of diarrhea. She has had six to eight stools per day, which are loose and foul smelling. On examination, she looks well. Which of the following viruses is the most likely cause of her illness?

(A) adenovirus
(B) enterovirus
(C) human herpesvirus, type 6
(D) respiratory syncytial virus
(E) rotavirus

Questions 21 and 22

21. A 10-year-old boy comes to your office in the winter with a sore throat he has had for 2 days. In addition, he has had fever, headache, and abdominal pain. He does not have any allergies to medications. On examination, he has a temperature of 38.6°C, an erythematous pharynx, and tender cervical adenopathy. Which of the following would be the most appropriate antimicrobial agent?

(A) erythromycin
(B) penicillin
(C) trimethoprim-sulfamethoxazole
(D) azithromycin
(E) cefaclor

22. The same child returns to your office the next day. He has taken the medication you prescribed. He is feeling a little better. His fever has resolved, but he has developed a rash. His examination is unchanged, except that he is afebrile and has a fine, papular rash over his body, which is accentuated in his axilla and groin. Which of the following is the most likely cause of his rash?

(A) allergic reaction to the antibiotic
(B) rash from the antibiotic seen in patients with mononucleosis
(C) scarlet fever
(D) serum sickness
(E) viral exanthem typical of enterovirus

Questions 23 and 24

An 8-year-old girl presents for a checkup. She is new to your practice. The mother states that she has always been small for her age; otherwise, she has been well. She is short and has a height age of 4 years, 4 months. You note some abnormalities in her general appearance (Fig. 3-1).

23. Which of the following is the most likely diagnosis?

(A) Marfan syndrome
(B) Noonan syndrome
(C) trisomy 21
(D) Turner syndrome
(E) Williams syndrome

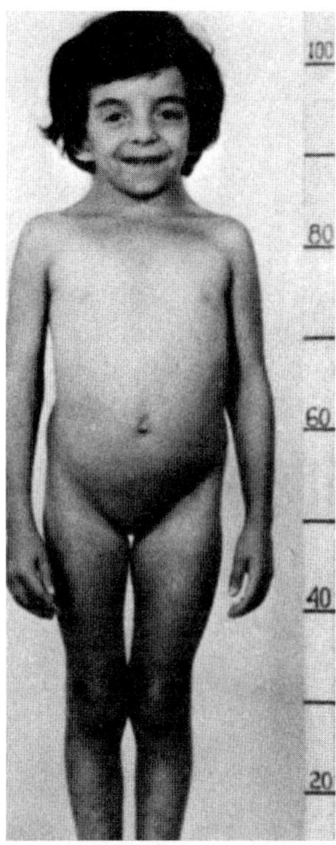

FIG. 3-1 *(From Grumbach, Barr. Recent Prog Horm Res 14:255, 1958.)*

24. As you continue your physical examination, you remember that congenital heart disease is common in this particular syndrome. Which of the following is the most likely congenital heart defect in patients with this syndrome?

(A) supravalvular aortic stenosis
(B) atrioventricular (AV) canal defects
(C) coarctation of the aorta
(D) pulmonary valvular stenosis
(E) mitral valve prolapse

Questions 25 and 26

A 12-year-old boy comes to the clinic for a sports physical. He is new to your practice. He comes with his foster mother, who states that he was recently placed in her care because of his mother's problems with drug abuse. Although a complete medical history is not available, she knows that he has not received regular care. He does not have any chronic medical problems. She also knows that his father died of heart disease when he was 35. On physical examination, the boy's height is greater than the 95th percentile. His arm span exceeds his height.

25. Which of the following is the most likely cause of his tall stature?

(A) Ehlers–Danlos syndrome
(B) Kleinfelter syndrome
(C) Marfan syndrome
(D) Noonan syndrome
(E) Williams syndrome

26. As you continue your physical examination, you remember that congenital heart disease is common in this particular syndrome. Which of the following is the most likely congenital heart defect in patients with this syndrome?

(A) supravalvular aortic stenosis
(B) AV canal defects
(C) coarctation of the aorta
(D) pulmonary valvular stenosis
(E) mitral valve prolapse

27. A 17-year-old girl comes to the clinic with several weeks of joint pain and rash. The joint pain is most prominent in the hands. She states that the pain is most severe in the morning and tends to improve over the day. She has noted some swelling of her fingers. She has also had a rash on her face that becomes more prominent when she is outdoors. She states that sunlight tends to bother her eyes. On further questioning, she states that she has not felt well for several months. She has had intermittent fever, has been more tired than usual, and has lost weight although she has not been restricting her diet. On physical examination, she looks tired. She has lost 5 lb since her last visit 1 year ago. She has an erythematous rash on her cheeks. She has several shallow ulcers in her mouth. She has fusiform swelling of her fingers and pain with movement of her fingers. Which of the following is the most likely diagnosis?

(A) systemic lupus erythematosus (SLE)
(B) dermatomyositis
(C) juvenile rheumatoid arthritis
(D) rheumatic fever
(E) Lyme disease

28. A 2-year-old girl has severe dental caries of the upper and lower incisors. Her teeth are brushed twice daily with a small amount of fluoride-containing toothpaste. What is the feeding practice most likely to result in this pattern of dental caries?

(A) drinking juice from a cup at snack time
(B) drinking juice from a bottle at snack time
(C) drinking milk from a bottle at meal time
(D) prolonged breast-feeding beyond the first year
(E) drinking a bottle of juice in bed

29. An 8-year-old Black boy is brought in for evaluation of a mass on the scalp. On examination, he is afebrile and nontoxic. There is a boggy mass on his scalp with alopecia. His posterior cervical lymph nodes are enlarged but nontender. Which of the following is the most appropriate treatment?

(A) incision and drainage
(B) oral amoxicillin
(C) IV naficillin
(D) selenium sulfide shampoo twice a week
(E) oral griseofulvin and selenium sulfide shampoo twice weekly

30. A 4-year-old child presents to your office in July with a history of a low-grade fever (38.1°C) and "sores" in his mouth for 2 days. He has been refusing to eat but has been drinking an adequate amount of liquids. On examination, he is afebrile and seems well hydrated. He has ulcers on his tongue and posterior pharynx, which are 4 mm in diameter. You also note a few vesicles on his hands and feet, which are 3–4 mm in size and mildly tender. Which of the following is the most likely diagnosis?

(A) herpes simplex virus (HSV)
(B) coxsackie virus
(C) aphthous ulcers
(D) Behçet syndrome
(E) traumatic ulcers

31. A 10-year-old boy comes to the office with fever and chills for 5 days and myalgia. He has recently returned from a 2-week vacation to New England with his family. On physical examination he has mild splenomegaly. Which of the following is the most likely cause of his symptoms?

(A) Kawasaki disease
(B) pneumococcus
(C) babesiosis
(D) leptospirosis
(E) psittacosis

32. A 6-year-old girl has a low-grade fever, headache, and nasal congestion. She has a flushed face and has developed a lacy reticular rash on the trunk and extensor surface of her arms and legs. Palms and soles are spared. Her mother has been ill with a low-grade fever and some joint stiffness and pain. Which of the following is the most likely diagnosis?

(A) rubella
(B) measles

(C) scarlet fever
(D) roseola infantum
(E) erythema infectiosum (fifth disease)

33. A 3-year-old boy has had fever for 4 days. On physical examination he has bilateral cervical lymphadenopathy, injected pharynx, and dry cracked lips. A throat swab is done and the rapid strep test is negative. The child is sent home and advised to follow-up if symptoms worsen. The child is brought back 2 days later with all previous findings including a maculopapular rash, swollen hands, and conjunctivitis. Which of the following is the most likely diagnosis?

(A) Scarlett fever
(B) Kawasaki disease
(C) toxic shock syndrome
(D) infectious mononucleosis
(E) erythema infectiosum

34. A 5-year-old febrile child presents with swelling of the right eyelid. Proptosis and limitation of ocular movements is noted. Which of the following is the most likely diagnosis?

(A) retinoblastoma
(B) orbital cellulitis
(C) periorbital cellulitis
(D) neuroblastoma
(E) hyphema

35. A 1-year-old Black infant is in for well-child care. He is primarily breast-fed. His parents do not give him much solid food because he has no teeth. He receives no medications or supplements. His parents are concerned about his bowed legs. On examination, you note some other bony abnormalities including frontal bossing, enlargement of the costochondral junctions, a protuberant sternum (pigeon chest), and severe bowing of the legs. You obtain x-rays to confirm your clinical diagnosis and also note a healing fracture of the left femur. Which of the following is the most likely diagnosis?

(A) osteogenesis imperfecta
(B) scurvy
(C) congenital syphilis
(D) rickets
(E) chondrodystrophy

36. A 14-year-old boy presents with sudden onset of pain and swelling of his right testicle. There was no history of trauma, he is not sexually active, and denies any history of penile discharge. On examination, the scrotum is swollen and tender. The cremasteric reflex is absent. A testicular flow scan shows a "cold spot" or absent flow to the affected side. Which of the following is the most likely cause?

(A) inguinal hernia
(B) hydrocele
(C) epididymitis
(D) testicular torsion
(E) torsion of the appendix testis

37. Otitis media occurring during the first 8 weeks of life deserves special consideration, because the bacteria responsible for infections during this time may be different from those that affect older infants and children. Which of the following organisms is the most likely to cause otitis media in these infants?

(A) *Chlamydia trachomatis*
(B) *Escherichia coli*
(C) *Neisseria gonorrhoeae*
(D) *Treponema pallidum*
(E) *Toxoplasma gondii*

38. Among the conditions that cause edema of the eyelids is orbital cellulitis. This is a serious infection that must be recognized early and treated aggressively if complications are to be avoided. Which of the following features is useful in differentiating orbital cellulitis from periorbital (preseptal) cellulitis?

(A) proptosis
(B) elevated WBC count
(C) fever
(D) lid swelling
(E) conjunctival inflammation

39. A 6-month-old infant is diagnosed with her first episode of otitis media. She does not have any allergies to medications. Which of the following medications would be the recommended initial therapy for this infant?

(A) amoxicillin
(B) amoxicillin–clavulanic acid
(C) cephalexin
(D) ceftriaxone
(E) erythromycin

40. A 5-year-old pedestrian is hit by a car in a mall parking lot and he is brought to the emergency department. There was loss of consciousness for less than 1 min. On evaluation, the child has no neurologic deficits and a CT scan of the head reveals no intracranial abnormalities and no obvious skull fractures. The parents want to know what possible long-term problems there might be. You remember that problems after head trauma may include the development of seizures and that the risk of developing posttraumatic epilepsy is increased by one of the following?

(A) a brief loss of consciousness
(B) an acute intracranial hemorrhage
(C) retrograde amnesia
(D) posttraumatic vomiting
(E) a small linear skull fracture

41. A 4-year-old previously healthy but unimmunized boy presents with sudden onset of high fever, inspiratory stridor, and refusal to drink. Of the following causes of inspiratory stridor, which best fits this clinical scenario?

(A) epiglottitis
(B) vascular ring
(C) croup
(D) foreign body aspiration
(E) laryngeal tumor

Questions 42 and 43

A 15-month-old Black male, who is otherwise healthy, is found to have a hemoglobin level of 8 g/dL on routine screening. The mean corpuscular volume (MCV) is decreased. His lead screen is within normal limits. You obtain a diet history, which reveals that he drinks about 30–40 oz of whole cow's milk a day. He eats no meat and some fruits and vegetables.

42. Which of the following is the most likely cause?

(A) sickle cell anemia
(B) thalassemia major
(C) lead poisoning
(D) iron-deficiency anemia
(E) anemia of chronic disease

43. The most effective next step in management would be to obtain which of the following?

(A) iron studies—serum iron, total iron binding capacity, ferritin
(B) reticulocyte count
(C) hemoglobin electrophoresis
(D) bone marrow aspirate
(E) a repeat hemoglobin in 1 month after empiric treatment with iron

44. A week-old infant presents blood in his stools. He was born at home, with the father assisting in the delivery; no physician or midwife was present. He has been breast-fed and has been nursing well. On examination, you also note some blood in his nose. He is not jaundiced; a rectal examination and guaic test of the stool confirms that blood is present. His examination is otherwise normal. He is on no medications. Which of the following is the most likely diagnosis?

(A) child abuse
(B) vitamin K deficiency
(C) breast milk allergy
(D) sepsis
(E) liver disease

Questions 45 and 46

A 6-year-old White female has breast enlargement (Tanner stage II) and coarse curly pubic hair. She is not yet menstruating. She is otherwise healthy and has normal growth parameters. There are no signs of virilization and her abdominal examination reveals no masses. Examination of the vaginal area shows signs of estrogenization.

45. Which of the following is the most likely preliminary working diagnosis?

(A) precocious puberty
(B) premature thelarche
(C) premature pubarche
(D) normal development
(E) precocious menarche

46. On laboratory evaluation, you find elevated levels of follicle-stimulating hormone (FSH), luteinizing hormone (LH), and pubertal levels of estradiol. The bone age is advanced beyond the height and chronologic age. The most likely cause is

(A) idiopathic
(B) central nervous system (CNS) tumor
(C) ovarian tumor
(D) functional ovarian cyst
(E) congenital adrenal hyperplasia

47. A 10-year-old boy is brought in with a chief complaint of multiple colds. On further questioning, you elicit a history of chronic, clear nasal discharge with no seasonal variation. Other symptoms include sneezing, itching of the nose and eyes, as well as tearing and occasional eye redness. Some relief is obtained with an over-the-counter cold medicine containing antihistamine and a decongestant. His history suggests which of the following?

(A) nasal foreign body
(B) immunologic deficiency
(C) rhinitis medicamentosa
(D) sinusitis
(E) allergic rhinitis

48. A full-term newborn develops cyanosis a few hours after birth. Oxygen administration does not improve color or oxygen saturations. Which of the following is the most likely diagnosis?

(A) atrial septal defect
(B) ventricular septal defect
(C) patent ductus arteriosus
(D) aortic stenosis
(E) pulmonary stenosis

49. A 4-year-old child was brought in for evaluation of sleep problems. He cried and screamed within an hour of falling asleep. He seemed disoriented and confused; he did not seem aware of his parents' presence. They were unable to arouse him to comfort him. This resolved spontaneously, and he had no recollection of the event the next morning. You informed the parents that he was most likely experiencing which of the following?

(A) nightmares
(B) night terrors
(C) somnambulism
(D) somniloquy
(E) narcolepsy

50. A 3-year-old boy was bitten while teasing a neighborhood cat. On examination, there are two puncture wounds on the right hand and some superficial scratch marks. There is erythema, warmth, and induration around the puncture sites. Which of the following organisms most likely caused the infection?

(A) *Pasturella multicoda*
(B) *Bartonella henselae*
(C) *Eikenella corrodens*
(D) *Peptostreptococcus* species
(E) alpha Streptococci

51. A 5-week-old bottle-fed boy presents with persistent and worsening projectile vomiting, poor weight gain, and hypochloremic metabolic alkalosis. Of the following diagnostic modalities, which would most likely reveal the diagnosis?

(A) ultrasound of abdomen
(B) barium enema
(C) evaluation of stool for ova and parasites
(D) testing well water for presence of nitrites
(E) serum thyroxine

52. Your next patient is a 4-month-old infant who is returning to have her ear checked. You diagnosed her with otitis media 2 weeks ago, and she has taken 10 days of amoxicillin. She is feeling well, and her mother's only concern is that she has developed a diaper rash over the last 3 days. The mother has been using emollient creams on it which have not helped. On physical examination, there are no abnormal findings except for the rash (Fig. 3-2). Which of the following is the most likely diagnosis?

(A) allergic dermatitis
(B) bullous impetigo
(C) *Candida* dermatitis
(D) irritant dermatitis
(E) seborrheic dermatitis

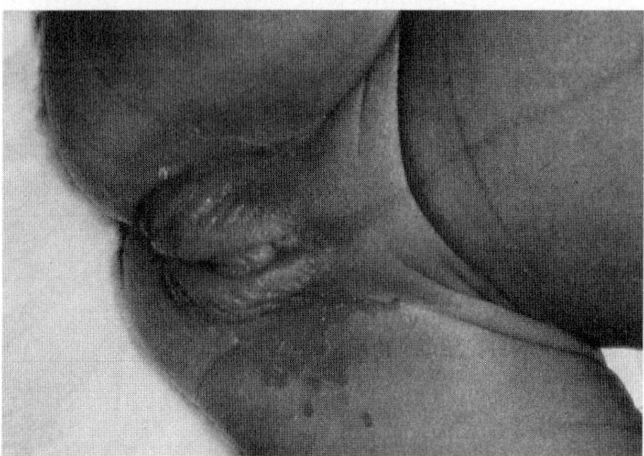

FIG. 3-2 *(Photograph courtesy of Neil S. Prose.)*

53. A 7-year-old boy presents with a rash. His mother states that he was well until 3 days ago when he developed fever and malaise. The next day, the rash started as papules on the trunk, which rapidly changed to vesicles. The lesions have spread all over the body. On physical examination, he has no fever and seems well. You note numerous vesicles all over the body, some of which have crusted over. Which of the following is the most likely diagnosis?

(A) chickenpox
(B) Kawasaki disease
(C) measles
(D) rubella
(E) staphylococcal scalded skin syndrome

54. A 10-year-old boy presents with a 1-day history of fever, cough, and chest pain. He has not been eating and has been listless. He does not have any previous history of health problems. On physical examination, his temperature is 40°C, and he is tachypneic. He looks ill. He has rales on his left posterior lower lung fields. You order a chest x-ray (Fig. 3-3). Which of the following organisms is most likely responsible for his pneumonia?

(A) *Haemophilus influenzae*
(B) *Mycoplasma pneumoniae*
(C) *Pneumocystis carinii*
(D) *Staphylococcus aureus*
(E) *Streptococcus pneumoniae*

55. An 18-month-old girl is brought to the hospital with a history of 6 days of bloody diarrhea. She has been drinking well but has not been wetting her diaper. She has been irritable. On physical examination, she has periorbital edema. She appears pale and is tachycardic. Her CBC shows a hemoglobin of 6 g/dL and a platelet count of 100,000/mm^3. Her blood urea nitrogen (BUN) is 50 mg/dL and creatinine is 5.5 mg/dL. Her urinalysis shows gross hematuria. Which of the following is the most likely causative organism for her clinical problem?

(A) *Escherichia coli* 0157:H7
(B) group A Streptococci
(C) group B Streptococci (GBS)
(D) *Staphylococcus aureus*
(E) the cause of this illness is not known

56. A 1-year-old child with ALL in remission is in the office for a health maintenance visit. He is due for multiple vaccinations including hepatitis B vaccine, inactivated polio vaccine (IPV), varicella vaccine *Haemophilus influenzae* B vaccine (Hib), and pneumococcal vaccine (PCV). You remember that some of these vaccines are live attenuated viruses and are contraindicated in immunocompromised patients. Which vaccine can you safely give to this patient?

(A) PCV
(B) varicella vaccine

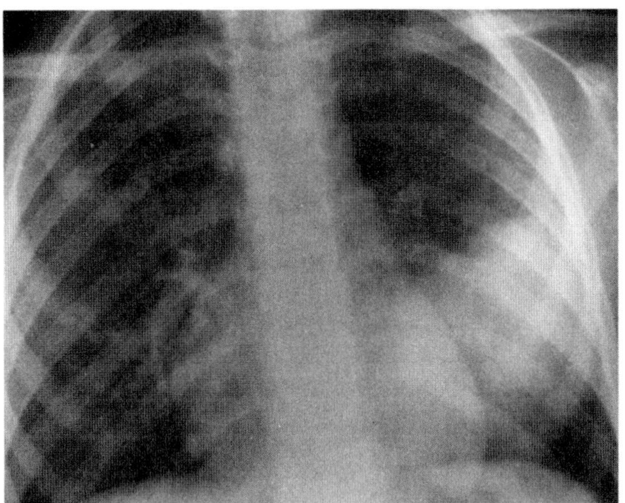

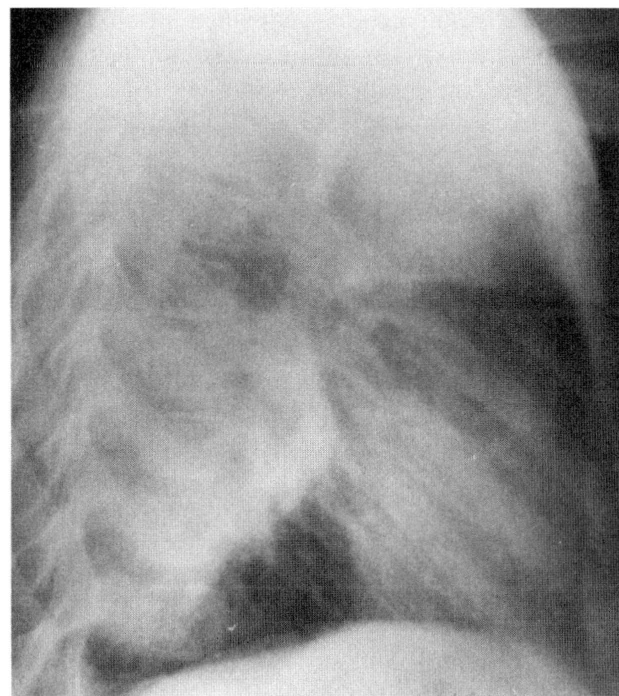

FIG. 3-3

(C) hepatitis B vaccine
(D) Hib
(E) IPV

57. A 9-year-old boy presents with a several-day history of progressive arm and leg weakness. He has been well except for an upper respiratory infection 2 weeks ago. The patient is alert and oriented. On repeated examination, the heart rate varies between 60 and 140 beats/min, and the blood pressure (BP) varies between 90/60 and 140/90 mmHg. Respirations are shallow, with a rate of 50/min. There is symmetric weakness of the face and all four extremities. Deep tendon reflexes are absent. Sensation is intact. Which of the following is the most likely diagnosis?

(A) polymyositis
(B) myasthenia gravis
(C) transverse myelitis
(D) Guillain–Barré syndrome
(E) viral encephalitis

58. An 18-month-old boy is brought to the clinic for a checkup. As part of his routine care, a serum lead level is obtained. It is 25 g/mL. Which of the following is the most appropriate next step in his management?

(A) chelation with CaEDTA
(B) chelation with succimer
(C) investigation of his home for lead hazards
(D) reassurance that this level is not a problem
(E) repeating the level in 6 months

59. An infant is due for her first dose of polio vaccine. Her parents have heard that there are two different types of vaccine for polio. They want to know why their daughter needs to get another shot rather than just taking the oral form of the vaccine. You tell the parents the major advantage of the injectable vaccine is

(A) lower cost
(B) increased mucosal immunity
(C) better efficacy
(D) avoidance of vaccine-associated paralytic poliomyelitis
(E) boosting herd immunity through secondary transmission

60. A 7-year-old child is scheduled for an elective tonsillectomy. The most important instruction to the parents should be to make sure that the child

(A) avoids contact with other children
(B) discontinues antibiotics 72 h before surgery
(C) avoids aspirin and antihistamines for 2 weeks before surgery
(D) does not drink from siblings' cups
(E) eats iron-laden foods for 3 weeks before surgery

61. Routine examination of an otherwise healthy kindergarten child with a history of asthma reveals a BP of 140/90 mmHg. Which of the following is the most likely cause of the hypertension?

(A) theophylline toxicity
(B) chronic lung disease
(C) renal disease
(D) coarctation of the aorta
(E) obesity

62. A 13-year-old girl presents with lethargy, fever, severe headache, and a stiff neck. On examination, a unilateral fixed, dilated pupil and papilledema are noted. Which of the following is the most appropriate initial step in managing this patient?

(A) administration of IV cefotaxime
(B) administration of IV mannitol
(C) CT of the head
(D) intubation and hyperventilation
(E) performance of a lumbar puncture

63. A newborn infant requires repeated resuscitation in the delivery room because of failure to breathe and cyanosis. During spells of crying, which appear to alleviate the cyanosis, his breath and heart sounds are normal, as is direct laryngoscopy. Vigorous respiratory movements appear ineffectual. Immediate management of this infant consists of which of the following?

(A) obtaining a chest x-ray
(B) obtaining an electrocardiogram (ECG)
(C) arterial blood gas determinations
(D) inserting an oropharyngeal airway
(E) administration of naloxone

64. A 4-month-old baby is in for a well-child check and routine immunizations. The baby had a fever of 39°C the day he received his 2-month immunizations. The parents have read about the vaccine on the Internet and express their concerns. Which of the following is an absolute contraindication to giving the Diptheria and tetanus toxoids and acellular pertussis (DTaP)?

(A) history of fever >38°C after previous vaccination
(B) history of local reaction after previous vaccination (redness, soreness, swelling)
(C) family history of seizures
(D) encephalopathy within 7 days of administration of previous dose of vaccine
(E) current antibiotic therapy

65. A 16-year-old male is brought to the emergency department with a crush injury due to a farm accident. His immunization status is unknown. The wound is heavily contaminated with soil, and you are concerned about tetanus. Which of the following is the most appropriate management step?

(A) administer a DTaP vaccination
(B) administer a Td vaccine only
(C) administer Td and tetanus immune globulin (TIG)
(D) administer TIG only
(E) await immunization records

66. Children with sickle cell anemia are at increased risk of developing overwhelming infection with certain microorganisms. Which of the following is the most reasonable step to prevent such infection?

(A) periodic injections of gamma globulin
(B) injection of VZIG after exposure to varicella
(C) withholding live virus vaccines

(D) prophylactic administration of oral penicillin daily
(E) early use of amoxicillin at home for episodes of fever

67. Varicella vaccination is a live virus vaccine. It is generally not recommended in immunocompromised patients. Which of the following is an exception to this rule?

(A) children on high doses of corticosteroids
(B) leukemia
(C) lymphoma
(D) congenital T-cell abnormalities
(E) asymptomatic children with HIV in CDC class 1 with $CD4^+$ T lymphocyte percentage >25%

68. A 1-year-old patient is in the office for a health maintenance visit and is ready for immunizations. The child has a mild upper respiratory infection and a low-grade fever. The mother does not want the child to receive vaccine because she has been told that the vaccine could make the illness worse. You tell her the only true contraindication to vaccination is which of the following?

(A) if the child has a skin rash
(B) if there is an immunosuppressed adult in the household
(C) if the child has hypersensitivity to a vaccine component
(D) if a pregnant woman is in the household
(E) if the mother is breast-feeding

69. A 4-day-old infant presents with yellow discoloration of the skin and sclera. The baby was born at term by a normal vaginal delivery. Pregnancy was uncomplicated; there were no risk factors for sepsis and no history of maternal alcohol or drug use. The baby is breast-fed and has been nursing every 2 h, about 10 min at each breast. The bilirubin level is 15 mg/dL (all unconjugated), the hematocrit is 45%, and the Coombs' test is negative. Which of the following is the most likely diagnosis?

(A) congenital biliary atresia
(B) isoimmune hemolytic disease
(C) Crigler–Najjar syndrome
(D) breast milk jaundice
(E) breast-feeding jaundice

70. A 7-month-old baby presents with a history of constipation for 1 month. He has one hard stool every week. He has been well otherwise. His physical examination is normal. Which of the following is the most likely cause of his problem?

(A) hypothyroidism
(B) lead poisoning
(C) functional constipation
(D) Hirschsprung disease
(E) hypocalcemia

Questions 71 and 72

A 10-year-old boy presents with a 3- to 4-day history of left ear pain. He is afebrile; he has had no symptoms of cold or cough. He has been swimming daily. On physical examination, there is pain on moving the pinna and the tragus. There is erythema and swelling of the ear canal; the tympanic membrane is obscured by thick white discharge.

71. Which of the following is the most likely diagnosis?

(A) otitis externa
(B) furunculosis
(C) otitis media with effusion
(D) mastoiditis
(E) foreign body in the ear

72. Which of the following is the most likely organism involved in this case?

(A) *Staphylococcus aureus*
(B) *Proteus mirabilis*
(C) *Candida*
(D) *Pseudomonas aeruginosa*
(E) Streptococci

73. A specific pattern of abnormalities has been identified among infants born to mothers who consume moderate-to-large amounts of alcohol during their pregnancies. Which of the following abnormalities is characteristic of these infants?

(A) cataracts
(B) developmental dysplasia of the hip
(C) gonadal dysgenesis
(D) neural tube defects
(E) mental retardation

74. A 4-year-old girl presents to the emergency department with fever and a petechial rash. A sepsis workup is performed, and IV antibiotics are administered. Gram-negative diplococci are identified in the CSF. Which of the following is true of this condition?

(A) Antibiotic prophylaxis of fellow daycare attendees is not necessary.
(B) The most common neurologic residual is seizures.
(C) The presence of meningitis decreases the survival rate.
(D) Shock is the usual cause of death.
(E) Vancomycin administered intravenously is the treatment of choice.

75. A 3-year-old boy suddenly begins choking and coughing while eating peanuts. On physical examination, he is coughing frequently. He has inspiratory stridor and mild intercostal and suprasternal retractions. Initial management should include which of the following?

(A) back blows
(B) abdominal thrusts
(C) blind finger-sweeps of the hypopharynx
(D) permitting him to clear the foreign body by coughing
(E) emergency tracheostomy

76. During a well-child visit, the grandmother of an 18-month-old patient is concerned because the child's feet turn inward. She first noticed this when her grandson began to walk. It does not seem to bother the child. On examining his gait, his knees point forward and his feet turn inward. Which of the following is the most likely cause of this condition?

(A) adducted great toe
(B) femoral anteversion
(C) Legg–Calvé–Perthes disease
(D) medial tibial torsion
(E) metatarsus adductus

77. A 13-year-old girl presents with parental concerns of poor posture. She has not had any back pain. On examination, she has unequal shoulder height, asymmetric flank creases, and a forward-bending test that shows rib asymmetry. The physical examination is otherwise normal. Which of the following is the most likely cause of her condition?

(A) congenital scoliosis
(B) leg length inequality
(C) idiopathic scoliosis
(D) postural roundback
(E) Scheuermann kyphosis

78. After 10 days of nasal congestion and rhinorrhea, a 3-month-old infant develops a severe hacking cough during which he repeatedly turns dusky and appears to choke on or to vomit profuse thick, clear nasopharyngeal mucus. For 7 days, the coughing continues unabated. On physical examination, he is afebrile and his lungs are clear. His chest x-ray is normal. His WBC count is 24,000/mm^3, with 15% polymorphonuclear cells, 82% lymphocytes, and 3% monocytes. Which of the following antibiotics should be used to treat this patient?

(A) amoxicillin
(B) amoxicillin–clavulanic acid
(C) erythromycin
(D) tetracycline
(E) no antibiotics are necessary

79. A 16-year-old girl presents with a history of primary amenorrhea. On examination, short stature and a short neck with a low posterior hairline are noted. Chromosomal analysis most likely would reveal which of the following?

(A) fragile X
(B) trisomy 18
(C) trisomy 21
(D) 45,XO
(E) XXY

80. A beekeeper's previously healthy 6-month-old son develops gradual onset of lethargy, poor feeding, constipation, and generalized weakness. On taking a history, you determine that the child has recently been placed on a homemade formula consisting of evaporated milk, water, and honey. Which of the following is the most likely explanation for this symptom complex?

(A) sodium intoxication
(B) Hirschsprung disease
(C) hypothyroidism
(D) spinal cord tumor
(E) botulism

81. A 12-month-old patient has allergies to multiple foods. The child's mother has eliminated the foods from the diet and wants to know if these allergies will be lifelong. You tell her that some allergies do get better if the food is eliminated for 1–2 years. In which of the following is the allergy most likely to resolve, with elimination of the food from the diet?

(A) peanuts
(B) milk
(C) nuts
(D) fish
(E) shellfish

82. A 4-year-old child manifests symptoms of fever, sore throat, and swollen lymph nodes. The spleen tip is palpable. Throat culture and rapid slide (Monospot) test results are negative. The next logical diagnostic procedure would involve which of the following?

(A) rapid streptococcal antigen test
(B) heterophil titer
(C) Epstein–Barr virus (EBV) titer
(D) chest x-ray
(E) bone marrow examination

83. A 2-year-old child is brought to the emergency department with sudden onset of unresponsiveness, miosis, bradycardia, and muscle fasciculations. These findings are most suggestive of poisoning with which of the following?

(A) acetaminophen
(B) organophosphates
(C) salicylates
(D) tricyclic antidepressants
(E) vitamin A

84. A 2-year-old boy presents with refusal to use his right arm for 1 day. He is otherwise well. His mother states she pulled upward on his arm the previous evening to keep him from tripping down the stairs. Which of the following is the most likely diagnosis?

(A) Colles' fracture
(B) fractured clavicle
(C) greenstick fracture of the humerus
(D) rotator cuff injury
(E) subluxation of the radial head

85. A 4-year-old child presents with an enlarged submandibular node that is 4 cm in diameter, nontender, and not fluctuant. The node has been enlarged for about 4 weeks, and there is no history of fever or contact with any person who was ill. A CBC is normal, and a Mantoux test with 5 tuberculin units of purified protein derivative shows 6 mm of induration. Which of the following is the most likely diagnosis?

(A) cat-scratch fever
(B) acute pyogenic lymphadenitis
(C) acute lymphoblastic leukemia
(D) tuberculous lymphadenitis
(E) atypical mycobacteria lymphadenitis

86. A 4-year-old child with grade III vesicoureteral reflux has recurrent urinary tract infections despite adequate antibiotic prophylaxis. Which of the following is the most appropriate next step in the treatment of this patient?

(A) IV antibiotic treatment for 2 weeks
(B) repeat renal scan
(C) renal arteriogram
(D) antireflux surgery
(E) addition of vitamin C (ascorbic acid) to the treatment regimen

87. A 2-week-old White male presents with constipation since birth. He was born full term via a normal vaginal delivery. He did not pass meconium till his 3rd day of life, after he was given a glycerin suppository. He has since stooled every 3–4 days, only with the help of a suppository. The stools are pellet like. He has had increasing abdominal distention. On rectal examination, tone appears normal and the ampulla contains no stool. Which of the following is the most likely cause?

(A) cystic fibrosis
(B) Hirschprung disease
(C) anal stenosis
(D) functional constipation
(E) hypothyroidism

88. Which of the following is the most appropriate evaluative procedure for an otherwise normal 7-day-old boy with perineal hypospadias?

(A) renal ultrasonography
(B) serum creatinine determination
(C) cystography
(D) circumcision
(E) intravenous pyelography (IVP)

89. A 2-week-old infant presents with hepatosplenomegaly and a thick, purulent, bloody nasal discharge. Coppery, oval, maculopapular skin lesions are present in an acral distribution. The neurologic examination is normal, including head circumference. Which of the following is the most likely cause of this congenital infection?

(A) cytomegalovirus (CMV)
(B) HSV
(C) GBS
(D) *Toxoplasma gondii*
(E) *Treponema pallidum*

90. A 7-month-old patient presents with a history of 3 days of fever to 104°F, which resolved the same day that an exanthem erupted. The exanthem is prominent on the neck and truck. It is macular, with discrete lesions 3–5 mm in diameter. Which of the following is the most likely diagnosis?

(A) erythema infectiosum
(B) measles
(C) roseola infantum
(D) rubella
(E) scarlet fever

91. A 3-year-old male presents after having a tonic-clonic seizure lasting about 1 min. On examination, the child now has no nuerologic abnormalities. He has a temperature of 40.3°C and has an obvious otitis media on the left but no other abnormalities on physical examination. You correctly counsel the family with which one of the following statements?

(A) The child will need hospitalization, a lumbar puncture, and antibiotics.
(B) An EEG and CNS imaging must be done.
(C) Anticonvulsants must be stated and continued for 6 months.
(D) There is a slight increase in risk for development of epilepsy.
(E) The child must be monitored carefully for long-term neurologic damage.

Questions 92 through 94

Children with sickle cell disease are at risk for certain conditions with characteristic presentation. Match the clinical scenario with the syndrome.

(A) acute chest syndrome
(B) acute splenic sequestration
(C) aplastic crisis
(D) hand-foot syndrome

(E) *Salmonella osteomyelitis*
(F) vasoocclusive crisis

92. A 12-month old patient presents with a 3-day history of lethargy and fever. He has also had rhinorrhea and a cough. On physical examination, he is pale, tachycardic, and has a left upper quadrant mass. His hemoglobin is 4 g/dL, platelet count is 100,000, and WBC is 15,000 with 50% segmented neutrophils. His reticulocyte count is 15%.

93. An 8-month-old patient with sickle cell disease presents with a 2-day history of painful, swollen fingers and toes.

94. A 5-year-old boy with sickle cell anemia presents with a 2-day history of increasing pain in both legs. He has had multiple admissions for similar episodes of pain. On examination, he has no swelling of the legs. There is diffuse tenderness along both legs. There is no joint involvement, and there is full range of movement.

95. A 1-day-old infant who received silver nitrate eye drops in the delivery room is suffering from bilateral purulent conjunctival discharge. Which of the following is the most likely cause of this child's condition?

(A) *N. gonorrhoeae* infection
(B) herpes simplex infection
(C) nasolacrimal duct obstruction
(D) chemical irritation
(E) *Pseudomonas* infection

96. A 2-year-old girl presents with fever of 39.3°C and irritability. She has had a upper respiratory tract infection for 4 days. On examination, the right ear is bulging and has poor movement on insufflation. Which of the following organisms is most likely responsible for these findings?

(A) *Streptococcus pneumoniae*
(B) *Staphylococcus aureus*
(C) *Mycoplasma pneumoniae*
(D) *Escherichia coli*
(E) group A *Streptococcus*

97. A few weeks after a presumed viral respiratory infection, a 4-year-old girl presents with bruising and petechiae. Bone marrow examination reveals increased numbers of megakaryocytes but is otherwise normal. Hb is 13.5 g/100 mL. Platelet count is 30,000/mm^3. Which of the following would be appropriate for this child at this time?

(A) daily prednisone
(B) a transfusion of packed RBCs and platelets
(C) IV gamma globulin
(D) splenectomy
(E) no specific therapy

98. A 4-month-old child presents with a 2-day history of vomiting and intermittent irritability. On examination, "currant jelly" stool is noted in the diaper, and a sausage-shaped mass is palpated in the right upper quadrant of the abdomen. Which of the following conditions is most likely to cause this?

(A) appendicitis
(B) diaphragmatic hernia
(C) giardiasis
(D) intussusception
(E) rotavirus gastroenteritis

99. During a routine yearly checkup, a 10-year-old boy is found to have 2+ proteinuria on urinalysis. Which of the following would be the most appropriate diagnostic test?

(A) electrolytes, BUN, and serum creatinine
(B) antistreptococcal antibodies
(C) IVP
(D) renal ultrasound
(E) a repeat urinalysis

100. An 18-month-old boy has received 5 days of amoxicillin for otitis media. He continues to have fever, and on physical examination, the right tympanic membrane is bulging with purulent fluid behind it. Which of the following is the best antibiotic to use?

(A) amoxicillin-clavulanic acid
(B) dicloxacillin
(C) cephalexin
(D) erythromycin
(E) penicillin

Questions 101 and 102

A 13-year-old boy presents for evaluation of short stature. His growth chart from ages 2 through 12 years is shown in Fig. 3-4. His growth in the first 2 years of life was typically at the 25th percentile. He has been healthy, has a good appetite, and is doing well in school. He lives with his parents and is an only child. His parents' heights are both at the 50th percentile. His father states that he grew several inches after he completed high school. A complete physical examination is normal. His Tanner stage is I.

101. Which of the following is the most likely cause of this patient's short stature?

(A) constitutional delay
(B) deprivational dwarfism
(C) familial short stature
(D) growth hormone deficiency
(E) hypothyroidism

102. Which of the following tests is the most appropriate next step in the care of this patient?

(A) bone age
(B) cranial imaging
(C) growth hormone stimulation
(D) thyroid function tests
(E) no tests are necessary

Questions 103 and 104

A 12-year-old girl presents with chest pain when she plays basketball. The pain is substernal, is associated with dyspnea, and occurs after she has been playing vigorously. The pain does not radiate. The pain and dyspnea resolve with rest. She does not have palpitations or any lightheadedness associated with the pain. She does not have pain or dyspnea at other times. There is no history of early cardiac deaths or unexplained deaths of young people in her family. Her physical examination is normal, except for a grade 2/6 systolic vibratory murmur heard at the left lower sternal border.

103. Which of the following is the most likely cause of her symptoms?

(A) angina
(B) asthma
(C) costochondritis
(D) esophagitis
(E) mitral valve prolapse

104. Which of the following tests should be ordered for this patient?

(A) chest x-ray
(B) echocardiogram
(C) pulmonary function tests
(D) 24-h Holter monitoring
(E) cardiac enzymes

105. A 10-year-old boy presents with red discoloration of the urine since the morning. He is healthy and otherwise asymptomatic. He denies dysuria, frequency, urgency, flank, or abdominal pain. His BP is normal. His examination is within normal limits including abdomen and genitourinary system. There is no rash or edema. His urine is pink in color; urinalysis is negative for hemoglobin or protein. No white cells, red cells, or bacteria are noted. Which of the following is the most appropriate next step?

(A) obtain a recent dietary and drug history
(B) obtain a urine culture
(C) test for myoglobin in the urine
(D) obtain a renal ultrasound
(E) obtain antistreptococcal antibodies

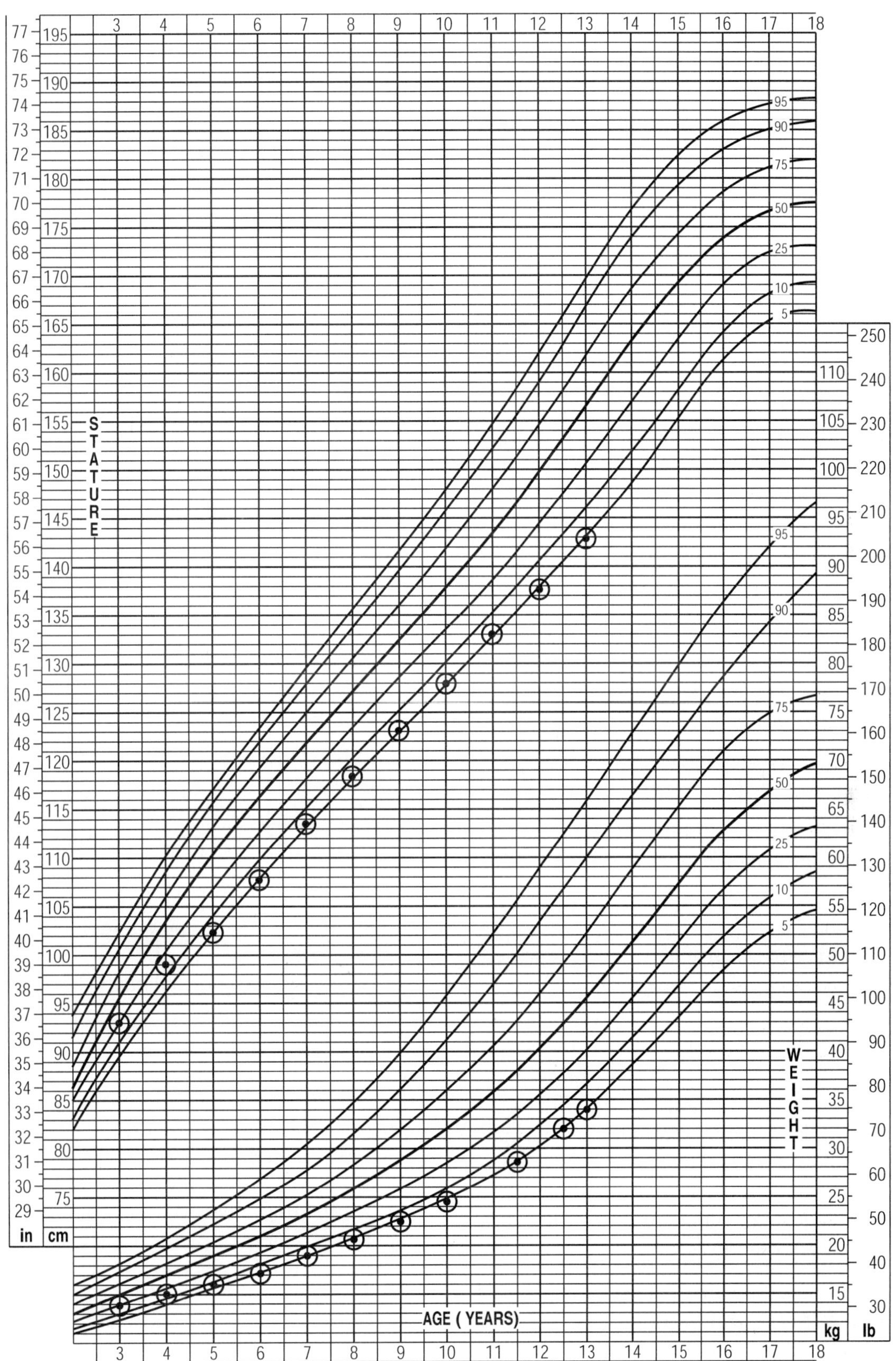
BOYS: 2 TO 18 YEARS
PHYSICAL GROWTH
NCHS PERCENTILE
STATURE
WEIGHT
AGE (YEARS)
in
cm
kg
lb

FIG. 3-4

106. A 12-year-old girl has had a sore throat over 2 days. She now has a fever of 39.5°C and has difficulty opening her mouth, swallowing, or speaking. Her throat can be visualized with difficulty, the right tonsil is significantly more enlarged than the left, and the uvula is displaced to the left side. Which of the following is the most likely diagnosis?

(A) retropharyngeal abscess
(B) acute uvulitis
(C) peritonsillar abscess
(D) acute pharyngitis
(E) lateral pharyngeal abscess

107. An 18-month-old boy presents with a history of fever to 39.0°C for 5 days. He has also been irritable and has not been drinking well. Associated symptoms include red eyes, a rash, and some trouble walking. On physical examination, he has a temperature of 39.5°C. He has bilateral bulbar conjunctivitis, a strawberry tongue, an inflamed oral pharynx, edema of the hands and feet, a morbilliform rash, and cervical lymphadenopathy. He is very irritable. His CBC shows a WBC of 15,000/mm^3 with 60% neutrophils, 35% lymphocytes, and 5% monocytes. His hemoglobin is 12.0 g/dL and platelet count is 500,000/mm^3. Which of the following is the most likely diagnosis?

(A) erythema infectiosum (fifth disease)
(B) Kawasaki disease
(C) rubella
(D) rubeola (measles)
(E) rheumatic fever

108. An athletic 12-year-old boy complains of left knee pain when he runs and plays sports. The pain resolves when he rests. He has otherwise been well. His physical examination is normal, except for swelling and increased prominence over the left tibial tubercle. A radiograph of the left knee is normal. Which of the following is the most likely diagnosis?

(A) Legg–Calvé–Perthes disease
(B) Osgood–Schlatter disease
(C) patellar subluxation
(D) popliteal cyst
(E) slipped capital femoral epiphysis

DIRECTIONS (Questions 109 through 113): For each item, select the ONE best lettered option that is most closely associated with it. Each lettered heading may be selected once, more than once, or not at all.

For each of the following patients with possible congenital heart disease, select the most likely diagnosis.

(A) aortic stenosis
(B) atrial septal defect
(C) AV canal defect
(D) carotid bruit
(E) coarctation of the aorta
(F) mitral stenosis
(G) mitral valve prolapse
(H) peripheral pulmonic stenosis
(I) pulmonic stenosis
(J) Still's murmur
(K) transposition of the great arteries
(L) tetralogy of Fallot
(M) truncus arteriosus
(N) venous hum
(O) ventricular septal defect

109. A newborn full-term infant develops cyanosis shortly after birth. On examination, the infant is in no distress, is well perfused, has a normal cardiac examination, including no obvious murmurs, and has no organomegaly. The pulse oximeter is 77%. The ECG is normal, and chest x-ray reveals a normal heart size with a narrow mediastinum and normal pulmonary vascularity.

110. A 4-year-old boy with normal growth, development, and physical activity is noted to have a murmur at a checkup. On examination, he has no abnormal findings except for a 2/6 musical systolic ejection murmur at the lower sternal border, which is softer when he sits up.

111. A 5-year-old boy with normal growth, development, and physical activity is in the clinic for a checkup. His physical examination is totally normal, except for a widely split second heart sound and a 2/6 systolic ejection murmur at the upper left sternal border that does not radiate.

112. A 2-month-old infant who is growing and developing normally is noted to have a murmur at a checkup. The physical examination is entirely normal, except for a 2/6 systolic ejection murmur heard over the entire chest, especially in the axilla and back.

113. An 18-month-old child who is growing and developing normally has a murmur noted at a checkup. The physical examination is entirely normal, except for a 2/6 holosystolic murmur at the left sternal border.

Answers and Explanations

1. **(B)** Generally, the interpretation of tuberculin skin test (TST) is the same regardless of BCG status. Induration >5 mm is considered positive in children in close contact with known or suspected cases of tuberculosis disease or children suspected to have tuberculosis disease. Induration >10 mm is considered positive in children at greater risk of disseminated disease (age <4 years; other medical conditions such as lymphoma, diabetes, chronic renal failure, or malnutrition) or children at greater risk of exposure to tuberculosis disease (born in, or parents born in high-prevalence regions, travel to these regions, exposure to adults at high risk, such as HIV infected, homeless, or drug abusers). Induration >15 mm is positive in children >4 years without any risk factors. Radiographic evaluation of all children with positive TST is recommended. Latent tuberculosis infection is defined as an infection in a person with a positive TST, no physical findings of the disease, and a chest radiograph that is either normal or reveals only granulomas or calcifications in the lungs or regional lymph nodes. Children with latent tuberculosis infection should receive prophylaxis, usually 9 months of INH. Those with symptoms, signs, and/or radiographic manifestations are said to have tuberculosis disease. There is no benefit to repeating the test in 3–6 months, and it will delay treatment. Sputum cultures are difficult to obtain in younger children. Gastric aspirate specimens obtained with a nasogastric tube are preferred. Culture material should be obtained in children with evidence of the disease in order to obtain information on drug susceptibility and resistance patterns. *(American Academy of Pediatrics, 2000a, pp. 593–613)*

2. **(C)** Transmission of perinatal hepatitis B virus (HBV) infection can be prevented in 95% of infants born to HBsAg-positive mothers by early active (immunization) and passive immunoprophylaxis (HBIG), preferably within 12 h of life. The immunization series should be completed by 6 months of life. The child should have serology testing 1–3 months after completion of the series. Testing for anti-HBs will establish if additional vaccine doses are needed; testing for HBsAg will identify infants who are chronically infected. Mothers whose HBsAg status is unknown should be tested as soon as possible; the first vaccine dose should be given within 12 h of birth. If the woman is found to be positive, HBIG should be given as soon as possible, not later than 7 days of age. *(American Academy of Pediatrics, 2000a, pp. 298–300)*

3. **(A)** Pityriasis rosea is a papulosquamous eruption consisting of multiple oval-shaped scaling lesions which are truncal in distribution. This eruption resembles the papulosquamous eruption of secondary syphilis, although the rash of secondary syphilis often involves the palms and soles. The etiology of pityriasis rosea is unknown, but is felt to be viral. It is a self-limiting illness lasting several weeks to a few months, and there is no adequate treatment other than symptomatic treatment of pruritus, when necessary. *(McMillan et al., p. 720)*

4. **(E)** Children with chickenpox may be infectious for 1 or 2 days before the appearance of the rash. Once skin lesions have crusted, the patient is no longer infectious. Susceptible individuals can contract chickenpox from patients with zoster. In the cases of both chickenpox and zoster, transmission is thought to occur by the respiratory route rather than by direct contact. The virus can travel long distances in the air and remain viable. Transmission from one hospital patient to other susceptible hospitalized patients has been reported to occur through air vents. VZIG should be given within 3 or 4 days of exposure to varicella-susceptible individuals who are immunocompromised.

(McMillan et al., pp. 1127–1223; American Academy of Pediatrics, 2000a, pp. 624–638)

5. **(A)** Prone sleeping is a major risk factor for sudden infant death syndrome (SIDS). Since the 1992 AAP recommendation that infants be placed to sleep on their backs, the frequency of prone sleeping has decreased from 70 to 20%, and the SIDS rate has decreased by >40%. Side sleeping has a slightly higher SIDS risk than supine but is still safer than the prone position. Other risk factors include maternal smoking, soft bedding, overheating, younger maternal age, prematurity, low birth weight, and male gender. Rates among Blacks and Native Americans are two to three times the national average. The issue of bed sharing or cosleeping is controversial. There are reports of overlying by adults leading to suffocation, especially when the adult uses drugs or alcohol. Bed sharing with multiple family members may be hazardous; there is increased risk of overlying, entrapment, rolling into prone position, and use of soft sleeping surfaces. Some studies show that infants have more arousals and less slow-wave sleep during bed sharing; however, there is no epidemiologic evidence that bed sharing is protective. *(American Academy of Pediatrics, 2000b, pp. 650–656)*

6. **(C)** Children, especially those in daycare, commonly are infected with the hepatitis A virus. Unlike adults, children most often are asymptomatic. Frequently, outbreaks of hepatitis A in a daycare center are not recognized until a daycare worker or parent of an attendee becomes ill. An elevated hepatitis A IgM is the most rapid and reliable confirmation of diagnosis. The incubation period is 15–50 days, with an average of 25–30 days. Household and sexual contacts who are exposed should receive immunoglobulin. *(American Academy of Pediatrics, 2000a, pp. 281–289)*

7. **(A)** Superficial corneal injuries expose underlying layers causing pain, photophobia, tearing, and decreased vision. Irrigation is recommended only if a foreign body is suspected. Abrasions are detected by instilling fluorescein dye and inspecting the cornea using blue-filtered light. Treatment consists of frequent applications of topical antibiotic ointment until the epithelium is healed. The use of a patch does not accelerate healing, and if improperly applied, may abrade the cornea. Referral to an ophthalmologist should be considered if there are significant changes in vision, or signs of deeper or more penetrating injury which often result in papillary abnormalities. *(Behrman et al., p. 1936)*

8. **(C)** The American Academy of Pediatrics recommends that children should face the rear of the vehicle until they are at least 20 lb and 1 year of age to reduce the risk of cervical spine injury in the event of a crash. Infants who weigh 20 lb before 1 year of age should ride rear facing in a convertible seat or infant seat approved for higher weights until 1 year of age. A car seat should never be placed in the front passenger seat. *(American Academy of Pediatrics, 1996, pp. 761–762)*

9. **(C)** Though infection must be considered as an etiology, acute trauma is more likely in this scenario. This case represents the classic picture of the shaken baby syndrome which produces intracranial trauma without obvious external findings. This infant is critically ill and lacks preceding illness or constitutional symptoms. The tense fontanels reflect increased intracranial pressure. A cranial CT scan may show diffuse edema or a localized lesion, such as a subdural hemorrhage. Metabolic causes of seizures do not cause increased intracranial pressure. Acetaminophen toxicity does not cause CNS symptoms. *(Kliegman et al., pp. 518–521; Rudolph et al., pp. 463–469)*

10. **(B)** The insect order Hymenoptera includes ants, bees, and wasps. Their venom usually only causes a local reaction. About 1–4% of the population is sensitized to the venom and at risk for immediate hypersensitivity reactions. Reactions may include urticaria, angioedema, wheezing, or hypotension. Severe reactions should be treated with IV fluids, oxygen, and epinephrine. Although the child responded well to diphenhydramine, because there was a systemic reaction, it is advisable to carry an

Epi-pen Jr at all times. Only children with life-threatening systemic reactions need to be referred for desensitization. Testing IgE or skin-prick test with Hymenoptera venom is not predictive of future systemic reactions. *(Behrman et al., p. 2177)*

11. **(D)** Children frequently insert foreign bodies into the nose. Initial symptoms are local obstruction, sneezing, and pain. Subsequently, there is swelling and infection leading to a purulent, malodorous, and often bloody discharge. The infection clears after removal of the foreign body. Nasal polyps cause obstruction of the nasal passages, hyponasal speech, and mouth breathing; gray, grape-like masses can be visualized on nasal examination. An upper respiratory infection is usually suggested by a careful history. Initial symptoms include a scratchy throat, followed by development of thin nasal discharge and sneezing. Myalgia, low-grade fever, headache, malaise, and decreased appetite may be present. By the 2nd or 3rd day, the discharge becomes thicker and more purulent. Cough is common. Symptoms usually resolve by 7–10 days. Adolescents with sinusitis may have classic symptoms of headache and sinus tenderness. In children, cough and nasal discharge are common; the cough is worse when supine. If upper respiratory infection symptoms persist without improvement for >10 days, sinusitis should be considered. A more acute form may occur, with a shorter duration and more severe symptoms such as fever >39°C, purulent nasal discharge, headache, and eye swelling. Children with allergic rhinitis present with sneezing, clear watery, rhinorrhea, and itching of the nose, palate, pharynx, and eyes. Itching, redness, and tearing of the eyes may be present. This occurs in response to exposure to an allergen such as pollen, mold spores, and animal or mite antigens. *(Behrman et al., pp. 1258–1264, 662–663)*

12. **(B)** Enuresis may be primary (75%) where nocturnal control was never achieved; secondary enuresis (25%) is when the child was dry at night for at least a few months. Nocturnal enuresis is more common in boys, and family history is positive in at least 50%. This may affect as much as 20% of children at age 5 years, and it spontaneously stops in at least 15% of affected children every year. Psychologic factors are often involved in secondary enuresis. A careful history should be obtained to rule out such organic factors as UTI (dysuria, frequency, urgency). Children with diabetes insipidus or diabetes mellitus have polydipsia and polyuria. Urinalysis should be considered to rule out an organic cause. In diabetes mellitus, urinalysis may reveal glycosuria and ketonuria. A urine-specific gravity of >1.015 makes diabetes insipidus unlikely. *(Behrman et al., pp. 1642–1643)*

13. **(E)** Active treatment should be avoided in children under age 6 years, as nocturnal enuresis is common. Parents should be reassured that the condition is self-limited. Fluid intake 1 h before sleep should be restricted. Simple behavioral reinforcement, such as a star or sticker chart to record dry nights, may be helpful. Punitive or humiliating measures should be discouraged. Bladder-stretching exercises and encouraging children to hold urine for longer periods during the day are usually not helpful. Pharmacologic therapy is not curative. DDAVP is a synthetic analog of antidiuretic hormone. It reduces urine production overnight. Hyponatremia has been reported with use of this drug. If used, it should only be for a limited time. Imipramine is a tricyclic antidepressant which was used more often in the past. It is effective in 30–60% of children, but side effects include anxiety, insomnia, and dry mouth. There is a poisoning risk, especially for younger children. Conditioning therapy may be considered in children older than 6 years. Success rates range from 30 to 60%. It involves the use of an alarm attached to electrodes in the underwear, which sounds when the child voids. Consistent use of the device is often helpful; it is more effective in older, more motivated children. A common complaint is that the alarm wakes up other family members but not the affected child. *(Behrman et al., pp. 551–552)*

14. **(D)** Gynecomastia is the enlargement of male breast tissue and occurs in approximately one-third of adolescent males during early- to

midpuberty. It usually resolves spontaneously and requires no further evaluation beyond a careful history and physical examination. Features include: breast tissue <4 cm in diameter and resembling female breast budding, and pubertal development between Tanner stage II and IV. Pubertal development signs precede gynecomastia by at least 6 months. It may be more noticeable in obese boys.

A drug and medication history should be obtained; these include estrogens, androgens, human chorionic gonadotropin (hCG), cardiovascular drugs (reserpine, methyldopa, digitalis), cytotoxic agents (busulfan, vincristine), antituberculosis drugs (INH), psychoactive drugs (tricyclic antidepressants, diazepam), ketoconazole, spironolactone, cimetidine, and phenytoin. Illegal drugs include marijuana, heroin, methadone, amphetamines, as well as alcohol.

If there is evidence of precocious puberty, hypogonadism or macrogynecomastia (breast tissue >5 cm diameter), laboratory testing should be done including dehydroepiandrosterone sulfate (DHAS), FSH, and LH, hCG, estradiol, and testosterone. Thyroid-stimulating hormone (TSH) may be obtained to rule out hyperthyroidism. Boys with Klinefelter syndrome have hypogonadism (testes <3 cm in diameter), delayed pubertal development, and gynecomastia. Laboratory tests reveal increased FSH and LH, and decreased testosterone; the diagnosis is confirmed by chromosome analysis. If DHAS, hCG, or estradiol levels are increased, an MRI of the head to exclude a CNS tumor and ultrasound of abdomen and testes to rule out an adrenal, liver, or testicular tumor should be considered. *(Mahony, pp. 1389–1404)*

15. (A) Wilms' tumor is a malignant embryonal neoplasm of the kidney. It is the second most common solid tumor of childhood. Girls are affected more frequently than boys (2:1). The incidence of Wilms' tumor peaks at 1–3 years of age. The classic presentation is a painless abdominal mass that is usually hard, smooth, and unilateral. Hematuria occurs in 12–25% of children with Wilms' tumor, and hypertension has been reported in up to 60% of patients. Aniridia or hemihypertrophy may be observed in patients with Wilms' tumor. *(McMillan et al., pp. 1515–1517, 2255)*

16. (A)

17. (B)

18. (B)

19. (D)

Explanations 16 through 19

Urine for urinalysis and culture must be properly obtained. Catheterization is the most reliable method of the choices offered. Suprapubic tap is considered the "gold-standard" but is not always technically feasible, especially in an outpatient office setting. A midstream, clean catch specimen would be acceptable in an older, toilet trained child. "Bagged" specimens are not recommended because of possible skin or fecal contamination of the specimen. Similarly, obtaining a sample from a diaper or potty would be unacceptable. Urinalysis includes dipstick method and microscopic examination. Leukocyte esterase (an enzyme in WBC) and nitrites suggest probable infection. Microscopic analysis of unspun urine for WBC (>10/high-power field) or bacteria is also predictive of infection. RBCs are often present in a urinary tract infection.

The patient is vomiting and dehydrated; this may indicate possible pyelonephritis. The most appropriate course would be IV hydration and empiric treatment with antibiotics (ceftriaxone) while awaiting cultures. Children with pyelonephritis are at increased risk of renal scarring, especially younger children, and should be treated early. *E. coli* is the most common organisms cultured; others include *Proteus, Klebsiella, Staphylococcus saprophyticus,* and *Enterococcus.* The occurrence of a urinary tract infection in a girl under age 3–5 years and in a boy of any age may be a marker for an underlying congenital anatomic abnormality, in particular, vesicourethral reflux. Radiologic investigation with renal ultrasound and VCUG is recommended. *(Behrman et al., pp. 1621–1625)*

20. **(E)** Because many childhood viral illnesses have seasonal presentations, the etiologic agent may be suspected on the basis of clinical and seasonal presentation. Yearly winter outbreaks of bronchiolitis and pneumonia are associated with respiratory syncytial virus. Summer outbreaks of gastroenteritis are associated with enterovirus, while winter outbreaks are associated with rotavirus. Although adenovirus can cause diarrhea, it more commonly causes respiratory symptoms. Human herpesvirus type 6 is the etiologic agent in roseola infantum. *(McMillan et al., pp. 1086–1088, 1102, 1124–1126, 1094–1098, 1147–1149)*

21. **(B)** Penicillin remains the drug of choice for treatment of streptococcal pharyngitis. Amoxicillin, macrolides, and cephalosporins are acceptable alternatives. *(McMillan et al., pp. 1016, 1297)*

22. **(C)** Scarlet fever is caused by toxins made by group A Streptococci. It is usually seen in patients with strep throat. The rash is papular and described as sandpaper-like. Sometimes it is easier to feel it than to see it. An allergic rash would be urticarial. More than 80% of patients with EBV infection develop a maculopapular rash if given amoxicillin. This patient's clinical course is not typical for EBV which presents more gradually, and patients often have posterior cervical adenopathy and splenomegaly. Patients with serum sickness often have urticarial rashes, sometimes progressing to angioedema. They may also have arthritis, myalgias, and lymphadenopathy. The rash in enteroviral infections is typically macular. *(Rudolph et al., pp. 996, 1225)*

23. **(D)** Patients with Turner syndrome have a 45,X karyotype. The classic physical features are illustrated in this case. Patients have short stature, a webbed neck, ptosis, triangular faces, prominent brow, hypertelorism, low-set ears, and pectus excavatum. *(Rudolph et al., p. 1785)*

24. **(C)** Turner syndrome is associated with coarctation of the aorta and aortic stenosis. Williams syndrome is associated specifically with supravalvular aortic stenosis. In Noonan syndrome, the cardiac defect most often is pulmonary valvular stenosis or an atrial septal defect. Marfan syndrome is associated with mitral valve prolapse and aortic root dilatation. Septal defects, primarily endocardial cushion defects, are the most common heart defects among children with Down syndrome. *(Rudolph et al., pp. 1781)*

25. **(C)** Marfan syndrome is a genetic disorder of connective tissue. It is transmitted in an autosomal-dominant manner. Patients have tall stature and skeletal disproportion, where the arm span exceeds the height. Other important clinical features include subluxation of the ocular lens which occurs in 50–80% of patients. Progressive dilatation of the aortic root and ascending aorta can lead to dissection or rupture. *(Rudolph et al., pp. 762–764)*

26. **(E)** Marfan syndrome is associated with mitral valve prolapse and aortic root dilatation. *(Rudolph et al., pp. 392–393)*

27. **(A)** SLE is an autoimmune disorder that affects multiple organs. The diagnosis is based on the presence of four or more major criteria. These include malar rash, oral ulcers, arthritis, and photosensitivity. This patient has all of these symptoms, as well as the systemic symptoms often seen at presentation. The disorder is predominately a disease of women and, in the pediatric population, is a disease of adolescence. Chronic renal disease is an important and common cause of morbidity and mortality among patients with SLE. *(Rudolph et al., pp. 847–850)*

28. **(E)** Organic acids produced by bacterial fermentation lower the pH of dental plaque causing demineralization and caries of the adjacent tooth. Nursing bottle caries is a pattern of caries involving the upper and lower incisors. It occurs because of prolonged contact of the tooth to a sugar-containing liquid (juice or milk). This is more likely to occur with overnight exposure or with use of a bottle. A similar pattern of caries may rarely occur with breast-fed babies who feed through the night. Cup feeding or drinks given during mealtimes

are less likely to cause prolonged contact to the teeth. *(Behrman et al., p. 1114)*

29. (E) A tender, boggy mass on the scalp is most likely to be a kerion. This is an inflammatory form of tinea capitis. Tinea capitis is more common in Black children and is the most common cause of alopecia in children. In the United States, a majority of cases are caused by *Trichophyton tonsurans; Microsporum canis* may also be involved. Tinea capitis may present with diffuse scaling, a black dot form, and as the inflammatory form—kerion. The recommended treatment is 8–12 weeks of oral griseofulvin. Shampooing with selenium sulfide shampoo is a helpful adjunctive therapy which decreases spore shedding. Topical therapy alone is ineffective. Incision and drainage or antibiotic therapy are not recommended in treatment of tinea capitis. *(Behrman et al., pp. 2036–2038)*

30. (B) Coxsackie A16 is the major cause of hand, foot, and mouth disease. This is a summer enteroviral illness presenting with classic lesions of the hand, feet, and mouth. Herpetic gingivostomatitis is the most common cause of stomatitis in children aged 1–3 years. There is often a high fever, fetor oris, refusal to eat, and irritability. The lesions are initially vesicular, and soon form ulcers ranging from 2 to 10 mm in diameter. The tongue, cheek, and gums are usually involved, and there may be submaxillary lymphadenitis. Aphthous ulcerations (canker sores) are painful ulcerations, which present as erythematous, indurated papules that erode to form circumscribed necrotic ulcers with gray fibrinous exudates and erythematous halo. They are 2–10 mm in diameter, heal spontaneously, and often recur. Behçet syndrome is a multisystem disorder characterized by recurrent oral and genital ulceration, iritis or uveitis, as well as other cutaneous, arthritic, neurologic, vascular, and gastrointestinal (GI) manifestations. It is rare in children. Traumatic oral ulcers may be seen in chronic cheek biters but do not involve extremities. *(Behrman et al., pp. 961, 968, 1119)*

31. (C) Kawasaki disease is an acute vasculitis of unknown etiology. Humans contract brucellosis by direct contact with infected animals or by drinking unpasteurized milk. babesiosis is transmitted by ticks. Leptospirosis is obtained from exposure to the urine of infected animals. Psittacosis is obtained from exposure to bird feces. *(American Academy of Pediatrics, 2000a, pp. 360–363)*

32. (E) Erythema infectiosum is a common childhood viral exanthem cause by parvovirus B19. It was the fifth in a classification system of childhood exanthems; the others were rubella, measles, scarlet fever, atypical scarlet fever, and roseola infantum. The rash classically presents early with flushed cheeks or a "slapped cheek" appearance. It is followed by development of a macular erythematous rash on trunk and extremities, which then shows central clearing, developing a lacy, reticulated appearance. The infection is often not clinically apparent. Adult and older adolescents, especially females, may develop arthropathy. The symptoms are usually self-limited. Parvovirus B19 is clinically significant in people with hemolytic anemias because it may induce a transient aplastic crisis. Immunocompromised individuals are also at risk for chronic infections accompanied by anemia, neutropenia, and thrombocytopenia. It may also induce fetal demise in case of primary infection of pregnant women. *(Behrman et al., pp. 964–966)*

33. (B) Centers for Disease Control and Prevention (CDC) criteria require fever of at least 5 days' duration for a clinical diagnosis of Kawasaki disease. According to these criteria, patients also must have at least four of five other findings, including bilateral conjunctival infection, one or more changes of the oral mucous membranes (e.g., pharyngeal erythema; dry, fissured, and erythematous lips; and *strawberry* tongue), one or more changes of the extremities (e.g., erythema, edema, and desquamation), rash, and cervical lymphadenopathy. Kawasaki disease occurs most commonly during the first 2 years of life. Thrombocytosis, rather than thrombocytopenia, is an almost invariable feature late in the course of illness. The most common serious complication of Kawasaki disease is coronary artery aneurysm formation which can result in thrombosis, aneurysmal rupture, or other cardiac effects. *(McMillan et al., pp. 924–932)*

34. (B) Orbital (also referred to as postseptal) cellulitis is a medical emergency. It is a bacterial infection of the orbit. It must be distinguished from periorbital (also referred to as preseptal) cellulitis by the presence of proptosis or limitations of extraocular movements. When orbital cellulitis is suspected, cultures of blood and CSF should be obtained, appropriate antibiotics should be administered intravenously, an ophthalmologist should be consulted, and CT films should be obtained to delineate the extent of the infectious process. Both retinoblastoma and battered child syndrome may present with lid edema. Typically, these children are afebrile and nontoxic in appearance. Hyphema is hemorrhage into the anterior chamber of the eye and is caused by trauma. Twenty percent of patients with neuroblastoma present with eye symptoms from metastasis. Proptosis is one of the possible presentations and can be of relatively acute onset. In general, other systemic symptoms are present and have developed more gradually. *(McMillan et al., p. 670)*

35. (D) Babies who are exclusively breast-fed for prolonged periods of time are at risk for developing rickets. Dark-skinned infants are at high risk, especially during winter months when they receive inadequate sunlight. Supplementation with vitamin D is recommended in children who are at high risk, as well as pregnant and lactating mothers. Clinical features include craniotabes, a thinning of the outer table of the skull. This may also occur in osteogenesis imperfecta. Enlargement of the costochondral junctions (rachitic rosary) may be seen in rickets, scurvy, and chondrodystrophy. Other features may include delayed primary teeth, enamel defects, and caries. There may be thickening of the wrists and ankles; bending of the femur, tibia, and fibula result in bowlegs or knock knees.

Greenstick fractures of long bones may occur without symptoms. Diagnosis is based on history of inadequate vitamin D intake and clinical features. Diagnosis may be confirmed by x-rays and chemistry; serum calcium is low or normal, serum phosphorus is low, serum alkaline phosphatase is elevated, and serum 25-hydroxycholecalciferol is decreased. Breast milk contains adequate vitamin C as long as the mother is not deficient. *(Behrman et al., pp. 186–187)*

36. (D) Testicular torsion is the most common cause of testicular pain in boys 12 years and older and is uncommon in those under 10 years. It may be sometimes related to trauma or injury but may occur spontaneously. If not diagnosed early, loss of blood flow to the testicle may result in permanent loss of testicular function. Torsion of the testicular appendix usually occurs between the ages of 2 and 11 years. The testicular appendix is a vestigial stalk at the upper pole of the testis. Torsion results in pain and swelling of the scrotum, but the onset of pain is more gradual. There is a 3- to 5-mm indurated, tender mass at the upper pole of the testis. It may sometimes be visible as a "blue-dot." Testicular scan may be helpful when this cannot be clinically differentiated from testicular torsion. A hydrocele is a painless collection of fluid in the tunica vaginalis. Transillumination confirms that the mass is filled with fluid. Hydroceles are present in 1–2% of male newborns and usually resolve by age 1 year. In older boys, a communicating hydrocele may be associated with an inguinal hernia. Inguinal hernias usually appear as a bulge in the inguinal area extending into the scrotum. Hernias are painless, and are more noticeable during crying or straining. They are painful only when strangulated or incarcerated. Epididymitis is an acute inflammation of the epididymis, and is more common in sexually active adolescents. Urinalysis shows pyuria and the etiology may be gonococcus or chlamydia but is often undetermined. *(Behrman et al., pp. 1650–1654)*

37. (B) *C. trachomatis* is considered an unusual cause of otitis media at any age. *N. gonorrhoeae* causes conjunctivitis in the newborn. Syphilis and toxoplasmosis cause congenital infections. *E. coli* is one of the neonatal pathogens that also causes otitis media in neonates. The symptoms of otitis media in newborns are often similar to those of sepsis; they are subtle and nonspecific and may include poor feeding, lethargy, vomiting, or diarrhea. Once the diagnosis is established, the initial therapy should be similar to that for neonatal sepsis, such as parenteral ampicillin and cefotaxime. Under ideal circumstances, the results of cultures obtained by tympanocentesis may then allow further treatment with a more specific antibiotic of low toxicity. Older infants may respond well to oral therapy but require frequent observation. *(Feigin and Cherry, pp. 908–909)*

38. **(A)** Proptosis and limitation of extraocular motility distinguish orbital cellulitis from periorbital cellulitis. Fever, lid swelling, redness of the eye, and leukocytosis generally are present in either condition. Orbital cellulitis (infection within the orbit) may follow directly from a wound near the orbit or may result from bacteremia, but the most common source involves extension from the paranasal sinuses. The organisms most frequently implicated as pathogens are *Haemophilus influenzae*, *Staphylococcus aureus*, group A beta-hemolytic Streptococci, and *Streptococcus pneumoniae*. The risk of complication is great, with extension resulting in cavernous sinus thrombosis, meningitis, or brain abscess. Prompt hospitalization and parenteral antibiotic therapy are indicated. *(McMillan et al., p. 670)*

39. **(A)** *H. influenzae*, *S. pneumoniae*, and *Moraxella catarrhalis* are the most common bacterial pathogens in otitis media of children. Amoxicillin is still the initial drug to use in uncomplicated otitis media because of its good coverage, except for beta-lactamase-positive organisms, and its excellent safety profile. The other drugs (except for erythromycin) are acceptable second-line medications. *(McMillan et al., pp. 1302–1304)*

40. **(B)** Late posttraumatic epilepsy is diagnosed when a seizure occurs for the first time more than 1 week after a head injury. Factors that correlate with an increased risk of developing posttraumatic epilepsy include presence of a depressed skull fracture, acute intracranial hemorrhage, cerebral contusion, or unconsciousness lasting more than 24 h. Because the risk of a subsequent seizure is approximately 75%, acute and chronic treatment with anticonvulsants is indicated. Loss of consciousness, retrograde amnesia, and vomiting are relatively common immediate consequences of head trauma. They are usually transient and are not highly correlated with a risk of subsequent posttraumatic seizures. *(Rudolph et al., pp. 2261–2265)*

41. **(A)** Croup and epiglottitis have similar presentations but need to be distinguished immediately. Croup usually results from a viral infection of the larynx and epiglottitis from a bacterial (*H. influenzae* type B) infection of the epiglottis. Children with epiglottitis tend to be toxic in appearance. Croup involves the airway, and epiglottitis involves the airway and the digestive tract. Children with croup usually will swallow and drink. Children with epiglottitis most often will refuse to drink and may even drool as a result of their refusal to swallow saliva. Patients with foreign bodies in their upper airways do not typically have fever. Patients with vascular rings and laryngeal tumors have more gradual onset of symptoms. *(McMillan et al., pp. 572, 1310)*

42. **(D)** Iron deficiency is the most common cause of microcytic anemia. In children it is often related to excessive consumption of cow's milk, which is low in iron content, and inadequate consumption of iron-rich foods. Allergy to cow's milk may also cause occult gastrointestinal blood losses. In thalassemia major, there is usually physical evidence of chronic anemia with signs of bone marrow expansion (frontal bossing) and severe anemia often requiring transfusions. Lead poisoning may cause microcytic anemias; it may also be associated with iron-deficiency anemia, which enhances lead absorption and, therefore, should always be excluded. Anemia of chronic disease (renal disease) may be microcytic or normocytic and should be excluded by history and examination. *(Behrman et al., pp. 1469–1471)*

43. (E) If iron deficiency is strongly suspected, it is reasonable to treat empirically with 3–6 mg/kg/day of elemental iron. An increase in hemoglobin of 1 g/dL within 2–4 weeks confirms the diagnosis. If laboratory confirmation is necessary because the child is at low risk for iron deficiency, confirmatory iron studies may be obtained. The serum iron is low, the total iron binding capacity high, and the ferritin is low. A reticulocyte count is helpful in hemolytic anemias where it is elevated. Bone marrow aspirate in iron deficiency is necessary if bone marrow infiltration is suspected (leukemia), but is overinvasive in this situation. Hemoglobin electrophoresis may be done if thalassemia or sickle cell anemia is likely. *(Behrman et al., pp. 1469–1471)*

44. (B) Neonates are routinely given intramuscular vitamin K at the time of birth. This is done to prevent the transient deficiency of vitamin-K-dependent factors, which occurs because of absence of bacterial intestinal flora which synthesize vitamin K. Hemorrhagic disease in the newborn because of vitamin K deficiency may result in gastrointestinal, nasal, subgaleal, and intracranial bleeding, or bleeding after circumcision. The prothrombin time (PT), partial thromboplastin time (PTT), and bleeding time are prolonged. These all correct after administration of vitamin K. Child abuse should always be considered with unusual bleeding, but the history reveals the etiology in this case. Babies are more likely to be allergic to formula than breast milk; however, it occurs rarely and may present with bloody stools. It does not, however, cause epistaxis. Neonatal sepsis may result in disseminated intravascular coagulation and bleeding; the infant is usually ill appearing, with associated acidosis or shock. Liver disease may cause factor deficiencies and should be excluded if there is no response to vitamin K. *(Behrman et al., pp. 526–527)*

45. (A) Precocious puberty has been redefined for girls as the presence of either pubic hair or breast development before age 6 for Blacks and age 7 for Whites. Premature thelarche is the isolated development of breasts, with no other secondary sexual development. Premature pubarche is the isolated development of pubic or axillary hair (sexual hair). Precocious menarche is a rare form of incomplete precocious puberty with cyclic menstruation but no other secondary sexual characteristics. *(Behrman et al., pp. 1688–1694; Kaplowitz and Oberfield, pp. 936–941)*

46. (A) The laboratory and radiologic studies indicate a form of central precocious puberty. It is most likely to be idiopathic; however, imaging of the head as well as a careful neurologic and visual examination is recommended to exclude a CNS lesion (tumor, trauma, hamartoma, and so forth). Estradiol secreting ovarian tumors and functional ovarian cysts may cause peripheral precocious puberty; however, the levels of FSH and LH are prepubertal. Congenital adrenal hyperplasia results in signs of virilization; these include excessive hirsuitism, deepening voice, acne, clitoromegaly, and muscle development. *(Behrman et al., pp. 1688–1694; Miller and Styne, 1999)*

47. (E) The symptoms are suggestive of perennial allergic rhinitis. Causative agents are usually those to which the child is exposed year round, such as house dust, mold spores, or pet danders. Seasonal allergic rhinitis is attributable to sensitization to pollens of trees, grasses, and weeds. Nasal foreign bodies usually result in a foul smelling, unilateral purulent, and occasionally blood tinged, discharge. Recurrent infections may rarely be attributable to immunologic deficiencies. Recurrent pneumonias are the most common complaint. Rhinitis medicamentosa occurs secondary to excessive use of vasoconstrictor nose drops or sprays, resulting in rebound nasal obstruction. Sinusitis is suggested by a bilateral purulent nasal discharge, often accompanied by fever, cough, headache, and sometimes sinus tenderness. *(Behrman et al., pp. 662–663)*

48. (E) Cyanosis in newborn infants is associated with major right-to-left shunts. Total anomalous pulmonary venous return results in a right-to-left shunting through an interatrial communication, usually a patent foramen ovale. Patent ductus arteriosus and atrial septal defect, when unaccompanied by other cardiovascular abnormalities, cause left-to-right shunts that do not produce cyanosis. Coarctation of the aorta does not typically cause symptoms in the newborn. Hypoplastic left heart presents with signs of failure in the newborn period. *(Rudolph et al., pp. 1774, 1800–1833)*

49. (B) Parasomnias or disorders of arousal include nightmares, night terrors, sleep walking (somnambulism), and sleep talking (somniloquy). This pattern suggests night terrors and is most common between ages 2 and 6 years. Nightmares occur at any age but peak between ages 3 and 5 years; they occur later in the night during rapid eye movement (REM) sleep. The child usually remembers the dream vividly, is upset on waking, but can be comforted by the parent. Sleep walking occurs, as do night terrors, during non-REM sleep. It is most common between ages 4 and 8 years; safety of the child is the main concern. Sleep talking is not specific to any stage of sleep and may occur in association with nightmares and night terrors. Narcolepsy is a rare disorder characterized by excessive daytime sleepiness. Confirmation requires referral to a sleep laboratory. *(Behrman et al., pp. 16, 74)*

50. (A) *P. multicoda* and *S. aureus* are organisms commonly associated with cat bites. The cat's sharp teeth and claws predispose the victim to puncture wounds. Wound infections are more common in cat bites than dog bites. *E. corrodens*, *Peptostreptococcus* species, and alpha Streptococci are more common with human bites. *B. henselae* causes cat-scratch disease, which presents with subacute lymphadenitis. *(Kliegman et al., pp. 973–975, 866–867)*

51. (A) The case presented is classic of pyloric stenosis. This results from hypertrophy and hyperplasia of smooth muscle in the stomach, causing a narrowed, even, obstructed outlet. Persistent projectile vomiting causes ongoing losses of calories and electrolytes, resulting in growth failure and hypochloremic metabolic alkalosis. Hyponatremia and hypokalemia may also be associated. Often, the diagnosis can be made by physical examination alone. However, if an olive-shaped mass is not palpated, an abdominal ultrasound may confirm the diagnosis. *(Behrman et al., pp. 1130–1131)*

52. (C) Diaper dermatitis is a very common problem in infants. The infant's rash is due to *Candida*. *Candida* dermatitis is red, without bullae, and has satellite lesions at the margins. It is common in infants, especially when they have been on antibiotics. In bullous impetigo, the skin is initially erythematous and then bullae develop. Allergic dermatitis and irritant dermatitis are the most prominent on the convex areas and are intensely red. In seborrheic dermatitis, children tend to have the rash on the scalp, neck, and face also. It is scaly and more prominent in the intertriginous areas. *(Hurwitz, pp. 34–38)*

53. (A) This is a typical presentation of chickenpox. A prodrome of fever and malaise is followed by the rapid eruption of papules that turn to vesicles and crust over. The rash in measles, rubella, and Kawasaki disease are macular or maculopapular. In staphylococcal scalded skin syndrome, a diffuse, tender erythroderma develops. *(Behrman et al., pp. 973–977)*

54. (E) This is a "round pneumonia," most commonly caused by *S. pneumoniae*. Onset of this disease is relatively acute. *H. influenzae* type B is an uncommon cause of systemic infections because of routine immunization. *Mycoplasma* is the most common cause of community-acquired pneumonia in this age group. Patients typically have a more gradual onset of symptoms. *Pneumocystis* does not cause pneumonia in otherwise healthy children. *S. aureus* can cause pneumonia in healthy children, but it is not as common as *S. pneumoniae* or *Mycoplasma*. *(McMillan et al., pp. 1227–1230)*

55. (A) The child most likely has hemolytic-uremic syndrome. This illness is most common in children under 2 years old. They present with a prodromal illness, bloody diarrhea, and then a sudden onset of lethargy and pallor when the hemolytic anemia occurs. Coincident with this is the development of acute renal failure, often with low urine output. *E. coli* 0157:H7 is the most common organism in this country. Group A Streptococci are associated with poststreptococcal acute glomerulonephritis. Thrombocytopenia and anemia are not seen in this disease. *(Rudolph et al., pp. 1696–1698)*

56. (B) Varicella vaccine is a live vaccine. All others are killed vaccines. Diphtheria and tetanus are both toxoids, the others are from killed microorganisms. *(American Academy of Pediatrics, 2000a, pp. 7–8, 632)*

57. (D) Progressive, symmetric motor weakness, areflexia, and autonomic instability, with mild or absent sensory signs, are typical features of Guillain–Barré syndrome. Frequently, there is a history of infection (often respiratory) in the several weeks preceding clinical onset of the syndrome. Supportive evidence for the diagnosis includes elevation of CSF protein concentration with a mild (10 or fewer cells/mL) mononuclear pleocytosis, and slowing of nerve conduction velocities. In polymyositis, deep tendon reflexes would be intact. Myasthenia gravis is characterized by weakness aggravated by repetitive movement. In transverse myelitis, sensation would also be lost. Viral encephalitis is characterized by mental status abnormalities. *(McMillan et al., pp. 1962–1963)*

58. (C) The CDC has identified lead poisoning as one of the most common and preventable childhood health problems in the United States. Recent data indicate that undesirable behavioral and cognitive deficits can occur at levels previously thought to be "safe." Screening all children aged 6–72 months, by questionnaire or blood-lead level, is suggested. Children at greatest risk for lead poisoning include young inner-city children who live in housing constructed before 1960; children living near lead processing smelters, battery recycling plants, or other industries that release lead; or children with siblings or playmates diagnosed with lead poisoning. Eliminating the lead source is the cornerstone of treatment. Chelation therapy generally is reserved for those children with blood-lead levels greater than 45 mcg/dL. *(CDC, pp. 51–65; Committee on Drugs, pp. 155–160)*

59. (D) In 1997, the expanded use of IPV in the United States began. Before this, the risk of vaccine-associated paralytic polio was 1 case per 2.4 million doses of oral polio vaccine (OPV); the rate after the first dose was 1 per 750,000 doses, including vaccine recipient and contact cases. This is the main disadvantage of the OPV vaccine. Although it is contraindicated in children or their contacts with immunodeficiencies, they are at high risk in case of inadvertent exposure, because there is feco-oral transmission of the virus for 4–6 weeks after the vaccine is given. The advantages of the OPV include lower cost, fewer "shots," and boosting herd immunity. The OPV vaccine is still recommended for global polio eradication. *(American Academy of Pediatrics, 2000a, pp. 467–470)*

60. (C) Aspirin and antihistamines have been shown to adversely affect platelet aggregation, leading to increased bleeding time. Moreover, this effect may persist for 7–10 days after discontinuing these medications. When possible, children undergoing surgery should not be receiving aspirin or antihistamines. The use of antibiotics would not be a contraindication to elective surgery. Children undergoing elective surgery should be free of respiratory infection. It is prudent to counsel the parents in ways to minimize infection, but avoiding social contacts and shared eating utensils would likely have little effect in the case described in the question. A child should be free of anemia before elective surgery, but eating iron-rich foods would not significantly elevate Hb in a short period of time. *(Rudolph et al., pp. 1244–1245; Champion et al., p. 335, 1559)*

61. (C) The most common causes of hypertension in young children are renal in origin. Polycystic kidney disease, congenital vascular anomalies, tumors, and infections all are causes. Urologic evaluation is imperative for the child described in the question. Theophylline toxicity that is severe enough to elevate BP significantly would be unlikely in the absence of jitteriness, nausea, or tachycardia. Chronic lung disease would not elevate the systemic BP in an otherwise healthy child. Coarctation of the aorta is a less common cause of hypertension in this age group. BPs taken on all extremities would be helpful in the diagnosis. *(Rudolph et al., p. 1879)*

62. (D) This case most likely represents an adolescent with meningitis who has developed increased intracranial pressure. Intubation and hyperventilation is indicated immediately. Hyperventilation is the most appropriate immediate, nonsurgical treatment of intracranial hypertension. By hyperventilating this patient, you will decrease the PCO_2, resulting in vasoconstriction in the CNS. Decreasing the PCO_2 5–10 mmHg will decrease intracranial pressure 25–30%. Administering antibiotics, preferably after blood cultures are obtained, is appropriate. Obtaining a CT scan of the head may reveal intracranial lesions which require additional therapy. Mannitol given intravenously also is a highly effective means for lowering intracranial pressure. Mannitol does not cross the blood-brain barrier.

It remains in the capillaries and creates an osmotic gradient, causing fluid to shift from intracellular spaces to the vasculature, thereby decreasing intracranial pressure. Although a lumbar puncture may be necessary eventually, it is contraindicated as initial management because of the possibility of brain stem herniation. *(McMillan et al., pp. 861–862)*

63. (D) The presence of a congenital membranous or bony septum between the nose and pharynx is called choanal atresia. Most newborns are obligatory nose breathers and breathe effectively only through their noses. Therefore, if choanal obstruction is unilateral, breathing difficulty may not occur until the first respiratory infection. On the other hand, those newborns with bilateral atresia who are also obligatory nose breathers will make vigorous attempts to inspire with sucking in of their lips, or may promptly become apneic and cyanotic, requiring resuscitation. Those who are able to mouth breathe may have difficulty when feeding or manifest persistent mouth breathing and cyanosis that is relieved by crying. Treatment consists of surgical correction. *(Rudolph et al., pp. 202, 1260)*

64. (D) Absolute contraindications to use of DTP/DTaP include history of anaphylactic reaction to the vaccine or history of encephalopathy. The following are precautions. These circumstances should be carefully reviewed, and if vaccine benefits outweigh the risks, the vaccine should be given. Precautions include any of the following after a prior dose of DTP/DTaP: temperature of >40.5°C within 48 h; collapse or shock-like state (hypotonic-hyporesponsive episode) within 48 h; seizures within 3 days; persistent inconsolable crying lasting 3 h within 48 h. Moderate or severe illness with or without a fever may be considered a precaution; however, a mild illness, such as an upper respiratory infection, is not a contraindication. Low-grade fevers and local reactions are common and are not contraindications; nor are antibiotic therapy or a family history of seizures. *(American Academy of Pediatrics, 2000a, pp. 755–758)*

65. (C) In patients with a clean, minor wound, Td vaccine is required if the patient has had <3 tetanus vaccinations or if the immunization status is unknown. In contaminated wounds (dirt, feces, soil, and saliva), puncture wound, avulsions, and wounds resulting from missiles, crushing, burns and frostbite, TIG and Td should be given. The DTaP vaccination is not recommended in children aged 7 or older because the DTaP produces more severe reactions in older children. Waiting for immunization records is not appropriate in an emergency situation. *(American Academy of Pediatrics, 2000a, pp. 565–568)*

66. (D) Children with sickle cell disease develop functional asplenia, presumably from repeated splenic infarction. This results in vulnerability to bacteremia and overwhelming infection, especially with encapsulated bacteria. The organism most commonly involved is *S. pneumoniae*. Daily prophylactic oral penicillin is indicated for young children. Because of the risk of bacteremia, these patients need careful medical evaluation when they develop fever. There are no data to support the use of gamma globulin in these children. They are not at higher risk for complications from live virus vaccines or from varicella. *(Rudolph et al., p. 1561)*

67. (E) Varicella vaccine should not be routinely given to children with T-lymphocyte deficiency, including lymphoma, leukemia, neoplasms affecting the bone marrow or lymphatic systems, and congenital T-cell abnormalities. One exception is children with ALL, in continuous remission for at least 1 year, with a lymphocyte count >700/mcL and a platelet count >100 × 10^3/mcL. Another exception is HIV-infected children in CDC class 1. These children are at increased risk of morbidity from varicella and herpes zoster; therefore, the benefits outweigh the risks in these limited circumstances. Children receiving high doses of steroids should not receive the vaccine. This is defined as >2 mg/kg/day of prednisone or its equivalent, or 20 mg/day, if their weight is >10 kg, for 14 days or more. The vaccine may be given a month after discontinuation of the therapy. *(American Academy of Pediatrics, 2000a, pp. 636–638)*

68. (C) Mild illness is not a contraindication to vaccination, nor is breast-feeding. Such live vaccines as MMR and varicella are not recommended for pregnant women, but may be safely given to their children. They are also not recommended in many immunocompromised children; however, it is recommended that household contacts receive the vaccinations to decrease the patient's chances of exposure. It is not necessary to restart a vaccine series if there has been a long gap between immunizations. *(American Academy of Pediatrics, 2000a, pp. 54–64)*

69. (E) The most common causes of neonatal cholestasis are extrahepatic biliary atresia and idiopathic neonatal hepatitis. Infants usually develop icterus by 2–6 weeks of age. They have conjugated hyperbilirubinemia, dark urine, and acholic stools. At time of presentation, there is usually hepatomegaly, as well as pruritis, splenomegaly, and ascites. The use of RhoGAM (anti-D gamma globulin) has reduced the incidence of Rh sensitization and resulting jaundice. ABO incompatibility can also cause a milder form of isoimmune hemolytic disease and jaundice. It is more common in infants with blood types A and B born to mothers with blood type O. Anemia is usually present; direct Coombs' test is weakly positive; and indirect Coombs' test is positive. Crigler–Najjar syndrome is autosomal recessive; there is usually marked hyperbilirubinemia (2–40 mg/dL) in an otherwise asymptomatic infant. The high levels result in kernicterus. Physiologic jaundice is the most common cause of unconjugated hyperbilirubinemia; it is characterized by peak bilirubin level of < 13 mg/dL on day of life 3–5, decrease to normal by 2 weeks. In breast-fed infants, this is often exaggerated, with levels >13 mg/dL. This occurs in 10–25% of breast-fed infants, as opposed to 4–7% of formula-fed infants. It is known as "breast-feeding" jaundice. "Breast-milk" jaundice, develops after the first week of life, peaking between the 2nd and 3rd week to 10–20 mg/dL. The cause of this has not been established. *(Kliegman et al., pp. 364–366)*

70. (C) Hypocalcemia is not a cause of constipation. On the contrary, it increases irritability of nerve cells and may result in diarrhea. Hypothyroidism, lead poisoning, and Hirschsprung disease all may be associated with constipation. Congenital hypothyroidism and Hirschsprung disease (a congenital disorder characterized by regional absence of ganglion cells from the myenteric plexus of the colon) present at birth. Lead poisoning is more common after the child becomes mobile. Functional constipation is the most common cause of constipation at this age. It is usually due to dietary factors. *(Behrman et al., pp. 1105, 1140)*

71. (A) Otitis externa is an infection of the external ear canal. Predisposing factors include excessive wetness (swimming), dryness (lack of protective cerumen), trauma (foreign body), and other skin pathology (eczema). It is characterized by pain, accentuated by moving the pinna and especially the tragus; edema and inflammation of the canal; and discharge. Furuncles usually cause a localized swelling or papule in the hair-bearing part of the canal. If the tympanic membrane is not visualized, otitis media is hard to differentiate from otitis externa. Otitis media does not cause pain with movement of the pinna. In severe otitis externa, the periauricular edema may push the pinna forward; this may be confused with mastoiditis.

In mastoiditis, however, the postauricular fold is usually obliterated. There is often a history of otitis media and hearing loss and tenderness over the mastoid antrum. *(Behrman et al., pp. 1948–1949)*

72. **(D)** *P. aeruginosa* is the most common agent involved in external otitis. The other organisms listed may also be isolated. *(Behrman et al., pp. 1948–1949)*

73. **(E)** The characteristics of fetal alcohol syndrome include: (a) persistent deficient growth affecting weight, height, and head circumference and beginning *in utero*; (b) such facial abnormalities as micrognathia, short palpebral fissures, and a thin upper lip; (c) cardiac abnormalities, commonly septal defects; (d) minor limb abnormalities with some restriction of mobility and some alteration in palmar crease patterns; and (e) mental deficiency ranging from mild to severe. There is a decided relationship between the extent of abnormalities and the degree of mental retardation. Affected infants may present with hypoglycemia and alcohol withdrawal symptoms which may last for 48–72 h. Immediate management of these infants consists of correction of the hypoglycemia. Ongoing monitoring of the child's development is essential. Prevention by restriction of alcohol consumption during pregnancy is advised. *(Rudolph et al., pp. 715–728)*

74. **(D)** Meningococcemia is a fulminant systemic rapidly progressing infection that results in shock and is followed by death in 20% of afflicted children. The presence of meningitis has been shown to increase the survival rate to approximately 95%. Sensorineural deafness is the most common residual following bacterial meningitis. Penicillin, ampicillin, or a third-generation cephalosporin would be an appropriate antibiotic to choose for treatment. Vancomycin's spectrum of activity is limited to gram-positive organisms. *(McMillan et al., pp. 982–983)*

75. **(D)** In the management of foreign body aspiration, it is generally felt that if the victim can speak, breathe, or cough, all interventions are unnecessary and potentially dangerous. When intervention is required, the first maneuver is a series of abdominal thrusts (for children >1 year of age) or back blows (for children 1 year of age or younger). When obstruction persists, foreign bodies sometimes can be removed from the oral cavity or pharynx if they can be seen, but blind finger sweeps of the hypopharynx are not recommended. Emergency tracheostomy, preferably performed by an experienced clinician, is employed only in cases of critical airway obstruction unrelieved by other maneuvers. *(McMillan et al., pp. 639–640)*

76. **(D)** Adducted great toe, metatarsus adductus, medial tibial torsion, and femoral anteversion can result in intoeing. In most cases, this is a benign condition that requires only observation. In this child, because the child's knees are straight, the rotational deformity is below this joint. In metatarsus adductus, the forefoot is adducted as compared to the hindfoot. Idiopathic avascular juvenile necrosis of the femoral head, or Legg–Calvé–Perthes disease, most commonly is seen in 4- to 8-year-old boys. Loss of hip medial rotation is an early sign. *(Staheli, pp. 30–35)*

77. **(C)** Idiopathic scoliosis is the most common back deformity in children. The incidence peaks in early adolescence and is much more common in girls. Screening for scoliosis should be part of every well check and sports physical in children at Tanner (II–V) stages. Congenital scoliosis is caused by failure of formation or fusion of the ossific nuclei of the vertebrae. It can present at any age, depending on the degree of curvature, and is much less common than idiopathic scoliosis. Patients with leg length inequality present with a limp. Patients with Scheuermann kyphosis usually present with back pain and have a sharp kyphotic angulation with forward bending. Postural roundback is an exaggerated kyphotic appearance often seen in adolescents. *(Rudolph et al., pp. 1241–1243)*

78. **(C)** Whooping cough, or pertussis, tends to have a prolonged course, with a 2-week prodrome of

undifferentiated upper respiratory infection followed by approximately 2 weeks of a paroxysmal, machine gun-like cough and nasopharyngeal mucus that is strangling, thick, and clear. The typical whoop, a stridorous inspiratory gasp at the end of each paroxysm, is often absent in infants younger than 6 months. Posttussive vomiting more likely will be found in this age group. The diagnosis should be suspected in children with a paroxysmal, harsh cough and absolute lymphocytosis. Specific inquiry into the history of a severe or long-lasting cough in adult caretakers should be sought. The diagnosis is made by culture of the organism (*Bordetella pertussis*) or by an immunofluorescent study of throat swab material. Erythromycin is the drug of choice. It has little effect on the illness course after paroxysms are established and is used primarily to limit spread of infection to others. *(American Academy of Pediatrics, 2000a, pp. 435–448)*

79. **(D)** Turner syndrome (usually 45,XO karyotype) occurs in 1 of 3000 live births. The hallmark of this genetic disease is gonadal dysgenesis. Although sexual maturation usually does not occur, a girl with Turner syndrome occasionally will have menstrual periods but rarely will be fertile. Treatment may include estrogen replacement or growth hormone usage. Psychosocial support is extremely important. *(McMillan et al., pp. 1775, 2231)*

80. **(E)** The child described in the question seems to be afflicted with infant botulism. *Clostridium botulinum* spores are commonly found in honey, and the toxin responsible for the symptoms described is produced in the infant's gastrointestinal tract. Therefore, children younger than 1 year should not be fed honey. Hypernatremic dehydration may show some similarities to infant botulism, but the skin and mucous membranes are characteristically dry. Serum sodium level is often greater than 160. Hirschsprung disease would explain constipation but not the other findings listed. Congenital hypothyroidism shows a more insidious onset, with prolonged constipation and weakness. In addition, developmental retardation would likely be present. *(Rudolph et al., pp. 917–918)*

81. **(B)** Cow's milk allergy may occur in 2–3% of infants and toddlers. After elimination from the diet, by age 3, 85% no longer have symptoms on food challenge. Older children and adults may also lose sensitivity to an offending food when it is eliminated from the diet for 1–2 years. The exceptions are IgE-mediated allergies to peanuts, nuts, fish, or shellfish. *(Behrman et al., pp. 1158–1159)*

82. **(C)** Infectious mononucleosis may affect children of all ages. The rapid slide (Monospot) test response is positive in approximately 90% of infected persons; however, younger children with mononucleosis may have a negative result. Moreover, many younger children have poor antibody response to the heterophil titer test. The specific serodiagnostic test for EBV, the agent responsible for most cases of infectious mononucleosis, confirms the diagnosis. A repeat throat culture, even if positive for beta-hemolytic *Streptococcus*, may be of only partial value, because both infectious mononucleosis and streptococcal pharyngitis may be present simultaneously. Bone marrow examinations potentially are painful and contribute little to the correct diagnosis. *(McMillan et al., pp. 1107–1112)*

83. **(B)** Organophosphate poisoning is a leading cause of fatal ingestions of nonpharmaceutical compounds. Common components of insecticides, organophosphates are readily absorbed across skin and mucous membranes. They bind irreversibly to cholinesterase, which results in prolongation of the effects of acetylcholine, centrally and peripherally. Symptoms include muscle fasciculations, paralysis (nicotinic effect) and miosis, salivation, diarrhea, bradycardia, lacrimation (muscarinic effect) and obtundation, seizures, or apnea (central effect). Acetaminophen ingestion can present with vomiting and then later signs of liver failure if it is severe enough. Patients with salicylate overdose present with hypoglycemia, respiratory alkalosis followed by metabolic acidosis, hypokalemia, and mental status changes.

Tricyclic antidepressants poisoning causes arrhythmias, mental status changes, and anticholinergic symptoms. Patients with acute vitamin A toxicity have mental status changes, nausea, and vomiting. *(Ellenhorn, pp. 184, 210–219, 622, 1021, 1615)*

84. (E) Nursemaid's elbow, or subluxation of the radial head, occurs in children following longitudinal traction on a pronated extended elbow. When attempting to restrain a child, an uninformed caretaker may jerk on a child's upper extremity. The result is a painful subluxed elbow that is easily reduced by simultaneous flexion and supination of the forearm. *(McMillan et al., p. 2123)*

85. (E) Nontuberculous lymphadenitis (atypical mycobacteria) is characterized by nontender lymphadenitis. Affected persons are usually afebrile, and the CBC is usually normal. Unlike tuberculous lymphadenitis, a history of contact with a tuberculous individual is lacking, and the reaction to 5 tuberculin units of purified protein derivative is almost always less than 10 mm of induration. Cat-scratch fever is characterized by tender, fluctuating nodes and low-grade fever. Acute lymphadenitis is characterized by tender nodes that may fluctuate. The WBC count is often elevated, and there is frequently a shift to the left on the differential. In addition, the sufferer is often febrile. Acute lymphoblastic leukemia may present as lymphadenitis, but the CBC is usually abnormal, with blasts present on the peripheral smear. *(Feigin and Cherry, pp. 220–230, 1085–1086, 1354–1356)*

86. (D) Vesicoureteral reflux is the most common anatomic abnormality associated with recurrent urinary tract infection in children. Many cases of reflux are the result of an inadequate length of submucosal ureter immediately proximal to its opening into the bladder lumen, a condition that sometimes requires surgical correction. However, in other children, reflux often seems to result from the direct effects of infection on ureteral tone and peristalsis. Thus, many children may outgrow mild degrees of reflux if they are maintained on prophylactic antibiotics. Moderate-to-severe degrees of reflux frequently require surgery. Failure of adequate antibiotic treatment to prevent infection is also a prime indication for surgery. Repeating an IVP or performing a renal arteriogram on an already diagnosed case would not be useful, although a radionuclide scan may be very helpful to determine the present degree of reflux with a minimum of radiation exposure. Vitamin C, although reportedly useful in acidifying the urine to help prevent infection, does not enhance adequate antibiotic prophylaxis. IV antibiotics would be necessary only if oral antibiotics were not successful in eradicating infection. *(Rudolph et al., pp. 1671–1672)*

87. (B) Hirschprung disease or congenital aganglionic megacolon is the most common cause of lower intestinal obstruction in neonates. Incidence is 1/5000 live births; males are four times as likely to be affected. Initial presentation is with delayed passage of meconium. Failure to pass stools leads to dilation of proximal bowel and abdominal distention. Diagnosis is by barium enema which reveals a small-caliber rectum with transition in the rectosigmoid to a dilated, obstructed proximal colon. Diagnosis is confirmed by biopsy. Meconium plugs and meconium ileus are often found in cystic fibrosis, which should be excluded. Anal stenosis may be diagnosed by rectal examination or endoscopy. Functional constipation usually presents in children older than 2 years. There may be some abdominal distention; anal tone is usually normal, and the rectal ampulla is often full of stool. Congenital hypothyroidism may present with constipation; neonatal screening tests usually allow early diagnosis. Other features include feeding difficulties, prolonged jaundice, sluggishness, a large abdomen with umbilical hernia, subnormal body temperature, myxedema, and developmental delay. *(Behrman et al., pp. 1139–1141; Kliegman et al., pp. 576–578)*

88. (A) Children with more severe cases of hypospadias have an increased incidence of concomitant urinary tract anomalies and require careful evaluation. Ultrasonography is a safe and noninvasive procedure that is sensitive in the diagnosis of neonatal urinary tract pathology. It is a better choice than either IVP or cystography which use contrast media and radiation. Serum creatinine determinations are a measure of renal function and are unnecessary in an otherwise healthy child. Circumcision is not indicated in children with hypospadias. In fact, it may be contraindicated in cases of second- or third-degree hypospadias, in which the prepuce can be used to construct an absent distal segment of urethra. *(Rudolph et al., p. 1739)*

89. **(E)** Transplacental passage of *T. pallidum* causes widespread disease in the fetus. Organs most severely affected include brain, bone, liver, and lung. Hepatosplenomegaly, rare in neonates with GBS or HSV infections, occurs in 90% of neonates with congenital syphilis. Mucocutaneous lesions produce a persistent, purulent, often bloody nasal discharge which is termed snuffles. This nasal discharge is highly infectious. Skin rash is uncommon in CMV and GBS infections. The acral distribution described is characteristic of congenital syphilis. Congenital toxoplasmosis characteristically presents with neurologic abnormalities. The classic triad includes hydrocephalus, chorioretinitis, and diffuse intracranial calcifications. *(McMillan et al., pp. 438–440)*

90. **(C)** Roseola infantum, or sixth disease, is a common acute illness of young children. Human herpesvirus 6 is the most common etiologic agent. The rash of erythema infectiosum presents initially on the face. It is intensely red with a "slapped-cheek" appearance. Rubella and measles are not commonly seen because of routine vaccination. The rash of scarlet fever is on the trunk and is described as sandpaper like. *(Feigin and Cherry, pp. 1789–1791)*

91. **(D)** Simple febrile seizures are common in children between ages 6 months and 5 years. They are usually brief, with bilateral clonic or tonic-clonic movement. They have a 30% likelihood of recurrence. The investigation should include a search for the cause of the fever, usually a viral infection, urinary tract infection, or following immunization. A lumbar puncture must be performed if there is suspicion of an intracranial infection and when features of the seizure suggest a focal or lateralized seizure. In these situations, EEG and imaging may also be considered. However, in most children with uncomplicated febrile seizures, these procedures are unnecessary. There is an increased risk for developing epilepsy in later life, as high as 7% in a study with mean follow-up of 18 years. When risk factors are present, the incidence of epilepsy rises to 49%. Risk factors include prior neurologic abnormality, prolonged seizures (>30 min), focal or lateralized seizure, and repeated seizure within 24 h. *(Kliegman et al., pp. 687–688)*

92. **(B)** This is the classic presentation of splenic sequestration which occurs in these patients in the first few years of life, before the spleen autoinfarcts. This often occurs following an acute febrile illness. Blood pools in the spleen, which becomes enlarged; signs of circulatory collapse may develop. In an aplastic crisis, a very low reticulocyte count would be expected, and there is no such splenic enlargement. *(Behrman et al., pp. 1478–1483)*

93. **(D)** Acute sickle dactylitis or hand-foot syndrome is often the earliest clinical syndrome seen in children with sickle cell anemia. There is painful, symmetrical swelling of the hands and feet. Roentgenograms usually reveal bony destruction only in the later phase, 1–2 weeks later. *(Behrman et al., pp. 1478–1483)*

94. **(F)** Acute painful episodes are the most common manifestation of sickle cell disease. Most patients experience some pain nearly daily. In younger children, this usually involves the extremities. In older children, head, chest, abdomen, and back pain may occur. *(Behrman et al., pp. 1478–1483)*

95. **(D)** Silver nitrate, the traditional prophylactic treatment for the neonate's eyes, is very effective against gonorrheal ophthalmitis. These drops are not effective against the most common cause of neonatal conjunctivitis, *C. trachomatis*, which requires erythromycin or tetracycline for eradication. Silver nitrate is commonly associated with the sterile purulent discharge of chemical conjunctivitis. HSV can cause neonatal conjunctivitis, but its occurrence on the first day of life would be unusual. *Pseudomonas* conjunctivitis generally is hospital acquired, occurring in ill infants receiving mechanical ventilation. Nasolacrimal duct obstruction is a transient structural anomaly that may be accompanied by persistent tearing and occasional purulent discharge. The condition is usually unilateral and clears within 6–9 months after birth. Rarely, duct probing or surgery is necessary because of persistent stenosis beyond 1 year of age or for repeated infections. *(McMillan et al., p. 670)*

96. (A) Nontypeable *H. influenzae*, *S. pneumoniae*, and *M. catarrhalis* are the most common bacterial pathogens in otitis media of children. *S. aureus*, *E. coli*, and group A Streptococci each account for 2% or less of all cases of otitis media in children beyond the neonatal period. *Mycoplasma* is thought to be an uncommon cause of otitis media. *(McMillan et al., pp. 1301–1304)*

97. (E) Most cases of idiopathic thrombocytopenic purpura (ITP) in children are preceded by viral infections and, in contrast to adults, the great majority of children recover spontaneously. Although not all patients require therapy, most authorities suggest treating when the platelet count is less than 20,000. Standard treatment has been oral prednisone. Recently, IV gamma globulin has been shown to be effective. However, this agent is expensive and less convenient than oral prednisone. The child described in the question might reasonably be treated with either agent. Because the child's Hb is 13.3 g/100 mL, there is no indication for transfusion of RBCs. Although the platelet count is very low, platelet transfusions are short lived and generally are indicated only in the presence of serious bleeding, as, for example, from the GI tract. Thus, platelet transfusions are not indicated in this patient. Splenectomy is reserved for the very rare child who does not respond to conservative therapy or who develops chronic ITP. *(Rudolph et al., pp. 1556–1557; Kliegman et al., pp. 917–918)*

98. (D) Intussusception, or telescoping of the bowel into a more distal section of bowel, is the most common cause of intestinal obstruction in infants aged 3–12 months. The case presented represents the classic presentation. Giardiasis presents less acutely and would not be associated with a mass. In gastroenteritis, frequent loose stools without blood would be the major symptom. Diaphragmatic hernia occurs in newborns, and the major symptom is respiratory distress. Although appendicitis can occur in infants, it is very unusual. *(McMillan et al., pp. 1652–1654)*

99. (E) Many healthy children have intermittent proteinuria. Transient proteinuria may occur with fever, strenuous exercise, and cold exposure. Testing for hematuria and RBCs and casts should be done. BP should also be checked. When proteinuria is intermittent and not accompanied by hematuria, chronic renal disease is unusual. A child who has proteinuria on a single specimen, thus, will need repeated urinalyses. If isolated proteinuria is present in three consecutive urinalyses, testing for orthostatic proteinuria should be considered. If this test is negative, qualitative measurement of proteinuria can confirm the diagnosis (>4 mg/m^2/h) and further evaluation may be considered. If proteinuria remains intermittent, most physicians do not perform invasive procedures such as a biopsy. Proteinuria alone is unlikely to be an indicator of urinary tract infection or structural kidney disease; thus, an IVP and renal ultrasound are unlikely to be helpful. Likewise, with isolated and intermittent proteinuria as the only abnormality, electrolytes, BUN, and creatinine levels are highly unlikely to be abnormal. *(Kliegman et al., pp. 413–420)*

100. (A) Patients with persistent otitis media after 5 days of amoxicillin likely have resistant *S. pneumoniae*, or a beta-lactamase-positive *M. catarrhalis* or *H. influenzae*. Cephalexin, erythromycin, dicloxacillin, and penicillin would not cover the beta-lactamase-positive organisms. Some would recommend that the patient would benefit from a higher dose of the amoxicillin component in the combination antibiotic to provide better coverage for resistant *S. pneumoniae*. *(Behrman et al., pp. 1950–1959)*

101. (A) Constitutional delay is a normal pattern of growth, characterized by a relatively late pubertal growth spurt. It is recognized most commonly in boys. Patients typically show a moderate degree of short stature in early to middle childhood. The growth pattern is often similar to one or both parents. Final adult height is within the expected genetic potential. The children are otherwise well. Familial short stature is also a normal growth pattern in a short but otherwise normal family. One or both parents are typically 1–2 standard deviations below mean height for adults. The growth pattern parallels the normal growth curve at a percentile consistent with genetic potential. Deprivational dwarfism is due to psychosocial factors. It typically presents at a younger age, and weight is affected more than the height so that these children are not proportionately small. Hypothyroidism can affect growth but would cause a decrease in growth velocity when it occurred. The patient's height curve would flatten out, instead of paralleling the normal curves. Short stature from growth hormone deficiency typically presents by 3 years. *(Kliegman et al., pp. 1096–1097)*

102. (E) Given that this is a classic case of constitutional growth delay, no diagnostic studies are indicated. Close monitoring of growth would be indicated. A bone age, if performed, would be less than chronologic age, demonstrating the growth potential for the patient. Cranial imaging would be indicated if the patient had evidence for onset of secondary hypopituitarism. *(Kliegman et al., pp. 1096–1097)*

103. (B) Chest pain in adolescents is a common problem. It is rarely associated with serious illness. In this patient, with onset with exercise, resolution with rest, and a family history of asthma, exercise-induced asthma is the most likely cause. Angina is a rare cause of chest pain in adolescents, and with a normal cardiac examination and no family history of cardiac disease, this is unlikely. Costochondritis is a common cause of chest pain but typically has an insidious onset and does not resolve with rest. Esophagitis is a common cause of chest pain but is typically impacted by eating, not exercise. Mitral valve prolapse can cause chest pain, although most pediatric patients with mitral valve prolapse are asymptomatic. On examination, they often have a systolic click. *(Kliegman et al., pp. 148–162)*

104. (E) In a patient with symptoms and signs consistent with exercise-induced asthma, a therapeutic trial of inhaled albuterol is the first line of therapy and diagnosis. If there is evidence of cardiac disease on history or physical examination, then one should proceed with the indicated tests. Pulmonary function tests could be used to confirm the diagnosis and are used in cases in which the diagnosis is uncertain or if patients fail the therapeutic trial. *(Kliegman et al., pp. 186–196)*

105. (A) There are many drugs and foods that cause red urine. These include azo dyes, beets, blackberries, ibuprofen, methyldopa, red food color, rifampin, phenolphthalein, pyridium, sulfasalazine, and many others. Dark brown or black urine can be associated with alanine, cascara, resocinol, and thymol. If the diet or drug history as well as dipstick are negative, porphyrinuria should be considered. A positive reagent strip (dipstick) indicates hemoglobin or myoglobin. Negative dipstick and normal urinalysis makes renal pathology unlikely. Because the urinalysis is negative, and the patient is asymptomatic, urine culture is not indicated at this time. Antistreptococcal antibodies should be done if poststreptococcal glomerulonephritis is suspected; it is characterized by proteinuria, hematuria, edema, and hypertension. *(Kliegman et al., pp. 425–429)*

106. (C) This is a classic presentation for a peritonsillar abscess. Development of a peritonsillar abscess is usually preceded by acute pharyngotonsillitis, followed by development of severe throat pain and trismus. It is usually caused by group A hemolytic Streptococci or oral anaerobes in preadolescent or adolescent patients. Speech is often with a "hot potato" voice. The affected tonsil is enlarged causing the uvula to be pushed to the other side. Antibiotics (penicillin) and incision and drainage are usually required. Retropharyngeal abscess is usually a complication of bacterial pharyngitis in younger children under age 3–4 years. It is caused by infection and further suppuration of nodes in the retropharyngeal area. Symptoms include high fever, difficulty swallowing, feeding refusal, hyperextension of the head, and drooling. There is bulging of the posterior pharyngeal wall; diagnosis can be confirmed by widening of the retropharyngeal space on x-ray. With lateral pharyngeal abscess there is bulging of the lateral pharyngeal wall. Acute uvulitis is caused by group A hemolytic Streptococci and *H. influenzae* type B, often in association with tonsillitis and uvulitis. *(Behrman et al., pp. 1264–1266)*

107. (B) Kawasaki disease is an acute febrile illness of unknown etiology that typically affects young children, usually those under 5 years of age. There are six clinical criteria used for diagnosing this disease. The presence of 5 days or more of fever, in addition to four of the five additional criteria, establishes the diagnosis. The five additional criteria are bilateral bulbar nonexudative conjunctivitis, rash, hand and foot changes (edema followed by desquamation), oral changes such as strawberry tongue and erythema, and cervical lymphadenopathy. Erythema infectiosum presents with a prodrome of malaise and myalgia and then with local erythema of the cheeks (slapped cheeks). Rubella and rubeola are unusual because of the MMR vaccination. Rubeola presents with the three "Cs"—cough, coryza, and conjunctivitis—followed by the oral inflammation and the pathognomonic Koplik spots, rash, and fever. Rubella is typically a mild disease characterized by low-grade fever and a maculopapular rash. Rheumatic fever is also unusual. It tends to present in children over 3 years of age after an infection with group A Streptococci, with transient migratory arthritis, carditis, chorea, rash, and nodules. Diagnosis is made according to the Jones criteria. *(Kliegman et al., pp. 1010–1011)*

108. (B) Osgood–Schlatter results from microfractures and inflammation of the tibial tubercle where the patellar tendon inserts. It is most commonly seen in young adolescents who are involved in athletics. Legg–Calvé–Perthes disease is idiopathic avascular necrosis of the capital femoral epiphysis and presents between the ages of 2 and 12 with a painless limp. Patellar subluxation is usually due to a congenital deficiency within the patellofemoral joint. On examination, these patients have tenderness over the inferior surface of the patella and terminal subluxation of the patella when the knee is fully extended. Popliteal cysts are usually asymptomatic and present with a fluid-filled mass in the popliteal fossa. The symptoms of slipped capital femoral epiphysis are variable but typically involve hip pain and limp. On examination, patients have limitation of motion in the hip. It is most common in obese adolescents. *(Behrman et al., pp. 2076, 2106)*

109. (K)

110. (J)

111. (B)

112. (H)

113. (O)

Explanations 109 through 113

Transposition of the great arteries is the most common cause of cyanotic heart disease in the neonate. Cyanosis usually appears in the first day of life. Cardiac findings are often otherwise normal, although patients may have a single S_2. The classic chest x-ray shows a normal heart size with a narrow mediastinum (egg on a string). Other causes of cyanotic congenital heart disease are tetralogy of Fallot and truncus arteriosus. The chest x-ray in truncus arteriosus shows increased pulmonary flow and in tetralogy of Fallot decreased pulmonary flow. Murmurs are commonly heard in children with normal hearts. This is particularly true in young children with relatively thin chest walls where the normal flow murmurs arising from the pulmonary and aortic roots are easily heard on the anterior chest. To label a murmur as normal, patients should be free of any cardiac symptoms. The rest of the cardiovascular examination should also be normal. One of the typical flow murmurs in young children is the Still's murmur. The murmur is musical or vibratory. It is a systolic ejection murmur and is usually heard best at the left lower sternal border. Atrial septal defect is one of the common congenital heart lesions with a left-to-right shunt. Patients are usually asymptomatic, and the problem is usually diagnosed when the murmur is detected. Murmurs are due to increased flow across normal valves. The systolic murmur is due to increased flow across the right ventricular outflow tract. The widely split second heart sound is due to the increased right ventricular diastolic volume and a prolonged ejection time across the pulmonary valve. Peripheral pulmonic stenosis is an ejection murmur heard best at the upper sternal border with transmission to the axilla and the back. It is caused by the sharp angle between the main pulmonary artery and its branches. It is heard in infants only and should disappear by 6 months of age. Ventricular septal defects are the most common congenital heart lesions. The most important characteristic about the murmur is that it begins early in systole, often obscuring S_1. Depending on the size of the defect, the murmur will be longer or shorter. AV canal detected after the newborn period can present with a similar sounding murmur. It is much less common than a ventricular septal defect but would be a strong possibility if the patient had Down syndrome. *(Kliegman et al., pp. 66–67, 136–138)*

REFERENCES

American Academy of Pediatrics. Committee on Injury and Poison Prevention. Selection and using the most appropriate car safety seats for growing children: guidelines for counseling parents. *Pediatrics* 1996;97(5):761–762.

American Academy of Pediatrics. *Report of the Committee on Infectious Diseases*, 25th ed. Evanston, IL: American Academy of Pediatrics, 2000a.

American Academy of Pediatrics. Task force on infant sleep position and sudden infant death syndrome. Changing concepts of sudden infant death implications for infant sleeping environment syndrome and sleep position. *Pediatrics* 2000b;105(3):650–656.

Behrman RE, Kliegman RM, Jenson HB. *Nelson Textbook of Pediatrics*, 16th ed. Philadelphia, PA: W.B. Saunders, 2000.

Centers for Disease Control and Prevention (CDC). *Preventing Lead Poisoning in Young Children*. Atlanta, GA, October 1991.

Champion LAA, Schwartz AD, Luddy RE, et al. The effects of four commonly used drugs on platelet function. *J Pediatr* 1976;89:653–656.

Committee on Drugs. Treatment guidelines for lead exposure in children. *Pediatrics* 1995;96:155–160.

Ellenhorn MJ. *Ellenhorn's Medical Toxicology: Diagnosis and Treatment of Human Poisoning*, 2nd ed. Baltimore, MD: Williams & Wilkins, 1997.

Feigin RD, Cherry JD. *Textbook of Pediatric Infectious Diseases*, 4th ed. Philadelphia, PA: W.B. Saunders, 1998.

Hurwitz S. *Clinical Pediatric Dermatology: A Textbook of Skin Disorders of Childhood and Adolescence*, 2nd ed. Philadelphia, PA: W.B. Saunders, 1993.

Kaplowitz PB, Oberfield SE. Re-examination of the age limit for defining when puberty is precocious in girls in the United States: implications for evaluation and treatment. *Pediatrics* 1999;104:936–941.

Kliegman RM, Greenbaum L, Lye P. *Practical Strategies in Pediatric Diagnosis and Therapy*. Philadelphia, PA: Elsevier, 2004.

Mahony CP (ed.). Adolescent gynecomastia. *Pediatr Clin North Am* 1990;37(6):1389–1404.

McMillan JA, DeAngelis CD, Feigin RD, et al. *Oski's Pediatrics: Principles and Practice*, 3rd ed. Philadelphia, PA: JB Lippincott, 1999.

Miller WL, Styne DM. Female puberty and its disorders. In: Yen SSC, Jaffe RB, Barbieri R (eds.), *Reproductive Endocrinology: Physiology, Pathophysiology, and Clinical Management*, 4th ed. Philadelphia, PA: W.B. Saunders, 1999.

Rudolph AM, Hoffman JIE, Rudolph CD. *Pediatrics*, 20th ed. New York, NY: McGraw-Hill, 2002.

Staheli LT. *Fundamentals of Pediatric Orthopedics*, 2nd ed. Philadelphia, PA: Lippincott Raven, 1998.

CHAPTER 4

Preventive Medicine

Leslie F. Martin, MD, MPH and Seira Kurian, MD, MS, MPH

Questions

DIRECTIONS (Questions 1 through 52): Each of the numbered items or incomplete statements in this section is followed by answers or by completions of the statement. Select the ONE lettered answer or completion that is BEST in each case.

1. A previously healthy male postal worker complains of fever, headache, myalgia, and cough for the past 3 days. He reports that several of his coworkers have also been ill with similar complaints. His leukocyte count is normal with a relative lymphopenia. A chest x-ray shows only enlarged hilar shadows. Which of the following is the most likely cause of this infection?

(A) influenza A virus
(B) Bacillus anthracis
(C) Francisella tularensis
(D) Yersinia pestis
(E) Clostridium botulinum

2. As a health officer, you have identified blindness among the elderly in your state as a cause of falls and resultant inability to perform activities of daily living. You try to prevent this by improving access to which of the following?

(A) residence in nursing homes
(B) corneal surgery for near vision
(C) cataract surgery
(D) treatment of glaucoma
(E) refractive correction

3. You participate in the global effort to eradicate poliomyelitis. A poliomyelitis outbreak has been identified in a community in Africa. You advise your outbreak investigation team that they must focus on transmission from which one of the following sources?

(A) green monkeys
(B) mosquitoes of the species *Aedes aegypti*
(C) contaminated vaccine
(D) polluted water sources
(E) poorly cooked food

4. A 20-year-old student asks to have his vaccinations updated. You recommend that he be vaccinated for typhoid fever under which of the following circumstances?

(A) Natural disasters destroy the local water and sewage systems.
(B) He takes a rural vacation in the southwestern United States.
(C) He travels in countries with endemic typhoid.
(D) He eats organic foods fertilized with raw cow manure.
(E) He lives in a community in which carriers are found.

5. A 50-year-old slaughterhouse worker complains of intermittent episodes of fever, malaise, weakness, and weight loss over the past several months. Several of his coworkers have experienced flu-like symptoms since last winter. Which of the following statements about his illness is correct?

(A) Each *Brucella* species produces its own distinct human illness.
(B) People who recover from brucellosis are more likely to become reinfected when they are reexposed to *Brucella* than they were before their initial infection.
(C) Person-to-person transmission of brucellosis is common.
(D) People with brucellosis generally have a chronic relapsing infection.
(E) Humans are the primary reservoir for *Brucella*.

6. You are asked by a company predominantly employing women to design an educational program to reduce morbidity and mortality due to cardiovascular disease. Which of the following statements should you include in this program to describe women's risk of cardiovascular disease?

(A) Men have fewer heart attacks than women.
(B) The underlying cause of heart disease in women is now well understood.
(C) The gender difference in vascular disease is greater in cerebral, aortic, and peripheral vessels than it is in the coronary arteries.
(D) Postmenopausal Hormone Replacement Therapy (HRT) is beneficial in reducing the risk of cardiovascular disease.
(E) In women, cardiovascular disease is more likely to present as angina than in men.

7. The health commissioner asks you to propose a primary prevention program for your community. Which of the following should you recommend?

(A) annual sigmoidoscopy
(B) routine immunization
(C) mammography
(D) prostate-specific antigen (PSA) testing
(E) isolation of disease contacts

8. Food-borne illness has been a recurrent problem in your community over the past year. As a result of this, you ask that the health department's registered sanitarian pay particular attention to which of the following during his inspection of restaurants?

(A) unhygienic food-handling methods
(B) improper storage of rodenticides
(C) inadequate cooking
(D) the use of unlabeled products
(E) use of old utensils

9. It is 2005. You are planning allocation of health department resources to meet the needs of a typical U.S. community over the next 10 years. You decide to allocate funding for each population group based on anticipated percent of population growth in each age group. The largest proportional increase in funding will go toward which age group?

(A) 0- through 10-year olds
(B) 55- through 64-year olds
(C) 65- through 74-year olds
(D) 75- through 84-year olds
(E) those over 85 years of age

10. It is reported that an alarming number of fractures are occurring among the elderly in your community. You are contacted by a local radio station for an interview on this subject. You explain that which of the following is the most likely cause of the high number of fractures?

(A) Alzheimer disease
(B) osteoporosis
(C) obesity
(D) Parkinson disease
(E) deteriorating eyesight

11. You counsel a 47-year-old smoker who says that she does not intend to quit smoking because she is not worried about the health risks of smoking. All of her relatives smoke, and none have developed lung cancer. You point out that the Framingham studies have indicated that disease of other organ systems is also associated with smoking, and her relatives have had such disease. The Framingham study found smoking to be associated with disease of which of the following?

(A) skeletal system
(B) spleen
(C) cerebrovascular system
(D) thyroid
(E) auditory system

12. Many patients you see in your practice live in homes built prior to 1977. In compliance with the Centers for Disease Control and Prevention (CDC) guidelines, at which of the following ages will you start the relevant routine lead screening of the children?

(A) birth
(B) 3 months of age
(C) 12 months of age
(D) entry to preschool
(E) entry to first grade

13. A young woman who works full time doing manual work in a factory, but who also has secretarial skills, is making her first prenatal visit to your office. Her work involves climbing high ladders, with the risk of falling. Which of the following is the best recommendation regarding this patient's job?

(A) Advise the patient not to work.
(B) Recommend that the patient seek alternative work.
(C) Recommend no change in employment but suggest avoiding risk.
(D) Suggest that you provide her with a restriction stating that she is not to work at unprotected heights.
(E) Write a note to the employer requesting reassignment of the patient to a secretarial position.

14. A study finds that the incidence of asthma in your community is higher than expected, and that 40% of the homes in your community are heated with forced air. Which of the following best describes this study design?

(A) ecological study
(B) cross-sectional study
(C) cohort study
(D) case-control study
(E) prospective study

15. A particular community is found to have high rates of dental caries. The health commissioner is attempting to institute a program to prevent further dental caries in his community. Which of the following is the most cost-effective method of preventing dental caries within a community?

(A) community fluoridation of the drinking water
(B) promoting dental hygiene
(C) instituting a universal sealant program in school children
(D) instituting dental hygienist visits to local schools
(E) instituting semiannual topical application of fluoride by a professional

16. A 1-year-old child in a large nursery school develops fever, irritability, confusion, a possible stiff neck, and a petechial rash, over the course of several hours. Which of the following agents is recommended for others in the nursery school who have had contact with the child, to control a possible outbreak?

(A) rifampin, ciprofloxacin or ceftriaxone
(B) gamma globulin
(C) group A meningococcal vaccine
(D) group C meningococcal vaccine
(E) quadrivalent meningococcal vaccine

17. A 16-year old male becomes ill with fever, chills, headache, myalgia, and arthralgia 6 days after hunting prairie dogs with his cousin at his uncle's farm. Examination reveals extremely large, painful, and tender inguinal lymph nodes and a couple of small papules around his ankles. Which of the following is the most likely diagnosis?

(A) influenza C
(B) bubonic plague
(C) tularemia
(D) cat-scratch fever
(E) West Nile virus

18. Schedules for the routine immunization of young children are developed jointly by the Advisory Commission on Immunization Practices (a federal commission) and the American Academy of Pediatrics. Which of the following vaccines is recommended for routine vaccination for all children in the United States?

(A) anthrax vaccine
(B) rabies vaccine
(C) Haemophilus influenzae b (Hib) vaccine
(D) hepatitis A vaccine
(E) typhoid vaccine

19. A health insurance company decides to market its services to a population that will not incur high charges. The use of health services in the United States is most strongly associated with which of the following characteristics?

(A) age
(B) sex
(C) race
(D) education
(E) income

20. A hurricane devastates your community. You decide to devote your attention to the aspect of disaster response that is most likely to be inadequate in coping with the disaster. Which of the following is most likely to hamper disaster response?

(A) lack of government resources
(B) failure to triage casualties
(C) failure of management
(D) lack of telecommunications
(E) lack of volunteer helpers

21. Repeated thunderstorms have resulted in overflow of municipal wastewater treatment plants by floodwaters. Volunteer sandbaggers downstream from the plants developed health concerns when the overflow became evident. As a public health officer you are asked to evaluate the situation. Which of the following is your most important recommendation to workers in order to prevent illness from exposure to the contaminated water?

(A) Do careful hand washing before meals and cigarette smoke breaks.
(B) Boil all water that is to be used for drinking or cooking.
(C) Offer hepatitis A vaccinations to all work crews prior to the next disaster.
(D) Start prophylaxis with a broad-spectrum antibiotic for all workers who do not have a contraindication.
(E) Offer oral polio vaccine to all eligible workers.

22. A father you are treating for hyperlipidemia brings his 23-month-old son into your clinic for a routine checkup. He reports that he and his wife are separated and that he is uncertain if the child has received appropriate medical care. The child has no known medical problems and is not a member of any high-risk population. The child is new to your clinic, but the father produces an immunization record which states the child has received the following vaccines: diphtheria, tetanus, and acellular pertussis at 2, 5, and 7 months; hepatitis B vaccine at birth, 2 months, and 7 months; *H. influenzae* type b at 2 and 5 months; inactivated poliovirus at 2, 5, and 7 months; and a measles, mumps, and rubella vaccine at 12 months. You tell the father that the child has received some of the recommended immunizations late, but that the child is adequately protected. The infant should receive varicella immunization in addition to which of the following vaccinations?

(A) hepatitis A vaccine now, and again in 6 months
(B) pneumococcus vaccine now, and again in 6 months
(C) oral polio vaccine now
(D) Diptheria, Tetanus, acellular Pertussis (DTaP) vaccine now
(E) oral typhoid vaccination now

23. A worker complains of paresthesias, numbness, and tingling that started distally in the lower extremities but that is starting to affect his hands. He is developing muscle weakness. He feels tired, and has a headache and complains of memory deficit. Electromyographic abnormalities suggest axonal degeneration and demyelination. Exposure to which of the following is the most suspect cause of this clinical picture?

(A) lead
(B) benzene
(C) zinc
(D) carbon disulfide
(E) vibration

24. A 20-year-old asymptomatic college student presents to your clinic for contraception. She states that she has been sexually active for 2 years with one partner, and that they usually use condoms. Along with a Papanicolaou (Pap) smear and pelvic examination, which of the following should you also recommend?

(A) self-breast examination
(B) screening for chlamydia
(C) screening for syphilis
(D) Thyroid-Stimulating Hormone (TSH) test
(E) screening for gonorrhea

25. You have performed annual examinations on a young mother for the last 3 years. She and her husband are considering having another child in 5 years, and she would like to restart oral contraceptive pills. You review her medical record and find that she had a normal Pap smear at last year's examination and also the year prior to that. You recommend that her next Pap smear be performed when?

(A) now
(B) in 1 year
(C) in 2 years
(D) in 3 years
(E) in 4 years

Questions 26 and 27

A 30-year-old asymptomatic male presents to your office because his father just had a heart attack. He is concerned that he may have inherited his father's condition because a cholesterol level test done at his work site last year was 220 mg/dL. You review his history and find that he smokes 25 cigarettes a day, eats mostly at fast food restaurants, sits at a desk job, and has no regular moderate intensity physical activities. His blood pressure is 130/85 mmHg and his body mass index is 26.

26. Which of the following is the best first recommendation?

(A) electrocardiography (ECG)
(B) ECG and an exercise treadmill test (ETT)
(C) a diet for weight loss
(D) commencement of a daily exercise routine
(E) antihypertensive medication

27. Which of the following is the most important next step to successfully help the patient quit smoking?

(A) smoking cessation counseling sessions
(B) nicotine patches
(C) bupropion hydrochloride
(D) physician recommendation to stop smoking
(E) identifying social supports to help quit

28. Jehovah's Witnesses usually refuse to consider a recommended blood transfusion. A 5-year-old child with hemophilia and dangerously low hemoglobin levels needs such a transfusion, but the Jehovah's Witness parents refuse to accept the recommendation. How are principles of autonomy best resolved?

(A) The hospital's representatives respect the parents' right to consent and support their refusal.
(B) The physician explains the need, in simple words, to the child who refuses the transfusion.
(C) The hospital requests a local court to exercise the rights of the child through the appointment of a surrogate guardian.
(D) The local court gives the physician the right to decide if the transfusion is warranted.
(E) The hospital Chaplain is usually given the final authority in these matters.

29. Age-adjusted cancer death rates for men and women reveal an increasing rate for which cancer over the last 20 years?

(A) prostate cancer
(B) lung cancer in women
(C) breast cancer
(D) colorectal cancer
(E) stomach cancer

30. You have decided to survey the population to establish a health risk profile for the population. Due to budget constraints, you must gather data using a stratified random sample. This approach is correctly described as which of the following?

(A) based on selecting individuals from a list at predetermined intervals (every *i*th individual)
(B) random sampling of separate segments of a population
(C) randomly grouping the population
(D) sampling a cluster of individuals
(E) removing outliers and sampling from remainder of group

Questions 31 through 35

You are examining the relationship between hypertension and myocardial infarction (MI) in your community. In order to do so, you send a questionnaire to the whole population in your community (1000 persons). All 1000 persons responded. The results obtained from that questionnaire are presented below in Table 4-1.

TABLE 4-1 ALL 1000 MEMBERS OF POPULATION "A": RESPONSES TO A QUESTIONNAIRE

	History of MI	
History of hypertension	**Present**	**Absent**
Present	15	185
Absent	5	795

31. What is the reported prevalence of hypertension in the population per 1000?

(A) 150
(B) 185
(C) 200
(D) 220
(E) 250

32. What is the prevalence of MI per 1000 hypertensive persons in the total population?

(A) 10
(B) 15
(C) 19
(D) 75
(E) 81

33. What is the prevalence of MI per 1000 persons in the community?

(A) 5
(B) 10
(C) 15
(D) 20
(E) 25

34. You randomly select a sample of 100 questionnaires in order to determine how representative your results would have been compared to the whole population if you had originally only sampled 100 individuals from your community. The results obtained are shown below in Table 4-2.

TABLE 4-2 SAMPLE OF 100 MEMBERS OF POPULATION "A": FINDINGS ON CLINICAL EXAM

	History of MI	
History of hypertension	**Present**	**Absent**
Present	4	36
Absent	1	59

Which of the following statistical tests could best be used to determine whether there is a significant increase in the history of MI among those persons who have hypertension in comparison with those without hypertension?

(A) *t*-test, single-tailed
(B) *t*-test, two-tailed
(C) test of variance
(D) *P* value
(E) chi-square test

35. If we compare the population sample examined with the whole population that responded to the questionnaire, which of the following statements accurately describes the available information?

(A) The sample group confirms the findings of the questionnaire.
(B) As expected, there is a higher "real" incidence of hypertension than reported.
(C) As expected, there is a higher "real" incidence of MI than reported.
(D) There is a statistical test that could be applied to assess the significance of the differences.
(E) The data as presented are not really adequate for further statistical examination.

36. A 45-year-old male living in a homeless shelter is exposed to TB from a fellow resident. He is found to have a 15 mm of induration on the Mantoux skin test. Which of the following risk factors will increase the man's likelihood of developing active TB subsequent to his infection?

(A) history of cough variant asthma
(B) silicosis
(C) chronic obstructive pulmonary disease (COPD)
(D) bronchitis
(E) siderosis

37. The causative organism of cholera, *Vibrio cholerae*, was first isolated by Koch in 1883. There have been seven pandemics of cholera, with the most recent subsiding only in the 1980s. With humans as the usual reservoir, the organism spreads as man travels. Which of the following is the most likely mode of spread?

(A) contaminated fomites
(B) specific strains of mosquitoes
(C) food cleaned in contaminated water
(D) person-to-person transmission via inhalation of droplet nuclei in crowded places
(E) the Phlebotomine fly (sand fly)

38. A 4-year-old child presents to his pediatrician with a complaint of a mild rash and fevers. His travel history is positive for a camping trip 2 weeks prior. The parents do not recall a tick bite on the child and do not remember if there were ticks in the area. No other members of the family complain of similar symptoms and the child does not attend day care. Physical examination is positive for a temperature of 100.9°F with an erythematous rash noted over the child's trunk. Which of the following factors would significantly increase the possibility that the child has Lyme disease?

(A) The camping trip occurred in an area endemic for the tick *Ixodes dentatus.*
(B) The camping trip occurred in Texas.
(C) The camping trip occurred in an area with a high indigenous population of lizards.
(D) The camping trip occurred in an area endemic for the white-footed mouse.
(E) The camping trip occurred in an area which had recently been sprayed with pesticides.

39. For which of the following circumstances would you consider initiating chelation, such as with CaEDTA, to treat workers for workplace exposure to lead and other heavy metals?

(A) as prophylaxis for all employees exposed to metal dust and fumes
(B) only after waiting for toxic effects of heavy metal exposure to resolve on their own
(C) only for patients with symptomatic disease
(D) when metal is being absorbed through the gastrointestinal (GI) tract
(E) when patients remain in a workplace where exposure occurs

Questions 40 and 41

Six hundred asymptomatic men with prostatic nodules are given a PSA test to screen for prostate cancer. With a cut off of 5 ng/mL, the PSA results are positive in 200 cases. Of these, 100 persons are confirmed on biopsy and follow-up testing to have the disease; however, 50 of the individuals who had negative test results are also shown to have the disease based on biopsy. You have been asked to screen another similar group of 50 men using the PSA test.

40. What proportion of persons having prostatic cancers will you correctly identify in the new group?

(A) 16.7%
(B) 22.2%
(C) 66.7%
(D) 77.8%
(E) 87.5%

41. What proportion of persons with no prostatic cancer will you correctly identify in the new group?

(A) 16.7%
(B) 22.2%
(C) 66.7%
(D) 77.8%
(E) 87.5%

42. Several members of a group of young adults camping, cooking, and traveling together in the developing world develop fever, malaise, nausea, and vomiting, and have dark urine. Two have yellow sclera. How could this best have been prevented?

(A) avoiding eating local foods
(B) washing hands before eating
(C) taking prophylactic Pepto Bismol
(D) getting vaccinations
(E) cooking all foods thoroughly and drinking boiled water

Questions 43 through 47

43. A group of male workers between the ages of 20 and 39 years are being screened for lung disease by spirometry. Nine subjects are examined. Their forced expiratory volume in 1 second (FEV_1) divided by forced vital capacity ($FEV_1/FVC\%$) results are 80, 76, 73, 61, 64, 79, 64, 64, and 78. What is the *mean*?

(A) 61
(B) 64
(C) 71
(D) 73
(E) 76

44. What is the *modal* reading?

(A) 61
(B) 64
(C) 71
(D) 73
(E) 76

45. What is the *median* value?

(A) 61
(B) 64
(C) 71
(D) 73
(E) 76

46. What is the *range*?

(A) 17
(B) 18

(C) 19
(D) 20
(E) 21

47. The variance of the set of values is 58.75. What is the standard deviation (SD)?

(A) 5.8
(B) 6.5
(C) 7.7
(D) 8.5
(E) 9.0.

48. The crude death rate in Sweden was 0.010 per year, while in Costa Rica it was 0.008 per year. All age-specific death rates, except those for the oldest-age category, were higher in Costa Rica than in Sweden. From these data, one can correctly infer which of the following?

(A) The difference is too small for any deductions to be made.
(B) It is healthier to live in Sweden than in Costa Rica.
(C) There is less cardiovascular disease in Costa Rica than in Sweden.
(D) A greater proportion of the Swedish population is in the older-age categories.
(E) There is unexplained progressive deterioration of health indicators in Costa Rica relative to those of Sweden.

Questions 49 through 51

A large segment of the population in your community smokes. In order to convince your patient population that it would be beneficial to quit smoking in order to prevent lung cancer, you conduct a case-control study of cigarette smoking and lung cancer. The results from that study can be found in Table 4-3.

TABLE 4-3 CIGARETTE SMOKING AND LUNG CANCER

	Lung cancer		
Cigarette smoking	**Cases**	**Controls**	**Totals**
Yes	75	25	100
No	25	75	100
Totals	100	100	200

49. What is the odds ratio (OR) in your study?

(A) 3
(B) 6
(C) 9
(D) 12
(E) 20

50. Using the same table, what is the relative risk?

(A) 3
(B) 6
(C) 9
(D) 12
(E) cannot be calculated

51. Which of the following is most true concerning ORs and relative risk calculations, as pertaining to this study?

(A) The overall size of the series is too large to estimate relative risk.
(B) If the number of controls were increased, the two ratios would be similar.
(C) The number of controls is twice as many as the cases.
(D) The OR is not appropriate for this series.
(E) The disease is rare.

52. An investigator in a community hospital decides to examine all patients for a problem with alcoholism to determine prevalence in the community. In addition to recall bias, which of the following is the most obvious error in selecting all patients admitted to a community hospital?

(A) observer bias
(B) selection bias
(C) detection bias
(D) interpretive bias
(E) calculation bias

DIRECTIONS (Questions 53 through 109): Each set of matching questions in this section consists of a list of lettered options followed by several numbered items. For each question, select the ONE best lettered answer that is most closely associated with it. Each lettered answer may be selected once, more than once, or not at all.

Questions 53 through 56

Workers in certain occupations are exposed to diseases for which animals are the reservoir. These workers may then become a source of infection to others. For each of the occupations listed, choose the infectious disease the workers are most likely to acquire and transmit.

(A) anthrax
(B) brucellosis
(C) Lyme disease
(D) murine (endemic) typhus
(E) salmonellosis

53. Butcher

54. Warehouse worker

55. Livestock worker

56. Rancher

Questions 57 through 59

The following questions identify health care planning methods used by various organizations. The answer options are strategies that may correspond to these methods. Select the strategy that best corresponds to each health care planning method.

(A) identifying what the market for services are and estimating future demands
(B) identifying mechanisms for carrying out established goals within specific program areas
(C) identifying financial resources to meet community needs
(D) identifying barriers to growth and the resources needed to overcome them

57. A local health department employs population-based planning in meeting the needs of its community.

58. A Health Maintenance Organization (HMO) employs institutional planning to identify its goals and objectives.

59. A maternal and child health care system employs program-based planning to address its goals.

Questions 60 through 64

For each of the diseases listed, select the arthropod vector responsible for its transmission.

(A) *Aedes aegypti*
(B) *Anopheles* species
(C) *Pediculus humanus corporis*
(D) *Dermacentor andersoni*
(E) *Sarcoptes scabiei*

60. Epidemic typhus

61. Malaria

62. Dengue fever

63. Colorado tick fever

64. Yellow fever

Questions 65 through 69

For each of the regulatory issues identified, select the corresponding regulatory agency.

(A) Food and Drug Administration (FDA)
(B) United States Department of Agriculture (USDA)
(C) Environmental Protection Agency (EPA)
(D) United Nations Food and Agriculture Organization (FAO)
(E) World Health Organization (WHO)

65. Which regulatory agency has the authority to control the use of pesticides in the United States?

66. A shipment of produce is identified as having a higher than allowable level of pesticide. Which of the following regulatory agencies retains the authority to remove the produce from the market?

67. Catfish caught in a freshwater stream in Florida has been identified as exceeding the action level for polychlorinated biphenyls in fish (PCBs). Which regulatory agency is responsible for defining these action levels?

68. Which regulatory agency enforces standards in the sale of meat?

69. Which of the following institutions is involved in mounting international control programs for the eradication of communicable disease?

Questions 70 through 73

For each organism causing food-related illness, choose the corresponding average incubation period.

(A) under 4 h
(B) 8–24 h
(C) 12–36 h
(D) 12 h to 6 days
(E) 1–3 weeks

70. *Clostridium perfringens*

71. *Clostridium botulinum*

72. *Staphylococcus aureus*

73. *Salmonella*

Questions 74 through 78

Several groups of organic compounds are associated with serious toxic effects when used as described. For each use, select the potentially toxic compounds employed.

(A) nitrosamines
(B) epoxy compounds
(C) PCBs
(D) formaldehydes
(E) organophosphorus compounds

74. Used in transformers because they withstand high temperatures

75. Used as insecticides and responsible for more deaths on a worldwide basis than any other group of insecticides

76. Highly toxic and dangerous as a solvent; used in the manufacture of rubber, dyes, and lubricating oils

77. Used in the production of resins, plasticizers, and solvents

78. Used in the manufacture of textiles and materials; often found in manufactured homes

Questions 79 through 83

For each of the following scenarios, select the gas exposure responsible for the signs and symptoms.

(A) carbon monoxide
(B) methane
(C) hydrogen sulfide
(D) ozone
(E) sulfur dioxide

79. A patient working with an electric arc noted a pungent odor, and now has signs of asthma or early pulmonary edema.

80. A sewer worker has acute onset of nausea, headache, and shortness of breath, and has anosmia.

81. A man has been pulled unconscious from a mine. No odors are noted, but an experienced miner says there was coal damp in the mine.

82. A garage worker turns on the ventilation system in the winter time while testing a motor, and now complains of a headache and vertigo.

83. A worker drilling for oil experiences acute tearing, mucous membrane irritation, and onset of a cough while repairing machinery.

Questions 84 through 88

For the screening tests listed below, select the screening schedule that is appropriate for women (as per the U.S. Preventive Services Task Force, 3rd ed.).

(A) do not routinely screen
(B) yearly over age 50
(C) at first prenatal visit
(D) every 1–2 years at age 40 and older
(E) every 1–2 years at age 50 and older
(F) every 3 years following an initial examination, but not after age 65
(G) every 3 years at age 50 and older

84. Mammography

85. Cervical cytology (Pap smear)

86. Fecal occult blood testing

87. Screening for hepatitis B

88. Palpation, ultrasound, or serologic testing of the abdomen to screen for cancer of the pancreas

Questions 89 through 93

For each of the clinical indications, choose an option for use of immune globulin (IG).

(A) indicated
(B) not proven effective
(C) not routinely indicated
(D) contraindicated
(E) compulsory

89. Hepatitis A prophylaxis

90. Hepatitis B prophylaxis

91. Hepatitis C prophylaxis

92. Measles prophylaxis

93. Rubella prophylaxis

Questions 94 through 100

For each of the infectious diseases of childhood, select the appropriate incubation period.

(A) 1–6 days
(B) 7–8 days
(C) 8–10 days
(D) 10–21 days
(E) 30–50 days
(F) 120–180 days

94. Diphtheria

95. Chickenpox

96. Infectious mononucleosis

97. Mumps

98. Pertussis

99. Tetanus

100. Rubella

Questions 101 through 109

For each of the conditions listed, select the organism associated with it.

(A) coagulase-positive *Staphylococcus aureus*
(B) beta-hemolytic *Streptococcus*
(C) respiratory syncytial virus
(D) *Mycoplasma pneumoniae*
(E) *Hemophilus pertussis*
(F) *Helicobacter pylori*
(G) *Escherichia coli*
(H) *Rickettsia prowazekii*
(I) *Giardia lamblia*
(J) *Clostridium perfringens*

101. A male student returns from traveling to a developing country, with a complaint of eructation, abdominal cramps, and diarrhea for the past 2 weeks, and has lost 10 lbs.

102. A 4-year-old child in late summer fell 1 week ago, and now has a crusty, mildly erythematous wound with regional lymphadenitis.

103. A parent of a 4-year-old child who goes to nursery school develops a chronic cough and low-grade fever.

104. Chronic diarrhea in a homosexual male

105. Nursery epidemics of watery diarrhea

106. Furunculosis

107. A 50-year-old man who reports drinking two or three alcoholic beverages per day complains of chronic, vague, intermittent dyspepsia.

108. A 2-year-old child is pulling on her earlobe and has a temperature of 39°C and a bulging eardrum.

109. Approximately 12 h after a banquet, most of those who ate stew report abdominal cramps and diarrhea which subsided after 1–2 days.

DIRECTIONS (Questions 110 through 136): Each of the numbered items or incomplete statements in this section is followed by answers or by completions of the statement. Select the ONE lettered answer or completion that is BEST in each case.

Questions 110 and 111

When making recommendations to a state general assembly against routine premarital screening, the State Health Commissioner used the following data to arrive at his conclusions. The state had a young adult population of 100,000. Their actual prevalence of human immunodeficiency virus (HIV) infection was 1 per 1000. The best screening test available had a sensitivity of 98% and a specificity of 95%.

110. How many people in this population would have screened false positive?

(A) 4995
(B) 98
(C) 2
(D) 100
(E) 5000

111. How many people would have screened as false negative?

(A) 4995
(B) 98
(C) 2
(D) 100
(E) 5000

112. Multiple disease outcomes associated with smoking can be assessed with which type of study?

(A) cross-sectional study
(B) randomized, controlled trial
(C) cohort study
(D) case-control study
(E) case series

113. You are reviewing a cohort (follow-up) study to determine whether dietary fiber reduces the risk of colon cancer. In the study, the population at risk at the beginning of the follow-up period should consist of which of the following?

(A) persons who all have diagnosed disease
(B) persons with diverse exposure levels and disease
(C) persons of comparable age, gender, and race
(D) persons with homogeneous disease probability
(E) persons who are susceptible but free of disease

114. Among the observational study designs, the prospective cohort design offers which of the following advantages?

(A) It provides a relatively quick answer.
(B) It allows one to take advantage of existing outcome data.
(C) It is easy to assemble a comparison group.
(D) It allows one to measure incidence.
(E) It is relatively cheap.

115. On January 15, 2005, a health survey was performed in an elementary school of a developing country. All the school children were examined for conjunctivitis, and 2% of the children were diagnosed with the disease. From these data, one can determine which of the following?

(A) the incidence of conjunctivitis
(B) the prevalence of conjunctivitis
(C) both incidence and prevalence of conjunctivitis
(D) neither the incidence nor prevalence of conjunctivitis
(E) the attributable risk

116. A new screening test for prostate cancer becomes available. You assess whether this will be useful to your practice by reviewing the operating characteristics of the test. The test's ability to correctly classify diseased persons as having disease is called what?

(A) specificity
(B) sensitivity
(C) positive predictive value
(D) negative predictive value
(E) reproducibility

117. The lab test has a sensitivity of 85% and a specificity of 70%. You want to have 1000 persons take the test. To estimate the positive predictive value of the test for this population, you need to know which of the following?

(A) disease incidence
(B) disease prevalence
(C) negative predictive value
(D) the cut off values for the test
(E) the latest period of the disease

Questions 118 through 120

Doing a retrospective chart review of unmatched cases and controls, you calculate an OR to make an initial assessment of whether women who have had induced abortions are more likely to develop breast cancer. Twenty of 100 women with breast cancer reported a history of induced abortion. Ten of 200 women without breast cancer reported a history of induced abortion.

118. What is the exposure odds among cases?

(A) 0.250
(B) 0.500
(C) 2.000
(D) 4.000
(E) 8.000

119. What is the exposure odds among controls?

(A) 3.973
(B) 1.682
(C) 0.184
(D) 0.053
(E) 0.009

120. What is the OR?

(A) 0.053
(B) 0.11
(C) 2.00
(D) 2.201
(E) 4.716

121. A 3-year-old child recovers from a severe episode of bloody diarrhea, hemolysis, and uremia. The child's case is linked to other cases across the country by statistical association with consumption of hamburgers obtained from a nationwide supplier of ground beef. Which of the following is the best method for preventing this illness in the general population?

(A) cooking ground beef to be well done, and thoroughly washing fruits and vegetables
(B) regulations enforcing worker hygiene in the workplace
(C) a testing program for enteric disease in livestock
(D) regulations enforcing sanitary conditions in slaughterhouses
(E) a ban on imported meats and produce

122. A study finds that the relative risk of stomach cancer after the consumption of a new sugar substitute is 3.5 with a 95% confidence interval of 1.1–5.3. Which of the following best describes the true relative risk?

(A) If repeated samples are taken from the population, 95% of the time the relative risk will fall between 1.1 and 5.3.
(B) If repeated samples are taken from the population and confidence intervals are found for each sample, 95% of the confidence intervals will include the true population relative risk.
(C) If repeated samples are taken from the population and confidence intervals are found for each sample, 95% of the confidence intervals will fall somewhere between 1.1 and 5.3.
(D) If repeated samples are taken from the population, 95% of the time the true relative risk for the population will fall between 1.1 and 5.3.
(E) Ninety-five percent of individuals from a particular sample will have a relative risk between 1.1 and 5.3.

123. You provide health services for employers in your community. The employers explain to you that they appreciate efforts to contain costs because their insurance premiums are experience rated. Which of the following describes why employers are concerned?

(A) An experienced management team has set new rates for the employers.
(B) The employers pay the cost of service as out of pocket expenses.
(C) Everyone in the community pays the same rate for insurance based on community charges and overhead.
(D) The employer pays a large deductible.
(E) An employer's rates reflect past utilization by the employer.

124. You assume care of a 28-year-old nursing home aide, who recently had a positive tuberculin skin test (TST). In the past, her tests have always been read as negative; this year, she developed a 20 × 25 mm induration. She feels well and has no cough. A baseline white blood cell count and liver function test is normal, and a recent HIV antibody test is negative. You order a chest x-ray, which is normal. Which of the following is the best next step in management?

(A) Begin three-drug antituberculosis therapy.
(B) Educate the patient on the symptoms of tuberculosis and repeat the chest x-ray in 1 month.
(C) Isolate her from her family and other close contacts.
(D) Immunize the patient with bacillus Calmette–Guérin (BCG) vaccine.
(E) Begin isoniazid, 300 mg daily.

125. You see a young mother whose child is in need of medical care. She has an income below the federal poverty level. She is eligible to receive cash payments under the Supplemental Security Income Program (SSI). As she has no heath insurance, you ask a social worker to help her enroll in a program funded with state and federal tax dollars, which provides complete medical care for her child. You ask that she be enrolled in which of the following programs?

(A) Medicaid
(B) Medicare
(C) Blue Cross/Blue Shield
(D) The Robert Woods Johnson Foundation
(E) Women, Infants, and Children program (WIC)

126. A young child finds a bat lying on the floor of his room. The child picks it up to show it to his mother, and it bites him on the hand. The bat then escapes, flying out an open window. Which of the following diseases poses the most serious threat to the child's health?

(A) rabies
(B) lacrosse encephalitis
(C) distemper
(D) tularemia
(E) tetanus

127. An outbreak of influenza occurs across the United States in the early winter. Of individuals contracting influenza, a large proportion had received vaccinations earlier in the fall. Which of the following is the most likely explanation?

(A) The vaccine was manufactured improperly.
(B) The vaccine used did not contain antigen specific to the outbreak strain.
(C) A systemic storage problem with a major shipper damaged the vaccine.
(D) Due to unusually cold weather, people were more susceptible.
(E) The virus was especially virulent.

128. A family is scheduled to move into a home that is 15 years old. Its water supply is a well, and sewage is discharged to an on-site septic system. In preparation for the move, they obtain a series of water tests from the well. All of the results show the presence of coliform bacteria. Which of the following is the implication of these data?

(A) They are at risk of acquiring a coliform bacterial infection.
(B) The well water has been mixed with untreated surface or groundwater.
(C) Nothing—this is a common finding in the country.
(D) The groundwater is extensively contaminated and the house is unlivable.
(E) They can live in the house but must seek medical care at the first sign of illness.

129. The mortality rates from two countries are being compared. Despite vast differences in wealth, level of public services, birth rates, and education, the difference in crude mortality rate is the opposite of what is expected: The more developed country has the higher crude mortality rate. Which of the following should you do to better understand this difference?

(A) Verify a difference in health status of residents by doing a health survey.
(B) Examine the causes of death to determine the reason for the difference.
(C) Recalculate the rates using 5-year aggregate data.
(D) Calculate an age-standardized death rate for each country.
(E) Compare the mortality rates for cities of equal size in each country.

130. An HMO has its annual medical directors meeting, and new treatments are discussed. A recent study has just clearly demonstrated that a new drug can lower blood pressure significantly, although monitoring tests for renal function are required. The directors consider adding the treatment to their list of approved treatments but feel handicapped. Which of the following is one of the real disadvantages of making treatment decisions based on clinical outcomes alone?

(A) Clinical tests cannot reliably tell which treatment works best.
(B) Clinical trials ignore the difference in costs between treatments.
(C) Results of clinical trials cannot possibly be applied to real-world situations.
(D) Effects noted in the study population will not show up in the general population.
(E) The advantages of improvement in clinical outcomes are always too significant to ignore.

131. The U.S. Preventive Services Task Force made recommendations for screening mammography and clinical breast examination every 1–2 years for women aged 40 years and older. Which of the following is the best explanation for why routine screening mammography was not recommended for women in the general population under 40 years of age?

(A) Screening mammography in women less than 40 is not as sensitive as in those over 40.
(B) Screening mammography in women less than 40 is more difficult due to tissue density.
(C) Women under the age of 40 are still likely to have high estrogen levels.

(D) Breast self-examination in the younger group is more sensitive in detecting cancers than mammography.
(E) The benefit of detecting cancers in the younger age group was outweighed by the risks screening caused in that age group.

132. In order to allocate health care resources in your community, you compare the health status of subpopulations by comparing infant mortality rates. Which of the following most accurately compares the infant mortality rates for children born to White mothers and for children born to Black mothers in 2001 in the United States?

(A) The infant mortality rate for children born to Black mothers was one-third the infant mortality rate for children born to White mothers.
(B) The infant mortality rate for children born to Black mothers was one-half the infant mortality rate for children born to White mothers.
(C) The infant mortality rate for children born to Black mothers was between one and two times the infant mortality rate for children born to White mothers.
(D) The infant mortality rate for children born to Black mothers was between two and three times the infant mortality rate for children born to White mothers.
(E) The infant mortality rate for children born to Black mothers was six times the mortality rate for children born to White mothers.

133. There is public alarm over the possible food-borne transmission of bovine spongiform encephalitis in your community. You decide to institute an active surveillance system to gather information on possible cases. In order to do this you should do which of the following?

(A) Collect information by gathering voluntary data reports from healthcare providers, laboratories, and others.
(B) Conduct a case-control study of individuals in your community with and without the disease.
(C) Organize the systematic calling of pathologists and neurologists from surrounding areas in an attempt to identify cases.
(D) Monitor disease in animal flocks.
(E) Collect billing reports to identify where the cattles were purchased from.

134. The National Center for Health Statistics collects information on chronic disease risk factors such as obesity, treatment for blood pressure, exercise, and alcohol use. These data are best captured using which of the following tools?

(A) health survey
(B) hospital records
(C) registries
(D) physician-based reports
(E) outpatient clinic records

135. An outbreak of fever, shock, and pulmonary edema without a known etiology is occurring in your community in the southwestern United States. The CDC sends a team of experts to the area for the purpose of finding the cause and stopping the outbreak. This is best done by using which of the following?

(A) active surveillance
(B) passive surveillance
(C) sentinel surveillance
(D) case-control study
(E) mandatory case reporting

136. Meningitis caused by type B *H. influenzae* is prevalent in a developing country. You advocate for health policy development to address this issue. Which of the following would be the most effective policy in reducing the number of cases?

(A) voluntary vaccination of children prior to school entry with Hib vaccine
(B) mandated reporting of cases of meningitis caused by type B *H. influenzae* to local health authorities
(C) mandated vaccination of all children prior to entry into day care or school with Hib vaccine
(D) active surveillance of cases of meningitis caused by type B *H. influenzae*
(E) passive surveillance of cases of meningitis caused by type B *H. influenzae*

DIRECTIONS (Questions 137 through 139): Each set of matching questions in this section consists of a list of lettered options followed by several numbered items. For each question, select the ONE best lettered answer that is most closely associated with it. Each lettered answer may be selected once, more than once, or not at all.

Questions 137 and 139

For each situation below, select the category of prevention it represents.

(A) primary prevention
(B) secondary prevention
(C) tertiary prevention
(D) selective prevention
(E) community prevention
(F) preventive therapy

137. A community hospital conducts a screening for hypercholesterolemia by setting up stations and testing blood samples. Persons with elevated cholesterol are referred for dietary counseling, exercise programs, and possible treatment.

138. State officials conduct a program providing public service messages outlining the dangers of smoking and urging adolescents not to start. The program is a success, in that surveys indicate fewer adolescents begin smoking.

139. A patient has severe respiratory disease as a result of years of smoking. He successfully quits smoking and improves his respiratory function.

DIRECTIONS (Questions 140 through 143): Each of the numbered items or incomplete statements in this section is followed by answers or by completions of the statement. Select the ONE lettered answer or completion that is BEST in each case.

140. A study that has been stratified for age finds a statistically significant association between alcohol use and socioeconomic status (SES). In reviewing the data, the investigators find that the relationship between alcohol and SES is greatest for those in the 40- to 50-year age group. In this scenario, age plays which of the following roles in the relationship between alcohol use and socioeconomic status?

(A) bias
(B) confounder
(C) effect modifier
(D) chance
(E) distractor

141. A 25-year-old welder is found to have diffuse small pulmonary opacities on a routine chest x-ray. He has no respiratory complaints and is found to have normal ventilatory function on lung function tests. Which of the following metals are most likely responsible for his "benign pneumoconiosis?"

(A) lead
(B) copper
(C) cadmium
(D) iron
(E) silver

142. An outbreak of cholera occurs in a village in South America. The source of the outbreak is thought to be a well used by the majority of the villagers. A public health worker is sent to determine the microbiological quality of the water source. Which of the following organisms is most often used as a measure of fecal contamination?

(A) coliform bacteria
(B) parvoviruses
(C) protozoa
(D) helminths
(E) amoebas

143. A private foundation wants certain protected health information such as names, addresses, and antibiotic which will be used to set up a new Tuberculosis Surveillance System. This is being done in an effort to track and monitor cases of multidrug resistance TB which seems to be on the rise in a particular community. According to the Health Insurance Portability and Accountability Act (HIPAA):

(A) This will be possible because only deidentified information is being used for the surveillance system.
(B) This will be possible because private foundations are not subject to privacy rules governed by HIPAA.
(C) This will not be possible because private foundations are only allowed to retrieve private health information under strict conditions which have not been met.
(D) This will not be possible because private foundations are not allowed to collect private health information under any circumstance.
(E) This will not be possible because tuberculosis information can only be collected by government.

Answers and Explanations

1. **(A)** Onset of influenza usually is abrupt, with fever, chills, fatigue, headache, myalgias, malaise, anorexia, scratchy throat, and nonproductive cough. Fever appears early and may reach 40°C (104°F). Myalgias affecting the back and legs, and retrobulbar headache are worse with high fever. There is a normal leukocyte count with relative lymphopenia. Chest x-ray may show enlarged hilar shadows. Fever lasts a few days. Upper and then lower respiratory symptoms become more prominent, and cough may persist for weeks. Respiratory anthrax is exceedingly rare. Initial symptoms may resemble influenza, but rhinorrhea is rare. X-rays generally show patchy lung infiltrate and mediastinal widening (due to enlarged hemorrhagic lymph nodes). Early treatment with antibiotics such as ciprofloxacin sometimes prevents death. *(Wallace and Doebbeling, p. 108; CDC website, 2004)*

2. **(C)** There is a markedly higher frequency of impaired vision of the elderly in nursing homes than in the community. While it is not frequently recorded as a reason for nursing home admission, people with impaired vision experience many other limitations. Cataract is the leading cause of blindness in both communities. Maximizing visual acuity by appropriate refraction obviously improves mobility and ability to function but is not effective if the patient has cataracts. *(Wallace and Doebbeling, pp. 1031–1033)*

3. **(D)** The virus is excreted in stools and pharyngeal secretions. Transmission occurs mainly by the fecal-oral route, particularly where sanitation and personal hygiene are poor, as in developing countries. The WHO, with the assistance of Rotary International, is progressing toward global eradication. There is no known reservoir for poliovirus except humans. By 2000, the Americans were polio free. *(Wallace and Doebbeling, pp. 123–125)*

4. **(C)** Vaccination against typhoid fever (caused by *Salmonella typhi*) is less effective than antibiotic treatment, with only 65–75% effectiveness. Transmission is via fecal-oral route, with humans as the reservoir. Most cases (62%) are contracted as a result of overseas travel to certain areas of the world where the incidence remains high. It is in such endemic areas that vaccine is still advised. There has been no indication that immunization after earthquakes or other cataclysmic disasters is either necessary or effective. *(Wallace and Doebbeling, p. 238)*

5. **(D)** Human illnesses caused by the various species of *Brucella* organisms tend to be quite similar. All tend to be chronic, relapsing infections. Reinfection rarely occurs in recovered patients, with immunity to subsequent *Brucella* infections in 90% of people. Infection is rarely airborne but can be encountered in laboratory and abattoir (slaughterhouse) workers. Person-to-person spread is rare. The primary reservoir is in animals. The mode of infection is principally from direct contact with infected animals or by the ingestion of infected unpasteurized milk. *(Wallace and Doebbeling, pp. 359–360)*

6. **(E)** Researchers have reported significant disparities between men and women in heart disease. An excess risk is documented in Western society through studies such as the Framingham study and studies in Finland. There appears to be relative protection from estrogens among younger women. However, the Women's Health Initiative demonstrated an increase in risk for heart disease in women using exogenous postmenopausal HRT. Cardiac disease is more likely to present as angina in women. Older women carry more cholesterol as high-density lipoprotein (HDL) than low-density lipoprotein (LDL) compared to younger women. The gender difference in vascular disease is less apparent in the aorta,

cerebral, and peripheral arteries than in the coronary arteries. In Eastern Europe, cardiovascular disease is increasing rapidly in women, while in the United States, the age-specific increase in cardiovascular disease is greater among women than men. *(Wallace and Doebbeling, p. 940; Lang and Hensrud, 2004)*

7. **(B)** Examples of primary prevention include routine immunization of individuals at risk for infectious disease, or healthy diet and exercise for persons at risk for diabetes; presymptomatic and clinical diseases are not present and are being avoided. Screening, such as by using Pap smears, colonoscopy, or mammography, typifies secondary prevention; disease is recognized earlier than it otherwise would be, making improved management of the disease possible. Efforts to reduce the consequences of existing recognized disease are termed tertiary prevention. *(Wallace and Doebbeling, p. 895)*

8. **(A)** The major hazards associated with food-borne illnesses are of biological origin. Although all of the phases of the food preparation process may present opportunities for contamination, the major problem is related to food handling rather than to the quality of the food itself. Poor personal hygiene and improper holding temperatures are the leading factors resulting in contamination with bacterial and viral pathogens. Commonly reported pathogens include *Salmonella, Staphylococcus aureus, Shigella, Clostridium perfringens, Escherichia coli*, hepatitis A, and Norwalk/Norwalk-like virus. *(Wallace and Doebbeling, p. 726)*

9. **(E)** Data from the National Center for Health Statistics show that the over 85 segment of the population is growing at the fastest rate. Disability and quality-of-life issues are very important for this age group. *(Wallace and Doebbeling, p. 1059)*

10. **(B)** There are many intrinsic factors that lead to falls in the elderly. Iatrogenic causes from medication prescribed commonly impair stability of gait. However, it is osteoporosis, particularly in the elderly female that results in the excess fractures, usually of the femur. A low BMI is associated with a higher risk of osteoporosis and therefore, fractures. Although the elderly are more likely to have Alzheimer and Parkinson diseases, and poor eyesight, these are not as important as osteoporosis in fractures among the elderly. *(Wallace and Doebbeling, p. 1063)*

11. **(C)** The Framingham study found no association between smoking and disease of the bones, spleen, thyroid, and auditory system. A number of studies have shown definite increased rate of diseases of the cerebrovascular system due to smoking. There may also be some increase in noise-induced hearing loss and some increased risk of fracture of the femur among smokers. *(USPSTF, 3rd ed.: Periodic Updates, Tobacco Use: Counseling, 2003)*

12. **(C)** Lead-based paint was banned from use in residential homes in 1977, and children exposed to environments built before that time should be screened for lead. The age at which children most frequently ingest the largest amounts of lead is during the crawling and walking stage, which is also the oral-anal stage of development that occurs between the ages of 6 months and 2 years. Until children are mobile, they are unlikely to come into contact with objects that might have been coated with lead-based paint. Current guidelines recommend screening beginning at 1 year of age in high-risk populations. Lead levels generally peak at about 2 years of age. After 2 years, children normally have less tendency to put unusual objects and soiled fingers in their mouths. *(Lane and Kemper, American College of Preventive Medicine, www.acpm.org)*

13. **(B)** The situation described in the question calls for clinical judgment. Restrictions should be specific and should pertain to what the patient may actually be asked to do. A company may not interdict a woman from performing a job just because she is pregnant. You should offer your best advice to a pregnant woman concerning her health and the health of the fetus. Advice should be given to patients and not to their employers. The vast majority of women can continue to do their jobs without restrictions. Telling a patient to simply avoid risk is impractical, difficult to interpret, and cannot be

applied effectively. Advise and offer to write task-specific restrictions, such as, "not to climb ladders and not to lift, push, or pull with more than 20 lbs of force," or "not to work at unprotected heights such as on high ladders." The patient is well advised to discuss her needs with her employer. The physician should not communicate directly with the employer unless that is requested by the patient. *(Wallace and Doebbeling, p. 696)*

14. **(A)** Ecological studies compare groups not individuals. The unit of observation in the above study was a community not individuals. A cross-sectional study design would have looked at the incidence of asthma in those who also owned the particular home heating system at a particular point in time. A cohort study would have taken disease-free individuals in the community who also owned the home heating system and followed them over time to see who developed disease. A case-control approach would have taken individuals with and without asthma and identified how many from each group also had the particular home heating system. *(Wallace and Doebbeling, pp. 18–19)*

15. **(A)** Community fluoridation is a very cost-effective method of preventing dental caries; in fact, it is actually a cost-saving practice. Implementation requires no additional effort on the part of the community in terms of health-care utilization and reimbursement. Promoting dental hygiene in and of itself has not been found to be effective in preventing dental caries. Therefore, regular visits to dental hygienists or having dental hygienists visit schools will not by itself prevent dental caries. Sealants are very effective in protecting against dental carries in populations who have deep pits and grooves on the dental surfaces. It is not as effective on smooth dental surfaces. Therefore, it is cost-effective but only in a subset of the population. Semiannual topical application of fluoride by a professional, although effective, will be an expensive program to institute especially in populations that do not have dental coverage. *(Wallace and Doebbeling, pp. 1096–1102)*

16. **(A)** Rifampin, ciprofloxacin, and ceftriaxone have been recommended for the chemoprophylaxis of close contacts of cases of meningococcal meningitis. Gamma globulin has not been shown effective for prevention of meningococcal disease. Most outbreaks are caused by strains of groups A, B, C, Y, and W-135. Most outbreaks in children less than 1 year old are caused by group B (for which there is no vaccine). A vaccine for groups A, C, Y, and W-135 is available but is used only when the source has been isolated and typed, which is rarely the case when prophylaxis must be started immediately. The immunogenicity of vaccines for groups A and C is poor, especially in children. Meningococcal vaccine has been reccomended for high-risk groups, including military troops and students living in dormatories. The search continues for a widely applicable vaccine. *(Wallace and Doebbeling, pp. 206–208; MMWR, June 30, 2000; MMWR, January 7, 2005)*

17. **(B)** Bubonic plague is uncommon in the United States. It is almost always contracted through a bite by an infected flea. A small local papule or vesicle, and sometimes a local ulceration, may occur at the site of the *Y. pestis* infecting bite. Mucous membranes and broken skin also can be entry sites. After an incubation period of 2–6 days, illness is manifested by fever, chills, headache, myalgia, and arthralgia. Eventually, there is painful enlargement (the bubo) of lymph nodes draining the inoculation site *(Wallace and Doebbeling, p. 312)*

18. **(C)** Hib vaccine is recommended for routine immunization of children. Introduction of the Hib conjugate vaccine in the late 1980s was followed by a spectacular decrease in the incidence of *H. influenzae* meningitis. Anthrax vaccine is used to vaccinate military troops in selected overseas deployment. Rabies vaccine is used for postexposure prophylaxis when children are bitten by potentially rabid mammals. Hepatitis A vaccine is used for children at special risk of such infection. Typhoid vaccine is not routinely recommended for use in the United States but may be indicated for travelers to areas in the developing world where typhoid fever is endemic. *(Wallace and Doebbeling, p. 117)*

19. **(A)** In 1990, there were 3 million persons in the United States aged 65 or more. In 2001,

there were 35 million, and by 2030 there may be 71 million. For the population as a whole, usage of health care is high at the time of birth and, to an even greater degree, in the period prior to death. *(Wallace and Doebbeling, p. 1066; Statistical Abstract of the United States, 2004–2005, Figs. 11 and 12)*

20. **(C)** Since the 1950s, the single most important failure in coping with disasters has been poor management by those in charge. There has been no significant problem with resources needed or with triage of casualties. Neither has there been evidence of poor response to the need for volunteer helpers. Telecommunications have improved continuously, especially with satellite communications available. *(Wallace and Doebbeling, pp. 1170–1173)*

21. **(A)** Public health sanitation measures in emergency conditions should reduce fecal contamination of food and water supplies. Communicable disease such as typhoid fever, cholera, bacillary and amoebic dysentery, hepatitis, polio, schistosomiasis, various helminthes infestations, and viral gastroenteritis can be transmitted through contact with human feces. Avoiding putting fecal material in the mouth is key to avoiding infection. *(Wallace and Doebbeling, p. 1171)*

22. **(D)** The fourth DTaP must be at least 6 months later than the third dose. Hepatitis A vaccine is recommended in some high-risk communities, but it is not recommended for all children. Pneumococcus vaccine for children not previously immunized by 23 months should receive two doses 8 weeks apart. Oral polio vaccine should not be used when inactivated poliovirus is available. *(Recommended childhood and adolescent immunization schedule United States, 2005)*

23. **(D)** Carbon disulfide causes sensorimotor peripheral neuropathy. Central nervous system (CNS) effects and optic neuritis are also common. Long-term exposure may increase cardiovascular risk. Lower sperm counts and more abnormal spermatozoa are observed than in unexposed subjects. *(Wallace and Doebbeling, p. 535)*

24. **(B)** The U.S. Preventive Services Task Force (USPSTF) strongly recommends that clinicians routinely screen all sexually active women aged 25 years and younger, and other asymptomatic women at increased risk for infection, for chlamydial infection. *(USPSTF 3rd ed.: Periodic Updates)*

25. **(D)** After two normal Pap smears, women with normal risk can be screened every 3 years. *(USPSTF, 3rd ed.: Periodic Updates)*

26. **(D)** The U.S. Preventive Services Task Force does not recommend ECG or ETT in asymptomatic patients. A BMI greater than 27 is associated with increased mortality. The U.S. Surgeon General recommends a program of moderate exercise most days of the week. *(USPSTF, 3rd ed.: Periodic Updates)*

27. **(C)** Whereas all of the interventions have a positive effect on smoking cessation, the bupropion hydrochloride has the greatest effect at 6-month follow-up. *(Hunt et al., pp. 1195–1202; USPSTF, 3rd ed.: Periodic Updates)*

28. **(C)** The law has generally recognized that the parents do not necessarily exercise autonomy appropriately on behalf of their child. It also recognizes that children cannot exercise autonomy for themselves, and that children should not be required to make complicated decisions about their own care. For children, and for adults who are unable to make medical decisions, a surrogate decision maker is normally named by a court of appropriate jurisdiction. *(Wallace and Doebbeling, pp. 35–36)*

29. **(B)** The age adjusted lung cancer mortality rate rose rapidly following adoption of smoking by women. This now has stabilized as the leading cause of cancer death in women. *(National Center for Health Statistics, Centers for Disease Control and Prevention, Health, United States, 2004. Table 29. www.cdc.gov/nchs)*

30. **(B)** Sometimes it is possible to identify subgroups or strata of a population. Randomly sampling these segments, called strata, may reduce sampling error. Systematic sampling, selecting every "*i*th" individual, is not necessarily random, depending on how lists are constructed. Random groups would presumably be based on random selection of individuals, and little benefit would derive from studying such groups. Random groups produce more hazards statistically than randomized strata. Clusters are somewhat different; they may be small groups of the population occurring in specific areas, such as families, villages, or wards. The characteristics of clusters are not necessarily those of the population, but more those of location. Cluster sampling may be useful but does not have the same outcome as a stratified sample. *(Greenberg et al., p. 97; Gordis, pp. 210–211)*

31. **(C)** Prevalence is the number of existing cases of a disease occurring in the total population at a given period of time. In this study, the prevalence rate is calculated based on reported figures (15 + 185 = 200 persons per 1000 persons surveyed report having hypertension). The actual figure, as demonstrated by the investigation of the sample, is likely to be higher. *(Greenberg et al., pp. 15–27)*

32. **(D)** In the tables that accompany the question, the number of hypertensive persons in the community is 200. The number of patients with hypertension who also report a history of MI is 15. The prevalence is therefore 15 in a population of 200, which may be translated as a rate of 75 per 1000. *(Greenberg et al., pp. 15–27)*

33. **(D)** In the study described in the question, the prevalence rate is the total number of cases occurring in the community, divided by the number of members in the community, multiplied by 1000. This is a point prevalence rate: the number of individuals who have had an MI at the time the questionnaire is administered. Thus, the prevalence is $(20/1000) \times 1000 = 20$. *(Gordis, p. 33)*

34. **(E)** The chi-square test is the most appropriate statistical test to determine whether series of frequencies or proportions are significantly different from each other. It is designed to describe with a single number how much the frequencies in each cell of a box of paired readings differ from the frequency we would expect if there were no relationship between the observed readings. If the observed readings are similar to expected readings, the chi-square will be a small number. If there is a greater difference, the chi-square will be larger. The mathematical equation is

$$\chi^2 = \sum \frac{(0-E)^2}{E}$$

(Wallace and Doebbeling, p. 25, Feinstein, p. 246)

35. **(E)** In a questionnaire relating to history, patients' knowledge as to whether or not they have hypertension or have had an MI might be sufficiently accurate to allow further statistical analysis. The data provided in this questionnaire are not adequate for more detailed statistical analysis. The questionnaire responses (Table 4-1) rely on memory recall, which at best is questionable, for comparison with an actual examination (Table 4-2). Criteria for establishing a diagnosis of MI and, if possible, actual blood pressure readings, as well as a definition of hypertension, are required. The crux of epidemiologic analysis is a detailed criterion for establishing a diagnosis. With this additional information, relevant statistical tests could be applied. In the absence of this information, any further statistical analysis is likely to lead to misleading results. *(Feinstein, pp. 2–3)*

36. **(B)** Silicosis is considered a risk factor for the development of active TB disease for those who have contracted the infection. HIV infection, malnutrition, IV drug use, alcoholism, leukemia and other cancers, poorly controlled diabetes, severe kidney disease, immune system suppression caused by medications such as drugs to prevent rejection of a transplanted organ, and living in crowded indoor conditions, are also considered risk factors for progression to active disease. Cough variant asthma and bronchitis are not included in this list. COPD can occur as a consequence of chronic TB disease and is not considered one of the risk factors. Siderosis results from accumulation of nonfibrogenic iron oxide particles in the lung and is not considered to predispose to TB. *(Wallace and Doebbeling, pp. 209)*

37. **(C)** Humans are the usual reservoir of *V. cholerae.* It tolerates exposure and drying poorly. It survives longest in water, especially if the water is at temperatures of 18–23°C (60–70°F). It does not spread on infected clothing (fomites). Direct person-to-person transmission probably does not occur. Contaminated water is the main source of infection (e.g., frequent exposure to polluted surface water through bathing, food preparation, and utensil washing). Although flies may transport small numbers of vibrios from excreta to food, lack of multiplication makes it unlikely that flies play an important part in transmission. Mosquitoes are not vectors. *(Wallace and Doebbeling, pp. 240–243)*

38. **(D)** The principal risk factor for Lyme disease in the United States is residence in an area with high infestation rates of infested ticks. In the coastal northeastern United States, the white-footed mouse is the most competent vertebrate reservoir of *B. burgdorferi*, the organism responsible for Lyme disease, with infection rates of up to 80%. Therefore, residence in an area where there is a large population of white-footed mice will also increase the likelihood of exposure to Lyme disease. The tick species *I. dentatus* has maintained cryptic cycles of *B. burgdorferi*, but it is not considered to be a public health risk because it rarely feeds on humans. Texas is not one of the endemic areas for Lyme disease. Lizards are actually considered to be a zooprophylactic host because they are an incompetent reservoir of *B. burgdorferi*, and they are also a preferential feeding source for immature stages of the tick. Pesticide spraying is actually protective against tick infestation and therefore will reduce the chances of tick exposure. *(Wallace and Doebbeling, pp. 327–332)*

39. **(C)** Chelating drugs are given as treatment for symptomatic poisoning by lead and other heavy metals. They should not be given prophylactically, since the agents themselves have some possible toxic side effects. These toxic effects may add to those already caused by ingestion of the metals and may actually increase absorption of the metal. For these reasons, advice should be given to workers to seek employment away from exposure to the offending agent while therapy continues. Removal from exposure is essential if levels are high. *(Rom, pp. 989–990)*

	Disease present	Disease absent	Totals
Test positive	100(TP)	100(FP)	200
Test negative	50(FN)	350(TN)	400
Totals	150	450	600

40. **(C)** Several concepts are important in determining the sensitivity of tests. The percentage sensitivity is the percentage of individuals with the disease (true positives [TP]) detected by the tests. False negatives (FN) are those who have the disease, but who were not detected by the test. The percentage sensitivity is calculated as $TP/(TP + FN) \times 100$. In the example given in the question, the calculation is $100/(100 + 50) \times 100 = 66.7\%$. *(Greenberg et al., pp. 78–79)*

41. **(D)** The percentage specificity of a test is the percentage of those persons without the disease (true negatives [TN]) who were correctly labeled by the test as not diseased. The false positives (FP) are those who were incorrectly labeled by the test as having the disease. The specificity is thus expressed as $TN/(TN + FP) \times 100$. In the example given in the question, the calculation is $350/(350 + 100) \times 100 = 77.8\%$. *(Greenberg et al., pp. 78–79)*

42. **(D)** Hepatitis A was first isolated in 1973. Since then, it has been demonstrated to be conveyed from person to person chiefly by the fecal-oral route. Humans appear to be the only natural host. Outbreaks attributed to food and water supplies are frequently reported. There were an estimated 61,000 new infections in the United States (particularly in the West) in 2003, continuing a trend downward. It does not cause chronic infection. Vaccination is effective and available for persons at risk, including travelers. Examples of where outbreaks occur include: among travelers, among young adults clustered together, and in day care environments. *(Wallace and Doebbeling, pp. 175–178; www.cdc.gov Viral Hepatitis Surveillance)*

43. **(C)** The mean, or average, is the total of all readings divided by the number of readings, or $(\Sigma x)/n$. In the example described in the question, the total of all readings equals 639; the number of readings is 9. Therefore, the mean is 639 divided by 9, or 71. *(Feinstein, pp. 31–34)*

44. **(B)** The modal reading is the most frequently occurring observation in a group of data. (On a graph of frequency of different observations, this would be where the peak is.) This reading generally is not very useful for statistical calculations, and when the series is small, no modal reading may even occur. When drawn in graph form, the determination of unimodal or bimodal distribution may be a helpful concept from which conclusions may be drawn. The distribution in the example that accompanies the question is unimodal. *(Feinstein, pp. 31–34)*

45. **(D)** The median is the observation that lies in the middle of the series, if the observations are tabulated in numerical order. Half of the observations are lower in numerical value than the median, and the remainder are higher. Clearly, this value is easily identified if the series contains an odd number of readings. Although not very frequently used as a statistic, the median has the advantage of not being affected by extreme observations. For example, if the lowest reading of those in the question had been 55 instead of 61, the median would be unchanged. *(Feinstein, pp. 31–34)*

46. **(C)** The range is the difference between the highest and lowest readings in a group of observations. The lowest reading is subtracted from the highest. Only one of these two readings is included in the range. If both were to be included, the range would be 20, as there are 20 possible values included in the limits of the data presented in the question. For simplicity, the first method is generally accepted. One disadvantage of the concept of range is that it may increase as the number of observations increases. *(Feinstein, p. 60)*

47. **(C)** The variance is the sum of the squares of the difference of each reading from the mean. This is a mathematical way of eliminating the opposing effects of negative and positive values. But the variance has a result that is of a different order than the original observations. The variance of 58.75 seems to have little relationship to a series of readings from 61 to 80. In order to determine a value that is the same order as the observations, the SD is calculated as the square root of the variance. This is mathematically represented as

$$\mathrm{SD}(x) = \frac{\sqrt{V(x)} \supseteq V(x) = \Sigma(x - x)^2}{n - 1}$$

Without using a calculator, it can be seen that the nearest correct answer (correct to 1 decimal place) is 7.7. *(LaDou, pp. 819, 822–825)*

48. **(D)** In a crude death rate, all deaths are in the numerator, and the total midyear population in the denominator. In age-specific death rates, the calculation is done using data from specific age intervals. Small differences in crude death rates may enable specific deductions to be made. A higher death rate in the older population may indicate that a more fragile population has successfully survived to that age. Of the statements listed, considering that age-specific death rates were greater in all age groups except the elderly, only the fact that a greater proportion of the population in Sweden is in the older age groups could account for the difference in crude mortality rate. *(Wallace and Doebbeling, p. 47)*

49. **(C)** The OR is used when the denominator data are missing. It is calculated using the following formula, comparing smokers and nonsmokers:

$$\frac{a \times d}{b \times c}$$

In this case, the mathematics is relatively simple: $75 \times 75/25 \times 25$. By reduction, this is $3 \times 3/1 \times 1$. *(Greenberg et al., p. 134)*

50. **(E)** A true risk ratio cannot be calculated from a case-control study. *(Gordis, pp. 135–136, 178–179)*

51. **(B)** For ease of calculation, to illustrate the concept, the numbers in the question were kept simple. If the numbers of controls were increased, the difference would be smaller. The ORs are a reasonable estimate when denominator data are missing. Relative risk is determined when denominator data are available. Few case-control experiments have denominator data. *(Gordis, pp. 184–185)*

52. **(B)** Bias is a systematic error that may be introduced, generally unwittingly, into an investigation. Selection bias is due to systemic differences between those selected and not selected for a study. When selecting all admissions to a community hospital, alcoholics may be overrepresented among hospital patients and not reflect the community base from which the patients were admitted. Further, the investigator has not chosen a control sample but only patients already in the hospital, which further invalidates any outcome. While other biases may creep into this study, the selection bias is the major problem with the study. *(Greenberg et al., pp. 144–151)*

Explanations 53 through 56

Note that each illness listed may be contracted by a person working with animals, animal products, and the associated rodents. The following answers refer to the most likely infections:

53. **(A)** Cutaneous anthrax is associated with a characteristic skin lesion, which becomes infected by the introduction of the bacillus through the skin. Occasionally, an infected carcass is not identified before butchering. A minor wound on the butcher may become infected. Human anthrax is secondary to the disease in animals, primarily mammals. In humans, the disease has three major clinical forms: cutaneous, inhalational, and GI. *(Wallace and Doebbeling, p. 357)*

54. **(D)** Rodents frequently infest granaries, despite strenuous efforts to control them. Murine (endemic) typhus has its principal reservoir in rodents and is conveyed to humans by flea bites. In the United States, murine or endemic typhus occurs mainly in the Southeastern and Gulf states. It is also common in parts of South America, Africa, and Southeast Asia. The disease generally follows a less severe course than epidemic typhus. *(Wallace and Doebbeling, p. 306)*

55. **(B)** *Brucella* infections in humans follow a varied and sometimes chronic or recurrent course. Chronic disease is rare in appropriately treated patients. Human infections generally occur through one of three routes: ingestion, direct contact, or inhalation. Cattle sheds become infected after abortion, a manifestation of the disease, or occasionally after normal parturition. Worldwide, ingestion of unpasteurized dairy products is the primary source of infection. *(Wallace and Doebbeling, p. 359)*

56. **(C)** Lyme disease was first comprehensively described in Connecticut in 1977. It is found in temperate North America and Eurasia. It may be identified some time after the initial illness, which may be a vague collection of symptoms. The vector is a tick found on the white-footed mouse, which is the reservoir. Persons who spend a significant amount of time in affected wooded areas are at risk for Lyme disease. *(Wallace and Doebbeling, p. 327)*

57. **(A)** Local health departments make plans for the entire population in the jurisdiction for which they have responsibility, whether it is a single county, city, or multicounty health department. Their planning is population based. This involves estimating health requirements, matching them with existing resources, and outlining a health strategy based on the deficit or surplus demonstrated. *(Wallace and Doebbeling, pp. 1155–1158)*

58. **(B)** A distinction is frequently made between what the patient wants (which would be used if available and money was no object), needs (services determined by professionals to be appropriate), and demands (services that are actually used in the current market situation). Planning for an HMO is based on that segment of the population or "market" for which the HMO is responsible. The population may or may not live in contiguous areas. The planning is designed to identify goals and objectives in institutional terms: What is the market for the

services the organization provides, and what is the estimate of future demands? The population need (as opposed to the population demand) is rarely a concern of institutional planners. *(Wallace and Doebbeling, pp. 1155–1158)*

59. **(D)** Program planning concerns itself with neither the fiscal need for a particular service nor its marketability. By definition, "the program" (e.g., maternal and child health care) will be developed and provided as directed by the state or local government. The planning is directed to carry out program goals for a targeted (select) population (pregnant women and their infants). This type of planning is necessary to implement government or private foundation-sponsored programs. *(Wallace and Doebbeling, pp. 1155–1158)*

60. **(C)**

61. **(B)**

62. **(A)**

63. **(B)**

64. **(A)**

Explanations 60 through 64

Epidemic typhus (classical typhus fever, or louse-borne typhus) has disappeared from most areas of the world but might reappear in conditions of famine, war, or other disasters. There are small areas where it is endemic. The responsible organism, a rickettsia, is conveyed from case to case by the human body louse, *Pediculus humanus corporis*. Malaria, in its various forms (*Plasmodium falciparum, Plasmodium vivax, Plasmodium ovale*, and *Plasmodium malariae*), is spread from human to human by females of the various *Anopheles* group of mosquitoes. Dengue fever has a worldwide distribution in tropical and subtropical areas. In addition to producing the classical fever with severe myalgia (breakbone fever), it can also cause a hemorrhagic fever. The causative agent, a group B arbovirus with four distinct serogroups, is virus-conveyed from case to case by the *A. aegypti* mosquito. Colorado tick fever occurs mainly in mountainous areas of the United States within the range of its vector, *Dermacentor andersoni*. The highest incidence is in May and June. Several hundred cases are recorded annually, but it is likely that the actual incidence is much higher. Avoidance of tick bites is the principal control measure. Yellow fever, the prototypical viral hemorrhagic fever, is African in origin but has spread to and remains endemic in equatorial regions of Central and South America. The vector, *A. aegypti*, has also spread worldwide, but surprisingly, cases have not been reported in India and Southeast Asia. The illness varies in severity from a mild, nonspecific fever to a more severe condition with hemorrhagic, hepatic, and renal manifestations. *(Wallace and Doebbeling, pp. 294, 295, 300, 305)*

65. **(C)**

66. **(A)**

67. **(C)**

68. **(B)**

69. **(E)**

Explanations 65 through 69

In the United States, the organization of food and water control is complex. Among the federal control agencies, the EPA is the most recent, and in many ways the most active and powerful. This agency has now set up an elaborate system of regulation and control of the use of pesticides (which until 1970 was the responsibility of the USDA) and has banned the marketing of chlorphenothane (DDT) for use in the home. The FDA has authority to remove food from the market if it contains pesticides (e.g., PCBs in fish) in excess of the action levels set by the EPA. The FDA also retains the authority to remove from the market any food with inappropriate additives, that contains substances harmful to human health, that is stored in unsanitary conditions, that has decomposed, or that is not fit for consumption. The USDA enforces wholesomeness standards that it sets for the production and sale of meat. International control is assisted by the WHO. This agency has mounted control programs for the eradication of communicable disease with conspicuous success in the case of smallpox. It also publishes the International Statistical Classification of Disease (ICD-9). *(www.hhs.gov key word organization chart; LaDou, p. 557)*

70. (B)

71. (D)

72. (A)

73. (C)

Explanations 70 through 73

Knowing the incubation period (average and range) of a pathogen can be important in determining the source of infection in food-borne disease. Knowing what food was eaten on the day of an attack of food poisoning may not help in establishing *C. botulinum* as the cause of illness, since certain strains of *S. aureus* cause food-borne disease by the production of enterotoxin. As no time is required after ingestion for the growth of colonies in the infected host, and the toxin affects the vagus nerve in the stomach, the incubation period is under 4 h. *Clostridium perfringens*, formerly known as *Clostridium welchii*, causes food-borne disease, after 8–24 h when enterotoxin is released when *C. perfringens* passes from stomach to intestine. Meat prepared in bulk for consumption at a banquet or in an institution is a possible source. Spores that survive incomplete cooking may start reproducing during cooling and may persist if subsequent rewarming is not completed to a temperature above 60°C (140°F) required to kill the organisms. *Salmonella* has an incubation time of 12–36 h. It may also survive in meat and other products if cooking is inadequate and heat does not penetrate below the surface of the food. The organisms multiply in the gut of the infected host, and low infective doses may therefore have longer incubation periods. *(Wallace and Doebbeling, p. 724).*

74. (C) PCBs were extensively used in the manufacture of electrical transformers until production was halted in the mid-1970s. The first sign of chronic exposure to these substances is the appearance of an acne-like eruption with inflammatory pustules. Other effects are eye irritation and gastrointestinal disturbance. The substances are persistent, and more than 25% of the population in the United States was discovered to have residues of greater than one part per million (ppm) in adipose tissue. Dietary exposure of the general population has been alleged to occur through milk, eggs, cheese, meat, and fish. *(Rom, pp. 1205–1217)*

75. (E) Organophosphorus compounds have been widely used since the 1950s as insecticides, both in national pest control programs and domestically. They have been responsible for many deaths on a worldwide basis, despite the lives initially saved by control of mosquitoes and malaria. From the point of view of the environmental toxicologist, it was perhaps fortuitous that many pests began to develop resistance to the substances fairly early in the use of these compounds. More recently, concern for environmental control has further limited their use; studies have attributed carcinogenic properties to several of these pesticides. *(Rom, pp. 1159–1163)*

76. (A) Nitrosamines are highly toxic and dangerous to handle when used as solvents. Toxic amounts may be absorbed without warning because danger signals such as specific odor or irritant effects are lacking. The manufacture of rubber, dyes, lubricating oils, explosives, insecticides, and fungicides, as well as the electrical industry, all have associations with these substances. Nitrosamines have animal carcinogenic properties and have been transmitted transplacentally in rats. *(Rom, pp. 1227–1238)*

77. (B) Epoxy compounds are used in the production of resins. They cause irritation of the skin and mucosa and have caused acute pulmonary edema. *(Rom, p. 499)*

78. (D) Formaldehyde commercial solutions contain up to 15% methanol. Formaldehyde has numerous industrial applications including, use as a base for urea formaldehyde resins. The gas is an irritant to the eyes and upper respiratory mucosa. The odors of products manufactured with formaldehyde products have been responsible for actions against manufacturers of tightly built manufactured homes. *(Rom, pp. 1115–1127)*

79. **(D)** Ozone is a colorless, pungent gas occurring naturally in the stratosphere, which can be produced by electric arcs. Ozone is generated by electrical storms and UV light and electric arcs and some forms of fuel combustion. In the stratosphere, it is protective by blocking solar radiation. At 10 ppm, it can cause pulmonary edema and tracheal pain and is believed to cause asthma. Based on animal tests and observations of gases trapped during inversions, an action level of 10 ppm has been set for workplace exposure. *(Wallace and Doebbeling, p. 577)*

80. **(C)** Hydrogen sulfide is a colorless gas that rapidly paralyzes the nasal receptors, and is found in sewers. Hydrogen sulfide produces nausea, headache, and shortness of breath. Because it paralyzes the nasal receptors at a concentration of 150 ppm and cannot be smelled shortly after exposure, it is highly dangerous, with instant death from a concentration as low as 1000 ppm. *(Wallace and Doebbeling, p. 577)*

81. **(B)** Methane is a colorless, odorless, flammable gas sometimes encountered in mines and wells. Methane (coal damp) is a frequent cause of death in inadequately ventilated mines and wells. It acts as an asphyxiant as well as being explosive. Miners used to take caged animals, especially birds, with them. The birds succumbed to the asphyxiants (methane and carbon dioxide) sooner than humans. *(Rom, p. 652)*

82. **(A)** Carbon monoxide is an odorless, colorless, tasteless gas produced by partial combustion of tobacco and fuels. The amounts produced by cigarette smoking are not insignificant. The gas combines with hemoglobin preferentially to form carboxyhemoglobin, which makes the patient appear pink. This diminishes the oxygen-carrying capacity of the blood. The resulting anoxia is the major hazard. The onset of symptoms is insidious. Individuals exposed to carbon monoxide may not voluntarily take the action necessary to remove themselves from the toxic fumes. *(Rom, pp. 1505–1507)*

83. **(E)** Sulfur dioxide is a colorless, pungent gas encountered in drilling for oil, paper production, treatment of fruit, and other processes. Sulfur dioxide is an irritant gas. It causes tearing, mucous membrane irritation, cough, and eventually pulmonary edema. In asthmatics it provokes bronchospasm at low doses. Like other irritant gases, in large quantities, it will damage alveoli and capillary endothelial cells. *(Rom, pp. 631–639)*

84. **(D)** The USPSTF (2004) recommends that women aged 40 and older have mammography with or without clinical breast examination, every 1–2 years. *(USPSTF, 3rd ed.: Periodic Updates)*

85. **(F)** The USPSTF (2003) strongly recommends screening for cervical cancer (Pap smear) at least every 3 years in women who have been sexually active or are 21 years old, and have a cervix. It recommends against screening after a normal hysterectomy, or after age 65, if recent Pap smears were normal and the woman is not at high risk. (Note: Although evidence is still considered insufficient, screening for human papilloma virus (HPV) infection shows promise as a part of cervical cancer prevention. Vaccination against HPV is expected to greatly decrease incidence of cervical cancer in the future.) *(USPSTF, 3rd ed.: Periodic Updates)*

86. **(E)** The USPSTF (2002) strongly recommends that men and women aged 50 or older be screened for colorectal cancer. Various methods exists, including fecal occult blood testing every 1–2 years, sigmoidoscopy perhaps every 5 years, colonoscopy perhaps every 10 years, and other tests. Digital rectal examination is not adequate. *(USPSTF, 3rd ed.: Periodic Updates)*

87. **(C)** The USPSTF (2004) strongly recommends screening pregnant women for hepatitis B at their first prenatal visit, but recommends

against screening the general population. *(USPSTF, 3rd ed.: Periodic Updates)*

88. (A) The USPSTF (2004) recommends against routine screening for pancreatic cancer in asymptomatic adults. *(USPSTF, 3rd ed.: Periodic Updates)*

89. (A)

90. (B)

91. (B)

92. (A)

93. (C)

Explanations 89 through 93

IG given before exposure or within 14 days of exposure is 75–85% effective in preventing symptomatic illness from hepatitis A. IG is produced from the plasma of normal adults and does not contain sufficient antibody to prevent hepatitis B infection. Hepatitis B immune globulin (HBIG) is prepared from plasma known to contain high antibody titers for hepatitis B surface antigen (HBsAg) and is specific for hepatitis B. Given immediately postexposure, and again 1 month later, it has a combined efficacy of about 75% in the prevention of hepatitis B. Postexposure IG has not been found effective in the prevention of hepatitis C infection; on the other hand, treatment of early hepatitis C infection is possible, and thus it is important to monitor exposed individuals to determine whether infection occurs. IG administered to individuals exposed to measles infection who are susceptible to the disease has been shown to be effective if given within 6 days of exposure. Recent use of IG is a contraindication to immunization with rubella vaccine. IG is not very effective at preventing *in utero* infection with rubella, and infants with congenital rubella syndrome have been born to women given IG shortly after exposure. IG is not routinely indicated, as it is indicated only if abortion is not elected. *(USPSTF, 3rd ed.: Periodic Updates; Wallace and Doebbeling, pp. 67, 184, 91, 97)*

94. (A)

95. (D)

96. (E)

97. (D)

98. (C)

99. (B)

100. (D)

Explanations 94 through 100

The incubation period for diphtheria is 1–7 days. The incubation period for chickenpox is 10–21 days, average 14. Infectious mononucleosis, caused by the Epstein-Barr virus, has an estimated incubation period of 30–50 days. The incubation period following infection by the mumps virus is usually 16–18 days but, like chickenpox, may vary from 14 to 25 days. Pertussis has a shorter incubation period, usually 7–10 days, with a variation of 4–21 days. The usual period from contamination with tetanus spores to clinical symptoms is generally 6–8 days. For rubella, the incubation period is from 14 to 21 days, but usually ranges from 16 to 18 days. *(Wallace and Doebbeling, pp. 105, 117, 190, 93, 98, 103, 95)*

101. (I)

102. (B)

103. (D)

104. (I)

105. (G)

106. (A)

107. (F)

108. (C)

109. (J)

Explanations 101 through 109

Giardiasis may cause cramping and a chronic diarrheal syndrome, with malabsorption and weight loss. Its distribution is worldwide, particularly where hygienic standards are not high. It also occurs sporadically in high-risk individuals. Streptococcal pyoderma, including erysipelas and impetigo, has been demonstrated to precede acute glomerulonephritis. Even when appropriate antibiotics are given in adequate dosage and duration for these conditions, renal damage may still result. Prevention thus consists of wound care, including cleaning wounds well and removal of crust. *Mycoplasma* infections are particularly common in families with younger children. They are frequently imported to the family by school-aged children, leading to a low-grade fever and persisting tracheobronchitis in the parents, or more acutely, an atypical pneumonia. *G. lamblia* is found in up to 20% of homosexual males, and may cause chronic diarrhea, although in these patients it tends to be asymptomatic. *E. coli* was first reported as a cause of watery diarrhea in nurseries in the 1940s. Although nursery epidemics with enteropathogenic serotypes had decreased in recent years in the United States, the increase of infant-child day care centers has resulted in their relatively frequent occurrence. Furunculosis is most frequently caused by coagulase-positive staphylococcal infections. The public health significance of this largely relates to the hazards of skin infections in food handlers and subsequent staphylococcal toxin in the food, leading to staphylococcal intoxication food-borne disease. *H. pylori* has been associated with gastric ulcer, but not with duodenal ulcer. Otitis media, whether acute or with effusion, commonly results from viral infection, such as by respiratory syncytial virus. Various other organisms maybe responsible including *Streptococcus pneumoniae, H. influenzae,* and others. *C. perfringens,* with rare exceptions, is transmitted in a meat dish prepared in bulk. Under propitious circumstances for the organism, especially on cooling of the food, bacterial multiplication can be very rapid. Symptoms begin to occur in the affected population in about 12 h. Epidemic typhus is a rickettsial illness. Man is the host and long-term reservoir. The vectors are body lice (*P. humanus corporis*). The rickettsia are not present in human excretions and cannot be transmitted by person-to-person contact. *(Wallace and Doebbeling, pp. 252, 201, 173, 252, 243, 265, 994, 116, 266, 305)*

110. (A)

111. (C)

Explanations 110 and 111

The following table was constructed using the data in the question. There would be 4995 FPs, 98 TPs, and 2 FNs. *(Greenberg et al., pp. 7–8, 78–79)*

	Disease		
	Present	**Absent**	**Totals**
Test			
Positive	98	4,995	5,093
Negative	2	94,905	94,905
Totals	100	99,900	100,000

112. (C) In a randomized, controlled trial, the determination of treatment group assignment is left to chance. The procedure maximizes the probability that the two groups are similar in important background characteristics. Thus, it avoids self-selection of study subjects to different exposure groups. In a cross-sectional study design, it is generally difficult to ascertain the antecendent-consequent aspects of the hypothesized relationship. In other words, since the exposure and outcome are measured at a given point in time, it is difficult to determine which came first. A cohort study classifies study subjects by exposure status and follows them forward in time to determine development of disease. More than one disease can be targeted as outcomes of interest. A case-control study defines cases and controls and retrospectively assesses the frequency of exposure. Multiple exposures can be assessed in connection with a specific disease. *(Gordis, pp. 115–128, 159–173, 149–157, 173–174)*

113. (E) The design of a cohort study requires a follow-up of a group of subjects who are susceptible but free of the disease of interest at the beginning of the study period. *(Gordis, pp. 149–157)*

114. **(D)** In a prospective cohort design, a group of subjects at risk of developing disease are followed over a specified period of time. This design permits the direct calculation of incidence by dividing the number of subjects who developed the disease of interest during the follow-up period by the population or person-time at risk. In contrast, incidence cannot be calculated directly from the other observational study designs (cross-sectional, case-control). *(Gordis, pp. 149–157)*

115. **(B)** The health survey was conducted in a defined population on a particular date. With this information, the prevalence of conjunctivitis can be determined, but not the incidence. Measuring incidence requires information on new occurrences of the disease from a follow-up study. *(Gordis, pp. 33–37)*

116. **(B)** By definition, sensitivity is the probability of testing positive if the disease is truly present. It indicates the percentage of persons with the disease of interest who have positive test results. Positive predictive value estimates the probability of disease in those who have positive test results. It indicates the percentage of persons with positive test results who actually have the disease of interest. *(Wallace and Doebbeling, pp. 907–908)*

117. **(B)** In order to calculate predictive value, it is necessary to know prevalence. To illustrate this, consider the extremes if prevalence is zero, positive predictive value will be zero, and negative predictive value will be 100%! *(Wallace and Doebbeling, pp. 907–908)*

118. **(A)** The problem can be represented by the following table:

	Breast cancer	
Abortion	**Yes**	**No**
Yes	20	10
No	80	190
Total	100	200

The odds of exposure among cases is calculated by dividing the probability that a case was exposed by the probability that a case was not exposed: (20/100)/(80/100) = 20/80 = 0.25. *(Greenberg et al., pp. 204–205)*

119. **(D)** The odds of exposure among controls is calculated by dividing the probability that a control was exposed by the probability that a control was not exposed: (10/200)/(190/200) = 10/190 = 0.053. *(Greenberg et al., pp. 204–205)*

120. **(E)** The OR for exposure is calculated by dividing the odds of exposure for cases by the odds of exposure for controls: OR = (20/80)/(10/190) = 4.716. (Note that an unmatched case-control study would be flawed by confounding [age] and bias [recall bias].) *(Greenberg et al., pp. 204–205)*

121. **(A)** The illness described is consistent with hemolytic uremic syndrome associated with *E. coli* 0157:H7 infection. *E. coli* 0157:H7 is the most common strain found of the enterohemorrhagic *E. coli* (EHEC) group. Although its most common reservoir is thought to be in cattle, it has been found in other livestock. The usual mode of exposure is contamination of beef. The problem is compounded significantly when beef is ground and mixed in bulk. Testing and elimination programs do not appear sensitive enough to eliminate exposure, although active research in the area continues. In addition, there are many other outbreaks associated with fresh vegetables, bean sprouts, and unpasteurized juices. It is hypothesized that these are due to contamination with human or animal waste. Since the organism is killed by heating, thorough cooking of ground beef products, avoidance of contamination of fresh foods with raw meat, and washing of produce intended to be served fresh is the most practical intervention. Currently, this remains the most practical advice to give the public. *(Wallace and Doebbeling, p. 726)*

122. **(B)** A confidence interval gives an estimated range of values which is likely to include an unknown population parameter, in this case the relative risk of stomach cancer with consumption of the sugar substitute. The estimated range is calculated from a given set of sample data. If independent samples are taken repeatedly from the same population, and a confidence interval calculated for each sample, then a certain percentage (termed the *confidence level*) of the intervals will include the unknown population parameter. *(Feinstein, pp. 195–197)*

123. (E) The insurance company charges premiums to the employer based on "experience rating," which means charges are based on past utilization of service. To control premiums in the future, control utilization now. Community rating would be different, in that risk would be spread across a broader community. Community rating makes insurance more affordable for individuals or groups that use a lot of health care, but removes incentive to control costs. *(Rom, p. 84)*

124. (E) The patient has a positive reaction to purified protein derivative (PPD). This indicates tuberculosis infection, but not necessarily clinical disease. Health care workers have a risk of acquiring tuberculosis that is 2–10 times the risk for the general public. Since conversion is recent (she had a negative test last year), the risk of progressing to disease is relatively large compared to the risk of hepatotoxicity from preventive treatment with isoniazid. Such preventive treatment is 65–80% effective in preventing progression to active disease. Note that new assays (ELISPOT, QuantiFERON) performed on a blood sample or oral swab are becoming available, and that they are more sensitive and specific for exposure to *Mycobacterium tuberculosis* than is the TST. *(Rom, p. 802; CDC website, 2004)*

125. (A) Medicaid and Medicare began under federal legislation in 1966. Medicaid is a state-run program funded with federal and state tax dollars. It was established to provide medical services to the poor, with special consideration to pregnant women and small children. Although eligibility varies greatly from state to state, persons who receive SSI welfare payments are categorically eligible. Medicare is a federal program, completely financed and run by the federal government. Its purpose is to provide medical care to citizens over 65. Blue Cross/Blue Shield is a private insurance that must be purchased; the Robert Wood Johnson Foundation is a large foundation that provides grants; and the WIC program is a food supplement program for needy mothers and children. *(Wallace and Doebbeling, p. 1128)*

126. (A) Transmission of rabies virus by a bat bite has been well documented, and in many areas of the country, bats are known to harbor the rabies virus. There are also well-documented cases of human rabies due to viral strains found in bats, but without a good history of being bitten. Therefore, presumptive treatment is recommended in the case of a bite (and in some cases for a possible bite) when the bat cannot be recovered and tested. Lacrosse encephalitis, distemper, and tularemia are not known to be transmitted by bats. Tetanus is unlikely because a child this age has probably been immunized. *(Wallace and Doebbeling, pp. 349, 350)*

127. (B) Manufacturing, storage, and shipping problems do occur. However, they have not been related to nationwide failures, although a major manufacturing problem in 2004 resulted in a major reduction in supply of vaccine. It is more likely that the vaccine in use is not completely protective against the prevalent viral strain. The WHO monitors influenza outbreaks worldwide. Based on strains present in outbreaks, and especially in the Pacific Rim, WHO makes a recommendation every spring regarding the antigens to use for the fall immunization campaign. Manufacturing then begins. Although their track record is good in this regard, antigen changes in influenza may reach the United States undetected or ahead of schedule. *(Wallace and Doebbeling, p. 110)*

128. (B) Testing for the presence of coliform bacteria is a standard bacterial test of water quality. Since coliform bacteria are ubiquitous in nature, their presence means only that the water has been contaminated with water from the ground surface or the septic system. It is only an indicator. Coliform bacteria are not the principal agents of disease. It is the other agents introduced into the water by the contamination that create the risk. The problem should be resolved before using the well water. A common cause of contamination is poor well construction, resulting in surface water moving down the outside of the well casing and into the water source. *(Wallace and Doebbeling, p. 745)*

129. (D) Crude mortality rates for a population are calculated using total deaths divided by total population. Differences in the age compositon of the population can make an enormous difference in crude mortality rates, since the elderly have a much higher mortality rate. Adjusting for age computes a hypothetical "adjusted" rate for each country based on their own age-specific mortality rates, but using standard population. The technique is called age adjusting, or standardization. It is used in other rate studies as well. For instance, the crude mortality rates for MI would be different for a largely middle-aged population than for an older population. Age adjusting allows comparison. *(Greenberg et al., pp. 51–53)*

130. (B) Although clinical trials can determine which treatment works best, they cannot determine the cost of this success. Unfortunately, they do not take into account costs and ultimate benefits, which would be the role of a cost-benefit study. If properly constructed, with study and control groups randomly drawn from the general population, the results should be applicable to the general population. In addition, they usually determine what works best by measurement of a clinical endpoint. In many cases, the treatment may achieve its objective, but the change in parameters may not be significant. It is worthy of note that the 3rd U.S. Preventive Services Task Force is now taking cost-effectiveness into account when making recommendations. *(USPSTF, 3rd ed.: Periodic Updates)*

131. (E) It is true that mammography for detection of breast cancer in older women is technically easier and probably more sensitive than in younger women. However, the burden of cost and mortality resulting from screening women less than 40 was the real reason that screening them was not recommended. For first mammograms of women aged 40–49, cancers were diagnosed at half the rate of women aged 50–59 years old, yet twice as many follow-up diagnostic tests were performed. Simply put, the cost in terms of dollars, mortality from testing, and mortality from radiation exposure for women under 40 were not considered to be worth the benefit. *(USPSTF, 3rd ed.: Periodic Updates)*

132. (D) In 2001, the infant mortality rate for children born to White mothers was 5.7 infant deaths/1000 live births. The infant mortality rate for children born to Black mothers was 14.0 infant deaths/1000 live births. *(http//www.cdc.gov)*

133. (C) Active surveillance is used in urgent situations, such as active and ongoing epidemics. Health agencies contact those data sources most likely to have current information regarding cases. The collection of data which has been voluntarily submitted is referred to as passive surveillance. Case-control studies are a form of investigation and represent a "next step" after surveillance. These studies seek to identify further information regarding the health problem by studying individuals with the disease. Surveillance systems on the other hand are used primarily to identify whether or not a problem exists and how it is changing through time. Monitoring disease in animal population or in other specific populations that are higher or earlier risk is referred to as senitnel data collection or surveillance. Identifying where cattle were purchased may help to identify the extent of disease spread in animals, but does not describe active surveillance of human cases. *(Wallace and Doebbeling, pp. 8–16)*

134. (A) The Behavioral Risk Factor Surveillance System is a health survey that uses telephone interviews to collect information about chronic disease risk factors such as obesity, treatment for blood pressure, alcohol use, and exercise. Review of hospital records may capture some of this information, but is not an efficient method of capturing information on multiple risk factors for chronic disease. Registries are primarily used to track clinical information regarding particular diseases or conditions. They do not tend to capture a large body of information on behavioral risk factors. Physican-based reports are usually generated as a consequence of state or federal mandates regarding the reporting of communicable disease, rather than behavioral risk factors for chronic disease. *(Wallace and Doebbeling, p. 12)*

135. (D) Surveillance systems focus on descriptive information that is analyzed to detect distributions and trends. Surveillance systems are used to detect whether or not a problem exists, and how it is changing. Case-control studies are used once a problem has in fact been detected, and help assess causation and how the problem may be controlled and prevented. *(Wallace and Doebbeling, pp. 8–9)*

136. (C) Infection with hemophilus type B is communicable and may cause meningitis. The most effective measure that can be employed to reduce the incidence of these infections is the use of mandated universal vaccination. Voluntary vaccination will not capture the entire population at risk and may allow for the continued spread of disease. Mandated reporting and active surveillance, will help to inform health officials regarding changes in the trends of disease, but will not directly help in containing or managing disease. *(Wallace and Doebbeling, pp. 12–13, 116–117)*

137. (B) This activity is secondary prevention since it identifies individuals with a risk factor for a disease and attempts to prevent the disease. It is important to note that the disease itself is not yet present, only the risk factor for its development. In this case, the risk factor for development of atherosclerotic vessel disease was high cholesterol, and the subjects of the intervention did not yet have any symptoms. *(USPSTF, 3rd ed.: Periodic Updates)*

138. (A) Primary prevention interventions prevent the development of risk factors or of disease. For instance, a program that reduces consumption of saturated fats in order to reduce hypercholesterolemia (risk factor), and thus the risk of developing coronary artery disease (disease) and a MI (disease) is primary prevention. *(USPSTF, 3rd ed.: Periodic Updates)*

139. (C) Tertiary prevention is the correction of a diseased state and prevention of complications that result from that state. In this case, the patient already had developed disease from smoking. Cessation of tobacco use is simply treating the disease. In this sense, most medical therapy is tertiary prevention. *(USPSTF, 3rd ed.: Periodic Updates)*

140. (C) An effect modifier changes the relationship between a risk factor and an outcome. In this example, the overall relationship between alcohol and SES has not changed, but its effects are greatest in a particular age group, and thus age is modifying the effect of the association between alcohol and SES. In this example, the study was stratified based on age, which would control for confounding effect based on age. Bias is seen when there is a systematic error in the manner in which age is distributed between the risk factor and outcome categories. Bias occurs when there is a systematic error in the design or conduct of a study. There is not enough information provided to determine whether bias may be present. Because the findings have been stratified and have been found to be statistically significant at each stratum, there is less of a possibility that chance is playing a role in the relationship between age and the exposure or outcome. Distractor is not a term commonly used to describe a variable's relationship to an outcome. *(Wallace and Doebbeling, pp. 24–25)*

141. (D) Iron siderosis is often referred to as a benign pneumoconiosis because only limited clinical effects are seen with iron inhalation. This term is used to label those pneumoconiosis which generally have a favorable prognosis because they are caused by relatively inert (i.e., nonfibrogenic) dusts, in contrast to those that may evolve toward debilitating pulmonary fibrosis. Findings are most often limited to radiologic findings such as those mentioned above. But workers are most often exposed to more than just iron dust, and combinations of iron with other substances such as asbestos or radon can cause significant lung damage. Iron siderosis is most commonly seen in welders, foundry workers, or grinders. *(Wallace and Doebbeling, p. 499)*

142. (A) Determination of whether coliform bacteria are present has been used as a measure of fecal contamination since the early twentieth century. Coliform bacteria, whether fecal or nonfecal, should not be present in significant numbers in any potable water supply. *(Wallace and Doebbeling, pp. 745–746)*

143. (C) Private foundations are regulated by HIPAA privacy rules. They are allowed to collect health information provided that (1) they have obtained a release of information from the patients, (2) the personal health information is deidentified (the information which is planned for use in the surveillance system has not been deidentified), (3) the personal health information is contained in a limited data set governed by a data-use agreement (this is not mentioned in the vignette), (4) release of the personal health information is in accord with the privacy rule's provisions for disclosure for research without authorization (this has not been clearly stated in the vignette). (*HIPAA Privacy Rule and Public Health Guidance from CDC and the U.S. DHHS, http://www.cdc.gov/mmwr/preview/mmwrhtml/m2e411a1.htm, 2004*

REFERENCES

Agency for Toxic Substances and Disease Registry. *Lead Toxicity. Case Studies in Environmental Medicine.* Atlanta, GA: U.S. Department of Health and Human Services, 2000. Available at: http://www.atsdr.cdc.gov/HEC/CSEM/

Centers for Disease Control and Prevention, 2004: http://www.cdc.gov/mmwr/preview/mmwrhtml/m2e411a1.htm.

Centers for Disease Control and Prevention. A-Z Index. Anthrax. 2004. Available at: www.cdc.gov/

Centers for Disease Control and Prevention. A-Z Index. Tuberculosis. 2004. Available at: www.cdc.gov/

Centers for Disease Control and Prevention. National Center for Health Statistics. Infant deaths, and infant mortality rates by race of mother and 130 selected causes of death: United States 2001 period data. Table 45. Available at: www.cdc.gov/nchs/data/dvs/LINK01WK45.pdf

Centers for Disease Control and Prevention. National Center for Health Statistics. Health, United States, 2004. Table 29: Age-adjusted death rates for selected causes of death, according to sex, race, and Hispanic origin: United States, selected years 1950–2002. Available at: www.cdc.gov/nchs

Centers for Disease Control and Prevention. National Center for Infectious Diseases: Viral Hepatitis Surveillance. Disease burden form Hepatitis A, B, and C in the United States, 2005. Available at: http://www.cdc.gov/ncidod/diseases/ hepatitis/resource/dz_burden02.htm

Centers for Disease Control and Prevention. Prevention and control of meningococcal disease. *MMWR* June 30, 2000; 49:RR07, 1. Available at: www.cdc.gov/mmwr

Centers for Disease Control and Prevention. Recommended childhood and adolescent immunization schedule–United States, 2005. *MMWR* January 7, 2005; 53(51):Q1–Q3. Available at: www.cdc.gov/mmwr

Dawson-Saunders EK. *Basic and Clinical Biostatistics*, 3rd ed. New York, NY: McGraw-Hill, 2000.

Department of Health and Human Services Organizational Chart. 2004. Available at: http://www.hhs.gov/about/orgchart.html

Feinstein AR. *Principles of Medical Statistics.* Washington, DC: Chapman & Hall, 2002.

Gordis L. *Epidemiology*, 3rd ed. Philadelphia, PA: W.B. Saunders, 2004.

Greenberg RS, Daniels SR, et al. *Medical Epidemiology*, 3rd ed. New York, NY: McGraw-Hill, 2001.

Hunt RD, Sachs DPL, Glover ED, et al. A comparison of sustained release bupropion and placebo for smoking cessation. *N Eng J Med* 1997; 337(17): 1195–1202.

Lane WG, Kemper AR. American College of Preventive Medicine. Practice Policy Statement. Screening for elevated blood lead levels in children. *Am J Prev Med* 2001;20(1):78–82. Available at: http://www.acpm.org/polstmt_blood.pdf

Lang RS, Hensrud DD. *Clinical Preventive Medicine*, 2nd ed. Chicago: AMA Press, 2004.

Last JM. *Public Health and Human Ecology*, 3rd ed. Stamford, CT: Appleton & Lange, 1998.

LaDou J. *Current Occupational & Environmental Medicine*, 3rd ed. New York, NY: McGraw-Hill, 2003.

McCunney RJ. *A Practical Approach to Occupational and Environmental Medicine*, 3rd ed. Philadelphia, PA: Lippincott Williams & Wilkins, 2003.

Rom WN (ed.). *Environmental and Occupational Medicine*, 3rd ed. Philadelphia, PA: Lippincott-Raven, 1998.

U.S. Census Bureau. *Statistical Abstract of the United States: 2004–2005*, 124th ed. Washington, DC, 2004. Figures 11-12. Available at: http://www.census.gov/statab/www/

U.S. Preventive Services Task Force. *Guide to Clinical Preventive Services*, 2nd ed. DHHS, 1996.

U.S. Preventive Services Task Force (USPSTF) Periodic Updates, 3rd ed. Washington, DC: DHHS, 2000–2004. (Note: USPSTF documents appear as periodic updates, accessible on the www at www.achpr.gov/.)

Wallace RB, Doebbeling BN (eds.). *Maxcy-Rosenau-Last Textbook of Public Health & Preventive Medicine*, 14th ed. Stamford, CT: Appleton & Lange, 1998.

CHAPTER 5

Psychiatry

Jon A. Lehrmann, MD

Questions

DIRECTIONS (Questions 1 through 5): Each of the numbered items or incomplete statements in this section is followed by answers or by completions of the statement. Select the ONE lettered answer or completion that is BEST in each case.

Questions 1 through 3

A 28-year-old woman with a 7-year history of chronic undifferentiated schizophrenia is hospitalized for an exacerbation of her schizophrenia, with an increase in auditory hallucinations. She has also developed the delusion that she is controlled by aliens from Mars. She has always been very sensitive to the extrapyramidal side effects (EPS) of antipsychotic medications.

1. Which of the following is an extrapyramidal side effect of antipsychotic medications most likely to be seen in the first few days of treatment with typical neuroleptic antipsychotics?

(A) pill-rolling tremor of the hands
(B) severe restlessness of the arms and legs
(C) involuntary lip smacking
(D) muscle spasm in the neck
(E) masked facies

2. This woman develops cogwheel rigidity and a pill-rolling tremor. Which of the following is the most appropriate treatment choice?

(A) benztropine
(B) propranolol
(C) haloperidol
(D) dantrolene
(E) L-dopa

3. She developed an acute restlessness in her legs and arms which her psychiatrist diagnosed as akathisia. Which of the following is the preferred treatment option?

(A) benztropine
(B) propranolol
(C) haldoperidol
(D) dantrolene
(E) fluoxetine

Questions 4 and 5

A 35-year-old man with no previous psychiatric history is referred by his family physician for psychiatric evaluation. The family physician has been following the man for mild hyperlipidemia, which is currently being successfully treated with dietary changes alone. The man reports that he has been happily married for 10 years and has two children. He has been working as an accountant and has generally enjoyed his job. About 2 months ago, with no obvious precipitating event, he says, the man began to feel very blue, with a drop in his desire to play with his children and to compete in his usual volleyball league games. He reports that he has lost most of his libido and is having difficulty sleeping, with early-morning wakening. He reports that his appetite has become very poor over the past 2 months, and he estimates that he has lost 10 lbs over that time.

4. Which of the following is the most likely diagnosis?

(A) Alzheimer disease
(B) schizophrenia
(C) major depressive disorder
(D) metastatic cancer to the brain
(E) systemic lupus erythematosus

5. Of the following, which would be the most appropriate initial treatment for this patient?

   (A) electroconvulsive therapy (ECT)
   (B) clozapine
   (C) diazepam
   (D) fluoxetine
   (E) buspirone

DIRECTIONS (Questions 6 through 10): For each numbered item, select the ONE best lettered option that is most closely associated with it. Each lettered option may be selected once, more than once, or not at all.

Identify the most likely diagnosis with the case descriptions below.

   (A) body dysmorphic disorder
   (B) conversion disorder
   (C) factitious disorder
   (D) hypochondriasis
   (E) malingering
   (F) pain disorder
   (G) panic disorder
   (H) somatization disorder

6. Despite repeated efforts to reassure a 40-year-old woman that the stomach pain she is experiencing is not cancerous, she continues to worry and fears that she will die.

7. A 23-year-old violinist reports to his neurologist that he thinks he has had a stroke. He is unable to feel anything with his left fingers and is barely able to hold down the violin strings with this same hand because of "paralysis." The numbness he describes reaches to his wrist only, and he "even feels a band" around the wrist delineating the sensitive from the insensitive areas.

8. A 35-year-old woman complains that she has been to multiple doctors, none of whom have been able to effectively treat or even diagnose the cause of her chronic stomach pain and diarrhea, repeated problems swallowing, headache, and recurrent back pain. The symptoms have been present on and off for most of her adult life.

9. A 55-year-old man requests "some kind of pain medication that really works!" to relieve the "extreme" pain in his foot. He walks with a cane. He angrily claims that his previous employer does not care about what happened to him in an accident 1 year earlier in which his foot was struck by an iron rod. No fracture was found. He claims his doctor said he had a "severe contusion" and then states "the doctor didn't know anything."

10. A 40-year-old woman is brought to the emergency department after she had frantically called the paramedics because she thought she would die. She was experiencing sharp chest pain, shortness of breath, racing heartbeat, and cold, sweaty chills. Cardiac assessment proved negative for myocardial ischemia.

DIRECTIONS (Questions 11 through 70): Each of the numbered items or incomplete statements in this section is followed by answers or by completions of the statement. Select the ONE lettered answer or completion that is BEST in each case.

Questions 11 and 12

A 70-year-old female with chronic paranoid schizophrenia presents to the ER acutely confused with visual hallucinations. Her skin is warm and dry and her heart rate is 110 beats per min. Her group home nurse tells you that the patient had been complaining of having a dry mouth and having difficulty initiating urination this past week.

11. Which of the following is the most likely cause for this presentation?

   (A) psychotic exacerbation of schizophrenia
   (B) urinary tract infection
   (C) Alzheimer dementia
   (D) anticholinergic delirium
   (E) myocardial infection

12. Which of the following is the treatment of choice for this patient's acute condition?

   (A) bethanechol
   (B) haldoperidol

(C) physostigmine
(D) bromocriptine
(E) dantrolene

13. A 25-year-old White man reports that he has gotten in trouble with the law as a result of his rubbing up against a woman he did not know in an elevator at work.

Recurrent, intense sexually arousing fantasies, sexual urges, or behaviors involving touching and rubbing against a nonconsenting person, such as a stranger in an elevator, which occur for at least 6 months and which cause significant impairment in an individual's functioning are best characterized as which of the following?

(A) exhibitionism
(B) fetishism
(C) frotteurism
(D) pedophilia
(E) sexual masochism

14. A patient reports that, on his way to the hospital, he saw a man feeding two squirrels in the park. He says that this means his future will be decided in 2 weeks. This man, he believes, is deliberately out to alarm him (the patient). One of the squirrels is scheming with the man; the other is innocent and trusting. Which of the following terms best describes what this man is experiencing?

(A) illusions
(B) hallucinations
(C) delusions
(D) loosened associations
(E) neologisms

Questions 15 and 16

A young mother seeks psychiatric help because she is unable to remember events surrounding her 3-year-old son's death after being struck by a car 2 months ago. She is worried that maybe she did something that put him at risk. Except for this brief time period, she is able to recall other events both before and after the tragedy.

15. Given the information above, which of the following is the most likely diagnosis?

(A) depersonalization disorder
(B) posttraumatic stress disorder
(C) dissociative amnesia
(D) dissociative fugue
(E) major depression

16. Of the following treatments, which is the most appropriate to help this patient regain her memory?

(A) electroshock therapy
(B) individual psychotherapy
(C) chlordiazepoxide
(D) sertraline
(E) thioridazine

17. A young mother brings her 2-year-old son to see his physician, and says he has become quite contrary recently. In Sigmund Freud's theory of the stages of psychosexual development, the period which extends roughly from 1 to 3 years of age and which is marked by intensification of aggressive drives and striving for independence and separation from dependence on and control by the parent is called which of the following?

(A) oral stage
(B) anal stage
(C) phallic stage
(D) latency stage
(E) genital stage

Questions 18 through 21

A 44-year-old man presents with fears that his mathematical abilities have been slowly sucked out of his brain for the last 4 years. He believes an "alien force disguised as a human being" is responsible. To avoid contacting this being, he has isolated himself in a room in a boarding house. His wife divorced him and left with their children. After 10 years teaching math at a local high school, he resigned about 3 years ago. He supports himself by "collecting cans." His affect is blunted. His appearance is disheveled, unshaven, and unwashed.

18. Which of the following is the most likely diagnosis?

(A) paranoid schizophrenia
(B) alcohol abuse and dependence
(C) major depression with psychotic features
(D) Alzheimer disease
(E) Huntington disease

19. Which of the following factors in this case would favor a more positive prognosis?

(A) presence of negative symptoms
(B) late onset
(C) being male
(D) being divorced
(E) experience in teaching mathematics

20. Which of the following hypotheses is the leading hypothesis to explain the patient's psychotic symptoms?

(A) serotonin hypothesis
(B) biogenic amine hypothesis
(C) acetylcholine hypothesis
(D) dopamine hypothesis
(E) gamma-amino-butyric acid (GABA) hypothesis

21. Considering the information learned thus far, which of the following would be an appropriate first-line treatment for this patient?

(A) thiamine
(B) olanzapine
(C) amitriptyline
(D) lithium carbonate
(E) fluoxetine

Questions 22 and 23

A 17-year-old girl is brought in by her parents because of their concerns about her weight loss. She is petite, and a normal weight for someone her height is 100 lbs, but she weighs 78 lbs. She reports menstrual irregularity. The patient believes she is obese. She does not believe she has a problem. Her mother reports that she found laxatives on her daughter's nightstand, and heard her vomiting in the bathroom yesterday after dinner.

22. Which of the following is the most likely diagnosis?

(A) bulimia nervosa
(B) pregnancy
(C) anorexia nervosa
(D) no diagnosis, normal presentation
(E) obesity

23. Which of the following is the best initial treatment?

(A) Have her return in 2 weeks for cognitive behavioral therapy.
(B) Initiate lithium as it often causes weight gain.
(C) Send her home telling her parents this is normal teen behavior.
(D) Start a prenatal vitamin.
(E) Admit her for inpatient psychiatric hospitalization.

Questions 24 through 26

A 70-year-old man is brought to his primary care doctor by the man's son. According to his son, who had not seen his father for about a year, the father seemed to have some personality changes. He was no longer interested in his hobbies and seemed apathetic. He seemed to forget easily, and he repeatedly asked the same already answered questions. On at least two occasions, the father wandered out of the house and was found by neighbors, who thought he was confused.

24. Which of the following is the most common cause of dementia in a 70-year-old man?

(A) Alzheimer disease
(B) Pick disease
(C) Parkinson disease
(D) vascular dementia
(E) subcortical dementia

25. Considering the information learned thus far, which of the following medications would be the most appropriate treatment here?

(A) donepezil
(B) fluoxetine
(C) aspirin
(D) amitriptyline
(E) ginkgo biloba

26. If this man had Pick disease, where would the preponderance of pathology be found?

(A) cerebellum
(B) caudate nucleus
(C) hippocampus
(D) frontotemporal areas
(E) parietotemporal areas

Questions 27 and 28

A 25-year-old male graduate student presents at a university hospital emergency department complaining of a sudden onset of a pounding in his chest, a feeling of choking, and shortness of breath. He reports that things somehow suddenly seem unreal, and he is afraid he is dying of a heart attack. An electrocardiogram (ECG) shows normal sinus rhythm and no abnormalities.

27. Which of the following is the most likely diagnosis?

(A) myocardial infarction
(B) panic attack
(C) hypochondriasis
(D) multiple sclerosis
(E) generalized anxiety disorder

28. If this patient continues to experience similar episodes over the next 2 months, with substantial apprehension about the episodes, which of the following drugs would be most appropriate for the treatment of this patient's condition?

(A) paroxetine
(B) buspirone
(C) olanzapine
(D) propranolol
(E) haloperidol

29. A 70-year-old woman was brought to the emergency department following her involvement in a minor car accident. She had sustained no injuries but was very upset and was, therefore, referred to a psychiatrist. After speaking at length about her part in the accident and sharing her reactions, she still remained tremulous, anxious, and tearful. You decide to use an anxiolytic to help her. Which of the following is the best choice?

(A) diazepam
(B) clorazepate
(C) lorazepam
(D) buspirone
(E) temazepam

30. Which of the following delusions would most likely be observed in a psychotically depressed person?

(A) "My mind's eye is perfused with a radiance of the gods."
(B) "I've been targeted by the FBI."
(C) "My body is rotting inside out."
(D) "I have been hand-picked to be the world's leader; I am awaiting the signal to bring the masses together."
(E) "All I need to do is clutch the book to myself and all the knowledge pours into me."

31. A fourth-year medical student on an emergency medicine clerkship is fascinated by the number of personality disordered patients who come to the emergency room on weekends. Which of the following personality disorders belongs to cluster A (odd, eccentric) in the DSM-IV-TR classification of personality disorders?

(A) schizoid personality disorder
(B) borderline personality disorder
(C) antisocial personality disorder
(D) avoidant personality disorder
(E) obsessive-compulsive personality disorder

32. A 5-year-old girl had been doing well at home and with her playmates until she started kindergarten 1 month ago. She cries whenever her mother and father go to drop her off at school, and she complains of fearing that she will never see them again. She complains of nightmares and refuses to go to school due to severe stomachaches. Which of the following is the most likely diagnosis?

(A) generalized anxiety disorder
(B) separation anxiety disorder
(C) social phobia
(D) specific phobia
(E) obsessive-compulsive disorder

33. A family brings in their 7-year-old boy because he has not been fitting in at school. The mother says he has not made any friends and tends to play mostly by himself. He exhibits repetitive hand flapping. When you interview him, he does not provide any eye contact, and the mother says this is typical for him. His speech seems age appropriate and per history has developed normally. This past year his IQ was tested to be normal. Which of the following is the most likely diagnosis?

(A) autism
(B) Asperger disorder
(C) Rett disorder
(D) attention deficit hyperactivity disorder
(E) borderline personality disorder

34. An 8-year-old boy suffers from compulsive eating, obesity, small stature, hypogonadism, and mental retardation. Which of the following is his most likely diagnosis?

(A) phenylketonuria
(B) Prader–Willi syndrome
(C) Down syndrome
(D) fragile X syndrome
(E) Cri-du-chat syndrome
(E) disorientation

Questions 35 and 36

You are called to the ICU to see a 65-year-old female who is 2 days status post hip surgery. The medical team is concerned because the patient is having visual hallucinations and did not sleep last night. She scored 21/30 on a Mini-Mental Status Examination (MMSE) with 5 points off for disorientation and 2 off for both concentration and short-term memory. The patient is restrained because she pulled out her IV last night. Records indicate she has no previous psychiatric history and that her cognitive functioning presurgery was normal.

35. Which of the following is the most likely axis I diagnosis?

(A) bipolar disorder manic phase
(B) schizophrenia, undifferentiated
(C) dementia NOS (not otherwise specified)
(D) delirium NOS
(E) psychosis NOS

36. Which of the following is not a predisposing factor for the above condition?

(A) cancer
(B) advanced age
(C) female gender
(D) dementia
(E) alcohol dependence

Questions 37 and 38

A 56-year-old man with a dual diagnosis of schizophrenia and alcohol abuse and dependency was arrested for "driving under the influence." After 2 days in jail, he was noted to be acting agitated and "crazy," claiming that the guards were going to kill him that night. When questioned about his profuse sweating, he claimed that he had just come in from his job working in the heat and humidity. He was distracted by various noises, claiming that these were made by people watching him and waiting for him. He appeared to watch things that seemed to be moving on the walls. On further examination, it was noted that he was very tremulous, unable to follow an object with his eyes only, and quite ataxic.

37. The working diagnosis at this point is most likely which of the following?

(A) acute exacerbation of schizophrenia
(B) alcohol withdrawal delirium
(C) alcohol-induced persisting dementia
(D) alcohol intoxication
(E) malingering

38. Which of the following benzodiazepines can reliably be given intramuscularly to this patient to help control his symptoms?

(A) diazepam
(B) chlordiazepoxide
(C) lorazepam
(D) alprazolam
(E) clonazepam

39. A 25-year-old woman presents with a recurrent depression, and says she has taken many antidepressant medications from several different classes of drugs in the past. Which of the following atypical antidepressants is a presynaptic alpha-2 receptor noradrenergic antagonist and a 5-HT_2 and 5-HT_3 receptor serotonergic antagonist?

(A) bupropion
(B) trazodone
(C) nefazodone
(D) venlafaxine
(E) mirtazapine

40. A 60-year-old man disappears from his home and travels 100 miles to a small town, where he opens a small grocery store using a different name. Six weeks later, he awakens in some agitation, uses his original name, and asks to know where he is. He wishes to return to his home. Which of the following is the most likely diagnosis?

(A) dissociative amnesia
(B) dissociative fugue
(C) dissociative identity disorder
(D) depersonalization disorder
(E) dissociative disorder not otherwise specified

Questions 41 and 42

A 35-year-old woman comes into the ER after cutting her wrists for the 10th time. She did this after her boyfriend of 2 weeks left her yesterday. She reports a history of unstable interpersonal relationships, chronic feelings of emptiness, impulsive sexual relationships, and problems with her sense of identity.

41. Which of the following is the most likely axis II diagnosis?

(A) histrionic personality disorder
(B) borderline personality disorder
(C) antisocial personality disorder
(D) dependent personality disorder
(E) avoidant personality disorder

42. The one psychotherapeutic technique to avoid would be

(A) physical holding sessions to help the patient feel in control
(B) clear roles and responsibilities of patient and therapist are established
(C) therapist conveys empathic validation
(D) flexibility
(E) patient and therapist mutually develop a hierarchy of priorities

Questions 43 through 45

A 58-year-old woman with a history of chronic paranoid schizophrenia, who has been continuously treated with antipsychotics for the past 20 years, lives in a community-based residential facility. She has recently suffered an increase in auditory hallucinations, and her haloperidol dose has been increased from 2.5 to 10 mg/day. Four days later, she is brought by a visiting nurse to the emergency room, where she presents with confusion, marked rigidity in her legs and arms, and a temperature of 103.5°F. Her blood pressure is 160/120 mmHg, her pulse is 120/min and irregular. As the on-call physician, you entertain the possibility of neuroleptic malignant syndrome as the diagnosis for this woman.

43. Which of the following is the most important laboratory test to evaluate the possibility of the syndrome?

(A) serum creatine phosphokinase (CPK) level
(B) serum sodium level
(C) serum potassium level
(D) serum glucose level
(E) serum calcium level

44. Which of the following is most likely to be an effective treatment for neuroleptic malignant syndrome in this patient?

(A) intramuscular haloperidol
(B) oral bromocriptine
(C) intramuscular diphenhydramine
(D) intramuscular benztropine
(E) oral propranolol

45. Which of the following is the most important risk of treatment of neuroleptic malignant syndrome with high-dose dantrolene?

(A) agranulocytosis
(B) tachycardia
(C) bradycardia
(D) hepatotoxicity
(E) drowsiness

Questions 46 and 47

A 31-year-old woman is being treated for her first psychotic break with oral haloperidol. Her auditory hallucinations and delusions are decreasing, but she seems very restless.

46. A common side effect of antipsychotic medications consisting of an unpleasant feeling of restlessness in the arms and legs, and the inability to sit still is called

(A) opisthotonus
(B) bradykinesia
(C) akathisia
(D) rabbit syndrome
(E) tardive dyskinesia

47. Which of the following is the most appropriate treatment for this side effect?

(A) increase haloperidol
(B) benztropine
(C) phenytoin
(D) propranolol
(E) physical restraints

48. A 37-year-old woman telephones to alert her psychiatrist that she has developed a severe pain in her right eye that has persisted for about 5 h. She has no history of migraine headaches. The psychiatrist is treating her with 150 mg imipramine for major depression. She denies any recent injury or infection in this eye. She wears corrective lenses for nearsightedness. Which of the following is the most appropriate step in management?

(A) Advise her to take an anti-inflammatory analgesic.
(B) Advise her to rest and call again in 8 h if the pain has not subsided.
(C) Consult immediately with her ophthalmologist.
(D) Plan to evaluate her eye at her next psychiatric appointment in 2 weeks.
(E) Decrease imipramine to 125 mg/day.

49. A 40-year old man has been treated for chronic paranoid schizophrenia for many years with a typical neuroleptic. To decrease his risk for tardive dyskinesia, his psychiatrist wants to change his medication to an atypical antipsychotic. Which of the following atypical antipsychotics is limited in its use by the risk of agranulocytosis, which occurs in 1–2% of all patients treated?

(A) olanzapine
(B) clozapine
(C) risperidone
(D) quetiapine
(E) ziprasidone

Questions 50 and 51

A 45-year-old homeless schizophrenic patient presents to you with suicidal ideation. You interview him and find out he is a divorced Roman Catholic. He recently lost his job after being caught a second time drinking on the job. He had attempted suicide impulsively 5 years previous by overdosing. He is not currently psychotic. He bought a handgun and ammunition recently and has been thinking about shooting himself in the head. He has gotten as close to acting on it as having loaded the gun and held it up to his head this morning. Someone walking by stopped him and convinced him to come see you. He is ambivalent about seeking help.

50. Which of the following is not associated with an increased suicide risk?

(A) Roman Catholic religion
(B) male
(C) divorced
(D) previous suicide attempt
(E) schizophrenia

51. Which of the following is the most appropriate immediate treatment recommendation?

(A) Start him on antidepressant medication.
(B) Send him home to live with his brother and ask the brother to keep the gun.
(C) Increase his antipsychotic medication.
(D) Prescribe a benzodiazepine to calm him down.
(E) Admit him to the inpatient psychiatric unit.

Questions 52 through 54

A 45-year-old woman, seen by her medical internist, has been experiencing fears that she may have a serious illness. She complains that after eating she experiences "a lot of gas" and abdominal pain, followed by diarrhea on occasion. Her heart at times seems to be beating rapidly, and she feels faint at times, has chest "discomfort," and wonders if she is having a heart attack. Multiple tests have identified only a mild irritable bowel syndrome. The woman's fears are not allayed by this. She makes repeated calls to be seen by her doctors as well as seeking consultation from other specialists. She insists that "there's something there" and believes the doctors are not taking her seriously.

52. Which of the following is the most likely diagnosis?

(A) factitious disorder
(B) major depression
(C) reaction psychosis
(D) hypochondriasis
(E) pain disorder

53. Which of the following is the most effective long-term management of this patient?

(A) Transfer her care to a psychiatrist.
(B) Prescribe alprazolam.
(C) Establish regular follow-up visits with regularly scheduled physical examinations.
(D) Refer for supportive group psychotherapy.
(E) Refer to a pain management clinic.

54. Which of the following most appropriately describes this woman's disorder?

(A) more frequently seen in women than in men
(B) 20–25% prevalence rate in a general medical practice
(C) course of disorder usually of short duration (2–3 months)
(D) associated with elevated erythrocyte sedimentation rate (ESR)
(E) absence of secondary gain is a favorable prognostic indicator

55. During the course of psychotherapy with a woman who has a severe phobia of cars, it is discovered that her first sexual experience, which was a humiliating one for her, took place in an automobile. The defense mechanism illustrated by this phobia is called

(A) acting out
(B) reaction formation
(C) displacement
(D) sublimation
(E) repression

56. A 65-year-old man is referred for a psychiatric evaluation by his primary care doctor. The doctor has noted that his patient seems less concerned about his personal hygiene, his clothes are mismatched, and he is no longer getting to his doctor's appointments on time. In addition, the patient seems depressed, cries, and "no longer enjoys a good joke." Which of the following is the most therapeutic opening question in interviewing this man?

(A) "Tell me about your depression."
(B) "Why are you crying?"
(C) "Tell me what's been happening that brings you here."
(D) "Your doctor tells me you don't match your clothes anymore—why not?"
(E) "Your doctor says you're depressed. How about an antidepressant to help you?"

57. A 30-year-old woman complains that she has had and sleep disturbances since the start of her depression 2 months ago. Which of the following is an accurate description of typical sleep abnormalities in depression?

(A) Sleep latency (the period of time between going to bed and falling asleep) is shortened.
(B) Rapid eye movement (REM) latency (the period of time from the onset of sleep to the first REM period) is shortened.
(C) Wakefulness is decreased.
(D) The arousal threshold is increased.
(E) Stage 3 and stage 4 sleep are increased.

Questions 58 through 60

A 25-year-old man presents in the emergency department for a 2-week problem of worsening urinary hesitancy. He has had problems getting his urine stream started and has noted a decrease in the force of the stream. Now it seems to just "dribble out." He denies any pain or burning, any medical problems, and any exposure to sexually transmitted diseases. For approximately 1 month, he has been taking thioridazine, 200 mg bid, and benztropine, 2 mg qid, and "sometimes one or two benztropine" prn.

58. Given the above information, which of the following is the most likely cause of this man's problem?

(A) anticholinergic side effects to the thioridazine and benztropine
(B) urethral stricture
(C) breakthrough of a psychotic delusion that he cannot urinate
(D) injury from a perverse sexual practice he is not admitting to
(E) infection of the urethra

59. After further evaluation, it is determined that there is no significant distention of the bladder at this time; there are no signs of trauma, infection, or other lesion on external inspection of the genitals, and no enlargement of the prostate. Which of the following is the most appropriate next step in this patient's management?

(A) give benztropine, 2 mg IM, for the side effect of thioridazine
(B) increase thioridazine to 200 mg tid
(C) administer bethanechol
(D) call in the urologist
(E) insert a urinary catheter

60. Which of the following is a safer choice of medication for this man?

(A) amitriptyline
(B) risperidone
(C) chlorpromazine
(D) mesoridazine
(E) imipramine

61. A 78-year-old woman is seen by a psychiatrist for depression. She is fairly cooperative in responding to questions. She admits to feeling blue; she "catnaps" throughout the day and is up at night; and her appetite is very poor. She thinks of death frequently but denies feeling suicidal. There is no past psychiatric history. On the MMSE, she obtains a score of 14. Her depressive symptoms have been present for "several days." Which of the following is highly suggested by the findings?

(A) impaired cognitive functioning
(B) psychosis not otherwise specified
(C) bipolar disorder—manic
(D) dysthymia
(E) changes secondary to normal aging

62. A 40-year-old man has been unsuccessfully treated for depression with two different medications for the past 3 months. He has a number of medical problems, and he recently was hospitalized after threatening suicide. His psychiatrist is considering the use of ECT for the patient. Which of the following is a relative contraindication to ECT?

(A) hypertension
(B) history of seizures
(C) clinically significant space-occupying cerebral lesion
(D) degenerative joint disease of the spine
(E) suicidality

Questions 63 and 64

A 40-year-old woman with no previous psychiatric history seeks help from her internist for a sleep problem. Initially, she is able to fall asleep but then sleeps fitfully, and finally around 4:00 a.m. decides to stay up. She averages approximately 3–4 h of sleep per night, and this has been occurring for the last 3 weeks. She finds herself quite tired and "blue" during the day but is unable to nap. Mornings are "the worst" for her, but she feels better toward the end of the day. There has been a 15-lb weight loss because "I'm just not hungry." She denies any physical problems except for constipation. As a grade-school teacher, she feels extremely stressed but sees no way out and no way to improve the situation. At times, suicide seems like a possible option, and she admits to spending long hours brooding on how to do it. A physical examination is unremarkable.

63. Which of the following is the most likely diagnosis?

(A) borderline personality disorder
(B) major depression
(C) dysthymia
(D) Alzheimer disease
(E) generalized anxiety disorder

64. Which of the following is the most appropriate treatment choice?

(A) olanzapine
(B) paroxetine
(C) alprazolam
(D) tranylcypromine
(E) ECT

65. Which of the following is considered a negative symptom of schizophrenia?

(A) anhedonia
(B) loose associations
(C) delusions of thought insertion
(D) incoherence
(E) stereotypic gestures

66. Which of the following medications may be appropriate for treating children with attention deficit disorder?

(A) lithium
(B) bupropion
(C) alprazolam
(D) propranolol
(E) perphenazine

67. A middle-aged man with depression requests help for his symptoms of low self-esteem and feelings that "life is bad no matter what you do." He prefers to use no medication and expresses the desire to not be in therapy "for years." There is no previous psychiatric treatment. Which of the following therapies would be the most helpful?

(A) psychoanalysis
(B) behavioral therapy
(C) cognitive psychotherapy
(D) supportive psychotherapy
(E) group psychotherapy

68. A 35-year-old woman is seen by her primary care physician for a physical examination. She tells him she has a twin brother who has bipolar disorder and has been worried that she will develop it. Which of the following would be most helpful for her to hear?

(A) "You're past the age when bipolar disorder develops, so don't worry about it."
(B) "There is no clear evidence that a bipolar disorder is genetically determined."
(C) "The concordance rate for bipolar disorder for dizygotic twins is 19%."
(D) "The concordance rate for bipolar disorder for dizygotic twins is 79%."
(E) "Prophylactic treatment with lithium is advisable."

69. Of the following, which is considered a cortical dementia?

(A) Huntington disease
(B) Pick disease
(C) Parkinson disease
(D) occult hydrocephalus (normal pressure)
(E) none of the above

70. A 42-year-old married woman reports being raped in an elevator 1 year ago. Her arms were fractured in the assault but have healed nicely. Still she reports difficulty sleeping, having nightmares of the attack several times per week ever since the assault. She avoids using the elevator and does not want to talk about the incident with anyone. She has been unable to return to work. Her husband feels she has been hypervigilant and irritable, and has been resistive to going out socially. She has a depressed mood. Her husband is encouraging her to seek disability.

Which of the following is the most likely diagnosis?

(A) major depression
(B) adjustment disorder with anxious and depressed features
(C) acute stress disorder
(D) malingering
(E) posttraumatic stress disorder

DIRECTIONS (Questions 71 through 114): Each set of matching questions in this section consists of a list of lettered options followed by several numbered items. For each item, select the ONE best lettered option that is most closely associated with it. Each lettered option may be selected once, more than once, or not at all.

Questions 71 through 75

For each clinical description that follows, select the diagnosis with which it is most likely to be associated.

(A) childhood depression
(B) childhood schizophrenia
(C) conduct disorder
(D) attention deficit hyperactivity disorder
(E) infantile autism

71. A 9-year-old boy has had persisting difficulties in language and interpersonal relationships since the age of 2 years, and, although he can barely read, he is able to perform arithmetic calculations at the fifth-grade level.

72. An 11-year-old girl has become uncharacteristically and markedly withdrawn in the past 8 months, staying in her room so that she can "talk to the ghosts in the attic."

73. An 11-year-old girl has become markedly withdrawn in the past 8 months and has complained of persisting abdominal pain and constipation, for which no organic cause has been found.

74. A 5-year-old boy is reported by his kindergarten teacher to be distractible, impulsive, in need of continual supervision, but not hyperactive.

75. A 3-year-old boy spends hours rocking in a chair or spinning the blades of a toy windmill; his parents say he never cries when he falls.

Questions 76 through 80

For each of the case vignettes below, identify the diagnosis that best describes the situation.

(A) major depressive disorder, recurrent
(B) bipolar I disorder
(C) bipolar II disorder
(D) cyclothymia
(E) dysthymic disorder
(F) mood disorder due to a general medical condition
(G) substance-induced mood disorder

76. A 35-year-old man comes into the hospital with deep sadness and suicidal thoughts. He reports having experienced similar episodes in the past; he says he has also experienced two periods of extremely elated mood, during which he talked nonstop, went without sleep, and believed he was God.

77. A 45-year-old woman comes to your office saying that she has once again gotten into a deep funk, losing sleep and weight, and feeling she is worthless. She reports this is the third time in her life that she has experienced such episodes, but she has never had periods of abnormally elevated mood.

78. A 24-year-old cocaine addict reports that he had been bingeing on cocaine for 2 months earlier in the year. He stopped using cocaine 2 months ago, and he has been very sad and tearful for the entire period since he stopped his cocaine use.

79. A 32-year-old woman reports that she has been feeling a low-grade, chronically depressed mood for more days than not for the past 3 years. She reports that she has never had a period of a severely depressed mood, but the low-grade feeling of sadness has not gone away for more than 2 or 3 days at a time over the past 3 years.

80. A 53-year-old man reports that he is currently in one of his "up" periods. He states that he feels very good, and he is quite talkative, but he reports that he is having no trouble keeping his job, and he is sleeping well. He has never had any periods of elevated mood that have substantially interfered with his working, and he has never needed hospitalization for his "up" periods. However, he has suffered two periods of severe depression, each requiring hospitalization for suicidal thoughts, the most recent having occurred 3 years ago.

Questions 81 through 84

For each patient's psychiatric symptoms, select the most appropriate medication. Presume no medical problems other than those mentioned.

(A) amitriptyline
(B) clozapine
(C) divalproex
(D) fluoxetine
(E) hypericum perforatum
(F) olanzapine
(G) lorazepam
(H) propranolol
(I) temazepam
(J) thiothixene

81. A 23-year-old university student has lost interest in his master's degree program. His two friends who bring him to the psychiatrist say he has been isolating himself in his room and has covered all electrical appliances and outlets with duct tape claiming that "electromagnetic waves are disturbing the microchip in my brain." He acknowledges that he once took a medication for the same problem with the "microchip," but then he became unbearably restless, could not sit still, and felt that he was "crawling" inside.

82. A 36-year-old man complains that he cannot sleep at night. "I just can't settle down; my mind is constantly working." He describes being able to complete a lot of work, being highly energized, and having a lot of fun. He is afraid that without sleep he will "crash." Once before, he took a medication for depression.

83. A 65-year-old woman with a history of cardiac problems complains that she has lost her appetite, she cries frequently, and has lost interest in her grandchildren, her gardening, and her craft making. She thinks maybe it is time to die.

84. A 50-year-old woman with a long history of taking trifluoperazine is noted to have repetitive chewing motions, and periodically protrudes her tongue. Her arms and shoulders seem to jerk fairly often, and there is a peculiar twisting movement in her right hand. She tried several of the "newer" medications that are not supposed to cause the movement problems, but then her auditory hallucinations started again.

Questions 85 through 89

Match the antidepressants below with the effect described.

(A) amitriptyline
(B) nefazodone
(C) paroxetine
(D) phenelzine
(E) venlafaxine

85. Primarily a selective serotonin reuptake inhibitor (SSRI)

86. Both a SSRI and serotonin type 2 (5-HT_2) receptor blockade

87. Strong sedation, strong serotonin effect, and norepinephrine effect

88. Little sedation, strong serotonin, and norepinephrine effect

89. Monoamine oxidase (MAO) inhibitory effect

Questions 90 through 95

For each clinical vignette below, select the pharmacotherapeutic agent which is most likely to be helpful to the patient.

(A) buspirone
(B) sertraline
(C) risperidone
(D) lithium carbonate
(E) naltrexone
(F) dextroamphetamine

90. A 35-year-old man has a history of alternating episodes of major depression and severe mania, several of which have required hospitalization.

91. A 40-year-old man has a history of severe alcohol dependence and is very interested in whatever help he can get to avoid relapsing in his alcohol use.

92. A 21-year-old male college student reports a 1-month period of intensely depressed mood, with marked anxiety, sleep disturbance, and weight loss. He has never before experienced an episode of a mood disorder.

93. A 41-year-old woman has a long history of chronic paranoid schizophrenia. She experiences auditory and visual hallucinations and has had difficulty maintaining a job.

94. A 45-year-old woman reports a 6-month history of free-floating anxiety, which makes her feel tense most of the time on most days.

95. A 7-year-old boy presents with his mother who reports he cannot pay attention and is having severe problems at school because of this and his hyperactivity.

Questions 96 through 100

Identify the following personality disorders with the symptoms listed below.

(A) antisocial
(B) avoidant
(C) borderline

(D) dependent
(E) histrionic
(F) narcissistic
(G) obsessive-compulsive
(H) paranoid
(I) schizoid
(J) schizotypal

96. is quick to perceive a slight as an attack or assault on one's character

97. seems to not care what others think or feel; is aloof

98. preoccupied with feelings of superstitiousness; has a sixth sense; seems odd

99. chronic feelings of emptiness, fear of abandonment; unstable self-image

100. unwilling to take personal risks; perceives self as inept, unappealing, inferior

Questions 101 through 105

Identify the following defense mechanisms with the descriptions below.

(A) acting out
(B) altruism
(C) displacement
(D) intellectualization
(E) passive-aggressive behavior
(F) projection
(G) rationalization
(H) reaction formation
(I) sublimation
(J) suppression

101. becoming angry with one's spouse at a party and deciding to wait until a more appropriate time to express it

102. becoming angry with one's spouse at a party and calling him or her a name in front of everyone

103. working as a nurse on a pediatric ward because one would like to have children but cannot

104. being afraid of one's rage and anger and presenting as unusually meek and mild

105. accusing another of being angry and jealous when the feelings belong to oneself

Questions 106 through 110

Match the antidepressant with the side effect or characteristic described.

(A) phenelzine
(B) venlafaxine
(C) trazodone
(D) fluoxetine
(E) mirtazapine
(F) nortriptyline

106. an SSRI with a half-life of 4–6 days

107. need to avoid tyramine with this med

108. can cause hypertension at higher doses, but is not an MAOI

109. can cause priapism

110. can cause prolonged QT on ECG (especially with high doses)

Questions 111 through 114

Match the medication with the potential blood dyscrasia side effect it can be associated with.

(A) leukocytosis
(B) thrombocytopenia
(C) agranulocytosis
(D) megaloblastic anemia
(E) lymphocytosis

111. Valproate

112. Lithium

113. Clozaril

114. Carbamazepine

Answers and Explanations

1. **(D)**

2. **(A)**

3. **(B)**

Explanations 1 through 3

Typical neuroleptic antipsychotic medications frequently cause unpleasant side effects, which occur at various times during treatment. The extrapyramidal side effect most likely to occur in the first few days of treatment is an acute dystonia, such as a muscle spasm in the neck. A pill-rolling tremor of the hands and masked facies are signs of Parkinsonian EPS, which tend to have their onset several weeks after treatment is begun; whereas severe restlessness of the arms and legs is caused by an unpleasant sensation called "akathisia," which also tends to have its onset several weeks after treatment is begun. Involuntary lip smacking is a sign of tardive dyskinesia, a sometimes irreversible motor syndrome that tends to occur after months or years of treatment with typical antipsychotics.

Anticholinergic medications such as benztropine are effective in treating dystonias and pill-rolling tremors. Propranolol is effective in treating akathisia. Haldoperidol would worsen EPS. Dantrolene uncouples muscle contractions and is used occasionally in severe neuroleptic malignant syndrome. L-Dopa would decrease the Parkinsonian EPS, but would worsen the psychosis and therefore is not used. Fluoxetine is an SSRI. *(Kaplan and Sadock, pp. 1057–1061)*

4. **(C)** The essential feature of a major depressive disorder is the development of a major depressive episode without a history of mania or hypomania. The hallmarks of a major depressive episode are a subjective sense of dysphoria and a loss of interest in previously enjoyed activities, also called anhedonia. Depressed patients often report decreased libido, sleep disturbance, and appetite disturbance. It would be important to rule out organic causes for this man's disorder, such as hypothyroidism or the relatively rare phenomenon of metastatic cancer to the brain in a 35-year-old. Given the patient's age and recent onset of symptoms, Alzheimer disease is unlikely. Schizophrenia generally has a gradual onset and is accompanied by psychotic symptoms such as hallucinations and delusions. *(Kaplan and Sadock, pp. 542–544, 556–557)*

5. **(D)** The most appropriate initial therapy for this man would be antidepressant medication with a medication such as fluoxetine, a SSRI with a relatively benign side effect profile in most patients. SSRIs produce antidepressant response rates approaching 70%. The addition of psychotherapy to help the patient get through his depression would likely be helpful. Although ECT is the most dependably effective treatment for major depression, it has significant side effects, such as short-term memory loss. The absence of severe suicidal tendencies in this patient means that ECT should be reserved for possible later use, should two different antidepressant medications fail. Clozapine, diazepam, and buspirone do little by themselves to alleviate depressive mood. *(Kaplan and Sadock, pp. 560–570)*

6. **(D)**

7. **(B)**

8. **(H)**

9. **(E)**

10. **(G)**

Explanations 6 through 10

Complaints involving both psychologic and medical conditions are difficult to diagnose and treat. At times, medically identifiable causes are present, but the psychologic factors contributing to the discomfort complicate the diagnosis and treatment and lead to frustration in both physician and patient. At other times, no identifiable cause for pain or other physical symptoms can be found; nevertheless, the patient still has the symptoms. Questions arise: Is the patient lying? Is there some deep psychologic problem? Could there be a medical disorder in the early stages of development that gives rise to physical symptoms but no clear physical signs to make the diagnosis? One group of psychiatric disorders addresses some of these issues—the somatoform disorders. Somatization disorder is an Axis I psychiatric disorder where a patient complains of multiple somatic complaints involving multiple organ systems, but which cannot be explained by physical and/or laboratory findings. Conversion disorder is another Axis I disorder where there is a disturbance of bodily function that does not conform to anatomical or neurological concepts, and it is due to psychological factors. Body dysmorphic disorder is a pervasive subjective feeling/belief that some aspect of the patient's appearance is ugly or deformed. Hypochondriasis is a persistent belief in the presence of one or two serious physical diseases despite medical assurance that one does not have the disease/illness. Pain disorder (Somatoform pain disorder) is a disorder w/ the presence of severe, distressing and persistent pain which cannot be explained adequately by evidence of a physiologic process or physical disorder.

Panic disorder is a kind of anxiety disorder. Discrete periods of extreme sympathetic nervous system symptoms occur, including tachycardia, sweating, shortness of breath, and others, during which time a person experiences extreme fear. Malingering is the deliberate manufacture of false or exaggerated symptoms for financial gain or to avoid an unpleasant situation such as jail time or military duty. In a fictitious disorder, there is the deliberate production of signs and symptoms of illness in order to assume the sick role. *(Kaplan and Sadock, pp. 651–653, 647–651, 643–647, 599–602, 897–898)*

11. **(D)** Acute confusion with visual hallucinations would be characteristic of a delirium. Warm and dry skin, tachycardia, dry mouth, constipation, and urinary retention are anticholinergic side effects. Many antipsychotics are anticholinergic, and when Parkinsonian extra-pyramidal symptoms present, anticholinergic meds are often added to reverse these side effects. These anticholinergic effects can be additive and can cause delirium. *(Kaplan and Sadock, pp. 878, 946, 981)*

12. **(C)** Severe anticholinergic reactions, such as delirium, should be treated with intramuscular or intravenous injection of physostigmine, 1–2 mg IV (1 mg every 2 min) or IM every 30–60 min. The first dose should be repeated in 15–20 min if no improvement is seen. Such peripheral anticholinergic side effects as urinary retention can be treated with bethanechol. Dantrolene and bromocriptine, not effective in the treatment of anticholinergic reactions, are two drugs that have been tried in the treatment of neuroleptic malignant syndrome, a rare but extremely dangerous neuroleptic-induced disorder. Haldol, having anticholinergic effects, is contraindicated. *(Kaplan and Sadock, pp. 1014, 1060)*

13. **(C)** Frotteurism is the term given to obtaining sexual gratification by rubbing. It is usually the only source of sexual gratification for the man involved, who rubs his penis against the buttocks or other bodily part of a fully clothed woman to achieve orgasm. Exhibitionism is the exposure of one's genitals to an unsuspecting person. Fetishism is the term for intense sexual fantasies and behaviors involving the use of nonliving objects, such as female undergarments. Pedophilia is the term for intense sexual urges toward children 13 years of age or younger, and sexual masochism is the term for sexual arousal involving the real act of being humiliated, beaten, bound, or otherwise made to suffer. *(Kaplan and Sadock, p. 721)*

14. **(C)** Delusions are false ideas that cannot be corrected by reasoning and that are not based on reality. Psychotic patients often experience ideas or delusions of reference and misinterpret incidents or events in the outside world as having direct personal reference to themselves. Delusions may occur in a variety of psychiatric disorders, including schizophrenia, paranoia, mania, depression, and organic brain syndromes. The bizarre nature of the delusion described in the question is more characteristic of schizophrenia than of other types of psychiatric ailments. Illusions are sensory misperceptions that occasionally may be experienced even by normal individuals. Psychotic persons may report hallucinations, which are sensory experiences that cannot be substantiated by normal observers. Loosened associations and neologisms are patterns of speech often noted in psychotic individuals. *(Kaplan and Sadock, pp. 283–284)*

15. (C) Dissociative amnesia is loss of ability to recall information occurring within a certain time period, usually related to a severely stressful event as occurred with this woman. In depersonalization disorder, a person feels detached from his or her own body or mental processes and feels as if he or she is standing apart and acting as observer. In posttraumatic stress disorder, there is a persistent reexperiencing of the traumatic event in a variety of ways, persistent avoidance of stimuli associated with that event, and persistent symptoms of arousal. It is possible for the arousal to be a part of this larger symptom complex. In dissociative fugue, the person forgets his identity, travels, and may even establish a new identity. Symptoms of major depression involve mood, inability to experience pleasure, appetite and sleep disturbance, fatigue, and other disturbances of affect and mood. *(Kaplan and Sadock, pp. 676–679)*

16. (B) Individual therapy, which would include exploring the events recalled surrounding the incident, reactions to the child's death, feelings about motherhood, as well as other issues, is considered the most effective treatment for dissociative amnesia. If other symptoms indicate another disorder (e.g., major depression, psychosis), then treatment would include appropriate drugs or ECT. In some cases, there is a role for hypnosis or sodium amobarbital interview to help recall. Benzodiazepines may be helpful to reduce anxiety. Integration through psychotherapy of the events of the traumatic episode into one's conscious state is important for recovery. *(Kaplan and Sadock, pp. 676–679)*

17. (B) Successful resolution of the anal phase, in Freudian theory, provides the basis for the development for personal autonomy; whereas, failure to master the anal phase is said to lead to a "fixation" on anal functions, which can be characterized by obstinacy, stubbornness, and obsessive-compulsive traits. The oral stage is the name given to the first 12–18 months of life, which is said to be focused on a trusting dependence on nursing and sustaining objects. The phallic stage lasts from about age 3 through age 5, and it provides an emerging sense of sexual identity. Latency stage lasts from about age 5 or 6 until about age 11 or 13, during which children are thought to develop a sense of industry. The genital stage is the period which extends from the onset of puberty through young adulthood, during which an individual strives for self-realization and satisfaction in the areas of work and love. *(Kaplan and Sadock, pp. 201–303)*

18. (A) The preoccupation with a rather well-developed delusional system and later age at onset suggest paranoid schizophrenia. A case can be made for undifferentiated schizophrenia because of the apparent disorganization in personal habits and the flattening of affect. There is no history of alcohol abuse and dependence to support the diagnosis. The long period of symptoms, bizarreness of paranoid delusion, and decline in functioning are more characteristic of schizophrenia. The time course of a major depression is much shorter. Usually, in major depression there is not the profound decline in functioning. No symptoms of memory impairment or loss of cognitive functioning has occurred that would suggest Alzheimer or Huntington dementias. In addition, in Huntington dementia, one would expect a prominent movement disorder seen in subcortical dementia. *(Kaplan and Sadock, pp. 471–504, 331–333, 333–334)*

19. (B) Features that weigh toward a good prognosis in schizophrenia include late onset, obvious precipitating factors, good premorbid functioning, mood disorder symptoms, being married, a family history of mood disorders, good support systems, and having primarily positive symptoms. *(Kaplan and Sadock, p. 485)*

20. (D) The dopamine hypothesis of schizophrenia grew from the observations that medications that block dopamine receptors have antipsychotic activity and medications that stimulate dopamine receptors (amphetamines) can induce psychosis. Serotonin abnormalities have been implicated in mood and anxiety disorders. The biogenic amine hypothesis of mood disorders was based on the finding that tricyclic and MAOI drugs are effective in alleviating the symptoms of depression. The GABAergic system has been implicated in anxiety disorders because benzodiazepines which are GABAergic have antianxiety effects. Acetylcholine abnormalities have been associated with dementia. *(Kaplan and Sadock, pp. 97–106)*

21. (B) The treatment of choice for patients with a schizophrenic disorder is an antipsychotic drug. Of the medications listed, only olanzapine is an antipsychotic drug. Olanzapine causes relatively fewer EPS than traditional neuroleptics, such as haloperidol, and seems to be substantially less likely to cause tardive dyskinesia than typical neuroleptics. Olanzapine blocks both dopamine D_2 receptors and serotonin 5-HT_2 receptors. Its use is often associated with some weight gain by patients. *(Kaplan and Sadock, p. 498)*

22. (C) Anorexia nervosa is an eating disorder that predominantly affects women in their teens and in early adulthood. It is defined as refusal to maintain a minimal normal weight, at least 85% of that weight considered normal for that person's age and height, and a morbid preoccupation with feeling obese. Common strategies to lose weight include avoidance of all fats and carbohydrates, self-induced vomiting, obsessive physical activity, and abuse of laxatives or diuretics or both. Despite apparent aversion to gaining weight, anorectics frequently take very special care in preparation and consumption of food and may delight in preparing gourmet feasts for others. Menstrual irregularity and amenorrhea are also commonly reported but are not essential factors in making the diagnosis. It is not yet clear whether such menstrual problems are simply secondary to starvation or whether they reflect a more pervasive endocrine dysfunction. Perhaps the most striking clinical feature of this disorder is the misperception of body image. Regardless of the method of confrontation, including use of mirrors or photographs, sufferers see themselves as overweight. The patient often refuses to agree that there is any problem whatsoever. Numerous factors, including developmental, family, endocrine, and gastrointestinal disturbances have been implicated in anorexia nervosa, but the etiology has yet to be clearly established. Most commonly, the course consists of a single episode followed by remission. Some patients may suffer a series of relapses and remissions. Mortality rates have been estimated to be as high as 20%. *(Kaplan and Sadock, pp. 739–746)*

23. (E) Generally speaking, anorexic patients who are 20% or more below their expected weight for their height are recommended for inpatient programs. Inpatient programs for anorexia nervosa usually use a combination of a behavioral management approach, individual psychotherapy, family education and therapy, and in some cases psychotropic medications. *(Kaplan and Sadock, p. 744).*

24. (A) Alzheimer disease is the most common form of dementia. Of persons with dementia, 50–60% will have Alzheimer. Vascular dementia is the second most common, accounting for about 15–30% of dementias. *(Kaplan and Sadock, pp. 328–329)*

25. (A) Donepezil is a cholinesterase inhibitor used for the treatment of mild-to-moderate impairment in Alzheimer disease. Fluoxetine is an SSRI antidepressant. Aspirin would decrease clotting. Amitriptyline is a tricyclic antidepressant and with its anticholinergic properties, it would worsen cognition. Ginkgo is an herbal medicine. *(Kaplan and Sadock, p. 1041)*

26. (D) Pathologic changes will be seen in the frontotemporal cortex in patients with Pick disease. Alzheimer, also a cortical dementia like Pick, has pathologic changes in the parietotemporal areas. *(Kaplan and Sadock, pp. 331–333)*

27. (B) Panic attacks most frequently have their onset sometime between the late teens and early thirties. Most patients describe their initial panic attack as coming out of the blue. They frequently suffer from palpitations, sweating, trembling, shortness of breath, a feeling of choking, chest pain, nausea, light headedness, derealization (feelings of unreality) or depersonalization (being detached from oneself), fear of going crazy, fear of dying, numbness, and hot flashes or chills. Individuals who suffer from recurrent, unexpected panic attacks with at least 1 month of persistent concern about the attacks or their implications, or a significant change of behavior related to the attacks suffer from panic disorder. If a patient with panic disorder avoids situations in which panic attacks have occurred or endures the situations, such as shopping in a mall, with marked distress or anxiety about having a panic attack, the patient is said to suffer from panic disorder with agoraphobia. This patient's negative ECG makes myocardial infarction an unlikely diagnosis. Hypochondriasis is the term given to a long-term preoccupation with fears of having a serious disease based on the misinterpretation of bodily symptoms; it does not generally present in the sudden manner in which panic attack presents. Multiple sclerosis usually causes many neurologic disturbances which vary across time. Generalized anxiety disorder is not typified by the sudden onset of severe anxiety characteristic of a panic attack. *(Kaplan and Sadock, pp. 599–602, 651–653)*

28. (A) If the patient continues to suffer panic attacks for a substantial period, he is said to be suffering from panic disorder. SSRIs, such as paroxetine, are frequently effective and generally safe drugs for the treatment of panic disorder. Despite its usefulness in treating generalized anxiety disorder, buspirone seems to be ineffective in treating panic. Beta-blockers such as propranolol may block symptoms of palpitations or tremor, but are generally not as effective against panic attacks as are SSRIs. Antipsychotic medications such as olanzapine and haloperidol are not appropriate medications for the first-line treatment of uncomplicated panic disorder. *(Kaplan and Sadock, pp. 1126–1127)*

29. (C) Lorazepam, because of its relatively short half-life, intermediate rate of onset, and absence of active metabolites, would be an appropriate medication for this elderly woman. Diazepam and clorazepate both have long half-lives as well as active metabolites. These properties lead to more severe side effects in older patients, such as prolonged sedation, respiratory depression, confusional states, and disorientation. Temazepam, although it has no active metabolites and a relatively short half-life, is very sedating and is used to promote sleep. Buspirone, a nonbenzodiazepine, is an effective antianxiety agent, but it may take up to a week to exert its effect. The woman in this case needs medication that will help her quickly. *(Kaplan and Sadock, pp. 1022–1029, 1031–1033)*

30. (C) Patients with severe psychotic depression will often have delusions that are mood congruent and reflect the depth of their despair and self-abhorrence. Patients with mania are more likely to have delusions that are mood congruent that would reflect their grandiosity, paranoid feelings, inflated self-esteem, and feelings of having special powers. *(Kaplan and Sadock, pp. 542–544)*

31. (A) Schizoid personality disorder is characterized by a pattern of pervasive social detachment with a narrow range of emotional expression. Schizoid persons seem to be fairly content with a lack of intimacy and are considered odd by persons around them. This contrasts with the picture in individuals with avoidant personality disorder, who long for social interaction, but feel inadequate and riddled with self-doubt in social situations. Like individuals with obsessive-compulsive disorder, people with avoidant personality disorder are categorized as having a cluster C (anxious, fearful) personality disorder; whereas, those with borderline personality disorder or antisocial personality disorder have problems characterized by engaging in impulsive behaviors and are classified as having a cluster B (dramatic, impulsive) personality disorder. *(Kaplan and Sadock, pp. 800–821)*

32. (B) Separation anxiety disorder is the name given to the problem of a child's developmentally excessive anxiety concerning separation from home and parents. Children who are more globally anxious may suffer from generalized anxiety disorder, while children who avoid playmates may suffer from social phobia. Children who have an unrealistic fear of, for example, dogs, have a specific phobia; whereas, those who suffer from intrusive anxious thoughts that lead them to spend much time performing rituals such as hand washing suffer from obsessive-compulsive disorder. *(Kaplan and Sadock, pp. 1259–1265)*

33. (B) Children with Asperger disorder show severe sustained impairment in social interaction, and restricted repetitive patterns of behavior. Unlike autistic disorder, in Asperger disorder language and cognitive development are not delayed. In Rett disorder a child shows deterioration of developmental milestones, head circumference, and overall growth. In Rett disorder, verbal abilities are usually lost completely. *(Kaplan and Sadock, pp. 1218–1219)*

34. (B) All of the listed syndromes cause mental retardation, but Prader–Willi syndrome is also typified by compulsive eating and obesity, hypogonadism, and small stature. It is thought to be due to a small deletion on chromosome 15. Phenylketonuria is an autosomal-recessive trait which can cause mental retardation in children who do not eat a low phenylalanine diet. Down syndrome, or trisomy 21, causes mental retardation and distinctive facies. Fragile X syndrome causes mental retardation, short stature, and postpubertal macroorchidism. Cri-du-chat syndrome, caused by a deletion on chromosome 5, is characterized by severe mental retardation, microcephaly, and a cat-like cry in infants due to laryngeal abnormalities. *(Kaplan and Sadock, pp. 1165–1167)*

35. (D) The hallmark of delirium is fluctuation in level of consciousness. Periods of lucency may be interspersed with periods of clouding and unresponsiveness. Impaired judgment, impaired memory, and disorientation are seen in both delirium and dementia. Disordered thought is seen in both and tends to be disorganized in delirium and impoverished in dementia. Another distinguishing feature is that the onset of delirium usually occurs within hours or days, whereas, the onset of dementia may be insidious throughout a period of weeks to months. *(Kaplan and Sadock, pp. 327–328)*

36. (C) Advanced age is a major risk factor for the development of delirium. Other predisposing risk factors include preexisting brain damage, a history of previous delirium, alcohol dependence, diabetes, cancer, dementia, sensory impairment, and malnutrition. Male gender is also an independent risk factor. *(Kaplan and Sadock, pp. 323–324)*

37. (B) According to the case study, this man can be presumed to have been without alcohol for at least the 2 days he has been in jail, and, therefore, the emerging symptoms would be most attributable to withdrawal and delirium. Withdrawal symptoms include autonomic hyperactivity, hand tremor, hallucinations, illusions, and agitation. Added to these are the signs of delirium, disorientation, irritability, agitation, disorganized thought, inability to focus and concentrate, and development of symptoms over a short time. A diagnosis of exacerbation of schizophrenia does not adequately explain these symptoms and their development shortly after the withdrawal of alcohol. The signs and symptoms are not consistent with dementia, in which one would expect a longer period for symptom development and a clouding of consciousness. Although malingering might be considered, especially for an incarcerated individual, the history of recent alcohol intoxication with abrupt withdrawal makes alcohol withdrawal delirium a more consistent diagnosis. *(APA, pp. 136–147, 739; Kaplan and Sadock, pp. 319–328)*

38. (C) Diazepam, chlordiazepoxide, and lorazepam can all be given parenterally, but only lorazepam is reliably absorbed after intramuscular injection. Alprazolam and clonazepam are not available in parenteral form in the United States. *(Kaplan and Sadock, pp. 403–406)*

39. (E) Mirtazapine is a tetracyclic antidepressant that has both presynaptic alpha-2 receptor noradrenergic antagonist properties and 5-HT_2 and 5-HT_3 receptor serotonergic antagonist properties, which, taken together, result in a net increase in both noradrenergic and serotonergic neurotransmission. Bupropion may exert its antidepressant effects by acting on the noradrenergic system, but its method of action is currently being investigated. Trazodone and nefazodone are combined serotonin reuptake inhibitors and 5-HT_2 serotonin antagonists. Venlafaxine is a combined norepinephrine and serotonin reuptake inhibitor. *(Kaplan and Sadock, pp. 1030, 1075, 1080, 1123–1124, 1135–1136)*

40. **(B)** Dissociative fugue is classically typified by a person's suddenly and unexpectedly traveling away from his or her home, assuming a new identity, and eventually recovering from the fugue or flight, unable to recall the events that took place during the episode. Dissociative amnesia is a more generalized term given to an inability to recall significant personal information. Dissociative identity disorder is the current diagnostic term for what was classically called multiple personality disorder. Depersonalization disorder is an alteration of experience in which an individual feels like an outside observer of his or her body or mental processes. Dissociative disorder not otherwise specified is a name given to other dissociative illnesses not specifically listed in DSM-IV-TR, such as dissociative states occurring in individuals subjected to brainwashing or indoctrination while held captive by terrorists. *(Kaplan and Sadock, pp. 679–685)*

41. **(B)** Recurrent suicidal behaviors, affective instability, unstable interpersonal relationships, chronic feelings of emptiness, and rejection sensitivity are all traits of borderline personality disorder. *(Kaplan and Sadock, pp. 808–810)*

42. **(A)** Physically holding a patient would be a boundary violation. Conveying empathic validation, having clear roles and responsibilities, being flexible, and developing a hierarchy of priorities are all common features of recommended psychotherapy for a patient with borderline personality disorder. *(Kaplan and Sadock, pp. 808–810)*

43. **(A)** Patients with neuroleptic malignant syndrome typically demonstrate tachycardia, labile blood pressure, severe muscle rigidity, and severe fever. Serum CPK levels, which can be elevated to more than 100 times normal levels as a result of muscle damage, are the most consistently noted abnormalities in patients with neuroleptic malignant syndrome. Although the white blood cell count may be elevated, and blood levels of calcium, iron, and magnesium may be decreased in patients with the syndrome, serum CPK is the most important laboratory study to obtain in a patient with suspected neuroleptic malignant syndrome. *(Kaplan and Sadock, pp. 993–994; Bernstein et al., pp. 130–133)*

44. **(B)** The most effective treatments for the extremely serious, potentially fatal complication of antipsychotic treatment called neuroleptic malignant syndrome are oral bromocriptine, a dopaminergic agonist, and intravenous or oral dantrolene, a skeletal muscle relaxant. A further increase in the patient's haloperidol dose would likely worsen her neuroleptic malignant syndrome, while the anticholinergic effects of diphenhydramine and benztropine, while they may alleviate some of the neuroleptic-induced muscular dystonia associated with the syndrome, are not likely to be life saving, and propranolol is not an effective medication in the treatment of neuroleptic malignant syndrome. *(Bernstein et al., pp. 130–134; Kaplan and Sadock, pp. 993–994)*

45. **(D)** Drowsiness and dizziness frequently occur with dantrolene, but are generally transient and mild. The most serious potential side effect of high-dose intravenous dantrolene is hepatotoxicity. *(Kaplan and Sadock, pp. 1045–1046; Bernstein et al., p. 132)*

46. **(C)** Akathisia is the name of the unpleasant feeling of restlessness that many patients on antipsychotic medications describe. Propranolol and benzodiazepines can be effective in controlling the feeling. Opisthotonus is an extreme dystonic reaction in which the back is arched. Bradykinesia is the name for the slowed movements that accompany the Parkinsonian syndrome, which may occur with antipsychotic use. The rabbit syndrome is a late effect of neuroleptic treatment consisting of fine rapid movements of the lips that mimic a rabbit's chewing. Tardive dyskinesia is a disorder that usually first occurs only after some months of an individual's treatment with antipsychotic medications and consists of involuntary movements of the face, trunk, or extremities. *(Kaplan and Sadock, pp. 993–996)*

47. **(D)** Propranolol and benzodiazepines can be used to effectively treat akathisia. Haldoperidol would worsen the akathisia. Benztropine is effective in treating Parkinsonian EPS, but not very effective with akathisia. Phenytoin is an anticonvulsant. Physical restraint would not be an appropriate treatment for akathisia. *(Kaplan and Sadock, p. 1026)*

48. **(C)** The onset of severe, persistent eye pain is always a cause for concern. In a patient medicated with a drug with anticholinergic side effects, such as imipramine, there is a potential for the development of narrow-angle glaucoma. A delay in the diagnosis and treatment of this will lead to irreparable harm to the eye. In this case, the psychiatrist would act immediately to facilitate appropriate evaluation and treatment which would best be provided by her ophthalmologist. *(Bernstein et al., pp. 170, 174; Kaplan and Sadock, p. 1014)*

49. **(B)** Olanzapine, clozapine, risperidone, quetiapine, and ziprasidone are all atypical antipsychotic medications. The use of clozapine, however, is limited because of the risk of potentially fatal agranulocytosis in patients taking it. Because the agranulocytosis is reversible, monitoring the blood count of patients on clozapine is recommended, usually starting on a weekly basis at the beginning of treatment. *(Kaplan and Sadock, pp. 1104–1113)*

50. **(A)** Historically, suicide rates among Roman Catholics have been lower than among Jews and Protestants. Being divorced, being male, and having a previous suicide attempt all increase the risk for suicide. Up to 10% of schizophrenics die from suicide. *(Kaplan and Sadock, p. 913–915)*

51. **(E)** Most suicides among psychiatric patients are felt to be preventable, as supported by the evidence that inadequate assessment or treatment is often associated with suicide. When to hospitalize patients with suicidal ideation is the most important clinical decision to be made. The absence of a strong support system, a history of past suicide attempt and impulsivity, and having a suicidal plan with intent would be indications for hospitalization. *(Kaplan and Sadock, p. 920).*

52. **(D)**

53. **(C)**

54. **(E)**

Explanations 52 through 54

Hypochondriasis is a somatoform disorder in which misperceptions or distortions of somatic signs and symptoms lead to preoccupation with fears of having a serious illness. In factitious disorders, one deliberately manufactures signs and symptoms to enter the sick role. The preoccupation with fear of serious illness is not part of factitious disorder. Major depression is characterized by symptoms of depression: sleep disturbance, appetite disturbance, and so forth. It may be complicated by hypochondriasis. In the case study, no supporting evidence for major depression (for which she would have been evaluated) is provided. This woman's symptoms as described are not of a psychotic level; thus, reactive psychosis would be inappropriate. In pain disorder, pain in a specific body site is the predominant focus, unlike the predominance of fear seen in hypochondriasis. Care of these patients is best managed supportively by developing a therapeutic alliance with them. Anticipating their needs by establishing regular office visits and physical examinations with them will help allay fears as well as reassure them of one's concern that if an occult condition becomes evident it will be diagnosed early. Certainly, regular consultation with other specialists is in order to manage these patients. Although the course of hypochondriasis tends to be chronic, there are indications that factor in for a good outcome. One of these is the absence of secondary gain.

This disorder is seen equally in both men and women. The prevalence in a general medical practice is approximately 4–6%. There is no relationship between hypochondriasis and increased ESR. *(Kaplan and Sadock, pp. 651–653)*

55. (C) In the defense mechanism of displacement, an emotion is severed from its original connection with a person or event and attached to a substitute person or object. With its origin thus disguised, the emotion may be more safely expressed. In the example described in the question, anxiety associated with sexual feelings is displaced onto the setting in which they occurred, with resulting phobic anxiety. *(Kaplan and Sadock, p. 198)*

56. (C) In starting an interview, generally an open-ended question will allow the patient the freedom to tell his or her story. Choice A assumes the person is depressed; the patient may object if he or she feels already diagnosed and hasn't had the opportunity to talk. Choices B and D may be seen as critical and do not directly address the issue of what brings this patient to the psychiatrist. The patient may experience these as unempathetic. Choice E is premature. As the consulting psychiatrist, you must perform a thorough evaluation to determine the nature and treatment of this patient's problem. *(Kaplan and Sadock, pp. 1–15)*

57. (B) One of the earliest findings in biological psychiatry was the abnormal sleep pattern of depressed patients. Electroencephalographic monitoring of sleep divides sleep into REM and non-REM sleep. Sleep latency is generally prolonged in depression, while REM latency is shortened. General wakefulness is increased, with a decreased arousal threshold. There tends to be a reduction in stage 3 and stage 4 sleep in depression. *(Kaplan and Sadock, pp. 539, 759)*

58. (A)

59. (C)

60. (B)

Explanations 58 through 60

Given the temporal relationship in the start of two anticholinergic drugs and the onset of the urinary hesitancy in an otherwise healthy young male, it would be reasonable to conclude that the drugs are causing the problem. Certainly, a rapid assessment regarding the possibility of other causes (e.g., infection, trauma, stricture) is important. Careful, attentive listening for any hint of psychotic delusion involving urination is important to screen for. The manner in which the patient describes his symptoms is invaluable in facilitating diagnosis. Also remember that a real medical condition can be described in bizarre, distorted terms, making assessment more difficult and complicated. Drug-induced urinary hesitancy may be treated by discontinuing the causative medications. In addition, bethanechol, 10–30 mg three to four times each day, may be administered. Bethanechol acts by stimulating the parasympathetic nervous system. The tone of the detrusor urinae muscle increases, producing a contraction strong enough to initiate micturition and emptying of the bladder. Giving benztropine, an anticholinergic, would only heighten the problem. Unfortunately, some patients understand that benztropine is "for the side effect" of their antipsychotic medication but do not understand the difference between the extrapyramidal effect and the anticholinergic effects. Increased thioridazine would also increase the urinary problem. Calling in a urologist would be indicated if the initial treatment failed to work or if the emergency department physician were not able to "get beyond" an extremely distorted, disorganized presentation by the patient. If the bladder were extremely distended and the patient very uncomfortable, insertion of a urinary catheter would be a reasonable course of action. In the patient described, the bladder is not distended.

Of the medications listed, risperidone is a reasonable and safe choice because its anticholinergic effects are low compared to the other drugs listed, and much lower than thioridazine. Chlorpromazine and mesoridazine have substantial anticholinergic effects. Amitriptyline and imipramine have substantial anticholinergic effects, and, in addition, they are tricyclic antidepressants, not antipsychotics. *(Kaplan and Sadock, pp. 982, 497–500)*

61. (A) One of the most significant findings here is that the woman, cooperative with the examination, has the score of 14 on the MMSE. A score of 25–30 indicates no cognitive impairment, 20–25 suggests possible mild impairment, and less than 20 is very strongly suggestive of cognitive impairment. This degree of change on the MMSE is not a normal sign of aging. In addition, there are no signs of psychosis or mania. Even if there were, in this woman with no previous psychiatric history, one would not likely consider psychosis not otherwise specified or mania. The time frame for dysthymia is not met by the "several days" length described here. *(Kaplan and Sadock, pp. 1320, 321)*

62. (C) ECT can be a life-saving tool in the treatment of depression, particularly in individuals who are very suicidal, because of its relatively quick onset of action. It is a relative contraindication to give patients with a clinically significant space-occupying cerebral lesion ECT because of the risk of brain stem herniation. ECT can be performed on patients with space-occupying lesions rarely, but the benefit needs to outweigh the risk, and it should be performed by experts. However, although hypertension and cardiovascular disease put patients at a higher risk for complications from ECT, they are not absolute contraindications to its use. With the use of muscle relaxants as part of the electroconvulsive technique, patients with degenerative joint disease of the spine can generally safely receive ECT. Seizures actually would typically decrease in frequency with the application of ECT. *(Kaplan and Sadock, p. 1140)*

63. (B) This woman's symptoms meet the criteria for a major depressive episode. She has had a depressed (blue) mood for at least a 2-week period, a significant weight loss, insomnia, fatigue and loss of energy, and thoughts of suicide. Because her symptoms seem to be limited to 3 weeks, dysthymic disorder would most likely not be considered. There are no indications for an organic mental disorder that would suggest Alzheimer disease. Generalized anxiety disorder is characterized by excessive anxiety and worry for about 6 months. For a diagnosis of borderline personality disorder, patterns of instability in relationships, self-image, affect, and impulsivity would have been present in early adulthood. None of that is described here. *(APA, pp. 349–356, 472–476; Kaplan and Sadock, pp. 542–544)*

64. (B) For a first, relatively acute episode of major depression, a tricyclic or SSRI is usually considered a first-choice drug. The SSRIs, considered as effective as the tricyclics, are often favored by clinicians because of their greater safety profiles and faster onset of action. Olanzapine is an example of an antipsychotic drug. Alprazolam is a benzodiazepine that does have some anxiolytic value in depression. Its addictive potential does not make it a drug of choice for depression. Tranylcypromine is an effective MAO inhibitor antidepressant selected for use after a depression has failed to respond to the tricyclics and SSRIs. ECT is also used after other treatments have failed. In very severe, debilitating depressions, however, a clinician may choose ECT as a first treatment. *(Kaplan and Sadock, pp. 565–570)*

65. (A) Negative symptoms of schizophrenia reflect the absence or deficiency of a mental function that is normally present. Anhedonia, or the inability to experience pleasure, is an example of such. Positive symptoms of schizophrenia reflect aberrance or distortion of mental functions. Loose associations, delusions of thought, insertion, incoherence, and stereotypic gestures are all examples of these distortions. *(Kaplan and Sadock, pp. 490–491)*

66. (B) The antidepressant bupropion has been found effective for treating some cases of attention deficit disorder and offers help to those children not responsive to the usual treatment with stimulants (methylphenidate, pemoline). The remaining choices have not been found useful in treating this condition. They are lithium, a mood stabilizer; alprazolam, a benzodiazepine anxiolytic; propranolol, a beta-blocker; and perphenazine, an antipsychotic. *(Kaplan and Sadock, pp. 1225–1226)*

67. **(C)** Cognitive psychotherapy would be helpful to this man to see and understand how cognitive distortions about himself, others, and the future bring about his depressive feelings. Psychoanalysis, a process lasting several years with a weekly commitment of three to four sessions, would require this person to be willing to explore and work through issues and conflicts that have their source in childhood. Behavioral therapy has as its goal the disruption of inappropriate behaviors with the substitute of more appropriate behaviors. It is intended for the treatment of phobias and various psychosomatic disorders (e.g., migraine, hypertension). Supportive psychotherapy could also be of some value. This is used frequently in conjunction with medication. Group therapy may be of some value after this patient has had the opportunity to work in a one-to-one situation in which understandings about himself have developed. Proper preparation is essential before entering group therapy. *(Kaplan and Sadock, pp. 956–960)*

68. **(C)** There is strong evidence for a genetic predisposition to bipolar disorder. Some of the evidence comes from twin studies. The concordance rate for monozygotic twin is 79%, but for dizygotic twin it is 19%. Advising the patient that she is past the age when bipolar disorders develop, using lithium to prevent the disorder, or saying that no genetic link has been determined is very misleading and clinically incorrect. *(Kaplan and Sadock, pp. 123–125)*

69. **(B)** Pick disease is considered a cortical dementia, with the preponderance of pathologic findings found in the frontotemporal area. Aphasia, apraxia, and agnosia are signs sometimes seen in these patients. Huntington and Parkinson diseases are caused by pathologic changes in the basal ganglia. Pathologic changes are seen in the ventricles in occult hydrocephalus. Signs seen in subcortical dementia more characteristically involve motor disorders: rigidity, tics, gait difficulties, and incoordination. *(Kaplan and Sadock, pp. 331–334, 1323)*

70. **(E)** The lifetime prevalence of posttraumatic stress disorder (PTSD) is approximately 8%. For PTSD to be diagnosed, the trauma has to be where serious injury or death were threatened or involved, and the traumatized individual experienced a sense of helplessness, fear, or horror, and has at least one reliving symptom (nightmares of the trauma, recurrent intrusive thoughts of the event, intense psychologic stress or physiologic reactivity to internal or external cues that symbolize or resemble an aspect of the trauma, or flashbacks), two or more symptoms of increased arousal (difficulty falling to or staying asleep, irritability, difficulty concentrating, hypervigilance, and exaggerated startle response), and three or more avoidance symptoms (efforts to avoid thoughts, feelings, or conversations about the trauma, efforts to avoid people, things or places that remind one of the trauma, inability to remember an important aspect of the trauma, diminished participation in activities, feeling detached or estranged from others, restricted range of affect, and/or sense of foreshortened future). The symptoms have to be recurring for at least a month. *(Kaplan and Sadock, pp. 626–627)*

71. **(E)**

72. **(B)**

73. **(A)**

74. **(D)**

75. **(E)**

Explanations 71 through 75

Infantile autism, called a pervasive developmental disorder in DSM-IV, typically is diagnosed when children do not demonstrate the acquisition of communication skills. Ability to form interpersonal relationships also is grossly impaired. Other behavioral manifestations of infantile autism include unusual repetitive mannerisms (e.g., spinning), marked anxiety during environmental changes, and high pain threshold. As to be expected, school performance is poor, though autistic children may display isolated areas (*islands*) of normal or superior intellectual functioning. Behavioral manipulation is useful in trying to contain the behavior of autistic children. Unlike infantile autism, childhood schizophrenia usually develops later in childhood and follows an intermittent course. Deterioration in social or school functioning is a characteristic presenting feature, along with hallucinations, delusions, and other manifestations of psychosis. Phenothiazine drugs offer effective treatment. Symptoms and signs of depression in children are similar to those in adults. However, children may not be able to recognize depressed feelings. Persistence of puzzling physical problems in association with apathetic, withdrawn behavior is a common presentation. The use of antidepressants is controversial; family and individual counseling often can be quite helpful. Attention deficit hyperactivity disorder once was called hyperactivity and minimal brain dysfunction. Characteristic signs include impulsivity, distractibility, inattention in school, and (usually but not universally) hyperactivity. A variety of pharmacologic agents, including imipramine, dextroamphetamine, and methylphenidate (Ritalin), have been recommended for treatment of attention deficit hyperactivity disorder. *(APA, pp. 70–75, 85–93; Kaplan and Sadock, pp. 1208–1231)*

76. (B)

77. (A)

78. (G)

79. (E)

80. (C)

Explanations 76 through 80

The criteria for mood disorders depend on the presence or absence and duration of depressive and hypomanic or manic symptoms as well as on their severity, and also on the presence or absence of a causative general medical condition or the ingestion of substances. Major depressive disorder, recurrent, is marked by the lifetime occurrence of two or more major depressive episodes without intervening hypomanic or manic episodes. A major depressive episode is a severe depression which has lasted at least 2 weeks. Bipolar I disorder is characterized by a history of at least one full-blown manic episode, during which the patient's mood has been abnormally and persistently elevated, expansive or irritable for at least 1 week with marked impairment in occupational functioning. Bipolar II disorder, on the other hand, is marked by a history of at least one major depressive episode and at least one hypomanic episode, during which a patient's mood has been elevated, but not to the extent of causing marked impairment in social or occupational functioning. A patient with bipolar II disorder may not, by definition, have had a full-blown manic episode. Cyclothymia is marked by periods of hypomanic symptoms alternating with depressive symptoms that do not meet the criteria for a major depressive episode. Dysthymic disorder is marked by a persistent, low-grade depression occurring more days than not for at least 2 years. A mood disorder due to a general medical condition is a prominent and persistent disturbance in mood that is judged to be the direct physiologic effect of a general medical condition, such as hyperthyroidism. A substance-induced mood disorder is a prominent and persistent disturbance in mood that is judged to be due to the direct effects of a substance, but which continues beyond the usual period of intoxication or withdrawal from a substance. *(APA, pp. 345–428)*

81. (F) This man's symptoms are psychotic in nature and somewhat bizarre. In addition, the information strongly suggests that he is very sensitive to the extrapyramidal effects of the traditional antipsychotics. Olanzapine, a new antipsychotic with very few extrapyramidal effects, would be a good choice here. *(Kaplan and Sadock, pp. 1105–1106)*

82. (C) A hypomanic state is described here. This is seen in bipolar I and bipolar II disorder. A treatment of choice is the mood stabilizer divalproex. If psychotic symptoms were present, the addition of an antipsychotic would be indicated. *(Kaplan and Sadock, pp. 570–572, 1131–1132)*

83. (D) This woman is exhibiting signs of severe depression. Because of her cardiac condition, avoiding an antidepressant with negative cardiac effect is important; therefore, amitriptyline would be eliminated. Fluoxetine, an SSRI, would be an appropriate choice. *(Kaplan and Sadock, pp. 565–566)*

84. **(B)** Signs of tardive dyskinesia are evident in this woman. She also was tried on several "newer" medications, one of which may have been olanzapine. This would have to be determined. Assuming this is so, a possible good choice is clozapine, which does not contribute to the development of tardive dyskinesia. *(Kaplan and Sadock, pp. 497–499, 1106–1107)*

85. **(C)**

86. **(B)**

87. **(A)**

88. **(E)**

89. **(D)**

Explanations 85 through 89

The drugs listed in this question are examples of the various classes of antidepressants. These classes include the tricyclics, the SSRIs, the MAOIs, the triazolopyridines, and the phenylethylamines. Understanding the site of action, neurotransmitter(s) involved, and side effects characteristic of these classes is helpful in selecting an antidepressant for a particular patient. SSRIs that are comparable in their antidepressant effects to the older tricyclics but significantly safer when taken in larger doses, as in suicidal overdose, are frequently used as the first choice in the treatment of depression. An example here is paroxetine. Drugs that both inhibit serotonin reuptake and block 5-HT_2 receptors are characteristic of the triazolopyridines. The overall effect of these actions is believed to decrease both depression and anxiety in patients. There are two drugs in this class: trazodone and nefazodone. Strong sedation caused by histaminergic and cholinergic activity is seen in the older antidepressants—the tricyclics. These also have both serotonin and norepinephrine effects that are important in decreasing depression. Amitriptyline is the drug example listed here. Drugs demonstrating little sedation and significant serotonin, norepinephrine, and dopamine effects are more characteristic of the phenylethylamines. They are effective in managing depression because there is no histaminergic activity and little sedation is seen. Venlafaxine is an example. MAOIs increase the concentrations of serotonin, norepinephrine, and dopamine by inhibiting their degradation. The MAOIs, although effective as antidepressants, are used relatively infrequently because of the potential development of a hypertensive crisis induced by consuming tyramine-containing foods while on the MAOI. An example here is phenelzine. *(Kaplan and Sadock, pp. 1093–1104, 1076–1081, 1123–1130, 1135–1136)*

90. **(D)**

91. **(E)**

92. **(B)**

93. **(C)**

94. **(A)**

95. **(F)**

Explanations 90 through 95

Lithium carbonate is an effective treatment for manic and depressive episodes due to bipolar I disorder, as well as for the prophylaxis of manic and depressive episodes in patients with bipolar I disorder. It can impede the release of thyroid hormone from the thyroid, and it can reduce the ability of the kidneys to concentrate urine; its use requires regular blood levels to ensure the avoidance of toxic blood levels that could cause tremor, dysarthria, ataxia, or death. Naltrexone (ReVia) is a pure opioid antagonist that decreases the craving for alcohol in patients with alcohol dependence. Sertraline (Zoloft) is a SSRI which is effective in the treatment of major depressive disorder, as well as in the treatment of panic disorder, obsessive-compulsive disorder, and posttraumatic stress disorder. Risperidone is an atypical antipsychotic that is effective in the treatment of psychotic conditions, including schizophrenia, and is associated with fewer serious long-term side effects, such as tardive dyskinesia, than traditional neuroleptics. Risperidone is a potent blocker of both 5-HT_2 serotonin receptors and D_2 dopamine receptors. Buspirone, a nonaddictive azapirone, acts as an agonist or partial agonist of 5-HT_1A serotonin receptors, and is effective in the treatment of generalized anxiety disorder. Dextroamphetamine is a stimulant and is an effective treatment for attention-deficit/hyperactivity disorder (ADHD). *(Kaplan and Sadock, pp. 1067–1069, 1102, 1085–1089, 1031–1033, 1111, 1308)*

96. (H)

97. (I)

98. (J)

99. (C)

100. (B)

Explanations 96 through 100

Persons with personality disorders are rigidly bound to the use of patterns of defense and various traits that distinguish the disorders. All have problems with interpersonal relationships. *(Kaplan and Sadock, pp. 800–821)*

101. (J)

102. (A)

103. (I)

104. (H)

105. (F)

Explanations 101 through 105

Defense mechanisms provide a means for dealing with anxiety and affect. The mechanisms chosen range from the very narcissistic and immature to mature. In suppression, a person makes a conscious decision to put the conflict aside until it can be dealt with more appropriately. On the other hand, in acting out, there is little or no attempt to contain the affect, and it is directly expressed, as in name calling. Sublimation provides a channel for the indirect expression of a need or affect. Its use is positive and socially acceptable. In reaction formation, the person acts as if the strong need or affect did not exist and acts out the opposing feeling. In projection, unacceptable feelings and thoughts are denied as part of the self and instead are "put on" the other person. *(Kaplan and Sadock, pp. 207–208)*

106. (D)

107. (A)

108. (B)

109. (C)

110. (F)

Explanations 106 through 110

Fluoxetine has the longest half-life of the current SSRIs, phenelzine is an MAOI and foods rich in tyramine can induce a hypertensive crisis. Venlafaxine can induce hypertension, especially at higher doses. Trazodone can rarely induce priapism (a painful sustained erection). Nortriptyline is a tricyclic antidepressant, and at high doses, it can cause arrhythmias. *(Kaplan and Sadock, pp. 1094, 1078, 1136, 1124)*

111. (B)

112. (A)

113. (C)

114. (C)

Explanations 111 through 114

Valproate can be associated with thrombocytopenia and platelet dysfunction especially at high doses. Leukocytosis is a common benign effect of lithium. Clozaril can cause agranulocytosis in 1–2% of patients. Agranulocytosis can be an idiosyncratic adverse event with carbamazepine. *(Kaplan and Sadock, pp. 1133, 1069).*

REFERENCES

American Psychiatric Association (APA). *Diagnostic and Statistical Manual of Mental Disorders*, 4th ed. Text Revision. Washington, DC: American Psychiatric Association, 2000.

Bernstein CA, Ladds BJ, Maloney AS, et al. *On Call Psychiatry*. Philadelphia, PA: W.B. Saunders, 1997.

Kaplan HI, Sadock BJ. *Synopsis of Psychiatry: Behavioral Sciences/Clinical Psychiatry*, 9th ed. Baltimore, MD: Williams & Wilkins, 2003.

CHAPTER 6

Surgery

Philip N. Redlich, MD, PhD and Andrea L. Winthrop, MD

Questions

DIRECTIONS (Questions 1 through 32): Each of the numbered items or incomplete statements in this section is followed by answers or by completions of the statement. Select the ONE lettered answer or completion that is BEST in each case.

1. A 32-year-old, previously healthy man is a victim of a drive-by shooting, sustaining a gunshot wound to the left lower extremity. The entrance wound is located over the medial aspect of the calf, with an exit wound over the anterior pretibial region. Neurovascular examination of the extremity is normal. There is associated soft-tissue injury from the blast effect and a severely comminuted tibial fracture demonstrated on radiographs. Appropriate management of this injury includes which of the following?

(A) local wound irrigation, closure of the soft-tissue defect, closed reduction, and immobilization in a long-leg cast
(B) local wound irrigation with antibiotic solution, closed reduction, and immobilization in a long-leg cast, with continued local wound care through an anterior cast window
(C) tetanus prophylaxis, intravenous (IV) antibiotics, and operative wound irrigation and debridement, with application of an external fixation device
(D) tetanus prophylaxis, IV antibiotics, operative wound irrigation with closure of the soft-tissue defect, closed reduction, and immobilization in a long-leg cast
(E) tetanus prophylaxis, IV antibiotics, long-leg splint for immobilization, and operative intervention during elective surgical schedule

Questions 2 and 3

A 16-year-old girl with a history of ulcerative colitis managed with steroid therapy presents to the emergency department with a 36-h history of nausea, crampy abdominal pain, and severe bloody diarrhea. On examination, the patient is febrile and pale, with a blood pressure of 90/60 mmHg and heart rate of 130 beats per min. Her abdomen is distended and diffusely tender. A complete blood count (CBC) demonstrates a leukocytosis with a left shift. The patient receives IV fluid resuscitation and nasogastric tube decompression.

2. Further therapeutic interventions should include which one of the following?

(A) 6-mercaptopurine
(B) azathioprine
(C) opioid antidiarrheals
(D) colonoscopic decompression
(E) high-dose IV steroids and broad-spectrum antibiotics

3. After 48 h, there is no clinical improvement. Which of the following is the most appropriate next step in management?

   (A) colonoscopic decompression
   (B) cyclosporine
   (C) abdominal colectomy and ileostomy and Hartmann's procedure
   (D) proctocolectomy with ileal pouch-anal anastomosis
   (E) abdominal colectomy with ileorectal anastomosis

Questions 4 and 5

A term infant is born at a small community hospital by cesarean section for failure to progress. The infant is noted to have the following abnormality at birth (see Fig. 6-1).

4. Which of the following is the most likely diagnosis?

   (A) umbilical hernia
   (B) omphalitis
   (C) omphalocele
   (D) gastroschisis
   (E) traumatic evisceration

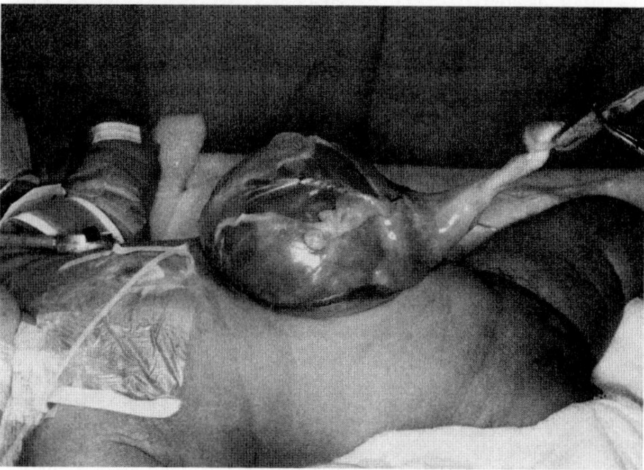

FIG. 6-1

5. Which of the following is the most appropriate initial management?

   (A) IV antibiotics alone
   (B) emergency surgery for reduction
   (C) monitor for spontaneous closure, with surgical intervention for persistent fascial defect
   (D) IV fluids, IV antibiotics, warm occlusive dressing, and transfer to a center with a pediatric surgeon
   (E) elective umbilical exploration

6. A 2-year-old child presents with a 2-day history of painless rectal bleeding. On examination, the child is pale with tachycardia. The abdomen is nondistended and nontender. There is dark blood on rectal examination. The child has the following imaging study (see Fig. 6-2). Which of the following is the most appropriate management?

   (A) surgical exploration
   (B) aggressive resuscitation followed by surgical exploration
   (C) colonoscopy
   (D) acid suppression therapy
   (E) IV steroids

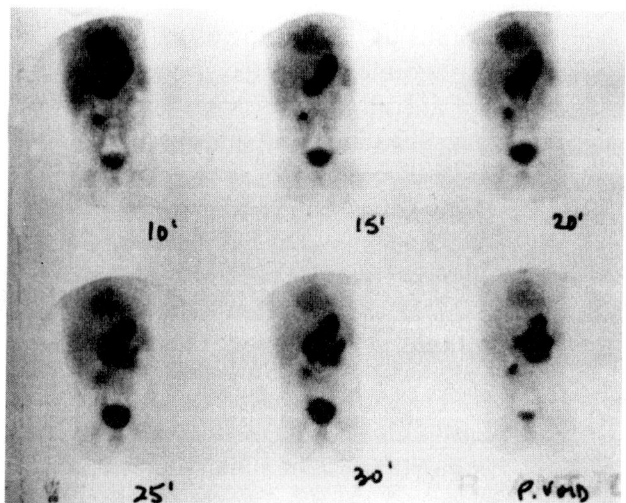

FIG. 6-2

Questions 7 and 8

A 55-year-old-woman presents to the physician's office for evaluation of mammographic findings on a screening mammogram. She denies any breast masses, nipple discharge, pain, or skin changes. Past history is pertinent for insulin-dependent diabetes. Family history is positive for postmenopausal breast cancer in her mother. She has a normal breast examination and no axillary adenopathy. A mediolateral oblique (MLO) view of the right breast is shown Fig. 6-3.

7. Which of the following is the most likely diagnosis?

   (A) milk of calcium
   (B) lobular carcinoma *in situ* (LCIS) with or without an invasive component
   (C) ductal carcinoma *in situ* (DCIS) with or without an invasive component
   (D) involuting fibroadenoma
   (E) phyllodes tumor

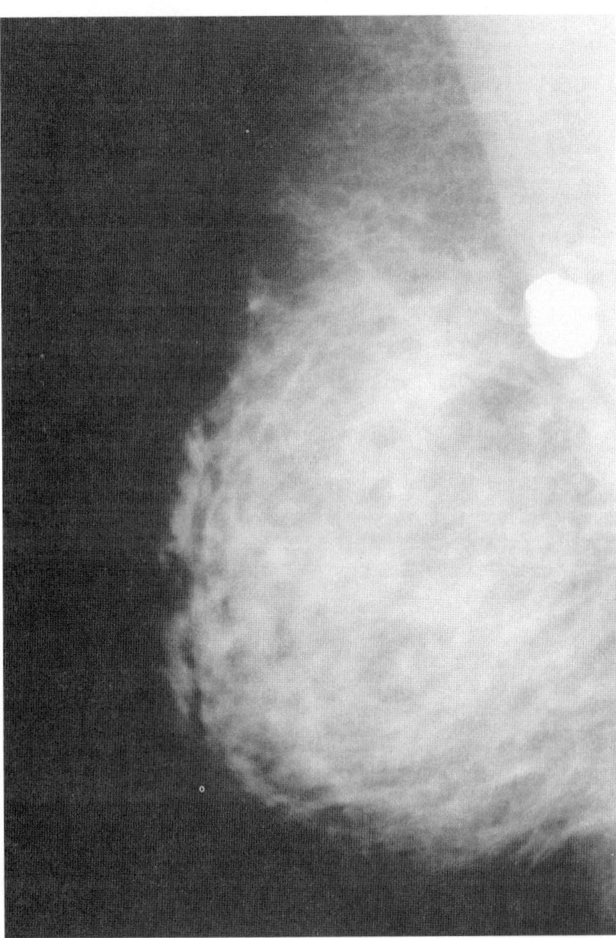

FIG. 6-3

8. Which of the following is the most appropriate next step in management?

   (A) observation, with repeat mammogram in 6–12 months
   (B) ultrasound
   (C) biopsy
   (D) lumpectomy, radiation therapy, and sentinel lymph node (SLN) biopsy
   (E) total mastectomy

Questions 9 and 10

A 51-year-old woman presents to the physician's office with a 2-month history of a right breast blood-tinged nipple discharge. Past history is unremarkable. Family history is positive for postmenopausal breast cancer in a maternal grandmother. Examination reveals no palpable masses or regional adenopathy, but a serous discharge is easily elicited from a single duct in the right breast. Bilateral mammograms show no abnormalities. Cytology from the discharge was not diagnostic. A ductogram was ordered, and the results are shown in Fig. 6-4.

9. Which of the following is the most likely diagnosis?

   (A) invasive carcinoma
   (B) intraductal carcinoma
   (C) intraductal papilloma
   (D) fibrocystic disease
   (E) duct ectasia

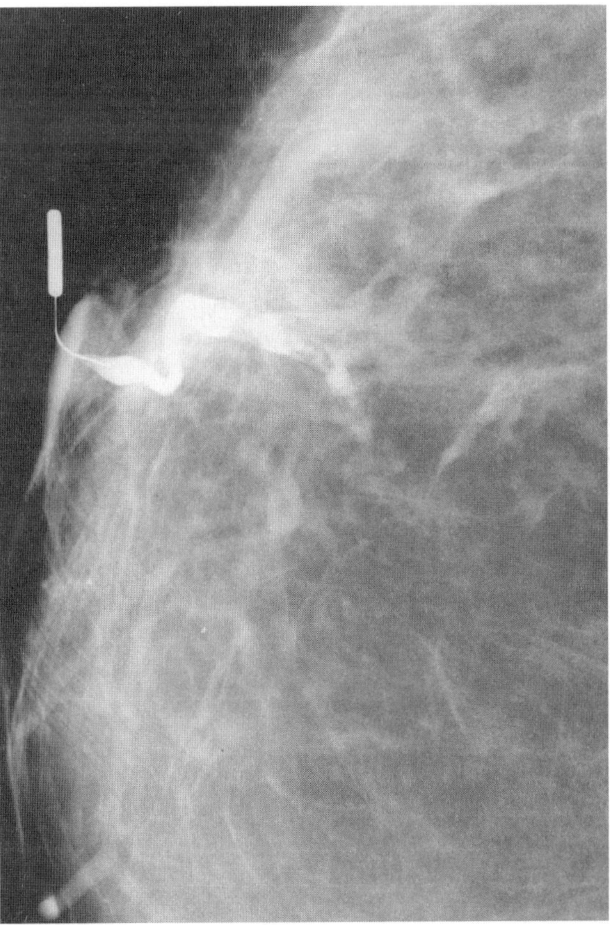

FIG. 6-4

10. Which of the following is the most appropriate next step in management?

(A) collection of discharge for repeat cytologic analysis
(B) observation, with repeat examination and imaging studies in 3–6 months
(C) modified radical mastectomy
(D) central lumpectomy (including removal of the nipple/areolar complex)
(E) terminal duct excision (microdochectomy)

Questions 11 and 12

An 85-year-old man presents to the emergency room with an acute onset of midepigastric pain, nausea, vomiting, and hiccups starting 2 days ago. He is unable to keep any food down. Past history is pertinent for a long-standing hiatal hernia, hypertension, and diet-controlled diabetes. Examination reveals vital signs of pulse rate 82/min, BP 100/52 mmHg, respiratory rate 16/min, and temperature 97.2°F. The patient is in no acute distress, but has epigastric tenderness without guarding. Laboratory analysis revealed a hematocrit of 46 and a normal white blood cell (WBC) count. A chest x-ray is shown in Fig. 6-5a. A fluoroscopically guided nasogastric (NG) tube was placed using contrast, and his stomach was decompressed. After adequate fluid and electrolyte resuscitation, an upper gastrointestinal (UGI) contrast study was obtained and is shown in Fig. 6-5b.

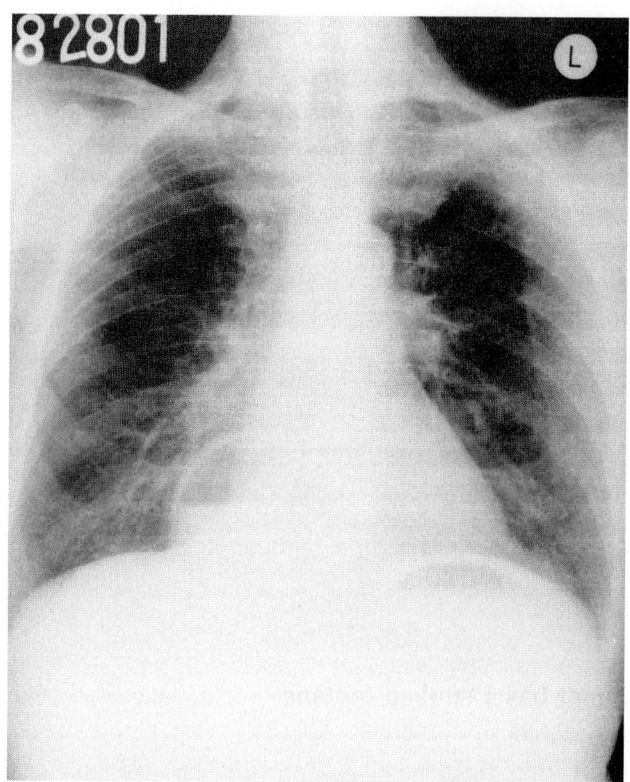

a

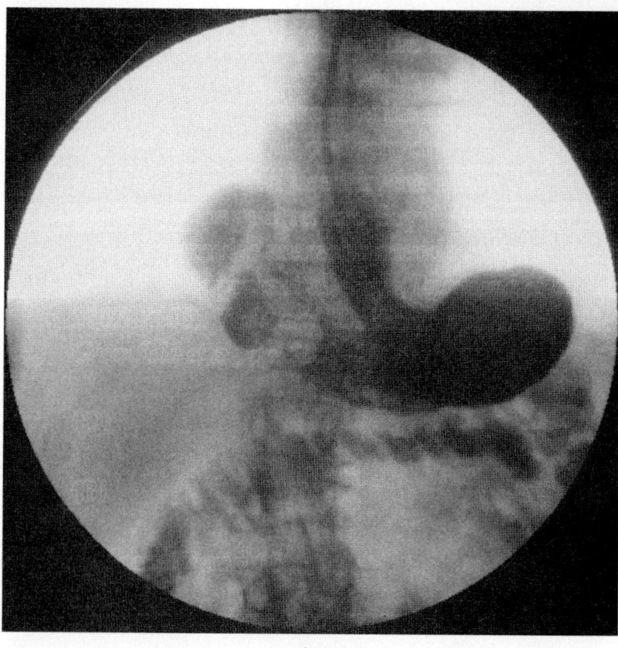

b

FIG. 6-5

11. Which of the following is the most likely diagnosis?

(A) sliding hiatal hernia
(B) hernia of Bochdalek (posterorlateral congenital diaphragmatic hernia)
(C) hernia of Morgagni (parasternal congenital diaphragmatic hernia)
(D) paraesophageal hernia
(E) eventration of the diaphragm (central diaphragm)

12. Which of the following is the most appropriate next step in management?

(A) laparotomy or laparoscopy and operative repair
(B) continued NG-tube decompression and initiation of total parenteral nutrition (TPN)
(C) thoracotomy or thoracoscopy and operative repair
(D) endotracheal intubation and initiation of ventilatory support
(E) upper endoscopy

Questions 13 through 16

A 5-week-old infant presents with a 1-week history of progressive nonbilious emesis, associated with a 24-h history of decreased urine output. The infant continues to be active and eager to feed. On examination, the infant has a sunken fontanelle and decreased skin turgor. The abdomen is scaphoid, and with a test feed, there is a visible peristaltic wave in the epigastrium.

13. Which of the following is the most likely diagnosis?

(A) viral gastroenteritis
(B) gastroesophageal reflux
(C) urinary tract sepsis
(D) pyloric stenosis
(E) milk protein allergy

14. The diagnosis is best confirmed by which of the following?

(A) abdominal ultrasound
(B) careful clinical examination with palpation of an epigastric mass
(C) UGI contrast study
(D) surgical exploration
(E) endoscopy

15. Electrolytes and a urinalysis are evaluated. Which of the following laboratory findings are most likely to be seen in this patient?

(A) Na 145, K 3.0, Cl 110, CO_2 17, urine pH 8.0
(B) Na 130, K 3.0, Cl 80, CO_2 36, urine pH 4.0
(C) Na 135, K 4.0, Cl 104, CO_2 23, urine pH 7.0
(D) Na 140, K 5.2, Cl 100, CO_2 16, urine pH 4.0
(E) Na 132, K 3.2, Cl 96, CO_2 25, urine pH 7.0

16. Which of the following is the most appropriate next step in management of this infant?

(A) immediate surgical exploration
(B) send the child home with an oral electrolyte rehydration solution
(C) change the infant's formula and feeding regimen
(D) IV fluid resuscitation, followed by surgical intervention
(E) initiate therapy with a prokinetic agent

Questions 17 and 18

A 40-year-old previously healthy man presents with sudden onset of severe abdominal pain that radiates from the right loin (flank) to groin. This pain is associated with nausea, sweating, and urinary urgency. He is distressed and restless, but an abdominal examination is normal.

17. Which of the following is the most likely diagnosis?

(A) torsion of the right testicle
(B) pyelonephritis
(C) appendicitis
(D) right ureteral calculus
(E) acute urinary retention

18. Which of the following is the most appropriate next step in management?

(A) insertion of a urethral catheter
(B) IV fluid hydration, IV analgesics, and nonenhanced computed tomography (CT) scan
(C) IV fluid hydration, IV analgesics, and arrangements for lithotripsy
(D) cystoscopy and retrograde pyelogram
(E) urine culture, followed by initiation of antibiotic therapy

19. A 25-year-old woman was involved in a motor vehicle crash and sustained a significant closed-head injury, a pulmonary contusion, and a pelvic fracture. She is unresponsive and is ventilated in the intensive care unit (ICU). Which of the following is the best initial approach to the management of this patient's nutritional needs?

(A) insertion of a subclavian venous catheter and initiation of central IV hyperalimentation
(B) wait for extubation and improvement of neurologic status, allowing institution of an oral caloric intake
(C) early institution of nasogastric or nasojejunal tube feeding with an elemental formulation
(D) wait for resolution of the associated gastrointestinal ileus, followed by delayed initiation of nasogastric tube feeding with a complex hypercaloric formulation
(E) peripheral IV hyperalimentation

20. A 26-year-old previously healthy man was pinned under a crane at a construction site. After a prolonged extrication, he was brought to the emergency department, immobilized on a back board and receiving 100% oxygen by mask. He is alert and complaining of chest pain with respiratory effort. On examination, he is found to have an oxygen saturation of 90% by pulse oximetry, shallow respirations at a respiratory rate of 35/min, heart rate of 120 beats per min, and a blood pressure of 85/60 mmHg. The trachea is deviated to the right. There is tenderness and crepitation over the left chest wall, asymmetric chest wall movement, and decreased air entry over the left lung field. Which of the following is the most appropriate next step in the initial evaluation and management of this patient?

(A) fluid resuscitation with 2 L of isotonic crystalloid
(B) needle decompression of the left chest, followed by insertion of a chest tube
(C) portable chest x-ray
(D) immediate intubation and assisted ventilation
(E) emergency department thoracotomy

Questions 21 through 23

A 4-year-old previously healthy girl presents to the emergency department with a 24-h history of rectal bleeding and dizziness. She has no other gastrointestinal symptoms. On examination, she appears pale. Her heart rate is 140 beats per min, and she has a 20 mmHg postural drop in systolic blood pressure. The child's abdomen is nondistended and nontender, and fresh blood and clots are in the rectal vault on rectal examination.

21. Which of the following is the most likely diagnosis?

(A) a bleeding Meckel's diverticulum
(B) juvenile rectal polyp
(C) hemorrhoids
(D) an anal fissure
(E) intussusception

22. Which of the following is the most appropriate diagnostic study to order for this patient?

(A) colonoscopy
(B) barium enema
(C) technetium scan
(D) UGI contrast study with small-bowel follow-through
(E) laparoscopy

23. Definitive management of this child should include which of the following?

(A) immediate exploratory laparotomy
(B) IV fluid resuscitation, transfusion with blood products as indicated, followed by a laparotomy with Meckel's diverticulectomy and ileal resection
(C) IV fluid resuscitation, followed by a colonoscopic polypectomy
(D) hemorrhoidectomy
(E) stool softeners and topical steroids

24. A 29-year-old nonhelmeted motorcycle driver is involved in a single vehicular crash, resulting in a significant closed-head injury. He is intubated in the field and transported to a level 1 trauma center. On arrival, he is oxygenating well with assisted ventilation and has a normal blood pressure and moderate tachycardia. His Glasgow Coma score is 7, and his pupils are equal and sluggishly reactive. After stabilization in the emergency department, the patient undergoes a CT scan of the head that demonstrates a small amount of subarachnoid blood and a right frontal lobe contusion with edema with no midline shift. CT scan of the abdomen is normal. The patient is transferred to the ICU. The optimal initial management of this patient's intracranial pressure (ICP) would be which of the following?

(A) craniotomy
(B) fluid restriction, hyperventilation, and osmotic diuresis
(C) fluid restriction, hyperventilation, and ventriculostomy
(D) hyperventilation and IV steroids
(E) normovolemia, normocarbia, sedation, and ventriculostomy

Questions 25 through 27

A 55-year-old woman presents with a 6-month history of weight loss, abdominal cramps, and intermittent nonbloody diarrhea. On examination, her abdomen is mildly distended and there is a palpable mass in the right lower quadrant. Stool cultures yield normal fecal flora. CT scan with oral contrast demonstrates an inflammatory mass in the right lower quadrant, with thickening of the terminal ileum and ileocecal valve.

25. Which of the following is the most likely diagnosis?

(A) ulcerative colitis
(B) appendicitis
(C) Crohn disease
(D) irritable bowel syndrome
(E) lactose intolerance

26. Which of the following is the best diagnostic test to confirm the diagnosis?

(A) repeat CT scan with delayed imaging
(B) ultrasonography
(C) sigmoidoscopy
(D) colonoscopy
(E) small-bowel radiography

27. Initial management should include which of the following?

(A) antibiotics and IV fluids
(B) lactose-free diet
(C) antispasmodics
(D) nutritional supplementation and systemic steroids
(E) laparotomy

28. A 13-year-old boy is brought to the emergency department at midnight with a 4-h history of right scrotal pain that was sudden in onset and associated with nausea and one episode of vomiting. On examination, he is in obvious distress. He has mild right lower abdominal tenderness, and high-riding, tender right testes. CBC and urinalysis are normal. Which of the following is the most appropriate next step in management?

(A) admit the patient to the hospital and place him on bed rest
(B) analgesics and a scrotal support
(C) antibiotic therapy
(D) schedule a testicular isotope scan
(E) urgent surgical exploration

29. A 70-year-old man presents with back pain and increasing difficulty with initiating a urinary stream. On rectal examination, he is found to have a hard, irregularly enlarged prostate. He has an elevated prostate-specific antigen (PSA), and osteoblastic lesions in the vertebral column and bones of the pelvis. A needle biopsy of the prostate shows well-differentiated adenocarcinoma. Which of the following is the treatment of choice?

(A) radical prostatectomy
(B) transurethral prostatectomy
(C) cytotoxic chemotherapy
(D) hormonal manipulation
(E) radiotherapy

30. A 25-year-old previously healthy man is scheduled for elective inguinal hernia repair under general anesthesia. After induction of anesthesia and initial inguinal incision, the patient develops tachycardia, muscle rigidity, fever of 38.5°C, and elevated end-tidal carbon dioxide. Which of the following is the most likely diagnosis?

(A) pneumonia
(B) atelectasis
(C) urinary tract infection
(D) myocardial infarction
(E) malignant hyperthermia

31. A previously healthy 19-year-old man presents to the emergency department with a penetrating wound to the right neck. There were reports of bleeding at the scene. The patient is talking, complaining of pain at the injury site and pain with swallowing. On examination, he has a normal respiratory rate, clear air entry on auscultation, blood pressure of 120/70 mmHg, and heart rate of 95 beats per min. There is a penetrating right neck wound in zone 2 (between the clavicle and the lower part of the mandible), with a surrounding hematoma. On probing, there is violation of the platysma. Which of the following is the best next step in the management of this patient?

(A) intubation and observation in the ICU
(B) admission to the ICU for close observation without intubation
(C) observation in the ICU only if carotid angiogram is normal
(D) observation in the ICU only if carotid angiogram, contrast esophagram, and bronchoscopy are normal
(E) neck exploration

32. A 45-year-old man is brought to the emergency department after being involved in an automobile crash. He is alert and oriented, with a normal neurologic examination. His respiratory rate is 20/min, with clear lungs, pulse rate of 120/min, and blood pressure of 60/0 mmHg. On examination, he is noted to have a distended abdomen, with decreased bowel sounds, and a fracture of the right ankle. IV access is established, and the patient receives a rapid infusion of 2 L of saline, without changes to pulse rate or blood pressure. Which of the following is the most appropriate next step in his management?

(A) abdominal CT scan
(B) insertion of a Swan–Ganz catheter
(C) exploratory laparotomy
(D) focused abdominal sonography for trauma (FAST)
(E) diagnostic peritoneal lavage

DIRECTIONS (Questions 33 through 51): Each set of matching questions in this section consists of a list of lettered options followed by several numbered items. For each item, select the ONE best lettered option that is most closely associated with it. Each lettered option may be selected once, more than once, or not at all.

Questions 33 and 34

Select the most likely diagnosis for each of the patients with polyuria.

(A) central diabetes insipidus (DI)
(B) nephrogenic DI
(C) water intoxication
(D) solute overload
(E) diabetes mellitus

33. A 25-year-old man was admitted to the ICU with severe head injury with a basal skull fracture. Eighteen hours after the injury, he developed polyuria. Urine osmolality was 150 mOsm/L and serum osmolality was 350 mOsm/L. IV fluids were stopped, and 1 h later urine output and urine osmolality remained unchanged. Five units of vasopressin were administered intravenously, and urine osmolality increased to 300 mOsm/L.

34. A 70-year-old man was admitted to the ICU with severe pancreatitis. During his ICU course, he underwent several CT scans with IV contrast and was also treated with an aminoglycoside for a urinary tract infection. The patient required a prolonged course of TPN, and developed *Candida* sepsis treated with amphotericin. He subsequently developed polyuria with urine osmolality of 250 mOsm/L and serum osmolality of 350 mOsm/L. After receiving 5 units of vasopressin intravenously, there is no change in urine osmolality or urine output.

Questions 35 through 39

For each patient with abdominal pain, select the most likely diagnosis.

(A) gastroenteritis
(B) regional enteritis
(C) acute appendicitis
(D) perforated peptic ulcer
(E) sigmoid diverticulitis
(F) acute pancreatitis
(G) acute cholecystitis
(H) superior mesenteric artery embolism
(I) ruptured abdominal aortic aneurysm
(J) ruptured ovarian cyst
(K) cecal volvulus

35. A 21-year-old previously healthy woman presents with abdominal pain of 48-h duration. The pain was initially periumbilical and on progression became localized in the right lower quadrant. The woman had nausea and a decreased appetite. She denied dysuria. Her last menstrual period was 2 weeks earlier. On examination, she was febrile (temperature 38.2°C), and was found to have localized tenderness in the right lower quadrant with guarding. Rectal examination was normal. Laboratory examination demonstrated mild leukocytosis.

36. A 40-year-old man with a history of alcohol abuse presents after an episode of binge drinking. He is complaining of epigastric pain, radiating to the back, associated with nausea and vomiting. On examination, he has marked tenderness in the epigastrium, with guarding, decreased bowel sounds, and moderate abdominal distention. Laboratory findings include leukocytosis and increased serum amylase and lipase. Abdominal roentgenograms demonstrate several dilated bowel loops in the upper abdomen.

37. A 65-year-old man presents with a 4-day history of worsening lower abdominal pain and constipation. On examination, he is febrile (38.5°C) and has lower abdominal tenderness that is most intense in the midline and left lower quadrant associated with a palpable fullness. Laboratory findings demonstrate a moderate leukocytosis and abdominal roentgenograms show an ileus pattern.

38. A 30-year-old man presents with sudden onset of severe epigastric pain 6 h ago. Examination reveals a low-grade fever, tender abdomen throughout, with rigidity of the abdominal musculature. Abdominal roentgenograms show pneumoperitoneum.

39. A 40-year-old woman presents to the emergency room with a 3-day history of worsening abdominal pain, with nausea and vomiting. Examination reveals a low-grade fever and abdominal tenderness in the right upper quadrant with guarding, especially during inspiration. Laboratory findings include a mild leukocytosis and a slightly elevated bilirubin.

Questions 40 through 46

For each patient with a neck mass, select the most likely diagnosis.

(A) thyroid carcinoma
(B) cystic hygroma
(C) acute suppurative lymphadenitis
(D) thyroglossal duct cyst
(E) lipoma
(F) carotid artery aneurysm
(G) mixed parotid tumor (pleomorphic adenoma)
(H) laryngeal carcinoma
(I) parathyroid adenoma
(J) branchial cleft cyst
(K) tuberculosis

40. A 3-year-old boy presents to the physician's office with an asymptomatic neck mass located in the midline, just below the level of the thyroid cartilage. The mass moves with deglutition and on protrusion of the tongue.

41. A 45-year-old man presents to the physician's office for evaluation of a posterior neck mass. The mass has been present for years, but has slowly enlarged over the last 2 years. Examination reveals a subcutaneous mass that is soft, nontender, and movable.

42. A 6-year-old boy presents to the emergency department with a cough, sore throat, and malaise of 4 days' duration. Examination reveals a temperature of 101.5°F, erythematous pharynx, and a tender right neck mass with overlying erythema.

43. An 18-month-old girl is brought to the physician's office for evaluation of left neck mass. Examination reveals a 2-cm soft, nontender, fluctuant mass in the left lateral neck. This is located at the anterior border of the sternomastoid, midway between the mastoid and clavicle.

44. A 50-year-old woman presents to the physician's office for evaluation of a right neck mass. The mass has been present for 3 years and is painless. On examination, a nontender, firm, 2.5-cm mass is noted slightly below and posterior to the angle of the mandible on the right.

45. A 35-year-old woman presents to the physician's office for evaluation of a left neck mass discovered 1 month ago on a routine physical examination. On examination, the mass measures 2 cm and is located anterolateral to the larynx and trachea. It is nontender and moves with swallowing. Past history is pertinent for a 15 pack-year smoking history and occasional alcohol intake.

46. A 55-year-old man presents to the physician's office with complaints of hoarseness and left neck fullness for the past month. On examination, a firm, movable, left submandibular mass is noted. Past history is pertinent for a 30 pack-year smoking history with occasional alcohol intake.

Questions 47 through 51

For each patient with jaundice, select the one most likely diagnosis.

(A) hepatitis A
(B) hemolysis
(C) choledocholithiasis
(D) biliary stricture
(E) choledochal cyst
(F) pancreatic carcinoma
(G) liver metastases
(H) cirrhosis
(I) pancreatitis

47. A 50-year-old man presents to the emergency department for increasing abdominal distention and jaundice over the last 4–6 weeks. Examination reveals mild jaundice, spider angiomas, and ascites. Enlarged veins are noted around the umbilicus.

48. A 75-year-old man is brought to the emergency department by his family for evaluation of jaundice. He complains of pruritus of 2 weeks' duration and a recent 10-lb weight loss. On examination, he is deeply jaundiced and has a nontender, globular mass in the right upper quadrant of the abdomen that moves with respiration.

49. A 75-year-old woman is brought to the emergency department from the nursing home for jaundice and mental confusion. The nursing home notes state that she has become less responsive and has developed jaundice over the last 2 weeks. Past history is pertinent for hypertension, diabetes, and prior colon resection for cancer at age 55. Examination reveals mild jaundice with vital signs of temperature 101.5°F, pulse rate 110/min, and BP 100/60 mmHg. She does not respond to verbal commands, but withdraws to pain. Abdominal examination reveals tenderness in the epigastrium and right upper quadrant.

50. A 65-year-old man presents to the physician's office with complaints of abdominal discomfort and jaundice for the past 3 weeks. Past history is pertinent for 30 pack-year smoking history, occasional alcohol intake, and a 5.5-mm ulcerating melanoma removed from his back $2\frac{1}{2}$ years ago. Examination reveals a mildly jaundiced patient with normal vital signs and a slightly distended abdomen with mild right upper quadrant tenderness and significant hepatomegaly.

51. A 54-year-old man presents to the emergency department on transfer from another hospital at the request of the family. He was admitted to the outside hospital 2 weeks ago with abdominal pain, nausea, vomiting, and fever. He was treated with antibiotics, nasogastric tube decompression, and TPN without significant improvement. He developed jaundice 2 days ago. His past history is pertinent for a 40 pack-year smoking history, chronic alcohol abuse, and diabetes. Examination reveals a mildly jaundiced patient with vital signs of temperature 100°F, pulse rate 95/min, and BP 110/60 mmHg. Cardiac examination is unremarkable, lung examination reveals decreased breath sounds at the bases bilaterally, and abdominal examination reveals fullness in the epigastrium with tenderness and voluntary guarding.

DIRECTIONS (Questions 52 through 113): Each of the numbered items or incomplete statements in this section is followed by answers or by completions of the statement. Select the ONE lettered answer or completion that is BEST in each case.

52. A 56-year-old woman presents to the physician's office with complaints of a new left breast mass. She denies any pain, nipple discharge, or skin dimpling. She has a prior history of breast cysts 5 years ago, treated by aspiration at that time. Her last mammogram was at age 53. Past history is pertinent for a 30 pack-year smoking history, prior total abdominal hysterectomy-bilateral salpingo-oöphorectomy (TAH-BSO) at age 54 for leiomyomas, and current use of hormone replacement therapy (HRT). Family history is negative for breast disease. Examination reveals a firm, well-defined, mobile, 1.5-cm nodule in the upper outer quadrant of the left breast without any regional lymphadenopathy. Which of the following is the most appropriate next step in management?

(A) fine-needle aspiration (FNA) biopsy
(B) discontinuation of HRT and reexamination in 4–6 weeks
(C) breast imaging
(D) open surgical biopsy
(E) core needle biopsy

53. A 56-year-old woman presents to the clinic for routine health screening. Her concern is the development of breast cancer. She has no current breast-related complaints. Past history is pertinent for fibrocystic changes with atypical ductal hyperplasia and a single fibroadenoma, both diagnosed by open biopsy 5 years ago. She smokes one pack per day and drinks one can of beer daily. Family history is positive for breast cancer in her mother, diagnosed at the age of 85. Current medications include a cholesterol-lowering agent, an antihypertensive, and HRT, which she has taken for 5 years. Physical examination is unremarkable. Mammograms show dense breasts, decreasing the accuracy of the study, but no suspicious findings were noted. Which of the following is the most common risk factor in evaluating women for breast cancer?

(A) fibrocystic changes with atypical ductal hyperplasia
(B) alcohol consumption
(C) positive family history
(D) HRT
(E) age

54. A 42-year-old woman returns to the clinic following an uneventful biopsy for a well-defined, mobile mass. The pathology report describes the mass as a fibroadenoma, but LCIS is identified in the breast parenchyma adjacent to the fibroadenoma and extending to the margin of resection. She has no current illnesses, is on no medications, and her family history is negative for breast cancer. Breast imaging studies show fatty breasts with no abnormal findings except for the fibroadenoma. Which of the following is the most appropriate management option?

(A) reexcision of the biopsy cavity to gain negative margins of resection
(B) ipsilateral mastectomy
(C) contralateral breast biopsy
(D) observation including examinations and mammography
(E) bilateral total mastectomies

Questions 55 and 56

A 35-year-old woman presents to clinic for a discussion on breast cancer risk. Her family history is pertinent for a grandmother who died of breast cancer at age 53, a mother who died of premenopausal breast cancer, and one of three sisters with breast cancer diagnosed at age 42. The sister with breast cancer underwent genetic testing and was found to have a BRCA1 mutation. Subsequently, the 35-year-old woman underwent genetic testing and was found to be a carrier of the same deleterious BRCA1 mutation.

55. Which of the following ranges represents the lifetime risk for breast cancer that should be quoted for this patient?

(A) 0–30%
(B) 10–40%
(C) 20–50%
(D) 50–80%
(E) 70%–100%

56. For this patient, which of the following strategies represent an accepted management option for her high-risk status?

(A) semiannual clinical breast examinations
(B) annual mammography
(C) chemoprevention with tamoxifen
(D) prophylactic bilateral mastectomy
(E) any of the above

Questions 57 and 58

A 65-year-old woman presents to the physician's office for a second opinion on the management options for recently diagnosed breast cancer. She presents with a 2.5-cm mass in the upper outer quadrant of the left breast associated with a palpable axillary node suspicious for metastatic disease. The remainder of her examination is normal. Mammography demonstrates the cancer and shows no other suspicious lesions in either breast. Chest x-ray, bone scan, and blood test panel, including liver function tests, are normal. Family history is positive for breast cancer diagnosed in her sister at age 65. Past history is unremarkable. The first physician recommended modified radical mastectomy.

57. Which of the following is the most appropriate management option for locoregional control yielding results equally effective as mastectomy?

(A) radical mastectomy
(B) lumpectomy, irradiation, and axillary node dissection
(C) lumpectomy and axillary node dissection
(D) irradiation of the breast and axilla
(E) quadrantectomy, irradiation, and axillary node dissection

58. The patient has read about SLN biopsy. She avidly wants to avoid the risk of lymphedema that her sister must endure. She asks the question "Am I a candidate for a SLN biopsy instead of a complete axillary dissection?" Which of the following is the most appropriate answer to her question?

(A) Yes, and if the SLN if positive, then a complete axillary dissection should be performed.
(B) Yes, and if the SLN is negative, then an axillary dissection can be avoided.
(C) No, because the success of SLN biopsy in patients over age 60 is decreased.
(D) No, because SLN biopsy is contraindicated when a palpable axillary node is suspicious for metastatic disease.
(E) No, because SLN biopsy is contraindicated for tumors greater than 2 cm.

Questions 59 and 60

A 65-year-old woman presents to the physician's office for evaluation of an abnormal screening mammogram. She denies any breast masses, nipple discharge, pain, or skin changes. Past history is pertinent for hypertension. Family history is positive for postmenopausal breast cancer in a sister. She has a normal breast examination and no axillary adenopathy. The remainder of her examination is unremarkable. An MLO view of the right breast is shown in Fig. 6-6a along with a magnification view of the craniocaudal (CC) film (Fig. 6-6b).

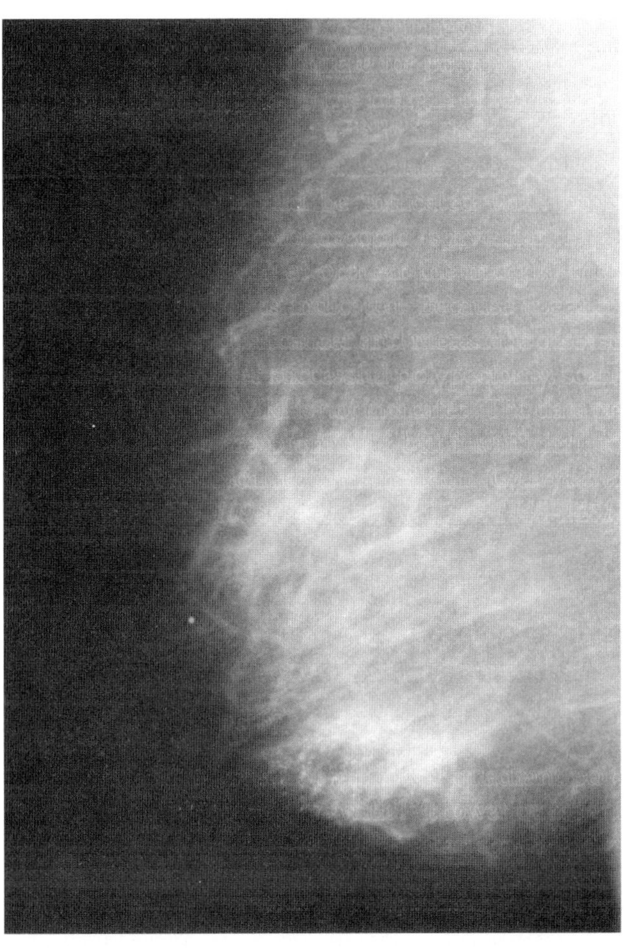

a

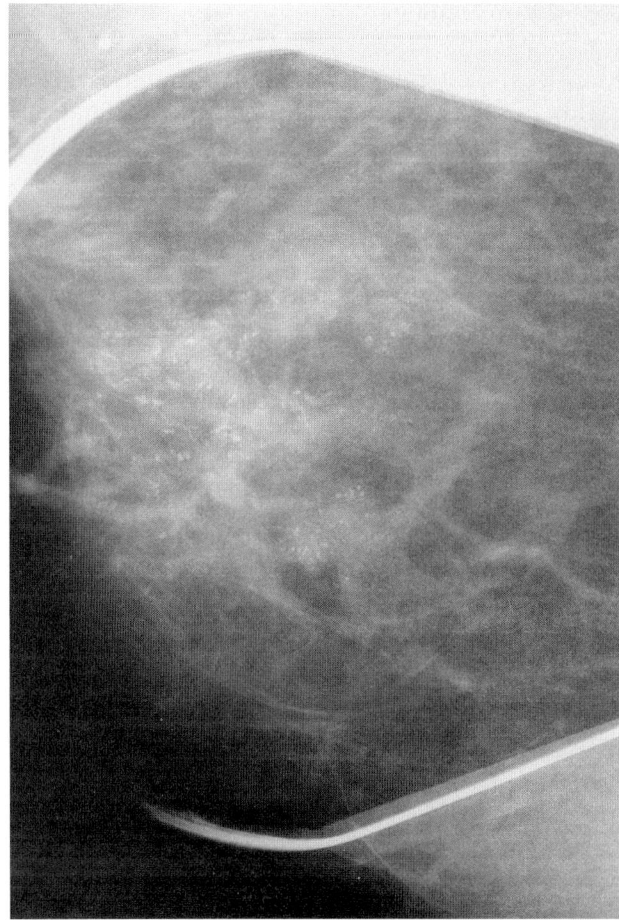

b

FIG. 6-6

59. Which of the following is the most likely diagnosis?

(A) milk of calcium
(B) LCIS with or without an invasive component
(C) DCIS with or without an invasive component
(D) involuting fibroadenoma
(E) phyllodes tumor

60. Which of the following is the most appropriate next step in management?

(A) observation, with repeat mammogram in 6 months
(B) observation, with repeat mammogram on an annual basis
(C) biopsy
(D) lumpectomy, radiation therapy, and SLN biopsy
(E) total mastectomy

Questions 61 and 62

An 83-year-old woman presents to a mammographic facility for a screening mammogram. The technician notices a mass in the lateral right breast. The patient denies any breast pain, nipple discharge, skin changes, or breast trauma. A right breast CC view is shown in Fig. 6-7.

61. Which of the following is the most likely diagnosis?

(A) papilloma
(B) invasive carcinoma
(C) cystosarcoma phyllodes
(D) DCIS
(E) fat necrosis

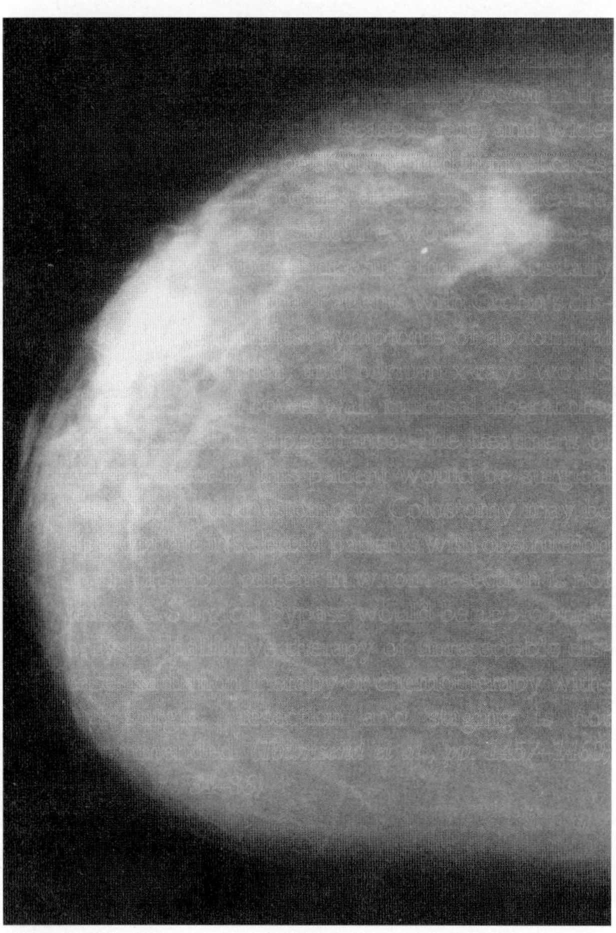

FIG. 6-7

62. Which of the following is the most appropriate next step in management?

(A) incisional biopsy
(B) needle biopsy
(C) lumpectomy, axillary dissection, and irradiation
(D) total mastectomy
(E) modified radical mastectomy

Questions 63 and 64

A 65-year-old woman presents to the physician's office with a 6-month history of epigastric discomfort, poor appetite, and 10-lb weight loss. Past history is pertinent for hypertension, diabetes, a 30 pack-year smoking history, and occasional alcohol intake. Examination is unremarkable except for mild epigastric tenderness to deep palpation. An abdominal ultrasound reveals cholelithiasis, and one view of a UGI x-ray series is shown in Fig. 6-8.

63. Which of the following is the most likely diagnosis?

(A) cholecystoenteric fistula
(B) duodenal ulcer
(C) gastric ulcer
(D) gastric diverticulum
(E) duodenal diverticulum

64. Which of the following is the most appropriate next step in management?

(A) H_2 blockers with reevaluation by UGI in 6 months
(B) vagotomy and pyloroplasty
(C) total gastrectomy
(D) endoscopy
(E) CT scan

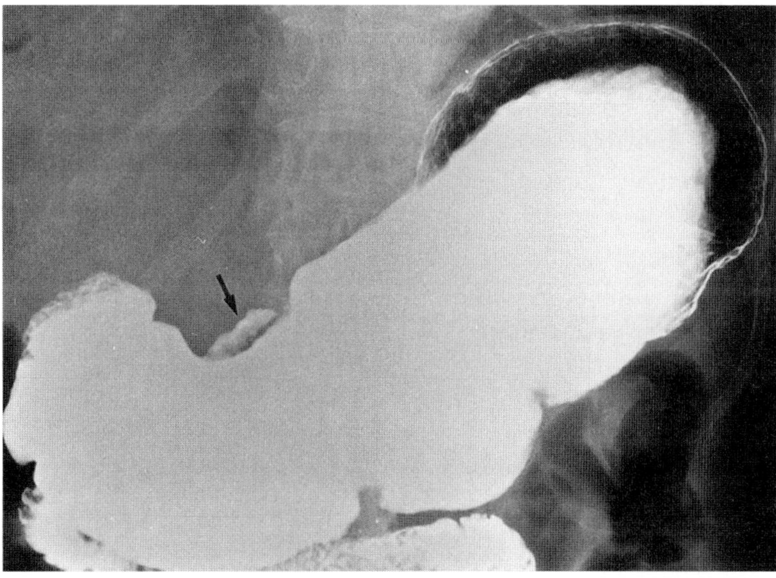

FIG. 6-8 *(Reprinted with permission from Zinner MJ.* Maingot's Abdominal Operations, *10th ed., vol. 1. Stamford, CT: Appleton & Lange, 1997.)*

65. A 55-year-old man presents to the physician's office for his yearly physical examination. He is asymptomatic. Past history is pertinent for hypertension. Family history is positive for breast cancer in his mother at age 70 and colon cancer in his father at age 65. His examination is unremarkable except for guiac positive stool. Barium enema shows a sigmoid colon polyp. Colonoscopy confirms a 3-cm pedunculated polyp in the sigmoid colon, and snare polypectomy is performed. Pathologic examination reveals an adenomatous polyp with a focus of invasive carcinoma in the head, with a 4-mm resection margin and no tumor noted in the stalk. Which of the following is the most appropriate next step in management?

(A) CT scan
(B) magnetic resonance imaging (MRI) scan
(C) surgical resection of sigmoid
(D) observation
(E) regular use of nonsteroidal anti-inflammatory drugs (NSAIDs)

Questions 66 and 67

A 55-year-old man presents to the emergency department with left lower quadrant abdominal pain. The pain has been present for 1 week, but has increased in intensity over the last 2 days associated with nausea, constipation, and dysuria. Past history is unremarkable. Examination reveals a temperature of 101°F, pulse rate of 95/min, BP of 130/70 mmHg, and normal heart and lung examinations. Abdominal examination reveals fullness and marked tenderness in the left lower quadrant, with voluntary guarding and decreased bowel sounds. Laboratory tests reveal a WBC count of 18,000 with a left shift and 20–50 WBCs in the urinalysis. A CT scan of the abdomen reveals a thickened sigmoid colon with pericolonic inflammation. He is admitted to the hospital for treatment.

66. Which of the following is the most likely diagnosis?

(A) colon cancer with contained perforation
(B) ischemic colitis
(C) pseudomembranous colitis
(D) diverticulitis
(E) pyelonephritis

67. Which of the following is the most appropriate management of this patient?

(A) NPO, IV fluids, and IV antibiotics for gram-negative and anaerobic coverage
(B) NPO, IV fluid hydration, followed by immediate sigmoid colon resection
(C) NPO, IV fluids, and anticoagulation
(D) NPO, IV fluids, evaluation of stool for *Clostridium difficile* toxin, and either metronidazole or vancomycin antibiotic therapy
(E) NPO, IV fluids, initiation of bowel preparation for elective sigmoid colon resection during the current hospitalization

Questions 68 and 69

A 75-year-old woman is brought to the emergency department from a nursing home for abdominal pain, distention, and obstipation over the last 2 days. Past history is pertinent for stroke, diabetes, atrial fibrillation, and chronic constipation. Examination reveals a temperature of 98.6°F, pulse rate 90/min and irregularly irregular, and BP 160/90 mmHg. Heart examination reveals irregularly irregular rhythm with no murmurs; lung examination reveals few bibasilar rales; and abdominal examination reveals a distended, tympanic abdomen with mild tenderness and no rebound tenderness. Plain abdominal x-rays reveal dilated loops of bowel, and a barium enema is obtained and shown in Fig. 6-9.

68. Which of the following is the most likely diagnosis?

(A) ischemic colitis with stricture
(B) diverticulitis with obstruction
(C) cecal volvulus
(D) sigmoid volvulus
(E) colon cancer with obstruction

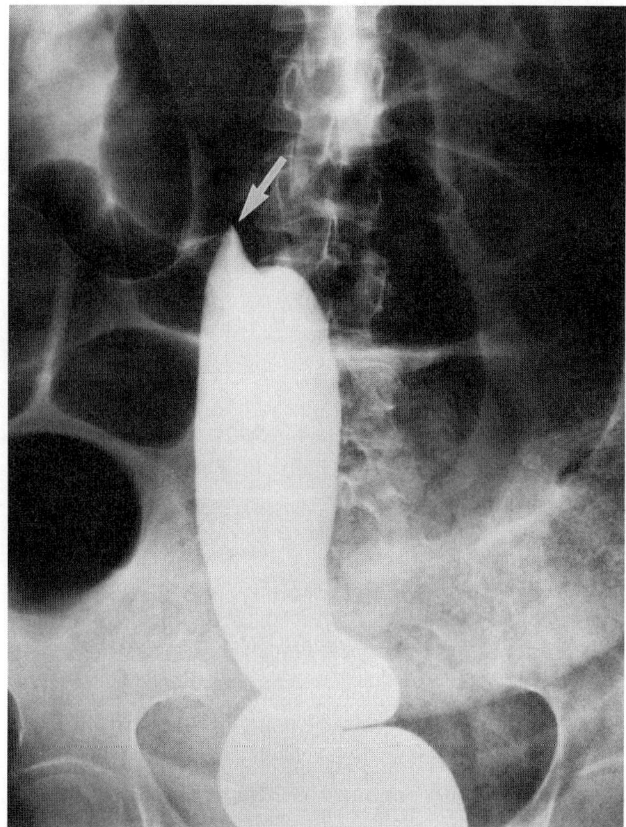

FIG. 6-9 *(Reprinted with permission from Zinner MJ.* Maingot's Abdominal Operations, *10th ed., vol. 1. Stamford, CT: Appleton & Lange, 1997.)*

69. Which of the following is the most appropriate next step in management following nasogastric tube decompression and resuscitation?

(A) urgent sigmoid resection
(B) nonoperative reduction by proctoscopy and rectal tube
(C) proximal colostomy
(D) urgent operative detorsion
(E) nonoperative reduction by passage of well-lubricated rectal tube

Questions 70 and 71

A 65-year-old man presents to the physician's office for his yearly physical examination. His only complaints relate to early fatigue while playing golf. Past history is pertinent for mild hypertension. Examination is unremarkable except for trace hematest-positive stool. Blood tests are normal except for a hematocrit of 32. A UGI series is performed and is normal. A barium enema is performed, and one view is shown in Fig. 6-10.

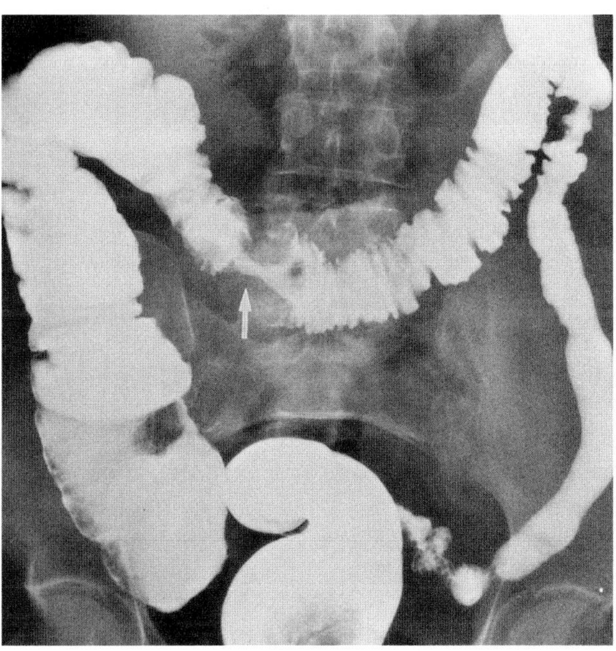

FIG. 6-10 *(Reprinted with permission from Zinner MJ.* Maingot's Abdominal Operations, *10th ed., vol. 1. Stamford, CT: Appleton & Lange, 1997.)*

70. Which of the following is the most likely diagnosis?

(A) diverticular disease
(B) colon cancer
(C) lymphoma
(D) ischemia with stricture
(E) Crohn's colitis with stricture

71. Which of the following is the most appropriate therapy following colonoscopy?

(A) proximal colostomy with mucous fistula
(B) radiation therapy
(C) chemotherapy
(D) surgical resection and primary anastomosis
(E) surgical bypass (colocolostomy)

Questions 72 and 73

A 54-year-old woman presents to her physician for an opinion regarding additional therapy following curative resection of recently diagnosed colon cancer. She underwent uncomplicated sigmoid resection for invasive colon cancer 4 weeks ago. The pathology revealed carcinoma invading into, but not through, the muscularis propria, with one of eight positive mesenteric nodes. There was no evidence of liver metastases at the time of operation. Preoperative chest x-ray and CT scan of the abdomen showed no evidence of distant disease. Preoperative carcinoembryonic antigen (CEA) level was normal. Past history is positive for diabetes and mild hypertension. Examination is unremarkable except for a healing abdominal incision.

72. Which of the following is the correct stage of this patient's colon cancer?

(A) stage 0
(B) stage I
(C) stage II
(D) stage III
(E) stage IV

73. Which of the following is the most appropriate recommendation regarding adjuvant therapy?

(A) no therapy indicated
(B) 5-fluorouracil chemotherapy
(C) 5-fluorouracil chemotherapy with leucovorin
(D) doxorubicin (Adriamycin) chemotherapy
(E) Adriamycin chemotherapy with methotrexate and cytoxan

Questions 74 and 75

A 62-year-old woman presents to the physician's office with complaints of constipation. She has had constipation for the last 6 months, which has worsened over the last month, associated with mild bloating. She noted that her stool has become "pencil thin" in the last month, with occasional blood, but she continues to have bowel movements daily. Past history is unremarkable. Examination reveals normal vital signs and heart and lung examination. Abdominal examination reveals mild fullness, especially in the lower quadrants. Rectal examination shows no rectal masses, but the stool is hematest positive. A barium x-ray is obtained, and one view is shown in Fig. 6-11.

74. Which of the following is the most likely diagnosis?

(A) Crohn disease
(B) ischemia with stricture
(C) rectal carcinoma
(D) sigmoid volvulus
(E) diverticulitis with colovesical fistula

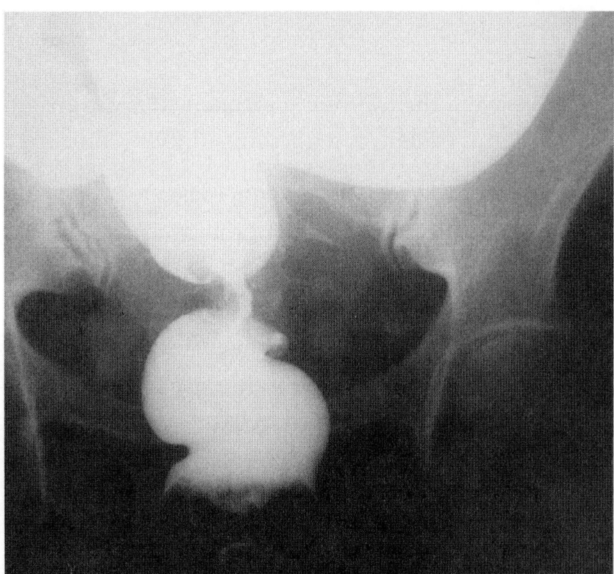

FIG. 6-11 *(Reprinted with permission from Zinner MJ.* Maingot's Abdominal Operations, *10th ed., vol. 2. Stamford, CT: Appleton & Lange, 1997.)*

75. Which of the following is the most appropriate next step in management?

(A) proctoscopy and passage of a rectal tube
(B) proctoscopy and biopsy
(C) colonoscopy
(D) endoscopic dilation of the stricture
(E) NPO, IV fluids, and antibiotics

Questions 76 and 77

A 45-year-old man presents to the physician's office for evaluation of a skin lesion on his abdomen. He states that the lesion has been present for 1 year, but has recently enlarged over the last 2 months. The mass is nontender, and he is otherwise asymptomatic. Past history is unremarkable. Examination reveals a 3-cm, pigmented, irregular skin lesion located in the left lower quadrant of the abdomen, as shown in Fig. 6-12. Heart, lung, and abdominal examination is normal. There are no palpable cervical, axillary, or inguinal lymph nodes. Chest x-ray and liver function tests are normal.

76. Which of the following is the most likely diagnosis?

(A) squamous cell carcinoma
(B) basal cell carcinoma
(C) Merkel cell carcinoma
(D) melanoma
(E) keratoacanthoma

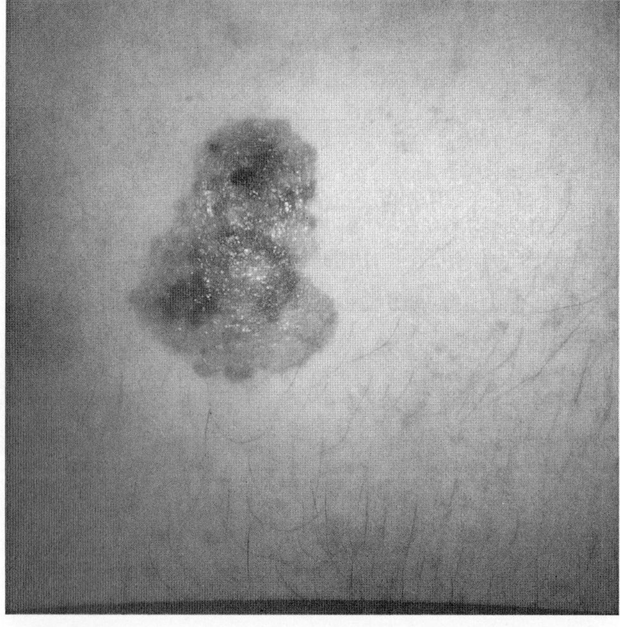

FIG. 6-12 *(Reprinted with permission from Hurwitz RM, Hood AF.* Pathology of the Skin: Atlas of Clinical–Pathological Correlation. *Stamford, CT: Appleton & Lange, 1998.)*

77. Which of the following is the most appropriate next step in management?

(A) wide excision with 2 cm margin
(B) wide excision with 2 cm margin and SLN mapping
(C) shave biopsy
(D) excisional biopsy with 1–2 mm margins
(E) Mohs' surgical excision

78. A 75-year-old woman is admitted to the hospital from a nursing home for abdominal pain and pneumonia. She was noted to be short of breath with increasing cough for 2 days before admission. Treatment, consisting of supplemental oxygen, IV antibiotics, and pulmonary toilet, is instituted, with improvement within 2 days. On the third hospital day, her abdominal pain worsens. Examination reveals a mildly distended abdomen with bowel sounds but no signs of peritonitis. Remainder of examination reveals a tender bulge in the medial left thigh below the inguinal ligament. Gentle pressure causes more pain but does not change the size or shape of the bulge. Abdominal films show a nonspecific bowel gas pattern. Laboratory analysis shows a WBC of 13,000, decreased from 18,000 at the time of admission. Which of the following is the most likely diagnosis?

(A) incarcerated direct inguinal hernia
(B) lymph node with abscess
(C) femoral artery aneurysm
(D) incarcerated indirect inguinal hernia
(E) incarcerated femoral hernia

Questions 79 and 80

A 65-year-old woman presents to the physician's office for her yearly physical examination. She has no complaints except for a recent 10-lb weight loss. Past history is pertinent for a 40 pack-year smoking history, hypertension, asthma, and hypothyroidism. Examination reveals a thin woman with normal vital signs and unremarkable heart and abdominal examinations. Lung examination reveals mild wheezing and a few bibasilar rales. A chest x-ray is obtained and is shown in Fig. 6-13. A chest x-ray obtained 3 years ago was normal. Yearly laboratory tests including a CBC, electrolytes, and lipid panels are normal.

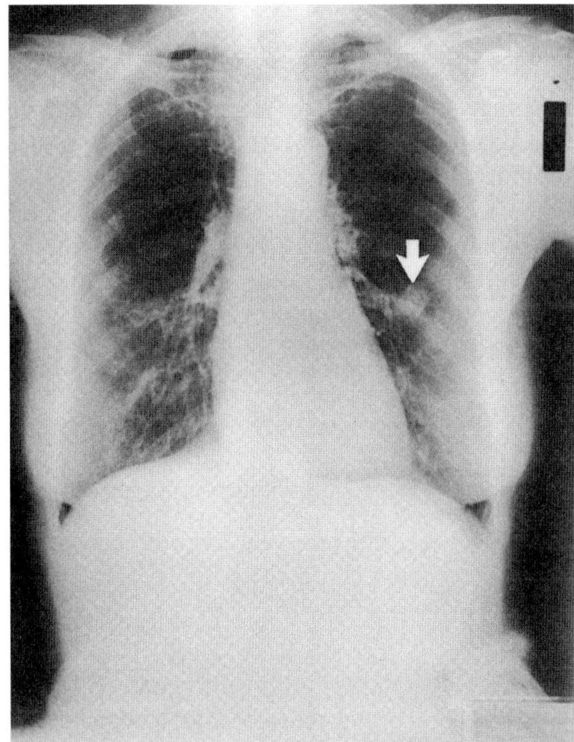

FIG. 6-13 *(Reprinted with permission from Niederhuber JE.* Fundamentals of Surgery. *Stamford, CT: Appleton & Lange, 1998.)*

79. Which of the following is the most likely diagnosis?

(A) small cell lung cancer
(B) tuberculosis
(C) nonsmall cell lung cancer
(D) hamartoma
(E) abscess

80. Which of the following is the most appropriate next diagnostic test?

(A) percutaneous needle biopsy
(B) CT scan
(C) pulmonary function tests
(D) mediastinoscopy
(E) bronchoscopy

Questions 81 and 82

A 75-year-old man is brought to the emergency department for severe pain in the left flank and back of 1 h duration. He has a prior history of a myocardial infarction and coronary artery bypass grafting 8 years ago. On examination, he is found to have a BP of 80/50 mmHg, pulse rate of 110/min, respiratory rate of 15/min, and a pulsatile, tender abdominal mass. He has had two large-bore IV lines placed by the paramedics. He is alert and oriented, and gives consent for surgery.

81. Which of the following is the most appropriate next step in management of this patient?

(A) immediate consultation with cardiology to assess cardiac risk for surgery, followed by transfer to the operating room
(B) resuscitation in the emergency department with IV fluids, transfer to radiology for a CT scan to assess for the location and degree of rupture, followed by transfer to the operating room
(C) resuscitation in the emergency department with IV fluids to achieve a systolic BP greater than 100, followed by transfer to the operating room
(D) immediate transfer to the operating room with concomitant resuscitation and laparotomy
(E) resuscitation in the emergency department with IV fluids, transfer to radiology for immediate aortic angiogram for assessment of the location of the rupture, followed by transfer to the operating room

82. On postop day 3, the patient develops dark-colored diarrhea but remains normotensive, on full mechanical ventilation, and is awake. Laboratory analysis reveals normal electrolytes, blood urea nitrogen (BUN), and creatinine; hematocrit of 30; and WBC of 15,000. Which is the most appropriate next step in management?

(A) stool for *C. difficile* toxin test and institution of metronidazole
(B) sigmoidoscopy
(C) air contrast barium enema
(D) CT scan
(E) abdominal x-rays

Questions 83 through 85

A 65-year-old man presents to the emergency department with sudden onset of pain and weakness of the left lower extremity of 2-h duration. Past history reveals chronic atrial fibrillation following a myocardial infarction 12 months ago. On examination, he is found to have a cool, pale left lower extremity with decreased strength and absent popliteal and pedal pulses. The opposite leg has a normal appearance with palpable pulses.

83. Which of the following is the most appropriate first step in management of this patient?

(A) echocardiography
(B) anticoagulation with heparin
(C) anticoagulation with warfarin
(D) arteriography
(E) alkalinization of the urine with IV sodium bicarbonate

84. Which of the following is the treatment of choice for this patient?

(A) streptokinase infusion following anticoagulation
(B) administration of vasodilators
(C) four-compartment fasciotomy
(D) thromboembolectomy
(E) anticoagulation and close observation

85. Following successful treatment for an embolus to the left femoral artery with no evidence of a reperfusion injury, which of the following long-term treatments would most likely decrease the chance of recurrent embolus?

(A) anticoagulation
(B) exercise program
(C) coronary artery bypass grafting
(D) aortofemoral bypass grafting
(E) placement of a vena cava filter

Questions 86 and 87

A 65-year-old man presents to the emergency department with an abrupt onset of excruciating chest pain 1 h ago. The pain is localized to the anterior chest, but radiates to the back and neck. On examination, the patient is afebrile, with a BP of 210/110 mmHg, pulse rate of 95/min, and a respiratory rate of 12/min. He appears pale and sweaty. Unequal carotid, radial, and femoral pulses are noted. An electrocardiogram (ECG) shows nonspecific ST-T segment changes. Chest x-ray shows a slightly widened mediastinum and normal lung fields.

86. Which of the following is the preferred modality in establishing the diagnosis?

(A) transcutaneous echocardiography
(B) transesophageal echocardiography
(C) CT scan
(D) coronary angiography
(E) aortography

87. Which of the following is the first step in management of this patient?

(A) treatment with thrombolytic agents
(B) systemic anticoagulation
(C) control of hypertension
(D) placement of an intraaortic balloon pump
(E) immediate operation

Questions 88 and 89

A 39-year-old woman presents to the physician's office for evaluation of a palpable nodule in the neck of 2 years' duration. Her past history is pertinent for Hashimoto's disease diagnosed 5 years ago, for which she takes thyroid hormone. She has a history of low-dose chest irradiation for an enlarged thymus gland during infancy. On examination, a 2.5-cm nodule is palpable in the left lobe of the thyroid and is firm and nontender.

88. Which of the following portions of her history increases the risk for thyroid cancer?

(A) age group of 20–40 years
(B) female gender
(C) low-dose irradiation during infancy
(D) chronicity of the nodule
(E) past history of Hashimoto's disease

89. Which of the following is the most appropriate next step in her management?

(A) ultrasound of the neck
(B) thyroid scintiscan
(C) MRI of the neck
(D) CT scan of the neck and chest
(E) FNA of the nodule

Questions 90 and 91

A 45-year-old man presents to the physician's office complaining of dysphagia and retrosternal pressure and pain of 2-year duration. The symptoms have worsened over the last 3 months. He has a 30 pack-year smoking history and drinks beer on weekends. Vital signs include a BP of 150/90 mmHg, pulse rate of 90/min, and respiratory rate of 12/min, with a normal temperature. Examination reveals a thin man with a normal heart, lung, and abdomen examination. An esophagogram reveals a 6-cm, smooth, concave defect in the midesophagus with sharp borders. Esophagoscopy reveals intact overlying mucosa and a mobile tumor.

90. Which of the following is the most likely diagnosis?

(A) esophageal carcinoma
(B) bronchogenic carcinoma with invasion of the esophagus
(C) benign esophageal polyp
(D) leiomyoma
(E) lymphoma

91. Which of the following is the most appropriate next step?

(A) repeat esophagoscopy with biopsy
(B) thoracotomy with extramucosal resection
(C) thoracotomy with esophageal resection
(D) radiation therapy
(E) chemotherapy

Questions 92 and 93

A 49-year-old woman presents to her physician with dysphagia, regurgitation of undigested food eaten hours earlier, and coughing over the last 6 months. She was hospitalized 1 month ago for aspiration pneumonia and successfully treated with antibiotics. Examination reveals a thin-appearing woman with normal vital signs and unremarkable chest, heart, and abdominal examination. A UGI contrast study is performed and reveals a pharyngoesophageal (Zenker's) diverticulum.

92. Which of the following statements is true regarding Zenker's diverticula?

(A) Cervical dysphagia is related to the size of the diverticulum.
(B) Pharyngoesophageal diverticula are of the pulsion type.
(C) Pharyngoesophageal diverticula are true diverticula.
(D) Pharyngoesophageal diverticula are congenital in origin.
(E) Upper esophageal sphincter function is usually normal.

93. Which of the following is the most important aspect of treatment?

(A) resection of the diverticulum
(B) cricopharyngeal muscle myotomy
(C) H_2 blockers
(D) elevation of the head of the bed
(E) diverticulopexy

94. A 55-year-old man presents to the emergency department at 5 a.m. complaining of vomiting blood. After binge drinking last night, the patient began to vomit repeatedly. After a number of episodes, the patient noted blood in the vomitus, followed by a melanotic stool 5 h later. His past history is pertinent for ethanol abuse and a 40 pack-year smoking history. Vital signs reveal a BP of 100/60 mmHg, pulse rate of 95/min, respiratory rate of 12/min, and temperature of 97°F. Examination reveals a thin man with normal chest, cardiac, and abdominal findings. Rectal examination reveals heme-positive stool. Laboratory data show normal electrolytes and a hematocrit of 30. A chest x-ray is unremarkable. Volume resuscitation, gastric lavage, and nasogastric tube decompression are initiated. Which of the following is the most appropriate diagnostic test?

(A) barium esophagogram
(B) water-soluble contrast esophagogram
(C) esophagoscopy
(D) CT scan
(E) angiogram

Questions 95 and 96

A 68-year-old man presents to the physician's office complaining of progressive dysphagia over the last 3 months associated with mild chest discomfort. He reports a 15-lb weight loss, a 30 pack-year smoking history, and occasional alcohol intake. The physical examination, including vital signs, is unremarkable. A chest x-ray was normal, and a barium esophagogram shows an irregular filling defect in the distal third of the esophagus with distortion and narrowing of the lumen.

95. Which of the following is the most likely diagnosis?

(A) esophagitis with stricture
(B) esophageal carcinoma
(C) lung carcinoma with invasion into the esophagus
(D) lymphoma
(E) achalasia

96. Which of the following is the most appropriate next step in management?

(A) CT scan
(B) esophagoscopy
(C) MRI scan
(D) surgical resection
(E) bronchoscopy

Questions 97 through 99

A 30-year-old man presents to the emergency department with sudden onset of severe epigastric pain and vomiting 3 h ago. He reports a 6-month history of chronic epigastric pain occurring nearly every day and relieved by antacids. On examination, he appears sweaty and avoids movement. Vital signs reveal a temperature of 100°F, BP of 100/60 mmHg, pulse rate of 110/min, and respiratory rate of 12/min. The remainder of his examination reveals diminished bowel sounds and a markedly tender and rigid abdomen. A chest x-ray and abdominal films reveal pneumoperitoneum.

97. Which of the following is the most likely diagnosis?

(A) small-bowel obstruction
(B) dead bowel
(C) perforated colon carcinoma
(D) perforated duodenal ulcer
(E) perforated gastric ulcer

98. Which of the following is the most appropriate next diagnostic test?

(A) CT scan
(B) UGI water-soluble contrast study
(C) lower GI water-soluble contrast study
(D) abdominal ultrasound
(E) none of the above

99. Which of the following is the most appropriate next step in management?

(A) immediate laparotomy
(B) nonoperative management with nasogastric decompression and antibiotics
(C) fluid resuscitation
(D) administration of H_2 blockers
(E) placement of a central venous line

Questions 100 and 101

A 55-year-old man presents to the physician's office complaining of upper abdominal pain of 2 months' duration. The pain is described as gnawing, localized to the upper midline, and associated with nausea. The pain is exacerbated by food, and there is an associated 20-lb weight loss over 2 months. His past history is pertinent for a 30 pack-year smoking history, occasional alcohol intake, and a prior history of a benign gastric ulcer 5 years ago. Physical examination reveals normal vital signs, mild epigastric pain with deep palpation, and mildly heme-positive stool. An evaluation for recurrence of a gastric ulcer is recommended.

100. Which of the following tests is the most reliable method for diagnosing a gastric ulcer?

(A) UGI barium x-rays
(B) fiberoptic upper endoscopy
(C) CT scan
(D) endoscopic ultrasound
(E) MRI

101. In this patient, a benign gastric ulcer was found, and he was placed on a proton-pump inhibitor and triple antibiotics for *Helicobacter pylori*. He returns to the physician's office 3 months later with similar complaints and, on reevaluation, the gastric ulcer was found to persist. Which of the following is the most appropriate next step in management?

(A) a second trial of proton-pump inhibitors with triple antibiotics and reevaluation in 2 months
(B) a trial of H_2 blockers with triple antibiotics and reevaluation in 2 months
(C) a trial of sucralfate and reevaluation in 2 months
(D) surgical management
(E) a trial of prostaglandins and reevaluation in 2 months

Questions 102 through 104

A 65-year-old man presents to the physician's office for his yearly examination. His past history is pertinent for a 40 pack-year smoking history and colon cancer 3 years ago for which he underwent a sigmoid colectomy. The most recent colonoscopic follow-up 3 months ago was negative. His physical examination is normal. Lab results show a normal CBC and electrolytes, markedly elevated cholesterol, and a CEA of 12 compared to values of less than 5 obtained every 6 months since colectomy. A repeat CEA 4 weeks later was 15, and liver function tests revealed a minimally elevated alkaline phosphatase, with normal transaminases and bilirubin.

102. Which of the following is the most appropriate next diagnostic test in this patient?

(A) Positron emission tomography (PET) scan
(B) radionuclide liver scan
(C) ultrasound
(D) CT scan
(E) MRI scan

103. The imaging studies demonstrate three lesions in the right hepatic lobe suspicious for metastatic disease, each measuring 3–4 cm in diameter. There was no evidence of extrahepatic disease. Which of the following is the most appropriate next step in management?

(A) systemic chemotherapy
(B) intraarterial chemotherapy through the hepatic artery
(C) surgical resection
(D) radiation therapy to the liver
(E) repeat imaging studies in 3 months to determine the growth rate of the disease

104. In your discussion with the patient regarding the risks and benefits of the different management options listed above, which of the following values should you quote regarding the expected 5-year survival rate following curative surgical resection?

(A) 5–10%
(B) 15–20%
(C) 25–35%
(D) 40–50%
(E) 60–70%

Questions 105 and 106

A previously healthy 45-year-old man presents with a 9-month history of a slow-growing, painless right neck mass. He is a nonsmoker and has no significant past medical history. On examination, there is a nontender, discrete, 3-cm mass over the angle of the right mandible. Facial muscle function and sensation are normal. An oropharyngeal examination is normal.

105. Which of the following is the most likely diagnosis?

(A) metastatic carcinoma
(B) infectious parotitis
(C) pleomorphic adenoma of the parotid
(D) Hodgkin disease
(E) reactive cervical lymphatic hyperplasia

106. Which of the following is the best next step in the management of this patient?

(A) antibiotics
(B) excisional biopsy
(C) observation with reevaluation in 2–4 weeks
(D) superficial parotidectomy
(E) chest x-ray

Questions 107 and 108

A 10-month-old infant presents to the emergency department with a 24-h history of low-grade fever and anorexia. The parents report several episodes in which the child has been suddenly inconsolable and crying, followed by periods of lethargy. He has had nonbilious vomiting and several loose stools. On examination, the infant is pale and mildly dehydrated. His abdomen is soft and nondistended, with fullness to palpation in the right upper quadrant. The child passed another stool in the emergency department (Fig. 6-14).

107. Which of the following is the most likely diagnosis?

(A) gastroenteritis
(B) intussusception
(C) midgut volvulus
(D) Meckel's diverticulum
(E) juvenile rectal polyp

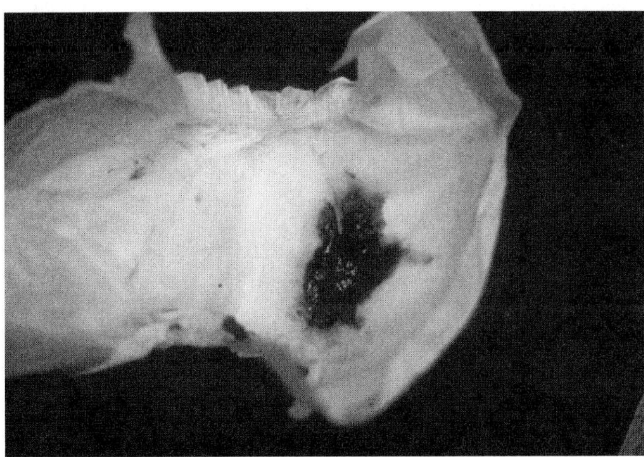

FIG. 6-14

108. Which of the following is the most appropriate next step in the diagnostic evaluation and management of this patient?

(A) proctoscopy
(B) oral rehydration and stool cultures
(C) IV fluid rehydration and a hydrostatic barium enema
(D) technetium scan
(E) IV fluid rehydration, nasogastric decompression, and a UGI contrast study

109. A 65-year-old diabetic man presents to the emergency department with a history of a penetrating wound to his buttock by a wooden stump while working in his garden 24 h earlier. On examination, he is febrile, the tissue around the wound is violaceous in color, and several bullae and crepitus are noted in the buttock. The drainage from the wound is foul smelling, watery, and grayish in appearance. The optimal treatment for this patient would include which of the following?

(A) high-dose IV penicillin G and broad-spectrum antibiotics
(B) high-dose IV penicillin G, broad-spectrum antibiotics, and local wound care with unroofing of bullae and culture of wound drainage
(C) high-dose IV penicillin G, broad-spectrum antibiotics, with surgical debridement only if and when there is no improvement with antibiotics
(D) radical surgical debridement
(E) high-dose IV penicillin G, broad-spectrum antibiotics, radical surgical debridement, and hyperbaric oxygen therapy

110. A 23-year-old man presents to the emergency department with a soft-tissue injury to the left lower extremity. The injury was sustained 8 h earlier in a motorcycle accident on a gravel road. On examination, the patient has a 7-cm deep laceration to the calf, with visible road debris. He had full tetanus immunization as a child and a tetanus booster immunization at age 15. Appropriate management of this injury would include which of the following?

(A) irrigation and debridement of the wound
(B) irrigation and debridement of the wound; tetanus toxoid and tetanus immune globulin
(C) irrigation and debridement of the wound; tetanus toxoid
(D) irrigation and debridement of the wound; IV antibiotics
(E) tetanus toxoid and IV antibiotics

111. A 6-year-old boy presents to the emergency department with a painful, markedly swollen elbow. While ice skating, he fell with his arm outstretched. Radiographs of the elbow demonstrate a displaced, supracondylar fracture of the humerus. On examination, there is pain on passive flexion at the wrist and a decreased radial pulse, with diminished capillary refill in the hand. Which of the following is the most appropriate management of this injury?

(A) admission to hospital for close observation, with immobilization of the elbow at 90° of flexion
(B) closed reduction with percutaneous pinning under general anesthesia
(C) open reduction and pinning under general anesthesia
(D) open reduction with pinning, and exploration of the brachial artery
(E) open reduction with pinning, exploration of the brachial artery, and decompression fasciotomy of the forearm fascial compartments

Questions 112 and 113

A 35-year-old woman is involved in a motor vehicle crash, sustaining a severe pelvic fracture, with disruption of the pelvic ring. In the trauma resuscitation room, she is confused and tachypneic, with a blood pressure of 90 mmHg systolic and a heart rate of 130/min. Laboratory investigations include serum electrolyte analysis, revealing a sodium of 139, a chloride of 103, and a bicarbonate of 14 meq/L.

112. This patient demonstrates which of the following?

(A) nonanion gap metabolic acidosis
(B) anion gap metabolic acidosis
(C) metabolic alkalosis
(D) respiratory acidosis
(E) normal serum electrolytes

113. Which of the following is the most appropriate management of this acid-base derangement?

(A) administration of sodium bicarbonate to correct the base deficit
(B) restoration of blood volume with aggressive IV fluid resuscitation
(C) IV hydrochloric acid
(D) intubation and hyperventilation
(E) this patient has no acid-base abnormality

DIRECTIONS (Questions 114 through 116): For each numbered item, select the ONE best lettered option that is most closely associated with it. Each lettered option may be selected once, more than once, or not at all.

For each newborn with vomiting and illustrated radiographs, select the most likely diagnosis.

(A) congenital hypertrophic pyloric stenosis
(B) annular pancreas
(C) duodenal atresia
(D) midgut volvulus
(E) intussusception
(F) imperforate anus
(G) Meckel's diverticulum
(H) meconium ileus
(I) Hirschsprung disease
(J) jejunal atresia

114. A 10-day-old infant presenting with bilious vomiting, paucity of gas on plain radiographs, and duodenal obstruction on UGI contrast study (Figs. 6-15 and 6-16)

115. A neonate with bile-stained vomiting, abdominal distention, dilated loops of bowel on plain radiographs, and a small-caliber colon on contrast enema (Fig. 6-17)

116. A 1-day-old infant with Down syndrome, feeding intolerance, bilious vomiting, and a double bubble on plain radiographs (Fig. 6-18)

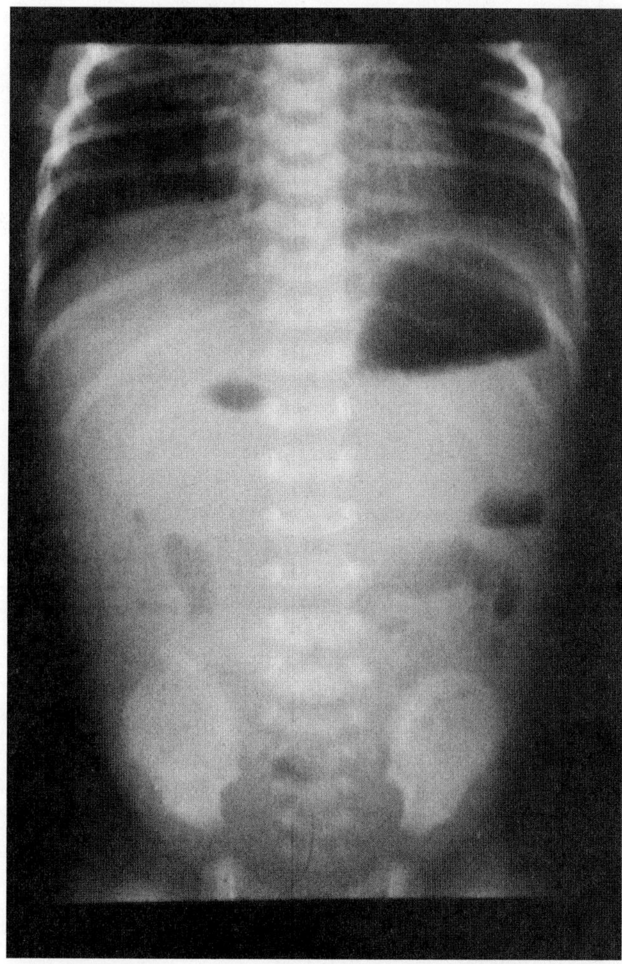

FIG. 6-15

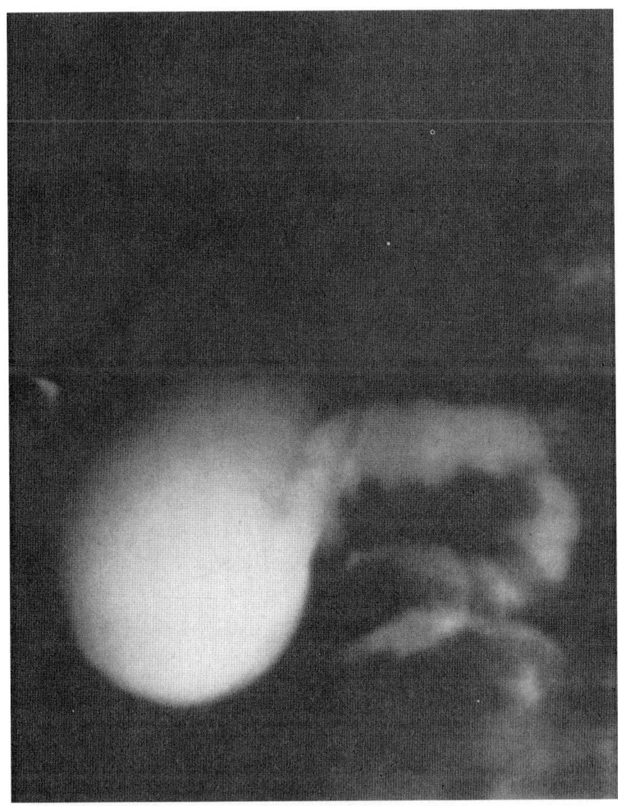

FIG. 6-16

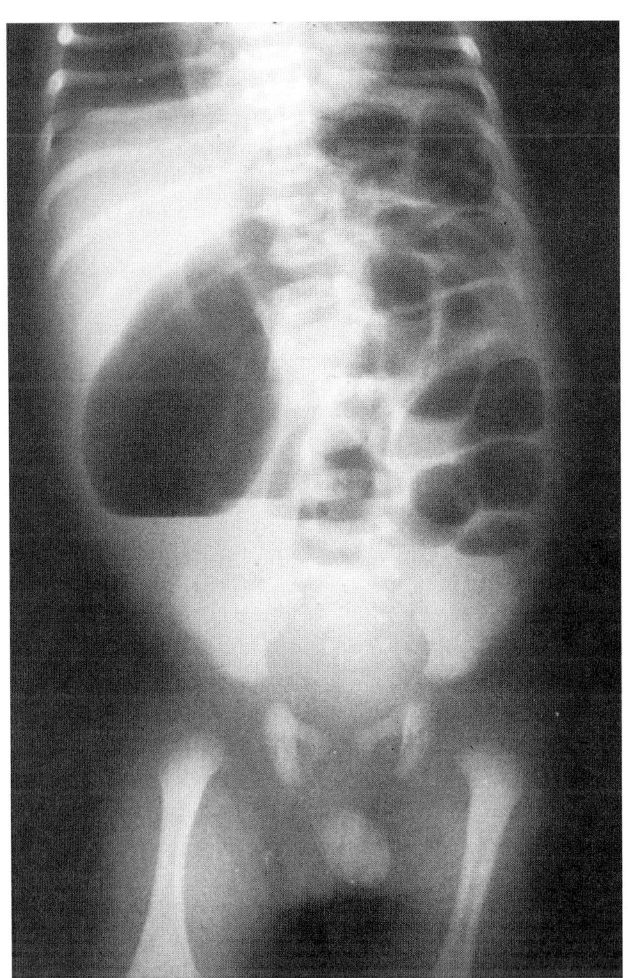

FIG. 6-17

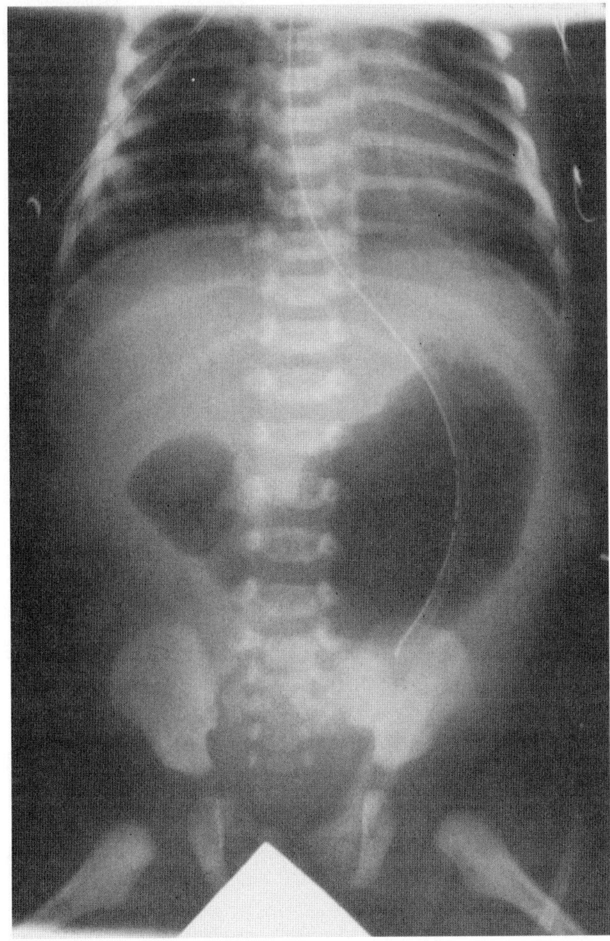

FIG. 6-18

DIRECTIONS (Questions 117 through 141): Each of the numbered items or incomplete statements in this section is followed by answers or by completions of the statement. Select the ONE lettered answer that is BEST in each case.

Questions 117 and 118

A 28-year-old man with a past history of bilateral orchiopexy for cryptorchidism presents with a painless, unilateral right scrotal enlargement. On examination, there is a palpable right testicular mass and enlarged inguinal nodes. Scrotal ultrasonography demonstrates heterogeneity of the testis, with an associated hydrocele. A CT scan of the abdomen and pelvis demonstrated right-sided retroperitoneal adenopathy. CT scan of the chest is normal.

117. Which of the following would help confirm the diagnosis?

(A) transscrotal needle biopsy
(B) transscrotal aspiration of the hydrocele for cytology
(C) radical orchiectomy through an inguinal incision
(D) transscrotal exploration and orchiectomy
(E) laparotomy with pelvic and retroperitoneal node dissection

118. Staging workup and surgery reveal a seminoma of the testicle, with positive inguinal and retroperitoneal nodes. Therapeutic management for this patient is which of the following?

(A) external beam radiotherapy
(B) multidrug combination chemotherapy
(C) combination radiotherapy and multidrug chemotherapy
(D) clinical surveillance
(E) laparotomy with pelvic and retroperitoneal node dissection

Questions 119 through 121

In a 6-month-old previously healthy male infant, an abnormality is revealed during a routine diaper change, as illustrated in Fig. 6-19. The parents have noted this finding on and off on several occasions over the last month. On each occasion, the child has been feeding well, and is content and playful.

119. Which of the following is the most likely diagnosis?

(A) noncommunicating hydrocele
(B) inguinal adenitis
(C) reducible inguinal hernia
(D) incarcerated inguinal hernia
(E) undescended testes

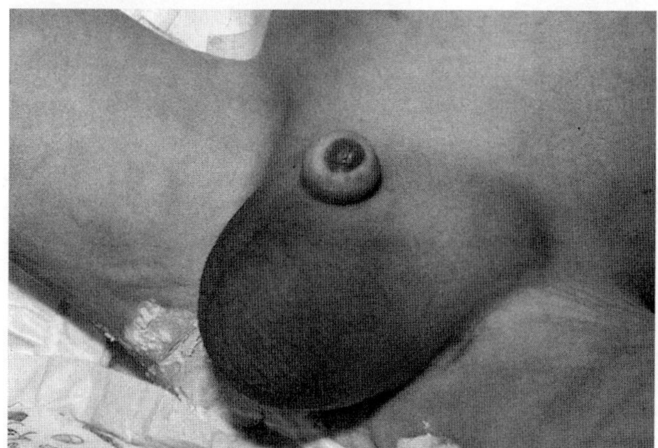

FIG. 6-19

120. Which of the following is the most appropriate management at this time?

(A) antibiotics
(B) reassurance to the parents that the abnormality will resolve without intervention
(C) referral to the emergency department for immediate surgical consultation
(D) referral for elective surgical repair
(E) scrotal support

121. Several weeks later, the child presents to the emergency department with a 4-h history of irritability. He has had one episode of nonbilious vomiting and has refused to breast feed. In the emergency department, the infant appears inconsolable. He is afebrile, and his abdomen is mildly distended but soft. On removal of his diaper, the same abnormality is documented (see Fig. 6-19). Which of the following is the most appropriate management at this time?

(A) urgent surgical exploration
(B) systemic antibiotics
(C) elective surgical repair
(D) sedation with manual reduction and arrangements for elective surgical repair
(E) sedation with manual reduction, admission, rehydration, and surgical repair within 24–48 h

Questions 122 and 123

A 70-year-old man with a 50 pack-year history of smoking presents with a 6-week history of intermittent, painless, gross hematuria and urinary frequency. There are no masses palpable on abdominal examination, and rectal examination is normal. Urinalysis confirms the presence of hematuria, and urine culture is negative.

122. Which of the following is the most appropriate initial diagnostic evaluation of this patient?

(A) plain abdominal radiographs and an intravenous pyelogram (IVP)
(B) voiding cystourethrogram
(C) cystourethroscopy
(D) abdominal ultrasound
(E) urine for cytology

123. The initial diagnostic evaluation does not reveal any abnormalities. Which of the following is the best next step in the diagnostic workup?

(A) an abdominal CT scan
(B) cystourethroscopy and urinary cytology
(C) a transrectal ultrasound
(D) exploratory laparoscopy
(E) reevaluation in 2–4 weeks, with repeat urinalysis and urine culture

124. A 7-week-old, breast-fed, term infant presents with increasing jaundice, abdominal distention, and abnormal stools (Fig. 6-20). Liver function tests demonstrate a conjugated hyperbilirubinemia, mildly elevated transaminases, and an elevated gamma-glutamyl transpeptidase. TORCH (congenital infection complex, including toxoplasmosis, rubella, cytomegalovirus, and hepatitis) serology and screening for inborn errors of metabolism are negative. As part of the diagnostic evaluation, the most sensitive imaging study in this clinical setting would be which of the following?

(A) radioisotope scanning
(B) radioisotope scanning with preimaging phenobarbital administration
(C) abdominal ultrasound
(D) CT scan of the abdomen
(E) MRI scan of the abdomen

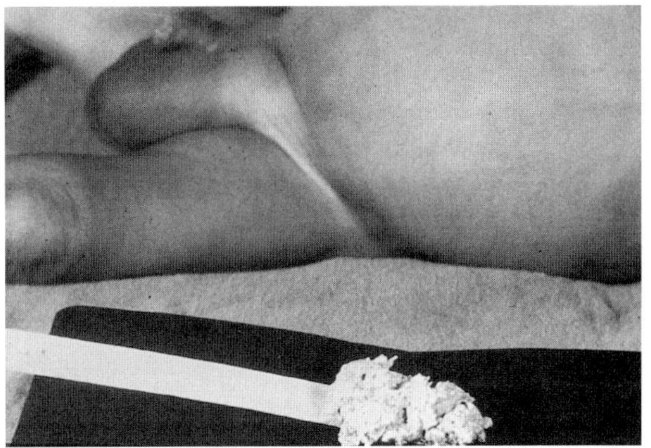

FIG. 6-20

Questions 125 and 126

During diagnostic evaluation, a 14-year-old girl with menorrhagia, frequent nosebleeds, and iron-deficiency anemia is found to have a low platelet count with a normal coagulation profile. Bone marrow biopsy reveals abundant megakaryocytes. On abdominal examination, no organomegaly is noted.

125. Which of the following is the most appropriate initial therapy for this patient?

(A) splenectomy
(B) platelet transfusion when peripheral platelet count drops below 50,000/mL
(C) systemic steroids
(D) chemotherapy
(E) expectant, with intervention only if the patient develops significant clinical bleeding

126. The patient has a satisfactory response to the initial therapeutic intervention, but over 6–12 months' time, the response is less dramatic and shorter in duration. There are signs and symptoms of increasing side effects from therapy. The next step in management should be to recommend which of the following?

(A) partial splenectomy
(B) splenectomy
(C) increase in steroid dose and frequency
(D) bone marrow transplant
(E) plasmapheresis

127. A 50-year-old man is admitted to the hospital with a UGI bleed from acute erosive gastritis, secondary to chronic nonsteroidal anti-inflammatory use. His hematocrit is 28%. With fluid resuscitation, his blood pressure normalizes, but he has a persistent hyperdynamic precordium, tachycardia, and flow murmur on auscultation. He complains of shortness of breath on ambulation. An ECG shows depressed ST-T segments. Which of the following is the next appropriate step in management?

(A) initiation of iron supplementation therapy
(B) supplemental oxygen
(C) continued IV fluid resuscitation
(D) initiation of a calcium channel blocker
(E) blood transfusion

128. A previously healthy 28-year-old woman develops significant postpartum hemorrhage, with a rapid drop in hematocrit to 18%. Despite aggressive IV fluid resuscitation, the patient has a persistent tachycardia, labile systolic blood pressure, and poor urine output. Ongoing resuscitation includes emergency transfusion with 2 units of O-negative packed red blood cells. During transfusion of the second unit, the patient develops chills, fever, vomiting, and hypertension. These symptoms are most likely the result of which of the following?

(A) a febrile nonhemolytic transfusion reaction
(B) an anaphylactic transfusion reaction
(C) ABO incompatibility with acute hemolytic transfusion reaction
(D) delayed hemolytic transfusion reaction
(E) acute bacterial infection transmitted in the blood product

129. A 22-year-old professional basketball player falls on his outstretched hand during a scrimmage game. He has mild swelling at the wrist and tenderness to palpation in the anatomic snuffbox. No fracture is visible on multiple radiographs of the wrist and hand. Which of the following is the most appropriate management of this patient?

(A) anti-inflammatory medication and application of ice
(B) elastic wrist support, analgesics, and restricted activity for 1–2 weeks
(C) presumptive diagnosis of a scaphoid fracture, with application of a wrist splint, and repeat x-rays in 10–14 days
(D) presumptive diagnosis of a scaphoid fracture, with application of a short-arm cast including the thumb
(E) presumptive diagnosis of a scaphoid fracture, application of a short-arm cast including the thumb, and removal of the cast, with repeat x-rays in 10–14 days

130. A previously healthy 45-year-old woman is involved in a motor vehicle crash, sustaining multiple rib fractures, a complex duodenal injury, and a fractured pelvis. She is ventilated in the ICU. Because of a persistent high-output duodenal fistula, the patient has required prolonged parenteral alimentation. During her ICU course, the patient develops diarrhea, mental depression, alopecia, and perioral and periorbital dermatitis. Administration of which of the following trace elements are most likely to reverse these complications?

(A) iodine
(B) zinc
(C) selenium
(D) silicon
(E) tin

Questions 131 and 132

A 70-year-old man is admitted to the ICU after repair of an abdominal aortic aneurysm. He has a prior history of hypertension and mild congestive heart failure, which were adequately controlled with digoxin and diuretics. To facilitate perioperative management, a Swan–Ganz (multilumen pulmonary artery) catheter was inserted in the operating room. During the first few hours postoperatively, the patient is noted to have a blood pressure of 140/70 mmHg, heart rate of 110/min, flat neck veins, a pulmonary arterial wedge pressure of 9 mmHg, and poor urine output.

131. Which of the following is the most appropriate next step in management of this patient?

(A) IV furosemide
(B) a bolus of IV crystalloid
(C) a dopamine infusion
(D) a nitroprusside infusion
(E) IV digoxin administration

132. Several hours after this intervention, the patient is reassessed. The blood pressure is 150/85 mmHg, heart rate is 90/min, neck veins are distended, and the pulmonary arterial wedge pressure is 17 mmHg. Urine output is still low in volume. At this point, management should be which of the following?

(A) IV furosemide
(B) a bolus of IV crystalloid
(C) a dopamine infusion
(D) a nitroprusside infusion
(E) IV digoxin administration

133. A 19-year-old previously healthy man is an unbelted driver of a motor vehicle involved in a front-end collision. On arrival in the emergency department, the patient is noted to have stridor, with marked respiratory distress, and an oxygen saturation of 88% despite 100% oxygen by mask. He has obvious extensive facial injuries, a flail chest, and poor chest expansion. Bag-mask-valve ventilation is ineffective. Which of the following is the most appropriate next step in management?

(A) orotracheal intubation
(B) nasotracheal intubation
(C) cricothyroidotomy
(D) tracheostomy
(E) placement of bilateral chest tubes

134. A 40-year-old alcoholic is brought to the emergency department with frostbite to both lower extremities. His core body temperature is 36°C. Which of the following is the most appropriate initial treatment for the patient's thermal injury?

(A) sympathectomy without any delay
(B) debridement of devitalized tissues
(C) slow rewarming at room temperature
(D) slow rewarming with dry heat
(E) rapid rewarming in warm water

Questions 135 and 136

A 50-year-old woman with a history of essential hypertension presents to the emergency department with sudden onset of a severe headache, nausea and vomiting, and photophobia. On examination, her BP is 160/100 mmHg. She is mildly confused and has nuchal rigidity, without focal neurologic signs.

135. Which of the following is the most likely diagnosis?

(A) meningitis
(B) ruptured cerebral aneurysm
(C) hemorrhagic stroke
(D) ischemic cerebrovascular accident
(E) transient ischemic attack

136. Once the diagnosis has been confirmed, which of the following is the next most important step in patient management?

(A) admission to the ICU, close monitoring, and aggressive treatment of hypertension
(B) urgent surgical intervention with aneurysm clipping
(C) admission to the ICU, close monitoring, and IV antibiotics
(D) serial lumbar punctures to drain cerebrospinal fluid (CSF)
(E) anticoagulation and antiplatelet therapy

137. During an elective laparoscopic cholecystectomy, the anesthesiologist reports that the patient has developed a sudden drop in systolic blood pressure, arterial desaturation, and an increase in ventilatory pressure. Which of the following is the most appropriate step in management?

(A) an IV fluid bolus
(B) decompression of the pneumoperitoneum
(C) insertion of a chest tube
(D) reevaluating the position of the endotracheal tube and obtaining a portable chest x-ray
(E) aborting the procedure and converting to an open cholecystectomy

Questions 138 through 140

A 55-year-old man with a history of diverticulosis presents with a 2-week history of dysuria, urgency, and pneumaturia. Furthermore, he has a 3-month history of vague, intermittent, left lower quadrant abdominal pain, and irregular bowel habits. On examination, he has fullness on palpation in the left lower quadrant, and urine culture demonstrates a polymicrobial infection. A CT scan demonstrates an inflammatory mass in the left pelvis.

138. Which of the following investigations is most likely to aid in diagnosis?

(A) voiding cystourethrogram
(B) CT scan with contrast
(C) air contrast barium enema
(D) colonoscopy
(E) laparoscopy

139. After confirming the diagnosis, the most appropriate initial steps in management of this patient include which one of the following?

(A) broad-spectrum antibiotics and insertion of an indwelling bladder catheter
(B) outpatient oral antibiotics and stool softeners
(C) clear fluids, magnesium citrate, and oral antibiotics
(D) urgent exploratory laparotomy
(E) proximal defunctioning colostomy

140. Which of the following is the optimal definitive surgical management for this patient?

(A) a proximal defunctioning loop colostomy
(B) sigmoid colon resection with primary anastomosis
(C) sigmoid colon resection with Hartmann's procedure
(D) abdominoperineal resection and permanent colostomy
(E) total abdominal colectomy and ileorectal anastomosis

141. An 80-year-old female resident of a nursing home presents to the emergency department with a history of sudden onset of crampy abdominal pain, vomiting, and abdominal distention. Her last bowel movement was 4 days before presentation, and she has not passed flatus since the onset of her symptoms. On examination, the patient is mildly dehydrated and afebrile, with a markedly distended but nontender abdomen. Barium enema is shown (Fig. 6-21). The patient receives IV resuscitation and nasogastric tube decompression. Which of the following is the most appropriate next step in management of this patient?

(A) urgent laparotomy
(B) admission to the hospital and serial abdominal examinations
(C) placement of a rectal decompression tube in the emergency department
(D) rigid proctoscopy and directed placement of a colonic decompression tube
(E) colonic enemas

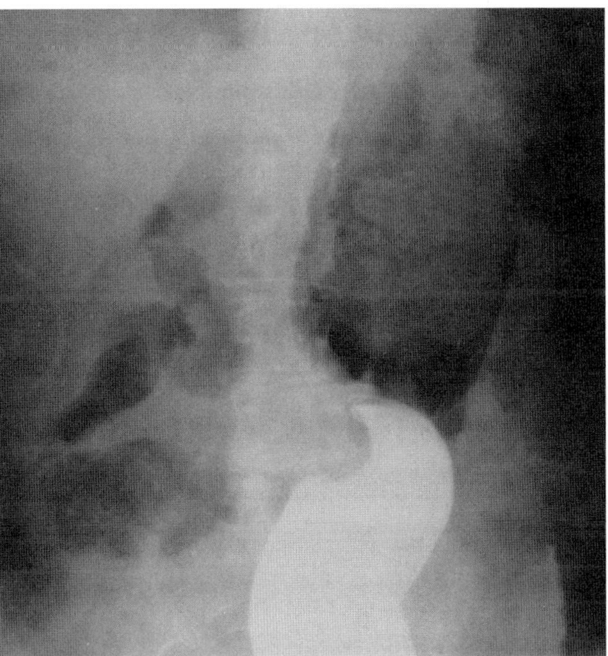

FIG. 6-21 *(Reprinted with permission from Zinner MJ.* Maingot's Abdominal Operations, *10th ed., vol. 2. Stamford, CT: Appleton & Lange, 1997.)*

Answers and Explanations

1. **(C)** This is an open fracture, and management constitutes an orthopedic emergency. Tetanus prophylaxis is indicated because the soft-tissue injury is a tetanus-prone wound. An open fracture is associated with a high risk of osteomyelitis. Systemic antibiotics should be started in the emergency department and continued postoperatively. Optimal local wound irrigation and debridement is achieved under general anesthesia. This fracture is severely comminuted and most likely unstable. Fracture stabilization can be accomplished with internal fixation or application of an external fixation device. The soft-tissue defect associated with an open fracture should not be closed primarily. It may require further debridement. With aggressive local wound care, delayed closure may be possible if the wound remains clean. Local wound irrigation and debridement may be limited by patient discomfort. The addition of antibiotics to the irrigation solution is of no additional benefit. Closed reduction would not be possible in this patient because the fracture is severely comminuted. Furthermore, a long-leg cast will not provide adequate immobilization of the unstable fracture fragments. *(Townsend et al., pp. 557–561)*

2. **(E)**

3. **(C)**

Explanations 2 and 3

This patient presents with an acute exacerbation of ulcerative colitis with systemic toxicity. Toxic megacolon is potentially life threatening and requires aggressive fluid resuscitation, bowel rest, and systemic antibiotics. High-dose steroids are initiated to treat the colonic inflammation. If there is no clinical improvement after 48 h of medical therapy, urgent surgery is indicated. Azathioprine and 6-mercaptopurine are immunosuppressive agents that may be beneficial in the treatment of steroid refractory colitis, but they are not indicated in the management of an acute toxic exacerbation. Opioid antidiarrheals are contraindicated, because they may increase colonic distention and increase the risk of perforation. Colonoscopy may also cause increased colonic distention with perforation. Urgent surgery in a patient with toxic megacolon should consist of abdominal colectomy, Hartmann's procedure (closure of the rectal stump), and ileostomy. Ileal pouch-anal anastomosis is a lengthy procedure, and is considered only for elective reconstruction. When performed in a systemically ill patient undergoing emergency colectomy of an unprepped colon, there are increased risks of anastomotic complications. Ileorectal anastomosis is no longer appropriate for the management of ulcerative colitis because of the retained diseased rectal mucosa, with concomitant risk of malignancy. *(Townsend et al., p. 1431; Way and Doherty, pp. 741–746)*

4. **(C)**

5. **(D)**

Explanations 4 and 5

This infant has an omphalocele. This is a result of failure of the abdominal muscles to close in the midline at the umbilical cord. The abdominal wall defect is therefore midline, with viscera enclosed in a sac composed of amniotic membranes. Children with omphalocele may have other associated anomalies. Infants with abdominal wall defects are at risk for fluid and temperature loss, and infection. Therefore, the initial management consists of measures to decompress the gastrointestinal tract, fluid resuscitation, IV antibiotics, and placing the viscera in a warm, moist occlusive dressing. An umbilical hernia results when the umbilical ring does not close, with viscera enclosed in a sac covered by peritoneum and skin. Many of these may spontaneously close on their own. Therefore, surgical intervention is restricted to those children with a persistent fascial defect. Omphalitis results from bacterial infection at the base of the cord and is well treated with antibiotics to cover skin organisms. Gastroschisis is a congenital evisceration, located to the right of the umbilical cord, and thought to be related to obliteration of one of the umbilical veins prior to birth. As with omphalocele, the child needs NG decompression, IV fluids and antibiotics, and a warm moist occlusive dressing. In gastroschisis, the bowel may be at risk of mechanical or vascular compromise, thus urgent surgical intervention is required. *(Townsend et al., pp. 2116–2117; Way and Doherty, pp. 1339–1340; Greenfield et al., pp. 1968–1971)*

6. **(B)** Meckel's diverticulum typically present in young children with painless rectal bleeding. The etiology of the bleeding is from ulceration of the adjacent ileum that is bathed by the acid produced from the ectopic gastric mucosa in the diverticulum. Bleeding may result in hypovolemia, requiring aggressive resuscitation before any surgical intervention. Diagnosis is made by technitium scan, with the child pretreated with H_2 blocks to increase the sensitivity. Colonoscopy is reserved for those children with a negative Meckel's scan. Acid suppression therapy is not indicated. At surgical exploration, the diverticulum and adjacent ileum are removed. *(Townsend et al., pp. 1366–1368; Greenfield et al., pp. 2010–2012)*

7. **(D)**

8. **(A)**

Explanations 7 and 8

The mammographic appearance of popcorn-like, coarse calcifications in the breast is characteristic of an involuting, or degenerating fibroadenoma in a postmenopausal woman. Mammographic followup is appropriate. A repeat study at 6 months would be considered if no prior films are available in order to assess stability of a new mammographic finding. Though ultrasound is often performed for solid masses, the amount of calcification in the mass would lead to artifact, making interpretation difficult. Biopsy would not be suggested based on the characteristic mammographic findings. Other surgical procedures would not be indicated. *(Greenfield et al., pp. 1345–1346; Donegan and Spratt, pp. 71–73, 294)*

9. **(C)**

10. **(E)**

Explanations 9 and 10

The most common cause of a nipple discharge is an intraductal papilloma. Galactography can often demonstrate a filling defect in the terminal ducts as is demonstrated in the figure. Duct ectasia may also cause a discharge, but the discharge is usually thick and pasty. Carcinoma is an uncommon cause of nipple discharge. The next step in management would be excision of the terminal duct containing the papilloma. Repeat cytology would not be useful because a negative result does not preclude biopsy. Observation would not be prudent, because a diagnosis of carcinoma must be excluded, and the papilloma may enlarge, requiring a more extensive operation at a later date. A more extensive operation, such as a central lumpectomy or mastectomy, would be unnecessary because the lesion is benign. *(Greenfield et al., pp. 1343–1344; Donegan and Spratt, pp. 95–97, 318–319)*

11. **(D)**

12. **(A)**

Explanations 11 and 12

The most likely diagnosis based on the chest x-ray and UGI contrast study is a paraesophageal hernia involving the gastric antrum and proximal duodenum. Although some contrast is seen in the transverse colon from that used during fluoroscopic placement of the NG-tube, most of the contrast in the UGI study does not leave the stomach and proximal duodenum, suggesting some degree of obstruction. A sliding hiatal hernia involves movement of the gastroesophageal junction into the mediastinum above the diaphragmatic hiatus. The figure shows the gastroesophageal junction below the diaphragmatic hiatus. Hernias of Bochdalek and Morgagni are congenital diaphragmatic hernias involving the posterorlateral and parasternal locations, respectively. Eventration is an attenuation of the central portion of the diaphragm with resultant upward displacement. The most appropriate treatment is laparatomy or laparscopy with reduction of the hernia and repair. Thoracotomy or thoracoscopy would not allow easy access to the abdominal contents and is associated with increased morbidity. Delaying surgery may result in strangulation and ischemia. Because the patient did not demonstrate any respiratory compromise, endotracheal intubation was not indicated. Endoscopy is useful to evaluate for mucosal erosions in the case of gastrointestinal bleeding. *(Townsend et al., pp. 1164–1166)*

13. (D)

14. (B)

15. (B)

16. (D)

Explanations 13 through 16

Infants with pyloric stenosis usually present after the third week of life with symptoms of progressive pyloric outlet obstruction secondary to increasing hypertrophy of the pyloric muscle. There are often clinical signs of dehydration, but the infant usually appears well and is eager to feed. Viral gastroenteritis and urinary tract sepsis may be associated with signs of such systemic illness as lethargy, poor feeding, and, in some cases, fever. Gastroesophageal reflux more typically presents with a history of regurgitation since birth. Milk protein allergy is often associated with colicky abdominal pain and diarrhea. The pathognomonic sign on clinical examination is a palpable "olive" in the epigastrium or right upper quadrant. Abdominal ultrasound is operator dependent, but with expertise in interpretation of the study, the thickened elongated pyloric channel can be demonstrated. A UGI contrast study may show the classic "shouldering" of the pyloric muscle, with a "string sign"; this also requires expertise in performing the examination, and other causes of pyloric outlet obstruction, such as pylorospasm may be misinterpreted as a positive study. Surgical exploration should be reserved for those patients in whom the diagnosis has been confirmed and only after the infant has received fluid resuscitation. Infants with gastric outlet obstruction develop a hypochloremic, hypokalemic metabolic alkalosis. This is secondary to the loss of chloride in the gastric contents, and the renal reabsorption of sodium in exchange for potassium and hydrogen. Carbonic anhydrase converts carbonic acid to hydrogen and bicarbonate ions, allowing hydrogen to be excreted in the urine, with retention of the bicarbonate. Hence, with the metabolic alkalosis, there is a "paradoxical aciduria." Hypernatremic, hyperchloremic, hypokalemic metabolic acidosis develops in infants with diarrhea. Infants with gastroesophageal reflux do not usually develop significant electrolyte derangements. Infants with pyloric stenosis will usually require a period of fluid resuscitation to correct hypovolemia as well as electrolyte and acid-base abnormalities. This is followed by a pyloromyotomy. Infants with vomiting and diarrhea from viral gastroenteritis are often successfully managed with oral rehydration. Prokinetic agents have been used in the management of gastroesophageal reflux. Soy formulas or elemental formulas are recommended for the infant with a milk protein allergy. *(Townsend et al., pp. 2107–2108; Way and Doherty, pp. 1315–1316; Greenfield et al., pp. 2007–2008)*

17. (D)

18. (B)

Explanations 17 and 18

The clinical signs and symptoms of a ureteral calculus are secondary to sudden obstruction of a hollow viscus, with visceral referred pain from loin to groin. The pain is severe and colicky in nature, with ureteral peristalsis against the obstruction. This is often associated with reflex vomiting mediated by visceral stretch and pain fibers. Typically, the patient is restless and cannot find a position of comfort. Urinary urgency and hematuria are common. Torsion of the testes produces sudden scrotal pain, and may have associated vague lower abdominal pain and vomiting. Pyelonephritis is associated with flank pain and costovertebral angle tenderness that is progressive in severity and constant in nature. Appendicitis will present with vague periumbilical pain, migrating to the right lower quadrant with the development of peritonitis. In the latter stages, the patient will lie quietly, as movement exacerbates the pain from peritoneal irritation. By increasing hydration and adequate analgesia, most patients will pass ureteral stones spontaneously. An imaging study should be obtained in all patients presenting with symptoms of urinary calculi. Nonenhanced CT scan will identify the location of the stone, size, and number of stones. This information assists with planning further management options, including referral for lithotripsy or cystoscopy and retrograde ureteroscopy. *(Townsend et al., p. 2299; Greenfield et al., pp. 2181–2185; Way and Doherty, pp. 1045–1046)*

19. **(C)** During the early catabolic phase after injury, nutritional support is essential in the management of the multiply injured patient. Elemental tube feeding can be initiated via the nasogastric route, or via the nasojejunal route if there is delayed gastric emptying. Enteral nutrition will aid in maintaining the integrity of the gastrointestinal mucosal barrier; thereby, reducing the risk of bacterial translocation and sepsis. The enteral route is less expensive than parenteral nutrition and does not subject the patient to the complications associated with an indwelling central venous catheter. *(Townsend et al., pp. 170–172, 628–629; Way and Doherty, pp. 170–174; Greenfield et al., pp. 55–56, 60–67)*

20. **(B)** This patient has a left tension pneumothorax, a diagnosis established based on symptoms and clinical examination. The patient is hypoxic, with respiratory distress, and demonstrates deviation of the mediastinum to the contralateral side. Hypotension is from the mediastinal shift that compromises venous return and not from hypovolemia. Therefore, aggressive fluid resuscitation is not indicated. A chest x-ray is unnecessary and will delay definitive life-saving intervention. The patient requires urgent decompression with a large-bore needle in the second intercostal space anteriorly, followed by insertion of a chest tube. Although assisted ventilation can improve oxygenation, positive pressure may increase the pneumothorax if initiated before adequate decompression. *(Townsend et al., p. 508; Way and Doherty, pp. 236–237; Greenfield et al., p. 326)*

21. **(A)**

22. **(C)**

23. **(B)**

Explanations 21 through 23

Hemorrhage associated with a Meckel's diverticulum classically presents with painless rectal bleeding in the absence of other gastrointestinal symptoms. The amount of hemorrhage may be enough to result in hypovolemia, with pallor, tachycardia, and postural hypotension. Abdominal examination is usually normal. Diagnosis is confirmed by technetium scan, with the isotope concentrated in the gastric mucosa of the diverticulum. Initial management should include IV fluid resuscitation and transfusion as needed, before laparotomy and diverticulectomy with resection of the adjacent ileum. Rectal polyps, hemorrhoids, and anal fissures may be associated with rectal bleeding. The bleeding is usually small in amount and often temporally related to defecation, typically on the surface of the stool or after defecation. Colonoscopy and proctoscopy are useful adjuncts to diagnosis. Bleeding associated with intussusception is described as "currant jelly" and is secondary to mucosal ischemia of the lead point. These children are most commonly between 2 months and 2 years of age, and often have a prodromal viral illness. They present with colicky abdominal pain and dehydration. Management includes hydrostatic reduction. *(Townsend et al., pp. 1366–1368, 2112–2113; Greenfield et al., pp. 2010–2012)*

24. **(E)** The guiding principle of management of closed-head injury is to maintain cerebral

perfusion and oxygenation; thereby, preventing secondary brain insult. Cerebral perfusion pressure (CPP) is dependent on systemic blood pressure, circulating blood volume, and ICP (i.e., CPP = mean BP – ICP). Normal CPP requires an adequate circulating blood volume with maintenance of normovolemia. Hypercarbia should be avoided because it leads to cerebral vasodilatation and increased ICP. Early insertion of a ventriculostomy is beneficial to permit controlled drainage of CSF as required to maintain a normal ICP. Fluid restriction and hyperventilation should be avoided in the early stages of management of a closed-head injury. Autoregulation of cerebral blood flow is disrupted in the early phases after head injury. Aggressive hyperventilation with resultant cerebral vasoconstriction may precariously compromise the perfusion to the injured brain and to the surrounding noninjured brain. In patients with deteriorating neurologic status and/or evidence of increasing ICP that is not well controlled with a ventriculostomy, osmotic diuretics and moderate hyperventilation may be useful adjuncts to therapy. The use of steroids in the management of closed-head injury is not indicated. Craniotomy is indicated for increased ICP attributed to a mass with a midline shift. *(Greenfield et al., pp. 299, 303–305; Way and Doherty, pp. 900–908)*

25. (C)

26. (E)

27. (D)

Explanations 25 through 27

Crohn's disease is a chronic inflammatory disease of the gastrointestinal tract that presents with intermittent crampy abdominal pain and diarrhea. It most commonly involves the terminal ileum and right colon. Because eating can exacerbate symptoms, oral intake may be decreased, contributing to the associated weight loss. Transmural inflammation leads to bowel wall thickening, and with adjacent mesenteric inflammation, the patient may develop a palpable mass. It may be difficult to differentiate Crohn's disease from ulcerative colitis on the basis of history and clinical examination. However, ulcerative colitis is a mucosal disease that is limited to the colon and nearly always involves the rectum. Diarrhea is usually bloody, and hemorrhage may be significant enough to require transfusion therapy. Complicated appendicitis may present with a right lower quadrant mass and diarrhea if there is perforation with abscess formation. The history is that of an acute illness in a previously well patient. Irritable bowel syndrome is associated with intermittent crampy abdominal pain, and diarrhea alternating with constipation. There is no inflammatory process, and weight loss is not a clinical feature. Evaluation of the small bowel is best accomplished with contrast radiography, such as a small-bowel follow-through study or enteroclysis. Radiographic abnormalities of small-bowel Crohn's disease are often distinctive and can demonstrate complications such as strictures and fistulae. CT scanning does not assist in confirming the diagnosis, but is helpful in detecting such complications as abscess. Ultrasonography has limited value. Sigmoido-scopy may not be useful, because Crohn's disease commonly spares the rectum and may be worse on the right side of the colon. Colonoscopy may be helpful when the colon is involved and when intubation of the ileocecal valve can be achieved; however, the disease may be limited to the small bowel resulting in a nondiagnostic examination. The principle of initial management of Crohn's disease is relief of symptoms, nutritional therapy, and suppression of the inflammatory process. Nutritional supplementation may require TPN in conjunction with bowel rest. Acute exacerbations of the disease are initially treated with systemic steroids. The use of antispasmodics may be effective in the treatment of irritable bowel syndrome. In Crohn's disease, however, antispasmodics may lead to an ileus or toxic bowel dilatation. Surgery in Crohn's disease is indicated for the management of complications, including fistula or abscess formation, stricture with obstruction, and perforation. *(Greenfield et al., pp. 813–820; Townsend et al., pp. 1342–1349; Way and Doherty, pp. 689–692)*

28. (E) Testicular torsion presents with acute onset of scrotal pain, reflex vomiting, referred abdominal pain, and an elevated tender testis. If there is a high index of suspicion based on history and clinical examination, the patient should undergo an urgent surgical exploration. Delay in definitive therapy increases the risk of testicular loss secondary to ischemia. Isotope scan may demonstrate absence of testicular blood flow in torsion, and increased flow in orchitis or epididymitis. Although useful in the differential diagnosis, these nuclear medicine studies may not be readily available, and definitive therapy should not be delayed awaiting imaging. Orchitis and epididymitis present with a more insidious clinical course associated with the progression of the inflammatory process. There may be a concomitant urinary tract infection, and therapy includes analgesics and antibiotics. *(Townsend et al., pp. 2297–2298; Way and Doherty, p. 1339; Greenfield et al., pp. 2052–2053)*

29. **(D)** This elderly patient has metastatic adenocarcinoma of the prostate, and management is, therefore, aimed at tumor control for palliation of symptoms. This is achieved with hormonal manipulation, either by orchiectomy or exogenous estrogen therapy. Radical prostatectomy is indicated only for patients in whom the malignancy is confined to the prostate gland. Transurethral prostatectomy is used to treat benign prostatic hypertrophy, and is not considered adequate surgical therapy for prostatic malignancy. Cytotoxic chemotherapy may be useful as an adjunct to radical surgical excision of localized disease. Chemotherapy is not indicated for the treatment of metastatic disease. Radiation therapy has been used for the management of localized disease, and there is some evidence that it affords equivalent survival when compared to surgical excision. In patients with bone pain that is not well palliated with hormonal manipulation, radiation therapy may be useful. *(Way and Doherty, pp. 1066–1069; Greenfield et al., pp. 2191–2194)*

30. **(E)** Malignant hyperthermia may occur after administration of certain inhalation agents for induction of general anesthesia or with succinylcholine for muscle relaxation. This is a result of a genetic defect in calcium release from the sarcoplasm of skeletal muscle. It often occurs within 30 min of induction, and in addition to fever, tachycardia, and muscle rigidity, there is a metabolic acidosis and hyperkalemia. The treatment is administration of dantrolene to block calcium release from the sarcoplasm and insulin/bicarbonate/dextrose infusion to treat the hyperkalemia. Diagnosis is confirmed by muscle biopsy. Pneumonia is an infective, inflammatory process; is not associated with muscle rigidity; and is not likely to have a rapid progressive onset after induction of anesthesia in a previously healthy patient. Atelectasis is unlikely under general anesthesia, particularly in patients receiving positive pressure ventilation. Although pyelonephritis may be associated with fever, it is not associated with muscle rigidity or metabolic acidosis and would be unlikely to become symptomatic after induction in an otherwise healthy patient. Myocardial infarction may be associated with tachyarrhythmias but would not account for the muscle rigidity, fever, or metabolic acidosis and, in the absence of risk factors, would be very unlikely in this healthy patient. *(Townsend et al., pp. 233, 304–305; Way and Doherty, pp. 201–202)*

31. **(E)** The anterior triangle of the neck is divided into three zones: zone I at the base of the neck and thoracic inlet, zone II in the midbody of the neck, and zone III above the angle of the mandible. Zone II, the most common area injured with penetrating trauma, encompasses the carotid artery, jugular vein, larynx, trachea, and esophagus. Patients with penetrating injuries to the neck that violate the platysma should be admitted to the hospital for further evaluation. This patient has a penetrating injury through the platysma, in zone II of the anterior triangle. He has signs of significant injury (i.e., external bleeding at the scene, odynophagia, and a neck hematoma on examination). This patient should undergo surgical exploration, without prior diagnostic studies. Observation in the ICU, with or without intubation, is not appropriate in a patient with obvious clinical signs of injury. Furthermore, extensive preoperative imaging studies are not necessary for zone II injuries because surgical exposure of vital structures in this area of the neck is easily achieved. All patients with clinical signs of injury should undergo surgical exploration. However, there is

controversy with respect to the management of patients without clinical signs of injury. There are two approaches: (a) mandatory surgical exploration; or (b) selective observation with or without imaging studies. *(Townsend et al., pp. 498–502; Way and Doherty, pp. 241–243; Greenfield et al., pp. 311–315)*

32. (C) This patient has a distended abdomen, with decreased bowel sounds, in the presence of shock that is unresponsive to aggressive fluid resuscitation. Intraabdominal hemorrhage from solid visceral injury (hepatic, splenic, or renal) is the most likely etiology. The patient should undergo an urgent exploratory laparotomy and damage control (packing) for control of the bleeding, in conjunction with ongoing resuscitation with infusion of IV fluids and blood products. Although hypotension can result from a cervical cord injury, it is unlikely in this case, in the presence of a documented normal neurologic examination. A Swan–Ganz catheter is not indicated in the initial evaluation and management of a patient presenting in hypovolemic shock from blunt trauma. Abdominal CT scan is indicated only for evaluation of blunt abdominal trauma in patients who are hemodynamically stable. FAST and diagnostic peritoneal lavage may be indicated in the evaluation of patients with hypotension in which the source of bleeding is unclear. In this patient, however, the presence of a distended abdomen suggests hemoperitoneum, and therefore, FAST and lavage are not necessary. *(Townsend et al., pp. 513–514, 528; Way and Doherty, pp. 249–252)*

33. (A)

34. (B)

Explanations 33 and 34

DI is a disorder due to impaired renal conservation of water. DI presents with polyuria and dilute urine in the presence of an elevated serum osmolality. This is either secondary to impaired production of antidiuretic hormone (ADH) from the posterior pituitary (central DI), or refractoriness of the distal renal tubules to ADH (nephrogenic DI). Central DI may complicate closed-head injury, and is considered a poor prognostic sign. These patients will respond to exogenous IV vasopressin, with resultant increase in urine osmolality and decrease in urine volume. Nephrogenic DI may be congenital, familial, or acquired. Acquired nephrogenic DI may occur in the setting of repeated renal tubular insults such as sepsis, IV contrast, and nephrotoxic drug therapy. With administration of vasopressin, these patients will have no change in urine osmolality or urine volume because the renal tubules are unresponsive. DI must be differentiated from other causes of polyuria. Water intoxication results from ingestion of a large volume of fluid, with resultant dilutional hyponatremia. If the patient has a normal diluting capacity, there will be polyuria, with a proportionally low serum and urine osmolality. Prolonged fluid restriction will result in appropriate rise in urine osmolality. Osmotic diuresis may occur from solute overload when the renal tubules are unable to reabsorb adequate quantities of filtered solutes. This is associated with administration of mannitol or, in the presence of glycosuria, from diabetes mellitus. *(Fauci et al., pp. 2004–2009; Townsend et al., pp. 81–84)*

35. (C)

36. (F)

37. (E)

38. (D)

39. (G)

Explanations 35 through 39

Acute appendicitis initially presents with periumbilical pain secondary to obstruction of the appendiceal lumen. This is mediated through visceral pain fibers, and because the appendix is from the embryologic midgut, the pain is referred to the umbilicus. With obstruction of a hollow viscus, there may be associated nausea. As the inflammatory process progresses to involve the visceral and parietal peritoneal surfaces, the pain becomes localized directly over the appendix in the right lower quadrant. Fever and leukocytosis are nonspecific signs of an inflammatory process. Gastroenteritis may be associated with nausea, anorexia, and low-grade fever. Periumbilical pain is colicky and secondary to increased peristalsis. Localized pain and signs of peritoneal irritation are uncommon. A ruptured right ovarian cyst may mimic appendicitis. Patients may exhibit right lower abdominal peritoneal irritation. However, the onset of pain is usually sudden, and the pain is initially felt in the right lower quadrant. These patients do not have anorexia or other gastrointestinal symptoms. The clinical picture of regional enteritis (Crohn's disease) is one of a chronic illness, often associated with weight loss, intermittent cramps, and diarrhea. Fever, tenderness, and a palpable right lower quadrant inflammatory mass may result from complications of ileal involvement. Sigmoid diverticulitis is more common in older patients, often with a prodromal history of irregular bowel habits. There may be left lower quadrant pain and tenderness, with a palpable left-sided inflammatory mass. A cecal volvulus presents with sudden onset of colicky abdominal pain and signs and symptoms of a bowel obstruction, including bilious emesis and abdominal distention. Alcohol-related acute pancreatitis presents with pain referred to the epigastrium, with radiation to the back mediated through the celiac ganglia. The patient may develop abdominal distention secondary to the associated paralytic ileus. Hyperamylasemia and an elevated serum lipase, in this clinical setting, are suggestive of pancreatitis. Perforated peptic ulcer and acute cholecystitis may also present with epigastric pain, and elevations of both serum lipase and amylase. Pain from a perforated ulcer, however, is sudden in onset and may be associated with shoulder-tip pain from diaphragmatic irritation. About 75% of patients with perforated duodenal ulcers have pneumoperitoneum on chest and abdominal radiographs. Acute cholecystitis will usually commence after a large meal and initially presents as colicky epigastric pain, progressing to pain localized in the right upper abdomen when transmural inflammation of the gallbladder wall produces peritoneal irritation. Acute mesenteric occlusion presents with sudden onset of severe but poorly localized periumbilical abdominal pain, associated with acidosis. There may be elevation of serum amylase and lipase. A ruptured abdominal aortic aneurysm will present with sudden onset of midabdominal pain, back pain, and hemodynamic instability. *(Townsend et al., pp. 1385–1387, 1651–1652, 1418–1420, 1284, 1611–1612; Greenfield et al., pp. 863–873, 1224–1236)*

40. **(D)** A thyroglossal duct cyst represents the remnants of the thyroglossal duct tract left over from descent of the thyroid gland from the foramen cecum. It is located in the midline and moves superiorly as the tongue protrudes because the tract communicates with the foramen cecum. *(Greenfield et al., pp. 1935–1936; Townsend et al., p. 2103; Way and Doherty, pp. 1302–1303)*

41. **(E)** Lipomas present as soft, subcutaneous masses that arise in all areas of the body. They are treated by simple excision. *(Greenfield et al., pp. 1236–1237)*

42. **(C)** Acute suppurative lymphadenitis is related to bacterial pathogens and most often accompanies an infectious illness, such as an upper respiratory tract infection. The nodes enlarge rapidly, are tender, and demonstrate overlying erythema of the skin. *(Greenfield et al., pp. 1936–1937; Townsend et al., p. 2104; Way and Doherty, pp. 1303–1304)*

43. **(J)** The location of this mass and its cystic nature are typical for a second branchial cleft remnant. Surgical excision is recommended, including the associated tract, which traverses between the carotid bifurcation and ends at the tonsillar fossa. *(Greenfield et al., pp. 1932–1935; Townsend et al., pp. 2102–2103; Way and Doherty, pp. 1300–1301)*

44. **(G)** Most tumors of the salivary glands present in the parotid, the most common of which is the pleomorphic adenoma. These occur most frequently in the fifth decade and present as a solitary painless mass in the superficial lobe of the parotid gland. Surgical treatment is complete excision with negative margins.

(Greenfield et al., pp. 650–652; Townsend et al., pp. 852–854; Way and Doherty, p. 293–295)

45. (A) The location of this neck mass and its movement with swallowing is strongly suggestive of a thyroid mass. The most common type of thyroid cancer is papillary carcinoma, which has an excellent prognosis under the age of 40. Needle biopsy should be performed as a diagnostic test, followed by operation. *(Greenfield et al., pp. 1273–1276; Way and Doherty, pp. 305–307; Townsend et al., pp. 961–965)*

46. (H) Laryngeal carcinoma is the most common malignancy of the upper aerodigestive tract in the United States. Presenting symptoms include hoarseness of the voice and, for supraglottic lesions, early metastatic disease to the neck. Risk factors include exposure to tobacco and alcohol. *(Greenfield et al., pp. 655–656; Townsend et al., pp. 844–846; Way and Doherty, pp. 290–292)*

47. (H) Chronic liver disease, such as cirrhosis, may be a cause of jaundice. Clinical features such as spider angiomas, ascites, and varices suggest cirrhosis. *(Townsend et al., pp. 1602–1604)*

48. (F) Pancreatic carcinoma occurs in the head of the gland in 75% of cases. About 75% of the patients with carcinoma in the head of the pancreas present with obstructive jaundice, weight loss, and, in the presence of advanced disease, abdominal pain. *(Townsend et al., pp. 1602–1604, 1668–1669)*

49. (C) Common duct stones (choledocholithiasis) may be the cause of acute bile duct obstruction without warning, resulting in jaundice, pain, and sepsis. The sepsis may manifest as fever, hypotension, and altered mental status. *(Townsend et al., pp. 1615–1617)*

50. (G) Liver dysfunction resulting in jaundice may be a manifestation of advanced metastatic disease to the liver. In a patient with a known malignancy at high risk for metastases (i.e., deeply invasive and ulcerative melanoma), metastatic disease must be considered in the evaluation of the jaundiced patient. Hepatomegaly found on abdominal examination is supportive of advanced metastatic disease. *(Townsend et al., pp. 1602–1604)*

51. (I) Pancreatitis may be the cause of jaundice by different mechanisms, resulting in compression of the common bile duct (CBD). Acute pancreatitis may cause edema of the head with resultant compression of the CBD; pancreatitis may lead to a pseudocyst in the head with compression of the duct; and chronic pancreatitis may lead to dense scarring around the duct with a resultant stricture. The clinical scenario of an alcohol abuser with acute abdominal pain; nausea; vomiting; jaundice; and a tender, palpable epigastric mass is most consistent with acute pancreatitis with CBD obstruction attributable to a pseudocyst. *(Greenfield et al., p. 875)*

52. (C) A new mass in a woman of this age group must be fully evaluated to rule out carcinoma. Though biopsy by fine needle, core needle, or open biopsy will be required to determine the etiology of the mass, they should not be performed until all necessary breast imaging studies have been performed. Imaging should include diagnostic mammography and possibly sonography to determine whether the mass is solid or cystic. An appropriate type of biopsy can be chosen (i.e., FNA for cystic lesions or core biopsy for solid lesions). Imaging should not be delayed, although the patient should discontinue HRT until the etiology of the mass is determined. *(Greenfield et al., pp. 1344–1349)*

53. (E) A number of breast cancer risk factors have been identified. These include family history, benign breast disease with atypical epithelial hyperplasia, alcohol consumption, and HRT. The most common and clinically useful risk factors are age and female gender. In most patients (70%) with breast cancer, however, no other major risk factor can be identified. *(Greenfield et al., p. 1352; Townsend et al., pp. 881–885)*

54. (D) LCIS is considered a marker for susceptibility of the breasts for malignant change. Lobular and ductal elements of both breasts are at risk. The risk for development of cancer is approximately 1% per year, equally divided between the two breasts. Therefore, reexcision to gain negative margins is not indicated, nor is ipsilateral mastectomy. There is no known added significance to bilateral LCIS; therefore, contralateral breast biopsy is not useful for determining appropriate management. Both breasts should be treated the same. For patients without any other identifiable risk factors, close observation with frequent physician examinations, monthly breast self-examination, and yearly mammography may be the best option. However, some patients may prefer bilateral total mastectomies as a personal preference or for situations in which they cannot adhere to close follow-up recommendations or whose risk for cancer is deemed too high. *(Greenfield et al., p. 1352; Donegan and Spratt, pp. 350–351)*

55. (D)

56. (E)

Explanations 55 and 56

Deleterious mutations in the BRCA1 and BRCA2 genes are associated with markedly elevated lifetime risks of breast cancer. The risk initially quoted was determined from families with high penetrance or expression of the disease, in the 80–90% range. A subsequent study, based on a larger population of gene mutation carriers, demonstrated a lower risk of 56%. Therefore, the risk generally quoted for mutation carriers is in the range of 50–80%. Management options for known mutation carriers, or other high-risk women, include intensive surveillance with monthly self-breast examinations, annual or semiannual clinical breast examinations, annual mammography starting 10 years prior to the earliest age of onset of breast cancer in a family member, chemoprevention with tamoxifen, and prophylactic mastectomy. The data supporting these options in BRCA-mutation carriers, however, is limited to small series. Evidence for imaging of these high-risk women using MRI as a screening modality is promising. *(Donegan and Spratt, p. 253, 260–262; Townsend et al., pp. 884–887).*

57. (B)

58. (D)

Explanations 57 and 58

Prospective randomized trials have addressed the issue of locoregional control of breast cancer. Conservative management consisting of lumpectomy (with negative margins), irradiation, and axillary node dissection is equally effective as modified radical mastectomy in patients with clinical stage I or II breast carcinoma. Although radical mastectomy yields equivalent survival to modified radical mastectomy, it is disfiguring and disabling and is rarely employed for treatment of primary operable breast cancer. Lumpectomy without irradiation leads to unacceptably high local recurrence rates. Irradiation without surgery is not as effective as surgery in the presence of gross disease. Quadrantectomy removes excessive tissue and leads to an inferior cosmetic result as compared to lumpectomy. If quadrantectomy is thought to be required to gain negative margins, mastectomy with reconstruction should be entertained. The use of SLN biopsy to stage the axilla in breast cancer is gaining wider acceptance as experience with the procedure grows. Trials are ongoing that will answer numerous questions regarding the accuracy and efficacy of SLN biopsy for breast cancer. There are contraindications to SLN biopsy that include palpable adenopathy that is suspicious for metastatic disease, locally advanced disease or tumor size >5 cm, multicentric disease, pregnant or lactating patient, and use of preoperative chemotherapy. Therefore, in this patient with palpable suspicious adenopathy, SLN biopsy would be contraindicated. Although age may influence success of SLN biopsy, increasing age does not preclude the procedure. *(Greenfield et al., pp. 1358–1363)*

59. (C)

60. (C)

Explanations 59 and 60

The mammographic appearance is most consistent with DCIS with or without an invasive component. The calcifications of DCIS are clustered, pleomorphic, irregular, and linear, and may be associated with a mass representing an invasive carcinoma. LCIS does not usually present with calcifications. Cystosarcoma phyllodes presents as a mass, often indistinguishable from a fibroadenoma. An involuting fibroadenoma often presents as a mass with large, coarse calcifications, indicating its benignity. Milk of calcium will often layer differently in the CC and mediolateral projections, suggesting fluid with calcium. The next step in management is to obtain a biopsy, preferably a core needle biopsy, for histologic confirmation and to evaluate for invasive disease. Observation is not recommended because these calcifications appear malignant. All other choices (i.e., lumpectomy or total mastectomy) are not indicated until a diagnosis by biopsy is obtained. *(Donegan and Spratt, pp. 293–298; Greenfield et al., pp. 1338–1342)*

61. (B)

62. (B)

Explanations 61 and 62

A new mass in an older woman must be evaluated for malignancy. In this case, the mammogram has characteristics of malignancy, which include a density or mass that is stellate or spiculated, irregular in size or shape, and possessing ill-defined borders. Other features suggestive of malignancy include clustered microcalcifications, asymmetric density, architectural distortion, and skin or nipple retraction. DCIS usually presents as calcifications without a definite mass. Cystosarcoma phyllodes presents much like a fibroadenoma as a well-defined mass with smooth margins. Papillomas are small and not usually palpable or noted by mammography. Fat necrosis can mimic the mammographic features of malignancy and is often associated with trauma. However, only when an oil cyst is noted, can an unequivocal diagnosis of fat necrosis be made. The next step is needle biopsy, by FNA, or core biopsy so a histologic diagnosis can be made and options for management (i.e., modified radical mastectomy or lumpectomy, axillary dissection, and irradiation) discussed. Needle biopsy is less invasive and less expensive than incisional biopsy and, therefore, is preferred. Excisional biopsy (not listed) is acceptable, but often requires a two-step procedure, the first to establish the diagnosis and the second for definitive treatment. A needle biopsy, especially a core biopsy that renders a histologic diagnosis, can often avoid the necessity of a second surgical procedure. *(Greenfield et al., pp. 1338–1349; Donegan and Spratt, pp. 289–293)*

63. (C)

64. (D)

Explanations 63 and 64

The symptoms of gastric cancer are nonspecific and may mimic those of such benign conditions as benign gastric ulcer. Pain, nausea, anorexia, and weight loss are common nonspecific symptoms. A UGI series shows a gastric ulcer that has characteristics of malignancy, including an intraluminal crater with nodular margins. A gastric diverticulum would extend as a protrusion beyond the gastric lumen. The duodenum is not well visualized in the x-ray, making the diagnosis of duodenal disease difficult. A fistula would be suggested by contrast filling of the gallbladder and biliary tree. Given the x-ray findings suggestive of malignancy, the next step would be to obtain a tissue diagnosis for confirmation by endoscopy. Once malignancy is confirmed, a CT scan would be helpful to evaluate for liver metastasis and extent of disease. Operative intervention may be determined at that time, usually a subtotal or total gastrectomy. Vagotomy and pyloroplasty would not be appropriate for gastric cancer. Medical therapy with H_2 blockers may improve the patient's symptoms but should not delay endoscopy and biopsy. *(Greenfield et al., pp. 774–782; Zinner, pp. 16–17)*

65. (D) The prevalence of adenomas without symptoms in patients over the age of 50 ranges between 20 and 40%. Screening studies suggest that 30% of patients without symptoms over the age of 50 who undergo colonoscopy for evaluation of positive fecal occult blood have a polyp detected. Polyps greater than 2 cm have a high potential for malignant degeneration. The polyp should be completely removed, preferably by snare polypectomy. Most studies indicate that polypectomy is adequate for polyps with carcinoma in the head if the margin of resection is 2 mm or greater, especially if the stalk is not invaded. Following adequate polypectomy, observation would be indicated with post-polypectomy colonoscopic surveillance. If cancer is present at or near the margin, then colon resection is indicated. Because the incidence of residual cancer and metastatic disease is very low after successful polypectomy, scanning by CT or MRI is not indicated. The data on NSAID use are promising but insufficient to support a clinical recommendation. *(Greenfield et al., pp. 1089–1098; Townsend et al., pp. 1448–1451)*

66. (D)

67. (A)

Explanations 66 and 67

The gradual onset of left lower quadrant pain over a number of days with left lower quadrant abdominal tenderness and CT scan showing sigmoid colon inflammatory changes is most consistent with diverticulitis. A contained perforation, either due to the diverticulitis or colon cancer, should be noted on the CT scan. There is no history of antecedent antibiotic therapy to suggest the diagnosis of pseudomembranous colitis. Though WBCs were present in the urinalysis, a diagnosis of pyelonephritis cannot be made on this basis alone, because pericolonic inflammation may be responsible for the WBCs. CT scanning is very accurate in diagnosing diverticulitis, so there is no need for any additional test. Barium enema and colonoscopy should not be performed in patients with suspected acute diverticulitis. The increased intraluminal pressure from either of these examinations may lead to free rupture of a contained abscess or phlegmon, leading to emergency surgery. However, either examination, or both, should be performed after complete resolution of diverticulitis (e.g., in 6 weeks' time) to evaluate for extent of disease, complications, and carcinoma. IVP and angiography are not indicated for diverticulitis. The appropriate management in this patient with his first episode of diverticulitis is medical management with IV antibiotics for gram-negative and anaerobic bacteria. Colon resection, either immediate or elective, should not be undertaken unless the patient's condition deteriorates or recurs. Bowel preparation cannot be performed safely in patients with acute diverticulitis. Anticoagulation has no role in therapy. Metronidazole or vancomycin therapy would be appropriate for pseudomembranous colitis, but not for diverticulitis. *(Townsend et al., pp. 1418–1420)*

68. (D)

69. (B)

Explanations 68 and 69

The diagnosis of sigmoid volvulus is based on the history, examination, and radiographs. Acute onset of abdominal pain, distention, and obstipation is suggestive of volvulus. Barium enema is diagnostic of sigmoid volvulus showing the characteristic tapering to a "bird's beak" pointing to the site of obstruction. Cecal volvulus would show complete filling of the left colon. Stricture as a result of ischemic colitis would show a long, narrowed segment of colon. Diverticulitis would be suggested by a different clinical presentation including fever, sepsis, and pain localized to the left lower quadrant. Obstruction from colon cancer would show an irregular narrowing of the colon segment rather than a smooth tapering. In patients who have no signs of bowel wall ischemia (e.g., rebound tenderness, sepsis, and so forth), nonoperative reduction should be attempted and would be expected to be successful in 70–80% of patients. The most widely used method of reduction is proctoscopy and rectal tube placement under direct vision. Blind passage of a rectal tube may lead to perforation and is contraindicated. Operation is indicated if nonoperative reduction is unsuccessful, with operative reduction preferred, followed by delayed resection and primary anastomosis rather than sigmoid resection. Operative reduction by detorsion alone is unacceptable because of the high recurrence rate and is, therefore, combined with sigmoidopexy or sigmoidostomy.

Proximal colostomy alone is contraindicated, because strangulation of the sigmoid or recurrent volvulus is not prevented. *(Townsend et al., pp. 1422–1424)*

70. (B)

71. (D)

Explanations 70 and 71

The clinical features of colon cancer are variable depending on the location. On the right, fatigue, as a manifestation of anemia, may be the predominant symptom; whereas, obstructive complaints may predominate for lesions on the left. In the figure, an annular or "apple core" lesion is noted, consistent with carcinoma. Radiography of diverticular disease would show numerous protrusions from the lumen, usually localized to the sigmoid colon. Lymphoma may occur in the colon, but this site of disease is rare, and widespread disease can be documented in most cases. Ischemia usually occurs at the splenic flexure, and the resultant stricture would produce a longer segment of narrowing than that usually seen with carcinoma. Patients with Crohn's disease would manifest symptoms of abdominal pain and diarrhea, and barium x-rays would show thickened bowel wall, mucosal ulcerations, and cobblestone appearance. The treatment of colon cancer in this patient would be surgical resection and anastomosis. Colostomy may be appropriate in selected patients with obstruction in an unstable patient in whom resection is not feasible. Surgical bypass would be appropriate only for palliative therapy of unresectable disease. Radiation therapy or chemotherapy without surgical resection and staging is not recommended. *(Townsend et al., pp. 1457–1460; Zinner, pp. 34–36)*

72. (D)

73. (C)

Explanations 72 and 73

The stage of colon cancer is based on the depth of invasion, nodal involvement, and distant metastases. Stage 0 represents carcinoma *in situ*, stage I invasion of the submucosa or muscularis propria without node involvement, stage II invasion through the muscularis propria or directly invading other organs without nodal involvement, stage III any depth of invasion with nodal metastasis, and stage IV any depth of invasion or nodal status with distant metastases. Adjuvant therapy has been shown to be beneficial in patients with stage III disease in randomized studies. The recommended regimen is 5-fluorouracil–based chemotherapy with leucovorin, rather than 5-fluorouracil alone. Adriamycin therapy, either alone or with other agents, has not been shown to be beneficial in patients with colon cancer. No adjuvant therapy would be indicated for patients with stage 0, I, or II disease, although some patients with stage II disease manifesting poor prognostic indicators may be candidates for adjuvant therapy. *(Townsend et al., pp. 1460–1462)*

74. (C)

75. (B)

Explanations 74 and 75

The history of decreasing caliber of the stool with evidence of bleeding is highly suggestive of rectal carcinoma. The barium x-ray shows a near-obstructing lesion of the rectum with an "apple core" appearance of cancer. Diverticulitis does not occur in the rectum due to the lack of diverticular disease at this site. Ischemia usually does not involve the rectum due to its more abundant blood supply than the colon. The barium enema findings of sigmoid volvulus would show a smooth, tapering, so-called "bird's beak" at the rectosigmoid junction, rather than an irregular lesion in the midrectum as shown in the figure. Crohn's disease would be expected to show fistulas, either by examination or radiography. The next step in management is to confirm the diagnosis by proctoscopy and biopsy. Colonoscopy may not be feasible given the degree of the stricture, and endoscopic dilation is not routine and would not be recommended. Experience with placement of stents is accruing, but endoscopic placement of stents is not yet widely available.

Because this process does not represent a volvulus, placement of a rectal tube is not required. Administration of antibiotics would be considered in the perioperative period, but not before making a histologic diagnosis. *(Townsend et al., pp. 1462–1463)*

76. (D)

77. (D)

Explanations 76 and 77

A multicolored brown or black pigmented lesion with irregular borders should raise the concern of melanoma. Squamous cell carcinoma usually presents as an erythematous papular nodule. The most common type of basal carcinoma presents as an ulcerative, well-circumscribed nodule, although occasionally it may be pigmented and confused with melanoma. Merkel cell carcinoma appears as red to purple papular nodules. Keratoacanthoma is a well-circumscribed keratotic lesion that may regress without treatment. The most appropriate next step is to perform an excisional biopsy with narrow margins to confirm the diagnosis and determine depth of invasion. Shave biopsy would yield a pathologic diagnosis, but would not allow appropriate staging and is never recommended. The margin of resection and determination of lymph node management would depend on the depth of invasion of the melanoma measured in millimeters. Therefore, wide excision is not recommended until the depth of invasion of the lesion is determined by excisional biopsy with narrow margins. Mohs' surgery should be considered for nonmelanoma tumors but is not recommended for melanoma. *(Greenfield et al., pp. 2239–2245)*

78. (E) The diagnosis of an incarcerated hernia must be considered in the differential diagnosis of a patient with abdominal symptoms and a nonreducible inguinal bulge. Femoral hernia presents as a bulge below the inguinal ligament medial to the femoral artery. Direct or indirect inguinal hernias would present above the inguinal ligament. An aneurysm of the femoral artery should be pulsatile. If there is concern for an aneurysm, a Doppler ultrasound examination may be diagnostic. A lymph node with abscess may present as a tender, nonreducible mass, but should be accompanied by additional adenopathy and a source of the infection. *(Townsend et al., p. 1211)*

79. (C)

80. (B)

Explanations 79 and 80

The finding of a new, irregular lesion in a patient with a long smoking history must be considered a lung carcinoma and should be managed accordingly. Nonsmall cell carcinoma is the most common lung neoplasm. Small cell carcinomas usually grow rapidly and disseminate widely by the time of diagnosis. Tuberculosis would present with systemic symptoms and apical disease on chest x-ray. Likewise, a lung abscess would be accompanied by systemic symptoms and may show air-fluid levels in the abscess cavity. A hamartoma presents as an extremely slowly growing nodule that may contain popcorn calcifications. The most appropriate test following suspicious findings on a chest x-ray would be a CT scan to evaluate further the nodule, evaluate the lymph node status, and triage subsequent diagnostic tests. If enlarged mediastinal nodes are seen, then mediastinoscopy may be indicated. Bronchoscopy may be helpful to assess for endobronchial lesions and to obtain tissue for diagnosis. Pulmonary function tests are necessary once a decision is made to consider operation. Percutaneous needle biopsy may be required to obtain tissue once CT scanning is performed. *(Townsend et al., pp. 1775, 1783–1784)*

81. (D)

82. (B)

Explanations 81 and 82

The clinical manifestations of ruptured abdominal aneurysm are back, flank, or abdominal pain; hypotension; and a pulsatile abdominal mass. The treatment should be immediate transfer to the operating room for laparotomy. Additional diagnostic tests, such as CT scan, angiography, or additional consultations delay immediate treatment, thereby putting the patient at risk for further rupture and death. Following successful treatment, diarrhea may suggest ischemic colitis, and urgent sigmoidoscopy is indicated. A delay in diagnosis of bowel ischemia caused by numerous other diagnostic tests may increase the mortality rate. If bowel ischemia is found, immediate colon resection should be undertaken. *(Greenfield et al., pp. 1807–1819)*

83. (B)

84. (D)

85. (A)

Explanations 83 and 85

The diagnosis of arterial embolism is suggested when the patient presents with an acute onset of severe pain, pallor, pulselessness, paresthesia, and paralysis (*five Ps*). The presence of atrial fibrillation is strongly suggestive of a cardiac source of the emboli. The first step in management is immediate heparinization to prevent propagation of the clot and maintain patency of collaterals. The cornerstone of treatment is thromboembolectomy. Thrombolytic therapy is reserved for treatment of irretrievable clots in small vessels. Fasciotomy, alkalinization of the urine, and mannitol diuresis are adjuncts to treatment, particularly if there is a delay in operation, increasing the risk of a reperfusion injury. Anticoagulation has been shown to reduce the rate of recurrent embolism. *(Greenfield et al., pp. 1568–1577)*

86. (B)

87. (C)

Explanations 86 and 87

The diagnosis of a dissecting aortic aneurysm is strongly suggested by the history of an abrupt onset of excruciating pain in the chest and back with variable radiation patterns, and a hypertensive, ill-appearing patient. A chest x-ray showing a widened mediastinum may be noted, but the radiograph may be normal. The differential diagnosis of an acute myocardial infarction must be entertained and an ECG performed. Though aortography has historically been the definitive diagnostic procedure and may be required in some patients, transesophageal echocardiography has become the preferred diagnostic modality. It can be performed in the emergency department, thus obviating the need to move an extremely ill patient. CT scan may also be helpful in establishing the diagnosis. Immediate drug therapy to control hypertension is mandatory, followed by definitive therapy, depending on the type of dissection. Thrombolytic therapy and anticoagulation are not indicated and may precipitate exsanguination. *(Greenfield et al., pp. 1781–1782)*

88. (C)

89. (E)

Explanations 88 and 89

Factors that increase the risk for carcinoma include exposure to low-dose irradiation, age under 20 or over 60, male gender (especially over age 40), and recent onset. An increased incidence of thyroid carcinoma in patients with Hashimoto's thyroiditis has not been substantiated. For diagnosis, FNA is highly accurate and has become the preferred diagnostic modality. FNA is the most important diagnostic test for selecting patients for operation, supplanting all other diagnostic tests. *(Greenfield et al., pp. 1273–1275)*

90. (D)

91. (B)

Explanations 90 and 91

Leiomyomas are the most common benign tumors of the esophagus. They are intramural, occur between 20 and 50 years of age, and may be symptomatic when over 5 cm. Symptoms may include dysphagia and retrosternal pressure and pain. Esophagogram shows characteristic features of a smooth concave defect with sharp borders. Esophagoscopy is indicated to rule out carcinoma. These tumors are mobile, with intact overlying mucosa. Biopsy should not be performed so that subsequent extramural resection can be performed without complication. Excision is recommended for symptomatic leiomyomas or those greater than 5 cm. *(Townsend et al., pp. 1116–1117)*

92. **(B)**

93. **(B)**

Explanations 92 and 93

Pharyngoesophageal (Zenker's) diverticulum is the most common esophageal diverticulum and typically occurs in the 30–50 age group and, therefore, is believed to be acquired. Its symptoms include cervical dysphagia, regurgitation of undigested food, and recurrent aspiration. It is categorized as a pulsion type, creating protrusion of mucosa, resulting in a false diverticulum. An underlying neuromotor abnormality exists, which is responsible for increased pharyngeal pressure. The most important aspect of treatment is a cricopharyngeal muscle myotomy, which can be combined with resection or diverticulopexy. *(Townsend et al., pp. 1106–1107)*

94. **(C)** Mallory–Weiss tear involves acute UGI hemorrhage that occurs after retching or vomiting and accounts for 5–15% of patients with UGI bleeding. The patient is often an alcoholic who vomits after binge drinking. Hematemesis follows vomiting without blood. After resuscitation, esophagoscopy is required to determine the source of bleeding and may be helpful in nonoperative management. Contrast studies are not helpful, and the use of barium would coat the stomach and preclude a diagnostic endoscopic examination. Most patients with Mallory–Weiss tears stop bleeding spontaneously. Angiography may be helpful in selected patients who continue to bleed and in whom the site of hemorrhage cannot be determined endoscopically. *(Greenfield et al., pp. 1152–1153)*

95. **(B)**

96. **(B)**

Explanations 95 and 96

Progressive dysphagia in an older adult warrants evaluation, especially with associated symptoms of weight loss, chest pain, or hematemesis. A barium esophagogram is the first study that should be obtained. The typical carcinoma demonstrates an irregular, rigid narrowing of the esophageal wall with distortion of the lumen. Achalasia demonstrates a narrow, tapering bird's beak appearance of the distal esophagus. Development of an esophageal stricture causes slowly progressive dysphagia, usually after a long history of gastroesophageal reflux disease (GERD). Esophagoscopy and biopsy are mandatory for evaluation of esophageal stenosis and yield a diagnosis of carcinoma in 95% of patients with malignant strictures. CT scanning is the standard technique for staging, once the diagnosis has been made. Bronchoscopy is helpful in patients with upper and middle third carcinomas to exclude invasion of the trachea or bronchi before esophagectomy. *(Townsend et al., pp. 1119–1120)*

97. **(D)**

98. **(E)**

99. **(C)**

Explanations 97 and 99

Perforated duodenal ulcer usually presents as a sudden onset of acute abdominal pain. Examination usually reveals severe abdominal tenderness with rigidity of the abdominal musculature (i.e., an acute abdomen). With a prior history of abdominal pain relieved by antacids, a chronic ulcer that has now perforated is strongly suggested. Perforated colon cancer occurs in an older age group, as well as gastric ulcer. Following plain radiographs that show pneumoperitoneum, no additional diagnostic tests are required and serve only to delay treatment. The treatment is laparotomy and either patch closure of the perforation or definitive operation, the latter being preferred, depending on operative findings. However, the patient must receive fluid resuscitation before laparotomy to avoid hypotension and its consequences.

Although nonoperative management for contained perforations has been suggested by some authors, an acute abdomen is an indication for operative management. *(Greenfield et al., pp. 761–762)*

100. (B)

101. (D)

Explanations 100 and 101

Gastric ulcers present with symptoms of abdominal pain, aggravated by food, and associated with nausea, vomiting, anorexia, and weight loss. The two principal means of diagnosing a gastric ulcer are UGI radiographs and fiberoptic endoscopy, the latter being the most reliable method. CT scan and endoscopic ultrasound may be helpful in staging gastric cancer, but are not routinely used with benign disease. The failure to respond to 12 weeks of medical management is an indication for surgical therapy to avoid potential complications and to exclude malignancy, despite biopsies obtained by endoscopy that show benign disease. *(Greenfield et al., pp. 762–763)*

102. (D)

103. (C)

104. (C)

Explanations 102 through 104

In a patient who has undergone surgical resection for colon cancer, elevated CEA, and liver function tests must be followed by an evaluation for metastatic disease, including the possibility of extrahepatic disease. The CT scan is the most useful examination to evaluate both intra- and extrahepatic disease. Various CT scans have been advocated for liver tumors, including dynamic and portography scans. PET scans may detect occult extrahepatic disease and studies are underway to define the role of this modality in metastatic colon cancer. MRI shows promise as a useful examination and can be useful to characterize lesions of uncertain significance. Radionuclide liver scans have been supplanted by more accurate scans. Surgical resection, if possible, is the treatment of choice for metastatic colorectal cancer to the liver. Chemotherapy is reserved for patients who are not surgical candidates or refuse surgical treatment. Radiation therapy is not usually used in these patients. Observation and repeat imaging delays the treatment for patients who may be resectable. The expected 5-year survival has been shown in multiple studies to be greater than 20%, usually in the range of 25 and 35%. *(Townsend et al., pp. 1554–1557)*

105. (C)

106. (D)

Explanations 105 and 106

The anatomic location of the mass suggests a parotid origin, and the lengthy history and absence of symptoms and signs of inflammation are consistent with a neoplasm of the parotid. The most common salivary gland neoplasm is a benign pleomorphic adenoma. Metastatic carcinoma from a head and neck primary tumor may first present as a neck mass, usually along the anterior or posterior cervical lymph node chain, and often in a patient with such risk factors as a history of smoking. Infectious parotitis may occur in the elderly or diabetic patient, usually presenting with a shorter history, with symptoms and signs of inflammation. Hodgkin's disease can present as a painless neck mass involving the anterior or supraclavicular lymph nodes. Reactive cervical lymphatic hyperplasia is associated with an inflammatory or infectious focus in the head and neck. The optimal management for a pleomorphic adenoma in the lateral lobe of the parotid is a superficial parotidectomy. IV antibiotics are not indicated in the absence of an inflammatory or infectious process. Although an excisional biopsy may be indicated for a mass arising from cervical lymph nodes, enucleation of a neoplastic parotid mass is insufficient and associated with an increased incidence of local recurrence. Observation and reevaluation are inappropriate in this patient. A chest x-ray would be indicated in the evaluation of a patient with suspected Hodgkin's disease. *(Townsend et al., pp. 852–854)*

107. (B)

108. (C)

Explanations 107 and 108

Intussusception most commonly occurs between 2 months and 2 years of age, often associated with a prodromal viral illness. Children will present with intermittent episodes of abdominal colic, secondary to peristaltic waves of the ileum against the partially obstructing ileocolic lesion. Reflex nonbilious vomiting is secondary to bowel distention and partial obstruction. There may be a palpable, right-sided, "sausage-shaped" mass, but in many patients, the abdominal examination is entirely normal. The classic "currant jelly" stool (see Fig. 6-14) is a late sign and is a result of ischemia and mucosal sloughing of the lead point. After the child has received IV fluid resuscitation, the management is hydrostatic reduction, either by contrast enema or air enema. Intussusception may occur during the clinical course of viral gastroenteritis. Bloody stools are more commonly associated with bacterial gastrointestinal infections, with characteristically loose, mucousy stools, and blood mixed with fecal material. Diagnosis is aided by obtaining stool cultures. A midgut volvulus can be associated with passage of a "currant jelly" stool secondary to small-bowel ischemia. However, these children usually present with bilious vomiting. Diagnosis may be confirmed with a UGI contrast study. Rectal bleeding from a Meckel's diverticulum is typically painless, without other associated gastrointestinal symptoms. Technetium scan is useful for diagnosis. Bleeding from a juvenile rectal polyp is usually small in amount and often occurs during normal stool passage. The children are clinically well, without other gastrointestinal symptoms. These polyps may be seen on proctoscopy. *(Townsend et al., pp. 2112–2113; Way and Doherty, pp. 1323–1324; Greenfield et al., pp. 2008–2010)*

109. (E) This patient presents with a rapidly progressive, necrotizing soft-tissue infection. The skin edema, purple hue, bullae, water drainage, and crepitus are classic findings in clostridial infections. Although culture of the wound drainage may be confirmatory, the diagnosis should be suspected on a clinical basis. Antibiotics alone are insufficient therapy. The mainstay of therapy is radical surgical debridement of devitalized tissues, in conjunction with high-dose IV antibiotics. Hyperbaric oxygen therapy may facilitate recovery. *(Townsend et al., pp. 264–266; Way and Doherty, pp. 123–125)*

110. (C) All traumatic soft-tissue injuries should be managed with aggressive local wound care. Because this injury is greater than 6 h old, contaminated, and greater than 1 cm in depth, it is a tetanus-prone wound. Therefore, in addition, this patient should receive tetanus toxoid, because it has been more than 5 years since his last immunization. He had full immunization as a child and, therefore, does not require additional passive immunization with tetanus immune globulin. Prophylactic antibiotics are controversial in the absence of an established wound infection. *(Townsend et al., pp. 261, 264; Way and Doherty, pp. 127–128)*

111. (E) This child has a displaced supracondylar fracture associated with vascular compromise of the forearm from associated brachial artery compression, distortion, or vessel injury. Decreased perfusion below the fracture in conjunction with pain on passive wrist flexion are signs of a developing forearm compartment syndrome. Management should include operative exploration of the brachial artery, open reduction and pinning of the fracture, and forearm compartment fasciotomy to limit progression of muscular ischemia. Immobilization of the elbow at 90° is suitable only for undisplaced fractures. For displaced fractures without neurovascular compromise, closed reduction and pinning may be adequate, but if adequate reduction cannot be achieved, open reduction may be required. *(Townsend et al., pp. 552–557; Way and Doherty, pp. 1134–1135)*

112. (B)

113. (B)

Explanations 112 and 113

This patient is acidotic, with a low serum bicarbonate (bicarbonate depletion defined as a serum bicarbonate less than 22 meq/L). She has hypovolemic shock from trauma and acute blood loss, resulting in decreased tissue perfusion and lactic acidosis. The resultant elevated anion gap (139 – [103 + 14] = 22 meq/L with a normal anion gap of 8–16 meq/L) is from the increased lactic acid. The tachypnea may be caused by the respiratory compensation with decreased P_{CO_2}. Correction of the acidosis should be aimed at improving tissue perfusion with aggressive IV fluid resuscitation. Metabolic alkalosis is associated with serum bicarbonate greater than 26 meq/L. Respiratory acidosis is related to primary carbon dioxide retention from decreased alveolar ventilation. Administration of sodium bicarbonate is indicated only in severe acidosis (pH < 7.2), and in patients with evidence of myocardial instability or arrhythmias. Hydrochloric acid is indicated only in life-threatening metabolic alkalosis that is not chloride responsive. Respiratory acidosis with alveolar hypoventilation may be corrected with assisted ventilation. *(Townsend et al., pp. 77–81; Way and Doherty, pp. 150–153)*

114. (D)

115. (J)

116. (C)

Explanations 114 through 116

Pyloric stenosis presents with nonbilious vomiting and gastric distention. An annular pancreas does not result in obstruction, except when it is associated with an underlying duodenal abnormality. Duodenal atresia is associated with Down syndrome. It results in early onset of bilious vomiting from complete duodenal obstruction distal to the ampulla. There is a "double bubble" sign on plain abdominal radiographs from air in the stomach and proximal duodenum. Midgut volvulus is a life-threatening complication of malrotation. It presents with acute onset of bilious vomiting, usually in infants in the first year of life. There is a paucity of gas on plain radiographs, with evidence of duodenal obstruction. UGI contrast study will confirm the abnormal position of the duodenal-jejunal junction and may demonstrate a corkscrew of the duodenum from volvulus. Intussusception is uncommon in newborns. Bilious vomiting is unusual at the outset, but may develop if the intussusception has been present for a significant time. Imperforate anus can be excluded by clinical examination. If unrecognized, the infant will develop a clinical picture of a distal bowel obstruction, with dilated small and large bowel. Meckel's diverticulum can present with obstruction secondary to volvulus around a Meckel's band, with a distal small-bowel obstruction. Contrast enema will demonstrate a normal-caliber decompressed colon, with proximal dilated small bowel. Meconium ileus is associated with cystic fibrosis. Obstruction occurs from inspissated meconium in the terminal ileum. Plain radiographs may demonstrate a "soap bubble" pattern in the right lower quadrant, with a decompressed colon on contrast enema. Hirschsprung disease presents with a distal bowel obstruction and delayed passage of meconium. A contrast enema may demonstrate a transition zone, with a narrow distal aganglionic segment, and proximal colonic dilatation. Jejunal atresia is a result of an intrauterine vascular accident. Infants present with bile-stained vomiting and abdominal distention early after birth. The colon is unused, and characteristically, on contrast enema, it is abnormally small in caliber (microcolon). *(Townsend et al., pp. 2107–2116; Way and Doherty, pp. 1315–1327)*

117. (C)

118. (C)

Explanations 117 and 118

Cryptorchidism increases the risk of developing a testicular malignancy. This patient has a solid testicular mass which should be presumed to be secondary to a testicular malignancy. Optimal surgical management is inguinal exploration, control of the spermatic cord, biopsy of the mass, and radical orchiectomy with high ligation of the cord, if tumor is confirmed. Transscrotal aspiration, exploration, or needle biopsy is contraindicated because of risk of tumor spillage, and risk of altering the lymphatic drainage of the scrotum. Laparotomy and retroperitoneal node dissection is not indicated until after confirmation of the diagnosis and excision of the primary tumor. This patient has seminoma with disease spread to ipsilateral regional lymph nodes. The tumor is very radiosensitive, and radiotherapy is the primary adjuvant therapy for local control. Chemotherapy is indicated in patients with nodal spread or disseminated disease. Radiotherapy is restricted to therapy for localized disease only. *(Townsend et al., pp. 2311–2316; Way and Doherty, pp. 1070–1072)*

119. (C)

120. (D)

121. (E)

Explanations 119 through 121

This patient has an inguinoscrotal mass from an indirect inguinal hernia. His initial presentation is one of a reducible inguinal hernia. Repair is indicated because of the risk of incarceration. He should be referred for early elective surgery. The second presentation several weeks later is at the time of incarceration of the hernia. This has resulted in pain, irritability, and reflex vomiting. Prolonged incarceration increases the risk of bowel ischemia. The appropriate management is sedation with manual reduction, admission with observation in hospital, and surgical repair within 24–48 h. Delaying repair after an initial episode of incarceration increases the risk of further episodes of incarceration, with potential bowel or testicular compromise. Failure to reduce an incarcerated hernia successfully mandates urgent surgical intervention. Testicular torsion is uncommon in this age group and presents with a tender, high-riding testicle. When suspected, urgent surgical exploration is indicated. Inguinal adenitis may be the result of an inflammatory focus in the diaper area, with resultant adenopathy, and secondary infection of the inguinal nodes with a gram-positive organism. The infant is usually febrile, with a tender inguinal mass. Therapy includes systemic antibiotics. An undescended testicle may present as an inguinal mass, with an empty hemiscrotum. It is usually asymptomatic. Management is elective orchiopexy at approximately 1 year of age. A noncommunicating hydrocele presents as an asymptomatic, fluctuant scrotal mass that transilluminates. Surgical intervention is not required, because most will resolve spontaneously by 1 year of age. *(Townsend et al., pp. 2117–2119; Way and Doherty, pp. 1336–1338)*

122. (A)

123. (B)

Explanations 122 and 123

Patients with gross hematuria require aggressive diagnostic evaluation. A careful, planned approach will yield the cause in the majority of patients. Painless hematuria is often the first sign of a urinary tract malignancy. After confirmation of hematuria, and exclusion of infection, all patients should have plain radiographs and IVP. This is the optimal initial diagnostic approach to aid in distinguishing between upper tract (renal) pathology and lower tract (lower ureteric and bladder) pathology. Further diagnostic evaluation will be guided by these noninvasive studies. A voiding cystourethrogram is invasive. It is a limited examination of bladder function and anatomy, and although advanced invasive bladder tumors may be demonstrated as a filling defect, it is not sensitive for lower stages of bladder neoplasms. Cystourethroscopy is invasive and is, therefore, not the initial examination in the evaluation of hematuria. It is indicated in the evaluation of gross hematuria in patients with a normal IVP. It is the optimal tool for evaluation of potential bladder pathology. An abdominal ultrasound or CT scan is indicated in patients with a suspected renal mass, either by clinical examination or demonstrated on IVP. Urine for cytology is useful for screening of patients with suspected urinary tract malignancy, but it is falsely negative in approximately 20% of patients and should not be used as the only diagnostic evaluation. A transrectal ultrasound may be helpful in evaluating the extent of invasion of a bladder or prostatic neoplasm. Abdominal CT scan is a superior imaging study for this purpose. *(Townsend et al., pp. 2305–2308)*

124. (B) This child presents with progressive cholestatic jaundice, as indicated by the elevated conjugated hyperbilirubinemia. Metabolic screening for inborn errors of metabolism and serologic evaluation for intrauterine infections are important to exclude these causes of intrahepatic cholestasis. Figure 6-20 depicts an acholic stool (absence of bile pigments), which is usually indicative of complete biliary tract obstruction. In this clinical setting, biliary atresia is the most probable diagnosis. The most sensitive imaging study is radioisotope scanning. Preimaging phenobarbital increases the diagnostic yield by stimulating hepatic microsomal enzymes. Abdominal ultrasound may show absence of the gallbladder, but this study is operator dependent and does not evaluate hepatocyte function and bile excretory pattern. CT or MRI scans may demonstrate hepatic parenchymal changes (e.g., extensive cirrhosis) and the presence or absence of bile duct dilatation, but do not evaluate and differentiate abnormalities of hepatocyte function or bile excretory pattern. *(Townsend et al., pp. 2123–2124; Way and Doherty, pp. 1333–1335)*

125. (C)

126. (B)

Explanations 125 and 126

This patient has idiopathic thrombocytopenic purpura (ITP), a disease characterized by a low platelet count, normal coagulation profile, increased megakaryocytes, and a normal-sized spleen. Patients with ITP will often demonstrate excessive bleeding in response to a minor injury. Circulating antiplatelet antibodies coat normal platelets, which are then sequestered by the spleen, with resultant platelet destruction. The majority of patients respond to initial therapy with systemic steroids. Splenectomy is indicated in patients who become steroid dependent with significant side effects or in patients requiring increasing doses of steroids to maintain a satisfactory platelet count. The entire spleen must be excised, including any accessory spleens found at surgery. Residual splenic parenchyma would result in persistent platelet sequestration. Splenectomy is not indicated in the initial management of ITP. Platelet transfusion is rarely required. Spontaneous bleeding is unusual unless the platelet counts drop below 20,000/L. When this occurs, if the patient is not responsive to steroids, platelet transfusion and urgent splenectomy is indicated. Antineoplastic chemotherapy is not used in the management of ITP. Expectant management is associated with significant risk, as the most life-threatening complication of ITP is spontaneous intracerebral hemorrhage. Bone marrow transplant is not indicated. ITP is a disease of peripheral platelet destruction, with normal or increased platelet production. *(Townsend et al., pp. 1682–1685; Way and Doherty, pp. 659–660)*

127. (E) This patient has symptomatic anemia. The decreased oxygen-carrying capacity has resulted in decreased tissue perfusion. The heart attempts to compensate with increased contractility and heart rate, in an attempt to improve cardiac output and oxygen delivery. In this patient, however, this is inadequate and has also placed excess metabolic demands on the myocardium with signs of ischemia. These changes can be ameliorated with a blood transfusion. Iron supplementation is indicated in the treatment of chronic iron-deficiency anemia. Restoration of iron stores and a normal red cell mass usually takes several months. Therefore, it is not appropriate in a patient with symptomatic anemia. Supplemental oxygen will not improve oxygen delivery in a patient with limited oxygen-carrying capacity and compensatory maximum oxygen extraction at the tissue level. IV fluid resuscitation will increase circulating blood volume, resulting in hemodilution and decreased red cell concentration. Calcium channel blockade is indicated for management of myocardial ischemia from primary coronary or myocardial pathology. *(Townsend et al., pp. 125–130)*

128. (A) A febrile nonhemolytic transfusion reaction is usually caused by an interaction between recipient antibodies and leukocytes in the transfused blood. Treatment is discontinuation of the transfusion and antipyretics. If further transfusion is required, further reactions can be prevented by filtration of blood products for leukocyte reduction. Anaphylactic transfusion reactions are rare. Patients develop urticaria, flushing, hypotension, and bronchospasm. O blood type is characterized by the absence of ABO antigens on the red blood cell surface. Therefore, type O blood is universally accepted as the donor type for transfusion therapy, making an acute hemolytic transfusion reaction from ABO incompatability impossible. Delayed hemolytic reactions usually occur 1–3 weeks after a first transfusion and are manifested by an unexplained drop in hematocrit, associated with unconjugated hyperbilirubinemia. Acute bacterial infection transmitted through blood products is extremely rare and has been reported only in association with platelet concentrates stored at room temperature. *(Townsend et al., p. 130; Way and Doherty, pp. 59–60)*

129. (E) Any patient with this history and point tenderness in the anatomic snuffbox must be assumed to have a scaphoid fracture. Undisplaced fractures may be difficult to visualize on initial radiographs, even when multiple views are obtained. The appropriate management is full immobilization of the scaphoid, which is achieved only with a cast that extends to include the thumb. X-rays should be repeated in 10–14 days, and if the fracture is confirmed, immobilization should be continued. Avascular necrosis is a common complication. Minor wrist injury with ligamentous sprain may be adequately treated with anti-inflammatory medication, application of ice, an elastic wrist support, and restricted activity. However, these are not adequate therapy for a suspected scaphoid fracture. Furthermore, a wrist splint does not provide adequate immobilization of the scaphoid. *(Townsend et al., p. 2218; Way and Doherty, p. 1146)*

130. (B) Symptoms of zinc deficiency include diarrhea, depression, alopecia, and perioral and periorbital dermatitis. Patients at greater risk for developing this syndrome include those with high gastrointestinal fluid losses, patients with multisystem trauma, and patients on prolonged parenteral nutrition. The symptoms resolve with zinc supplementation. Iodine deficiency results in hypothyroidism. Deficiency syndromes for selenium, silicon, and tin have not been described. *(Townsend et al., p. 156; Way and Doherty, p. 163)*

131. (B)

132. (D)

Explanations 131 and 132

In the initial postoperative period, the patient has a low pulmonary artery wedge pressure and poor urine output. Renal perfusion is compromised by hypovolemia, with subsequent inadequate preload and decreased cardiac output. The appropriate therapeutic intervention at this time is further IV fluid resuscitation. Diuretics are contraindicated in the patient with hypovolemia and are unlikely to improve urine output in the face of inadequate renal perfusion. A dopamine infusion or digoxin may improve cardiac contractility but will not result in improvement in cardiac output unless there is adequate preload. In a hypovolemic patient, nitroprusside will result in a significant drop in blood pressure. After receiving a fluid bolus, the patient develops distended neck veins and an elevated pulmonary wedge pressure, indicating biventricular dysfunction with increased left ventricular end-diastolic pressure, and increased left ventricular end-systolic volume. Cardiac output is low, and urine output has not improved. In a patient with a history of hypertension, this clinical picture is often caused by increased afterload. Afterload reduction can be obtained with a nitroprusside infusion. *(Townsend et al., pp. 310–316, 617–622)*

133. (C) This patient has an obstructed airway from maxillofacial trauma. The patient is stridorous, hypoxic, and cannot be ventilated with bag and mask. Immediate cricothyroidotomy is lifesaving. In the presence of severe facial trauma, orotracheal intubation is likely to be difficult because of distortion of landmarks and excessive oropharyngeal secretions. Nasotracheal intubation is contraindicated in this setting. A definitive tracheostomy is more time consuming than a cricothyroidotomy and requires specific surgical expertise. Stabilization of the airway is the first resuscitation priority, before placement of chest tubes to relieve potential pneumothoraces. *(Townsend et al., pp. 490–491, 502; Way and Doherty, pp. 232–234, 236)*

134. (E) Frostbite is produced by formation of ice crystals in the tissue, with cessation of tissue perfusion. Appropriate initial treatment is rapid rewarming in warm water, to minimize further tissue damage. Dry heat can cause further tissue damage. With reperfusion, there is continued progression of tissue injury because of progressive microcirculatory thrombosis. Therefore, nonviable tissue should be allowed to demarcate over several weeks, with delayed debridement. A sympathectomy is not indicated acutely, because the vasculature in frozen tissue is already maximally dilated. *(Townsend et al., p. 2216; Way and Doherty, pp. 279–280)*

135. (B)

136. (B)

Explanations 135 and 136

Ruptured cerebral aneurysms often occur in the setting of hypertension. The severe headache, nausea and vomiting, photophobia, and nuchal rigidity are the result of meningeal irritation from subarachnoid blood. Subarachnoid hemorrhage is visualized on CT scan, with definitive diagnosis of the aneurysm and its location by cerebral angiography. Early surgical clipping is the current neurosurgical approach because of the significant risk of rebleeding in the first 24 h after initial presentation. Hydrocephalus may occur as a late complication of subarachnoid hemorrhage and require serial lumbar puncture to drain CSF and control ICP. A hemorrhagic stroke can occur in association with malignant hypertension and may have concurrent subarachnoid hemorrhage. Focal neurologic signs are usually present. Meningitis will produce similar signs of meningeal irritation, but usually with other systemic signs of infection and a clinical prodrome suggesting an infectious etiology. Lumbar puncture is diagnostic, and if a bacterial source is suspected, systemic antibiotics are initiated pending culture of CSF. Ischemic cerebrovascular accidents and transient ischemic attacks are not associated with subarachnoid hemorrhage and, hence, do not present with signs of meningeal irritation. Focal neurologic signs are usually present. Evaluation of a possible cause includes Doppler examination of the carotid arteries. Management includes anticoagulation and antiplatelet therapy. EEG measures brain electrical activity and is indicated in the diagnostic evaluation of seizures. *(Townsend et al., pp. 2135–2139; Way and Doherty, pp. 937–943)*

137. (C) This patient has developed a tension pneumothorax from dissection of carbon dioxide into the pleural space, either via an unrecognized defect in the diaphragm or via the retroperitoneal and retropleural spaces. Treatment is immediate decompression with a chest tube. Hypotension associated with a tension pneumothorax is secondary to decreased venous return from mediastinal shift. IV fluids are indicated only if there is associated hypovolemia. Release of the pneumoperitoneum may prevent further carbon dioxide accumulation, but chest tube decompression is still required. A tension pneumothorax is a clinical diagnosis and does not require a chest x-ray for confirmation. Once the pneumothorax is adequately decompressed and the patient is stabilized, the laparoscopic procedure may continue. *(Townsend et al., pp. 452–454, 508)*

138. (B)

139. (A)

140. (B)

Explanations 138 through 140

This patient with diverticular disease has developed a colovesical fistula from diverticulitis, with localized sigmoid perforation into the adjacent bladder. Patients will present with signs and symptoms of a urinary tract infection, with air in the urinary stream and multiple fecal organisms on urine culture. CT scan is most useful in the diagnostic evaluation, and will often demonstrate air within the bladder. An air contrast barium enema may show evidence of diverticular disease and is useful to exclude other pathology. The diagnostic yield of cystography and colonoscopy are approximately 20%. Diagnostic laparoscopy is not indicated. This patient should be managed with broad-spectrum antibiotics and bladder drainage. When the acute inflammatory process has resolved, definitive surgical therapy can be performed electively. These patients will tolerate a gentle bowel prep and can then undergo a sigmoid colon resection and primary anastomosis. Outpatient management is not optimal, and oral antibiotics are insufficient therapy. Clear fluids, magnesium citrate, and oral antibiotics are components of a surgical bowel prep. This should only be undertaken after treatment of the urinary tract sepsis and a period of bowel rest. A colovesical fistula is not a surgical emergency. Management of the complications of diverticular disease by proximal defunctioning colostomy is reserved for patients who are profoundly ill and require diversion of the fecal stream to control continued intraabdominal and pelvic sepsis. This is not definitive therapy for a colovesical fistula, because it leaves a column of stool above the fistula, with continued fecal contamination of the urinary tract. A resection with Hartmann's procedure has the disadvantage of requiring a second major laparotomy to reestablish intestinal continuity. An abdominoperineal resection is not required for the management of diverticular disease. Diverticular disease does not involve the rectum. The sigmoid colon is the most common location for symptomatic diverticular disease resulting in a colovesical fistula. A total abdominal colectomy is therefore rarely indicated. *(Townsend et al., pp. 1417–1422; Way and Doherty, p. 735)*

141. (D) This patient presents with signs and symptoms of a sigmoid volvulus. Most commonly, this occurs in the elderly debilitated patient with a history of chronic constipation, resulting in the development of a long, redundant, mobile sigmoid colon. Patients present with a clinical picture of an acute colonic obstruction. Abdominal radiographs will show a large dilated loop of colon originating in the left lower abdomen, and extending to the right upper abdomen. Management includes decompression with a rigid proctoscope, which will usually result in detorsion of the bowel. Placement of a sigmoid decompression tube is necessary to prevent recurrence. Urgent laparotomy is indicated in patients with fever, abdominal tenderness, and metabolic acidosis, suggesting colonic ischemia. Patients admitted to the hospital who do not undergo urgent decompression are at risk of developing colonic ischemia from the closed-loop obstruction. A rectal decompression tube is insufficient for decompression because the tip is located distal to the obstruction. Colonic enemas are ineffective in the face of a complete obstruction and may, in fact, further increase colonic distention. *(Townsend et al., pp. 1422–1424; Way and Doherty, pp. 738–740)*

REFERENCES

Donegan WL, Spratt JS (eds.). *Cancer of the Breast*, 5th ed. Philadelphia, PA: W.B. Saunders, 2002.

Fauci AS, Braunwald E, Isselbacher KJ, et al. (eds.). *Harrison's Principles of Internal Medicine*, 15th ed. New York, NY: McGraw-Hill, 2001.

Greenfield LJ, Mulholland M, Oldham KT, et al. (eds.). *Surgery: Scientific Principles and Practice*. Philadelphia, PA: Lippincott-Raven, 2001.

Townsend CM Jr, Beauchamp RD, Evers BM, et al. (eds.). *Sabiston Textbook of Surgery: The Biologic Basis of Modern Surgical Practice*, 17th ed. Philadelphia, PA: W.B. Saunders, 2004.

Way LW, Doherty GM (eds.). *Current Surgical Diagnosis and Treatment*, 11th ed. New York, NY: McGraw-Hill, 2003.

Zinner MJ. *Maingot's Abdominal Operations*, 10th ed., Vols. I and II. Stamford, CT: Appleton & Lange, 1997.

CHAPTER 7

Practice Test 1

Questions

DIRECTIONS (Questions 1 through 28): Each of the numbered items or incomplete statements in this section is followed by answers or by completions of the statement. Select the ONE lettered answer or completion that is BEST in each case.

Questions 1 and 2

A 68-year-old man comes to the emergency department with complaints of watery diarrhea, crampy abdominal pain with distention, and low-grade fever of 3 days' duration. He underwent coronary artery bypass surgery 10 days previously and was discharged on postoperative day 5 on an oral first-generation cephalosporin for wound cellulitis that has since resolved. Physical examination reveals a temperature of 100°F, pulse rate 95/min, blood pressure (BP) 110/60 mmHg, respiratory rate 12/min, and a mildly distended abdomen with mild left lower quadrant pain with guarding, no rebound tenderness, and heme-positive stool on rectal examination. Pertinent laboratory tests reveal an elevated blood urea nitrogen (BUN) and creatinine, and white blood count (WBC) of 25,000.

1. Which of the following tests is most likely to yield a definitive diagnosis?

(A) chest and abdominal x-rays
(B) stool for ova and parasites
(C) stool for *Clostridium difficile* toxins
(D) stool for enterotoxigenic *Escherichia coli*
(E) computed tomography (CT) scan of the abdomen

2. Which of the following is the most appropriate next step in management of this patient?

(A) intravenous (IV) fluids in the emergency department and discharge to home on an oral cephalosporin with instructions to return for increasing symptoms or fever greater than 101.5°F
(B) IV fluids, admittance to the hospital, and institution of third-generation cephalosporin antibiotics
(C) IV fluids, admittance to the hospital, discontinuation of cephalosporin, and colonoscopy
(D) IV fluids, admittance to the hospital, discontinuation of cephalosporin, and institution of metronidazole
(E) IV fluids in the emergency department and discharge to home on an oral cephalosporin with an appointment to return for an air contrast barium enema

3. A 40-year-old man calls your office asking for a chest x-ray. He is worried because a friend was just diagnosed with lung cancer. Both he and his friend smoke two packs of cigarettes a day and have chronic coughs. He admits he seldom goes to the doctor unless he has a serious injury. You order an x-ray, and it is normal. Which of the following is the most appropriate course of action at this point?

   (A) Advise the patient that he really needs a CT scan, since x-rays can miss early cancers.
   (B) Reinforce his concern by showing him pictures of victims of lung cancer and emphysema.
   (C) Assess his readiness to quit smoking.
   (D) Advise him that smoking makes it about 15 times more likely that he will develop cancer of the lung.
   (E) Advise him that he should quit smoking now.

4. A 1-day-old infant has persistent vomiting. He has not had any stools. He was born at term and has not had any respiratory difficulties. A nasogastric tube is easily placed into his stomach. An abdominal film is ordered and is shown in Fig. 7-1. Which of the following is the most likely diagnosis for this infant?

   (A) adrenogenital syndrome
   (B) pyloric stenosis
   (C) duodenal atresia
   (D) esophageal atresia with distal tracheoesophageal atresia
   (E) cystic fibrosis

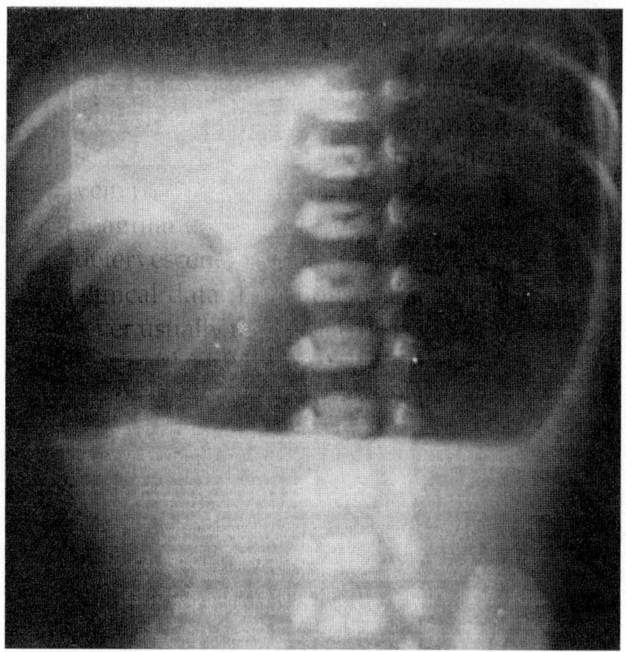

FIG. 7-1

Questions 5 through 7

A 22-year-old college student is evaluated by a psychiatrist for the onset of paranoid delusions, command auditory hallucinations, and an overwhelming sense that his thoughts are being drawn out of his brain by "negative electromagnetic waves." There is no prior psychiatric history. His parents, who accompany him, report that 2 months ago he had moved back home with them, isolated himself in his room, and become increasingly careless about his personal appearance. He was described as a quiet but friendly person with several good friends. In both high school and college (except for the last 2 or 3 months), he was a good student and seemed to enjoy his studies as well as participating in soccer and track. It seemed to his parents that he was worried about graduation and fears of finding a job. The patient denied the use of illicit drugs. It was noted that a paternal uncle had a diagnosis of schizophrenia.

5. Which of the following is the best initial drug to treat this man?

   (A) buspirone
   (B) bupropion
   (C) fluvoxamine
   (D) clomipramine
   (E) quetiapine

6. The sense that thoughts were being drawn out of his brain by "negative electromagnetic waves" is an example of which of the following?

   (A) projection
   (B) loose association
   (C) delusion
   (D) hallucination
   (E) heightened sensitivity to environmental stimuli

7. Which of the following supports the possibility of a good prognosis for this patient?

   (A) uncle with schizophrenia
   (B) history of good achievement in school
   (C) being single
   (D) insidious onset
   (E) no clear precipitating factors

8. A worker complains of paresthesias, numbness, and tingling that started distally in the lower extremities but that is starting to affect his hands. He is developing muscle weakness. Electromyographic abnormalities suggest axonal degeneration and demyelination. Which exposure is the most suspect cause of this clinical picture?

   (A) lead
   (B) *n*-hexane
   (C) benzene
   (D) cadmium
   (E) carbon disulfide

9. A 59-year-old woman with no children had 3 days of vaginal bleeding 1 month ago, the first episode of vaginal bleeding since menopause at age 53 years. She has a history of alcoholic cirrhosis. Her body mass index (BMI) is 39 kg/m^2. She has taken a combination estrogen-progestin for hormone replacement therapy (HRT) for 4 years. She currently has three sexual partners. Her pelvic examination is normal, and her Pap smear is subsequently read as normal. Which of the following is the most appropriate next step in management?

   (A) office endometrial biopsy
   (B) colposcopy
   (C) transvaginal ultrasonography
   (D) serum Ca-125 measurement
   (E) vaginal hysterectomy

Questions 10 through 13

A 22-year-old man presents to the physician's office with the complaint of a new nodule in the neck noted 1 month ago. He is the oldest of five children ranging in age from 8 to 22. His family history is pertinent for thyroid carcinoma, hypertension in his paternal grandparents, and an unknown type of tumor in the abdomen of his father, now deceased. On examination, he has a normal appearance and body habitus. He is afebrile, with a BP of 145/90 mmHg and pulse rate of 70/min. Neck examination reveals a firm, 2-cm thyroid nodule. Fine-needle aspiration of the nodule reveals thyroid carcinoma.

10. Which of the following is the most likely type of thyroid carcinoma?

    (A) papillary
    (B) follicular
    (C) Hürthle cell
    (D) medullary
    (E) anaplastic

11. Screening for which one of the following diseases must be undertaken before treatment of the thyroid carcinoma?

    (A) an adrenocorticotropic hormone (ACTH)-producing tumor
    (B) Zollinger–Ellison syndrome
    (C) pituitary adenoma
    (D) pheochromocytoma
    (E) ganglioneuroma

12. Which of the following is the minimal treatment for the patient's thyroid carcinoma?

    (A) ipsilateral subtotal lobectomy
    (B) ipsilateral lobectomy and isthmectomy
    (C) subtotal thyroidectomy and isthmectomy
    (D) total thyroidectomy
    (E) total thyroidectomy and parathyroidectomy

13. Screening for abnormalities in which protooncogene should be offered to his siblings?

(A) myc
(B) ret
(C) ras
(D) myb
(E) erbB

14. An infant recently had a sweat chloride test because her private physician was concerned about her having cystic fibrosis. The test was positive. She has been referred to you for further diagnostic testing and counseling. She is the first child of a married couple. No one in either family has ever been diagnosed with this disease. Which of the following advice should you include in your initial session with this patient and her family?

(A) The sweat chloride test is a screening test, but further tests should be done to confirm the diagnosis.
(B) Pulmonary complications are severe and serious but fortunately are uncommon.
(C) Glucose intolerance is common in the first year of life.
(D) Current therapy does not provide a cure for this disease but can prolong life considerably.
(E) The disease is clearly genetic but does not follow a definite autosomal or recessive pattern.

15. In a patient with diabetes, which of the following is the ideal low-density lipoprotein (LDL) cholesterol?

(A) >100
(B) >130
(C) <130
(D) <100
(E) >160

16. Which of the following medications is most useful in a patient with diabetes who is hypertensive and has evidence for microalbuminuria?

(A) metoprolol
(B) enalapril
(C) clonidine
(D) nifedipine
(E) reserpine

17. A Puerto Rican woman, treated for depression, is reported to be pulling out her hair. In evaluating her, you note that her eye lashes are missing and her head hair is very thin, with patches of no hair evident. She repetitively pulls on her hair, but at least for the moment appears not to pull any out. She reports that she has engaged in this behavior for almost a year. Which of the following is the most likely diagnosis?

(A) catatonic schizophrenia—excited form
(B) trichotillomania
(C) ghost sickness
(D) mal de ojo
(E) autism

18. Thromboangiitis obliterans (Buerger disease) is characterized by which of the following?

(A) typically occurs in smokers
(B) occurs most often in young females
(C) typically affects large arteries
(D) noninvolvement of veins
(E) highest worldwide prevalence in the southern United States

19. Labor is induced with a dilute IV oxytocin infusion at 39 weeks' gestation in a 29-year-old woman whose pregnancy was uncomplicated. Labor and delivery occur without complications. Which one of the following is a contraindication to the use of oxytocin?

(A) oligohydramnios
(B) nonreactive nonstress test (NST)
(C) prior stillbirth at 41 weeks' gestation
(D) prior low transverse cesarean section
(E) prior classical cesarean section

20. A 22-year-old nulligravid woman had monthly menses without pain until approximately 18 months ago. In the past 18 months, she has noted progressively more painful menses for which she misses 2 days of work each month. She has no urinary or intestinal symptoms.

She has never had sexual intercourse and has had no gynecologic surgery. The pain is partially relieved by nonsteroidal anti-inflammatory medication. Which of the following is the most likely cause of her secondary dysmenorrhea?

(A) endometriosis
(B) pelvic infection and adhesions
(C) pelvic congestion syndrome
(D) cervical stenosis
(E) irritable bowel syndrome

21. A 23-year-old woman has a positive urine ligase chain reaction (LCR) test for chlamydia. She is 8 weeks pregnant. Which of the following is the appropriate next step in diagnosis and treatment?

(A) Repeat the LCR test.
(B) Prescribe a 7-day course of doxycycline.
(C) Prescribe a 7-day course of amoxicillin or erythromycin, or a single dose of azithromycin.
(D) Order a culture to confirm diagnosis and determine sensitivity of the organism before starting treatment.
(E) Order a polymerase chain reaction (PCR) test to confirm the diagnosis before starting treatment.

Questions 22 and 23

A 25-year-old woman presents to the physician's office with a 2-week history of right breast pain. The pain is localized to the nipple areolar complex and surrounding skin and is associated with redness and swelling. The pain does not change with the menstrual cycle. On examination, vital signs are normal, and there is induration, erythema, and tenderness involving the nipple areolar complex of the breast, with a subareolar mass. Axillary examination reveals slightly tender ipsilateral nodes. Ultrasound examination suggests the presence of a subareolar complex fluid collection.

22. Which of the following is the most likely diagnosis?

(A) inflammatory carcinoma of the breast
(B) periductal mastitis with abscess
(C) Paget's disease of the nipple
(D) Mondor's disease (thrombophlebitis)
(E) intraductal papilloma

23. Which of the following is the most appropriate next step in management?

(A) aspiration of the fluid and antibiotics
(B) central lumpectomy, axillary node dissection, and radiation therapy
(C) incision and drainage
(D) antibiotics alone with reevaluation in 1 week
(E) excisional biopsy

24. A 24-year-old G2P2 woman engages in unprotected intercourse on the 14th day of her menstrual cycle. Two days later, she requests emergency contraception. Which of the following is effective contraception?

(A) one triphasic oral contraceptive tablet daily for 21 days starting on cycle day 16
(B) methotrexate, 50 mg/m^2 intramuscularly (IM)
(C) diethylstilbestrol (DES), 5 mg orally one time
(D) danazol 200 mg orally taken once
(E) levonorgestrel 0.75 mg orally every 12 h for two doses

25. A thin, White 53-year-old woman who had her last menstrual period 2 years ago complains of hot flashes for 1 year, vaginal dryness, and sleep loss from night sweats. You offer hormone replacement with combination estrogen-progesterone therapy, explaining that it will do which of the following?

(A) increase her risk of endometrial carcinoma
(B) increase her risk of breast cancer
(C) increase orgasmic ability
(D) increase bone mineral density
(E) increase her risk of colon cancer

26. A 12-month-old infant, previously in good health, develops an illness characterized by 3 days of fever followed by defervescence and the development of a maculopapular rash on the trunk. No other signs or symptoms are present. Which of the following is the most likely diagnosis?

(A) erythema infectiosum (fifth disease)
(B) Kawasaki disease
(C) roseola infantum (exanthem subitum)
(D) rubeola (measles)
(E) scarlet fever

27. Which of the following would be the most helpful in the management of the terminally ill patient?

(A) withholding information about prognosis and treatment of side effects so as not to burden the patient
(B) asking the patient how much she or he would like to know about the illness
(C) trusting that families and friends will provide the emotional support the patient needs
(D) administering analgesic medications on a strict schedule so the patient will get the medication regularly
(E) not referring for group therapy, which is of little value for this population

28. A 2-week-old infant is brought to the emergency department with vomiting for 1 day. On physical examination, the baby is very lethargic, is poorly perfused, and appears moderately dehydrated. His electrolytes are sodium, 115; potassium, 6.0; and carbon dioxide, 15. His glucose is 40. Which of the following is the most likely diagnosis?

(A) congenital adrenal hyperplasia
(B) duodenal atresia
(C) gastroenteritis
(D) pyloric stenosis
(E) tracheoesophageal fistula

DIRECTIONS (Questions 29 through 35): For each numbered item, select the ONE best lettered option that is most closely associated with it. Each lettered option may be selected once, more than once, or not at all.

For each patient with gastrointestinal bleeding, select the most likely diagnosis.

(A) diverticulosis of the colon
(B) ulcerative colitis
(C) Meckel's diverticulum
(D) ischemic colitis
(E) aortoenteric fistula
(F) peptic ulcer
(G) carcinoma of the colon
(H) esophageal varices
(I) gastric ulcer

29. A 60-year-old man is brought to the emergency department following a fainting episode at home. He complains of bright red blood per rectum for the last 6 h. He denies abdominal pain or vomiting. Examination reveals a pulse rate of 110/min; BP of 95/50 mmHg; and no significant heart, lung, or abdominal findings. He has gross blood on rectal examination.

30. A 56-year-old woman presents to the emergency department following an episode of melanotic stool 48 h ago. She underwent resuscitation at another facility before transfer. She has no current complaints. The melena has not recurred. Past surgical history is pertinent for appendectomy at age 25 and abdominal aortic aneurysm repair 2 years ago. She has a 30 pack-year smoking history and drinks alcohol socially on weekends. Upper gastrointestinal (UGI) endoscopy to the duodenal bulb is normal, as well as colonoscopy.

31. A 65-year-old woman presents to the emergency department complaining of severe fatigue and weakness over the last week. Past history is pertinent for hypertension, diabetes, and coronary artery disease. Medications include a calcium channel blocker, insulin, and daily aspirin. She has a 40 pack-year smoking history and drinks a moderate amount of alcohol. Examination reveals pulse rate of 90/min, BP of 105/65 mmHg, and unremarkable heart and lung findings. She has fullness and mild tenderness in the right lower quadrant. Blood tests reveal a hematocrit of 21.

32. A 65-year-old man is transferred to the emergency department from an outside facility for evaluation of hematemesis and melena. Past history is pertinent for recently discovered cholelithiasis, for which he has not yet received a surgical consultation. He has complained of abdominal pain for the last 3–4 weeks and has been taking ibuprofen four times daily for 3 weeks as well as alcohol for the pain. Examination reveals a pulse rate of 100/min and BP of 100/60 mmHg following resuscitation. Abdominal examination reveals tenderness in the right upper quadrant and epigastrium. Rectal examination reveals melanotic stool.

33. A 50-year-old man presents to the emergency department following an episode of hematemesis. Past history is pertinent for a 40 pack-year smoking history and chronic alcoholism. Examination reveals a pulse rate of 120/min, BP of 90/60 mmHg, and an unremarkable heart and lung examination. Skin examination reveals spider angiomata and palmar erythema. Abdominal examination reveals a nontender abdomen that is distended.

34. A 35-year-old man presents to the emergency department with abdominal pain, hematemesis, and black, tarry stools. He complains of abdominal pain for 2 weeks, for which he has taken antacids with partial relief. Past history is pertinent for hypertension, 20 pack-year smoking history, and occasional alcohol intake. Examination reveals a pulse rate of 110/min, BP of 95/60 mmHg, tenderness in the epigastrium, and melanotic stool on rectal examination.

35. A 35-year-old woman presents to the emergency department with a 1-week history of bloody diarrhea. She complains of intermittent abdominal pain for 1 month that is now constant and weight loss of 10 lbs. Past history is unremarkable. Examination reveals a temperature of 101°F, pulse rate of 85/min, and BP of 110/60 mmHg. Heart and lung examinations are unremarkable. Abdominal examination reveals diffuse abdominal tenderness.

DIRECTIONS (Questions 36 through 135): Each of the numbered items or incomplete statements in this section is followed by answers or by completions of the statement. Select the ONE lettered answer or completion that is BEST in each case.

36. A 25-year-old nullipara consults you because she has stopped menstruating. Her menses were monthly until 1 year ago, when they became less frequent. She also complains of hot flashes, vaginal dryness, and discomfort with intercourse. The most appropriate first step in her evaluation is measurement of which of the following?

(A) serum thyroid-stimulating hormone (TSH) concentration
(B) serum prolactin concentration
(C) human chorionic gonadotropin (hCG) concentration
(D) serum estradiol-17 concentration
(E) serum testosterone concentration

37. A 37-year-old obese (BMI = 32 kg/m^2) woman who smokes a half pack of cigarettes daily requests oral contraption. She has a history of migraine headaches relieved with medication, cholelithiasis, adult onset diabetes mellitus, and 10-week size uterine fibroids. Which of the following is an absolute contraindication to oral contraceptives?

(A) women over 35 who smoke
(B) migraine headaches
(C) cholelithiasis
(D) diabetes mellitus
(E) uterine fibroids

38. The parents of an infant born at term are concerned about the possibility of their child having developmental dysplasia of the hip (DDH). Which of the following historical factors would make this diagnosis more likely?

(A) The baby is a boy.
(B) The baby is delivered in the breech position.
(C) The baby is delivered vaginally.
(D) The baby is their third child.
(E) The family is Black.

39. A 25-year-old man is hospitalized after weeks of worsening psychosis. He is begun on the antipsychotic drug thiothixene. Five days later, he develops a fever of 39.8°C. In addition, he has become delirious, is lying stiffly in his bed, and is uncommunicative. His family reports he had been physically well at the time of admission. The admission physical examination confirmed this. Which of the following is of most immediate concern at this point?

(A) worsening psychotic state
(B) pseudoparkinsonism reaction
(C) ruptured cerebral aneurysm
(D) unsuspected opioid dependence
(E) neuroleptic malignant syndrome (NMS)

40. You screen a 30-year-old woman for chlamydia with a nucleic acid amplification test that has a sensitivity of 90% and a specificity of 95%, and the result comes back positive. What is the likelihood that she has chlamydia?

(A) You cannot tell without knowing what the likelihood is that other women like her have chlamydia.
(B) There is about a 95% chance that she has it.
(C) There is about a 5% chance that she has it.
(D) You cannot tell without knowing the reproducibility of the test.
(E) You can't tell without obtaining the results of a PCR test to make a definitive diagnosis.

Questions 41 through 43

A 22-year-old, previously healthy, 176-lb man was rescued from a house fire, after being trapped in a small bedroom of the house for several hours. When brought to the emergency department, he is noted to be combative and disoriented. His lungs are clear to auscultation bilaterally. His respiratory rate is 30/min, BP 100/70 mmHg, and heart rate 115/min. He has sustained 15% second- and third-degree burns on the lower extremities, with a circumferential full-thickness injury below the right knee.

41. Which of the following is the most appropriate initial step in management?

(A) sedation with IV midazolam
(B) IV morphine for analgesia
(C) administration of 100% oxygen by face mask
(D) debridement of the lower-extremity burns
(E) IV fluid bolus of 20 mL/kg

42. The patient improves and is transferred to the intensive care unit for further management. Which of the following is the appropriate initial fluid resuscitation?

(A) IV dextrose/0.5 normal saline at 150 mL/h
(B) IV lactated Ringer's at maintenance rate per hour, with boluses of albumin as required
(C) IV lactated Ringer's at twice maintenance rate per hour
(D) 4800 mL of lactated Ringer's, given at 200 mL/h
(E) IV maintenance fluids plus an additional 4800 mL of lactated Ringer's, one-half given over the first 8 h and the remainder given over 16 h

43. Within several hours of admission, the patient begins to complain of pain in the right foot. He is noted to have swelling of the foot and ankle, decreased capillary refill of the right toes, and decreased sensation. Which of the following is the treatment of choice?

(A) elevation of the affected extremity
(B) initiation of antibiotics
(C) hyperbaric oxygen
(D) administration of 100% oxygen by face mask
(E) escharotomy

44. A 55-year-old woman refuses to take HRT because she fears that she will develop breast cancer. You discuss the use of a selective estrogen receptor modulator (SERM) such as raloxifene (Evista). Which of the following statements is supported by data?

(A) Bone mineral density is increased after 24 months.
(B) High-density lipoprotein (HDL) concentrations are increased within 6 months.
(C) Hot flashes are relieved.
(D) Endometrial thickness increases after 12 months.
(E) Breast cancer risk is increased.

45. A 15-year-old girl comes to the emergency department 4 h after ingesting aspirin. After obtaining the history, you estimate that she has ingested approximately 150 mg/kg of aspirin. Her physical examination is entirely normal. Which of the following treatments would be most useful in her management?

(A) induced emesis
(B) administration of *N*-acetylcysteine
(C) administration of a cathartic
(D) administration of IV fluid to increase urine output
(E) no medical intervention is necessary

46. An asymptomatic sexually active woman aged less than 25 sees you in clinic for a Pap smear. She tells you that she is in a monogamous relationship. Which of the following best describes correct advice to her concerning sexually transmitted diseases?

(A) I recommend that you get a chlamydia test.
(B) You should consider getting a chlamydia test.
(C) If you are pregnant, you should be screened for chlamydia.
(D) If you have burning with urination, I definitely recommend that you be screened for chlamydia.
(E) Screening for chlamydia is of uncertain benefit.

47. A 50-year-old woman presents with weakness of her right hand, accompanied by a tingling sensation on awakening each morning. She is found to have hypesthesia of the thumb, index, and middle fingers, along with atrophy of the thenar muscles. Which of the following is the most likely diagnosis?

(A) compression of the digital nerve to the thumb
(B) compression of the median nerve in the hand
(C) compression of the median nerve in the carpal tunnel
(D) compression of the median nerve by the pronator teres
(E) compression of the median nerve in the axilla

48. A 24-year-old gravida 1 woman received magnesium sulfate for preeclampsia and oxytocin to induce labor at 39 weeks' gestation. Labor and delivery were uneventful until 1 h postpartum when she had severe postpartum hemorrhage that required vigorous fundal massage and ergotamine to control the bleeding. Although she wished to breast feed her son, she was unable to do so because she never formed milk. Six months later, you see her because she has yet to menstruate since the delivery. Which of the following is the most likely diagnosis?

(A) polycystic ovary syndrome
(B) premature ovarian failure
(C) endometrial sclerosis (Asherman syndrome)
(D) cervical stenosis
(E) Sheehan syndrome

49. A 2-year-old toddler refuses to move his left arm and is holding it flexed at the elbow, with the forearm pronated. His father had been swinging him by the forearms; there is no other history of trauma. Which of the following is the most likely diagnosis?

(A) fractured clavicle
(B) Salter type IV fracture of the distal humerus
(C) dislocation of the radial head
(D) torus fracture of the distal radius
(E) contusion of the ulnar nerve

50. A 14-year-old boy comes to the clinic for a checkup. His only concern is that he has developed acne. On physical examination, he has moderate facial acne and is Tanner stage 3. Which of the following is the best next step in his management?

(A) Advise him to wash his face vigorously four times per day.
(B) Advise him that it should resolve as he continues to progress through puberty.
(C) Ask him to decrease his intake of chocolate, starches, and oily or fried foods.
(D) Reassure him that no treatment is necessary unless he develops cystic acne.
(E) Treat him with topical benzoyl peroxide and tretinoin.

51. Which of the following groups of disorders is most common as a cause of syncope?

(A) psychiatric
(B) arrhythmias
(C) neurally mediated
(D) medication related
(E) gastrointestinal

52. In 1990, a study was conducted to determine the relationship between outdoor air pollution and bronchitis in postal workers employed during the period 1970–1980. Information on the occurrence of bronchitis since employment and other relevant factors were gathered from the medical records of 2500 letter carriers delivering mail outdoors as well as those of 500 comparable post office employees who had worked indoors. The risk of bronchitis was found to be higher among those working outdoors. Which of the following describes this study design?

(A) ecologic study
(B) historical cohort
(C) cross-sectional
(D) prospective cohort
(E) randomized, controlled trial

53. A 19-year-old student at a rural state university is admitted to a hospital with rapid onset of fever, headache, photophobia, and a stiff neck. The student soon develops an extensive purpuric skin rash and becomes obtunded. Gram stain of the cerebrospinal fluid (CSF) shows numerous gram-negative diplococci. Within 3 days, two other students are admitted with fever, headache, and stiff neck. Gram stains of their CSF also show gram-negative diplococci. One of the students had attended a seminar with the first student. The third has no known relationship with the others. You are the public health officer for the area, and school officials are calling you for advice. There are 2 months of school left. Which of the following do you recommend to control the outbreak?

(A) Administer rifampin, 500 mg twice daily for 2 days, to all students and faculty.
(B) Close the school and send the students home until new cases cease to appear.
(C) Conduct a mass immunization for meningococcal disease.
(D) Identify the source of infection using a quick case-control study.
(E) Conduct a mass media campaign on the signs and symptoms of meningitis.

Questions 54 and 55

A 26-year-old, previously healthy man is brought to the emergency department with a stab wound to the fifth left intercostal space in the midclavicular line. He is found to have a pulse of 140/min, systolic BP of 80 mmHg, and respiration of 20/min. His trachea is midline, heart sounds appear distant, and breath sounds are equal bilaterally.

54. Which of the following is the most likely diagnosis?

(A) transected descending aorta
(B) cardiac tamponade
(C) massive left hemothorax
(D) tension pneumothorax
(E) phrenic nerve paralysis

55. Which of the following is the most appropriate next step in management?

(A) insertion of a left chest tube
(B) emergency department thoracotomy
(C) pericardiocentesis
(D) rapid infusion of an IV fluid bolus
(E) intubation and assisted ventilation

56. An infant is born to a mother treated late in pregnancy for primary syphilis. After birth, the infant is evaluated for evidence of congenital syphilis. Which of the following statements is true?

(A) Mean infant birth weight is increased because of fetal hydrops.
(B) Congenital syphilis is more common when the mother had late syphilis versus primary syphilis.
(C) The stillbirth rate is significantly increased.
(D) Evidence of congenital syphilis is usually present at birth.
(E) The false-negative rate of serologic tests for syphilis is increased in human immunodeficiency virus (HIV)-infected women.

57. A patient had an uncomplicated cesarean section 6 days previously. She has been on a regimen of ampicillin, gentamicin, and clindamycin for 5 days, but still has temperature spikes of 39.4°C (103°F). Physical examination is normal. Which of the following is the most likely cause of her fever?

(A) a pelvic abscess
(B) septic pelvic thrombophlebitis
(C) endometritis
(D) pyelonephritis
(E) breast engorgement

58. Over the course of an evening, 10 individuals present to an emergency department complaining of abrupt onset of severe nausea, vomiting, and abdominal cramps. Many were prostrate with sweats and dizziness. Some of the individuals developed diarrhea. On examination, they were afebrile. All of them noted the onset of symptoms within 1–3 h of eating at the same restaurant, and all of them had eaten minced barbecue from the restaurant buffet. The health department conducted an inspection the next day. Which of the following findings is most likely associated with the illness?

(A) obtaining a history of vomiting and diarrhea from the food handler preparing the barbecue
(B) inadequate reheating of previously refrigerated food
(C) an infected cut on the hand of a food handler who prepared the barbecue
(D) an outbreak of gastroenteritis among restaurant staff 1 week ago
(E) the meat for the barbecue came from a supplier previously implicated in an *E. coli* O157:H7 outbreak

59. A 17-year-old female is brought to the emergency department because she ingested vitamins that contained iron. Which of the following symptoms you might see early in the course of acute iron poisoning?

(A) bleeding diathesis
(B) gastrointestinal hemorrhage
(C) liver failure
(D) prolonged QT interval
(E) respiratory failure

60. A 12-year-old girl with malaise, fatigue, sore throat, fever, hepatosplenomegaly, and generalized lymphadenopathy is diagnosed as having Epstein-Barr virus-related mononucleosis. Which of the following complications is most likely in this patient?

(A) azotemia
(B) chronic active hepatitis
(C) encephalitis
(D) leukopenia
(E) pancreatitis

61. A 55-year-old woman is referred for psychiatric consultation for depression. She is 60 days post bone marrow transplant. Her husband says that she "just cries," barely says anything, sleeps very restlessly if at all, and has lost interest in him and their children, as well as in her housework and hobbies. The oncologist who referred her wants you to "give her something for her depression." Which of the following is the next appropriate step?

(A) prescribe sertraline
(B) prescribe lorazepam
(C) interview the woman
(D) have a family conference
(E) electroconvulsive therapy (ECT)

62. You are in a shopping mall and you notice two people next to a trash container. One is lying on the ground with involuntary twitching. The other is on her knees, in obvious physical distress, including respiratory difficulty, and is starting to exhibit involuntary movements of the extremities. Which of the following is the most appropriate action to take?

(A) Call others for help, get someone to call 911, check airways, breathing, and pulse.
(B) Check airways, breathing and pulse, then call for help and call 911 if needed.
(C) Call 911 and then check airways, breathing, and pulse.
(D) Leave them where they are, tell everyone to evacuate the area, leave the area yourself, and call 911.
(E) If possible, quickly transfer the two people to a protected area where they can be cared for without interference.

63. Which of the following is a side effect or toxic effect of cisplatin?

(A) renal toxicity
(B) leukopenia
(C) atopic dermatitis
(D) hemorrhagic cystitis
(E) decreased visual acuity

64. A pharmaceutical company sponsors the development of a new screening tool for asthma and plans to test it in a clinic where there are a large number of asthmatics. The high prevalence rate of asthma in the test population will have an effect on which of the following characteristics of the screening tool?

(A) sensitivity
(B) specificity
(C) positive predictive value
(D) accuracy
(E) reliability

65. A 19-year-old primipara at 38 weeks' gestation has a BP of 150/106 mmHg, hyperreflexia, and 3+ proteinuria. Which of the following statements is correct?

(A) The risk of eclampsia increases with increasing systolic BP.
(B) Delivery of the infant is the treatment for this woman.
(C) A beta-blocker is contraindicated in pregnancy.
(D) The risk of placenta previa is increased in this woman.
(E) Perinatal mortality is increased slightly in hypertensive pregnant women.

66. After a 12-h first stage, a 45-min second stage, and a 10-min third stage of labor, a healthy primigravid woman delivers a 7.9-lb boy with

Apgar scores of 9 at 1 min and 10 at 5 min. Which of the following statements about labor is correct?

(A) Labor is defined by the presence of regular uterine contractions at an interval of 5 min or less.
(B) The first stage begins with the onset of regular uterine contractions and ends with full dilatation of the cervix.
(C) The first stage of labor is prolonged in this patient.
(D) The second stage is from complete cervical dilation to the delivery of the placenta.
(E) The third stage of labor begins after delivery of the placenta and ends when the episiotomy is repaired.

67. Which of the following statements about paclitaxel (Taxol) is true?

(A) It is extracted from the roots of the western yew.
(B) Myelosuppression is the major dose-limiting effect.
(C) It acts by preventing microtubule assembly.
(D) It is used to treat advanced cervical cancer.
(E) Nausea and vomiting are uncommon side effects.

68. A high-risk cardiac patient has been counseled repeatedly by his physician to alter his currently unhealthy diet. He considered changing his diet in the past, but thought that it would be too difficult. At his last routine health visit, he was told that he had gained an additional 10 lbs. The patient realizes that his lifestyle is a problem and makes a commitment to make a change within the next 6 months. According to the transtheoretical model of behavior change, which of the following stages best fits this patient?

(A) precontemplation
(B) contemplation
(C) preparation
(D) action
(E) maintenance

69. A 19-year-old G1 whose last menses began 9 weeks ago comes to the emergency department because of heavy vaginal bleeding and lower abdominal cramping for 3 h. Her BP is 146/96 mmHg, and her pulse rate is 84min. A lower abdominal mass is palpable halfway between her symphysis and umbilicus. The cervix is closed, and there is active bleeding through the cervical os. On bimanual examination, the uterus is approximately 16 weeks' size. Fetal heart tones could not be heard, and a fetus is not seen by abdominal and transvaginal ultrasonography. Her serum hCG concentration is 80,000 mIU/mL, significantly higher than normal for a 9-week pregnancy. Which of the following is the most likely diagnosis?

(A) multiple gestation
(B) tubal pregnancy
(C) blighted ovum
(D) singleton pregnancy in a myomatous uterus
(E) hydatidiform mole

70. A 5-month-old child has a history of 2 days of rhinorrhea and 1 day of fever and worsening cough. She has been well prior to this time and has not previously had similar symptoms. On physical examination, she has inspiratory stridor. Which of the following should be considered in the differential diagnosis?

(A) acute bronchiolitis
(B) acute laryngotracheobronchitis
(C) a foreign body in the upper airway
(D) laryngomalacia
(E) peritonsillar abscess

Questions 71 through 73

A 7-year-old girl is brought to your office by her mother because she is having problems in school and at home. She is having temper tantrums, and is frequently oppositional. Her teachers noticed she was behind the other children last year and placed her in special education classes. Neuropsychiatric testing confirmed a below average intelligence quotient (IQ) with a full scale score of 66.

71. Which of the following syndromes/disorders is unlikely to be the cause of this child's mental retardation?

(A) Down syndrome
(B) fragile X syndrome
(C) fetal alcohol syndrome
(D) Turner syndrome
(E) Cri-du-chat syndrome

72. You obtain further historical information from her mother. She was hypotonic at birth. She has simian creases on her hands and is short is stature. You notice she has slanted palpebral fissures and a flat wide nasal bridge. She had a congenital heart defect repaired when she was 3 years old. What is the most likely cause of her condition?

(A) Down syndrome
(B) fragile X syndrome
(C) fetal alcohol syndrome
(D) Klinefelter syndrome
(E) Cri-du-chat syndrome

73. Which of the following is the most widely accepted and useful test for the assessment of intelligence in children?

(A) Stanford–Binet Test
(B) Metropolitan Achievement Test
(C) Wechsler Intelligence Scale for Children (WISC)
(D) Bellevue–Wechsler Scale
(E) Vineland Social Maturity Scale

Questions 74 and 75

A premenopausal woman complains of a thick, white, malodorous discharge. The pH is less than 4.5. There is no amine odor when potassium hydroxide is added to the discharge on a slide. There are no clue cells on wet smear. The microscopic appearance of the discharge is shown in Fig. 7-2.

74. Which of the following is the most likely cause of the discharge?

(A) *Gardnerella vaginalis*
(B) *Trichomonas vaginalis*
(C) *Chlamydia trachomatis*
(D) *Candida albicans*
(E) *Treponema pallidum*

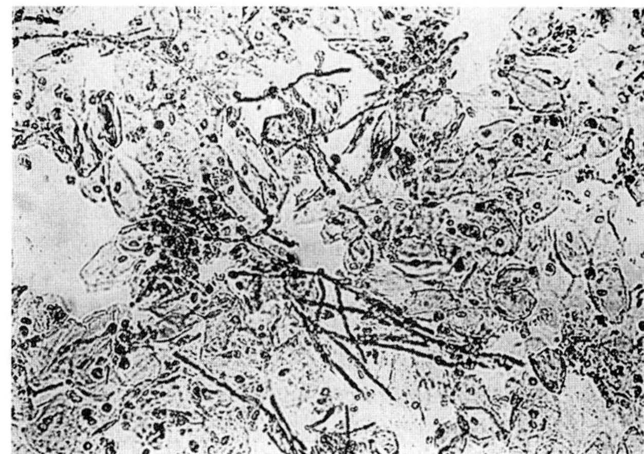

FIG. 7-2

75. Which of the following is the most appropriate treatment for the discharge seen in Fig. 7-2?

(A) oral metronidazole
(B) oral ketoconazole
(C) IM ceftriaxone
(D) oral azithromycin
(E) oral clindamycin

76. A 16-year-old girl comes to the clinic for a checkup. Her parents are concerned about her weight. Over the past year, she has lost 20 lbs. She has not been ill. She is an excellent student and active in many after-school activities. On physical examination, she is emaciated, hypothermic, and bradycardic. Which of the following is the most likely diagnosis?

(A) anorexia nervosa
(B) bulimia
(C) hyperthyroidism
(D) diabetes mellitus
(E) depression

77. A child is diagnosed with acute lymphoblastic leukemia (ALL). Which of the following is a favorable prognostic factor in ALL in childhood?

(A) age >7 years
(B) female gender
(C) initial WBC of 10,000
(D) presence of a mediastinal mass
(E) platelet count of 100,000

Questions 78 and 79

A 22-year-old man is brought to the emergency room of a general hospital by police. They report that he disturbed services at a church by walking in and announcing that he was Jesus Christ. The patient's mother comes to the emergency room soon after the patient's arrival and reports that her son had an episode of severe depression 2 years ago, but that he has never exhibited symptoms like his current ones. When the patient is examined, he talks rapidly and incessantly, insisting that he is the Messiah.

78. Which of the following is this patient's most likely diagnosis?

(A) bipolar I disorder
(B) bipolar II disorder
(C) paranoid schizophrenia
(D) hyperthyroidism
(E) hypothyroidism

79. Which of the following medications is most likely to be effective in the treatment of this patient?

(A) valproic acid
(B) fluoxetine
(C) clonazepam
(D) bupropion
(E) venlafaxine

Questions 80 through 82

A 19-year-old woman has never menstruated, although breast growth began about the age of 11 years. Pubic hair first appeared 6–12 months later. There are no affected family members. Her BP and pulse rate are 106/68 mmHg and 68/min, respectively. Her breasts and pubic hair are developed to Tanner stage 5. The vagina is very short and there is no cervix seen by speculum examination. A uterus cannot be palpated, despite an adequate bimanual examination.

80. Which of the following is the most appropriate next step in evaluating the cause of her amenorrhea?

(A) pelvic ultrasound
(B) CT scan of her pituitary
(C) laparoscopy
(D) serum estradiol
(E) karyotype

81. Which of the following is the most likely diagnosis?

(A) anorexia nervosa
(B) gonadal dysgenesis
(C) Müllerian agenesis
(D) testicular feminization
(E) 17α-hydroxylase deficiency

82. Which of the following is the best treatment for this woman's condition?

(A) surgical removal of her gonads
(B) HRT with estrogen alone
(C) hormone replacement with estrogen plus progestin
(D) glucocorticoid replacement
(E) creation of a vagina

83. A 78-year-old female presents to your office with a 2-year history of a cognitive decline which includes an impairment in short-term memory. Her husband brought her in because he is very worried about her. This past week she became lost coming home from the neighborhood grocery store. Which of the following is the most likely diagnosis?

(A) vascular dementia
(B) alcohol-related dementia
(C) Alzheimer dementia
(D) delirium NOS (not otherwise specified)
(E) Pick disease

84. A 15-year-old presents with a 3-week history of headache, drowsiness, and fever. On physical examination, there is mild nuchal rigidity and a third cranial nerve palsy on the left. A lumbar puncture is performed and shows an elevated white blood cell count with primarily monocytes, a protein of 750 g/100 mL, and a low glucose. The most likely organism is which of the following?

(A) *Mycobacterium tuberculosis*
(B) *Neisserria meningitis*
(C) *Streptococcus pneumoniae*
(D) *Haemophilus influenzae*
(E) *Salmonella typhimurium*

Questions 85 through 87

A 38-year-old married woman, the mother of two children and a medical social worker, is hospitalized with a diagnosis of breast cancer. She is anticipating surgery and then possible radiation and chemotherapy. Since arriving, she has been demanding, hostile, and uncooperative. She complained bitterly to the nurses about their insensitivity and rudeness. Her husband tried to reassure the nurses that "really, she is not like this at all," but then he left when his wife told him to "get out!" The nursing staff requested a psychiatric consult to medicate this "unreasonable, uncontrolled woman."

85. This patient's behavior is most likely

(A) indicative of borderline personality disorder
(B) the result of premenstrual syndrome (PMS)
(C) regression and acting out
(D) due to metastasis to the brain, giving rise to behavioral changes
(E) due to major depression with agitation

86. The nurses' anger is best described as an example of which of the following?

(A) acting out
(B) transference
(C) countertransference
(D) reaction formation
(E) splitting

87. Which of the following is the major goal of a psychiatrist evaluating this woman?

(A) determine the need for restraints
(B) determine the need to transfer her to another hospital
(C) set firm limits to her shouting and complaining
(D) help her identify and talk about her fears
(E) get specific information about specific nurses in order to file a grievance

Questions 88 and 89

A 27-year-old woman complains of progressive facial hirsutism and menstrual intervals that vary from 26 to 90 days. Her hirsutism and oligomenorrhea began shortly after menarche at the age of 13 years. She takes no medications with androgenic effects. Her family history is negative for hirsutism or oligomenorrhea. Her BP is normal. She has no galactorrhea, and her pelvic examination is normal except for a male pubic hair pattern. Her vagina contains rugae, and abundant clear mucus is present in the cervical canal.

88. Which of the following is the most appropriate diagnostic test?

(A) a pelvic ultrasound
(B) measurement of serum 17-hydroxyprogesterone
(C) an ACTH stimulation test
(D) a dexamethasone suppression test
(E) measurement of serum follicle-stimulating hormone (FSH)

89. The patient's serum 17-hydroxyprogesterone level is normal. In addition, her serum prolactin concentration is 13 ng/mL (normal, <20). Which of the following is the most likely diagnosis?

(A) polycystic ovary syndrome
(B) attenuated 21-hydroxylase deficiency
(C) pituitary adenoma
(D) Sertoli-Leydig cell tumor
(E) adrenal adenoma

Questions 90 through 92

A 52-year-old schoolteacher presents to the emergency department for evaluation of a tender, swollen, red left thigh. She just returned from spring break, during which she drove for 9 h one way to visit her parents. She is a smoker whose only medications are estrogen and progesterone. Her vital signs, including respiratory rate, are normal. Other than her leg, her examination is unremarkable.

90. Which of the following is the best initial step in her evaluation?

(A) ventilation-perfusion (VQ) scan
(B) pulmonary angiography
(C) duplex scanning of her left leg
(D) venogram
(E) pulse oximetry

91. After finding that she has thrombosis of the left femoral vein, she is admitted for IV heparin treatment. After 5 days of therapy, her platelets are noted to be 45,000. Admission platelets were 375,000. You make the diagnosis of heparin-induced thrombocytopenia (HIT). Which of the following is true about this syndrome?

(A) It usually occurs within hours after beginning heparin.
(B) Risk usually is dose-dependent and increases with higher doses.
(C) It usually produces marked thrombocytopenia with counts less than 20,000.
(D) There is an IgA antibody that binds to a complex of heparin and platelet factor 4.
(E) Risk is higher with use of porcine rather than bovine heparin.

92. Which of the following is the most common complication?

(A) bleeding
(B) arterial thrombosis
(C) deep venous thrombosis (DVT)
(D) stroke
(E) skin necrosis

93. An 11-month-old infant presents with poor growth, alopecia, large volume stools, and skin rash. You recall that this is consistent with acrodermatitis enteropathica. The findings in this disorder are caused by an inability to absorb which of the following?

(A) zinc
(B) vitamin K
(C) vitamin B_{12}
(D) copper
(E) iron

94. An 18-month-old boy presents with a 2-day history of intermittent vomiting and irritability. On physical examination, he looks uncomfortable, has right lower quadrant fullness, and a "currant jelly" stool in his diaper. Which of the following is the most likely diagnosis?

(A) constipation
(B) gastroenteritis
(C) intussusception
(D) Meckel's diverticulum
(E) volvulus

95. A 3-day-old infant is brought to the clinic because she is constipated. She was born at term and went home within 24 h. She has not had any stools since she was born. She has been breast feeding well and has not had any vomiting. Her mother thinks that her abdomen is bloated. On physical examination, her weight is equal to her birth weight. Her abdomen is distended, and there are no other abnormal findings. Which of the following is the most likely diagnosis?

(A) duodenal stenosis
(B) esophageal atresia
(C) functional constipation
(D) Hirschsprung's disease
(E) breast-feeding failure

96. A 6-month-old boy is brought to the clinic with a 1-day history of rectal bleeding. He has not had any pain or discomfort and has had no other symptoms. On physical examination, he looks well. His abdominal examination is normal. The diaper that the parents brought in is filled with dark red blood. Which of the following is the most likely diagnosis?

(A) anal fissure
(B) intussusception
(C) Meckel's diverticulum
(D) milk allergy
(E) volvulus

97. A 3-year-old boy is scheduled for a tonsillectomy. As part of his preoperative evaluation, coagulation studies are obtained. They are normal except for an increased bleeding time and a prolonged partial thromboplastin time (PTT). Which of the following is the most likely diagnosis?

(A) idiopathic thrombocytopenia purpura
(B) von Willebrand disease
(C) classic hemophilia
(D) deficiency in factors II, VII, IX, and X
(E) deficiency in factor IX

98. A 1-week-old infant is brought to the emergency department with a 1-day history of fever. He has also been irritable and been eating less than usual. On physical examination, he has a temperature of 39°C. He is irritable and inconsolable. Which of the following diagnostic studies should be done?

(A) complete blood count (CBC)
(B) CBC, blood culture
(C) CBC, blood culture, urinalysis (UA)
(D) CBC, blood culture, UA, urine culture
(E) CBC, blood culture, UA, urine culture, spinal tap

99. The appropriate diagnostic studies are obtained. Which of the following organisms is most likely to cause systemic infection in this infant?

(A) group A *Streptococcus*
(B) group B *Streptococcus*
(C) *Haemophilus influenzae*, type B
(D) *Listeria monocytogenes*
(E) *Staphylococcus aureus*

100. Which of the following organisms is most likely to cause acute cervical adenitis in an 8-month-old child?

(A) group A *Streptococcus*
(B) group B *Streptococcus*
(C) *Haemophilus influenzae*, type B
(D) *Pasteurella multocida*
(E) *Streptococcus pneumoniae*

101. An unmatched case-control study of the relationship between colon cancer and exposure to ionizing radiation reported the following data:

Ionizing radiation	Colon cancer Cases	Colon cancer Controls	Total
Yes	11	35	46
No	50	209	259
Total	61	244	305

These results indicate which of the following?

(A) The lifetime risk of colon cancer in the total population is approximately 20%.
(B) Among those without colon cancer, the odds of ionizing radiation exposure are about 1:5.
(C) Among those who were exposed to ionizing radiation, the estimated risk of colon cancer is 20.8%.
(D) The relative risk of colon cancer associated with exposure to ionizing radiation is approximated by an odds ratio of 1:3.
(E) The risk of colon cancer in the control group is 14.3%.

102. A 9-year-old girl with a history of intermittent wheezing for several years is brought to the pediatrician. The child has not been on medications for some time. Physical examination reveals a febrile child who is agitated and has perioral cyanosis. Intercostal and suprasternal retractions are present. The breath sounds are quiet, and wheezing is audible bilaterally. Which of the following is the most appropriate initial intervention?

(A) Prescribe IV aminophylline.
(B) Obtain a chest film.
(C) Prescribe nebulized cromolyn sodium.
(D) Obtain a CBC and blood culture.
(E) Prescribe nebulized albuterol.

103. A 4-year-old girl is brought to the office 2 days after she was bitten by her neighbor's cat. The bite is on her hand and occurred when she was teasing the cat. On physical examination, there are two closed puncture sites with erythema and induration around the wound. Which of the following organisms is most likely to cause the infection in this wound?

(A) *Rochalimaea henselae*
(B) *Eikenella corrodens*
(C) *Pasteurella multocida*
(D) *Francisella tularensis*
(E) *Spirillum minus*

104. A 26-year-old G1P0 woman presents to you for her first prenatal visit at 4 weeks gestation. The height and weight of the patient are measured, and you calculate her BMI to be 31. Which of the following recommendations concerning target weight gain for her pregnancy is most appropriate?

(A) You should limit weight gain to about 15 lbs.
(B) You should limit weight gain to about 40 lbs.
(C) You should roughly maintain your prepregnancy weight.
(D) You should attempt to lose a moderate amount of weight during the course of your pregnancy.
(E) You should not worry about weight gain or loss.

Questions 105 and 106

A 45-year-old man is involved in a motor vehicle accident after drinking heavily. He is brought to a general hospital, where he is treated for a fractured left femur. About 6 h after being admitted to the hospital, he begins to demonstrate tremulousness, which progresses to a pronounced tremor. He goes on to develop full-blown alcohol withdrawal delirium (delirium tremens) on the third day after admission. He becomes disoriented and diaphoretic, with a pulse rate of 120/min and BP of 220/140 mmHg. He reports seeing terrifying bugs in his room.

105. In addition to tremulousness and the clinical picture of delirium tremens outlined above, which of the following is a frequent complication of alcohol withdrawal?

(A) generalized seizures
(B) persistent stupor
(C) hyperglycemia
(D) hypernatremia
(E) hypermagnesemia

106. Which of the following medications can help prevent alcohol-induced persisting amnestic disorder (Wernicke's encephalopathy followed by Korsakoff syndrome) in patients such as this one?

(A) IV glucose
(B) IV thiamine
(C) IV lorazapam
(D) IV diazepam
(E) IV haloperidol

107. A 68-year-old woman with chronic obstructive pulmonary disease (COPD) is admitted in January with right middle lobe pneumonia. She lives at home with her husband, has two cats and two birds. Which of the following is the most likely cause of her pneumonia?

(A) *Staphylococcus aureus*
(B) *Chlamydia psittaci*
(C) influenza
(D) *Haemophilus influenzae*
(E) *Streptococcus pneumoniae*

108. A 30-year-old man tells you that he believes his headaches are a result of exposure to an aerosolized adhesive at work. Which of the following questions is most important to ask to determine whether the exposure caused the headaches?

(A) Are the headaches worse when you use more of the adhesive?
(B) What is in the adhesive (request the Material Safety Data Sheet corresponding to the product)?
(C) Do any coworkers have similar symptoms?
(D) When did the symptoms start?
(E) Do you have the headaches on days off?

109. Several people in a village in a developing nation have contracted brucellosis. You recommend that pasteurization be used to eliminate *Brucella* sp. from milk products consumed in the community. Which of the following best describes this sort of preventive measure?

(A) primary prevention
(B) secondary prevention
(C) tertiary prevention
(D) prophylactic prevention
(E) quaternary prevention

110. A 65-year-old woman presents to the physician's office for evaluation of depression. Past history is pertinent for passage of a kidney stone 1 month ago. Physical examination is unremarkable. Screening blood tests reveal a calcium of 12.8 and albumin of 4.0. Parathyroid hormone (PTH) assay reveals an elevated value of 328. Which of the following is the most likely etiology of her symptoms?

(A) parathyroid adenoma
(B) parathyroid hyperplasia
(C) multiple endocrine neoplasia type I (MEN I)
(D) multiple endocrine neoplasia type IIa (MEN IIa)
(E) parathyroid carcinoma

111. An envelope containing a fine powder was opened by a secretary in an office area. She fears that it may contain anthrax spores. Which of the following is true about anthrax as a weapon of mass destruction?

(A) Inhalation of spores is followed by a symptom-free incubation period of 1–6 days and then without warning, the sudden onset of a catastrophic illness, including hemoptysis, that generally results in death.
(B) The spore form is commonly found in the intestines of cattle, which generally are not made ill by anthrax.
(C) A person with inhalational anthrax is contagious, and respiratory isolation of potentially infected persons is an essential aspect of infection control.
(D) Immunity following recovery from anthrax is life long, and applies to all known strains.
(E) Inhalational anthrax is treatable with doxycycline or ciprofloxacin or amoxicillin if administered early.

112. An 8-month-old child has a temperature of 38.7°C. Physical examination reveals a non-toxic appearing child with no focal signs of infection on physical examination. A blood culture is obtained and is positive in 35 h. Which of the following organisms is most likely to be found in the blood culture?

(A) *Escherichia coli*
(B) *Haemophilus influenzae*
(C) *Staphylococcus aureus*
(D) *Streptococcus pneumoniae*
(E) *Neisseria meningitidis*

Questions 113 through 116

A 37-year-old woman is being evaluated for possible multiple sclerosis (MS). She began noting paresthesias in both legs intermittently several months ago and now has symptoms of urinary incontinence.

113. Which of the following physical findings is characteristic of MS?

(A) memory loss
(B) constipation
(C) internuclear ophthalmoplegia
(D) intention tremor
(E) bilateral upgoing toes

114. Which of the following is the best initial step in establishing the diagnosis?

(A) brain CT scan
(B) brain MRI
(C) EEG
(D) visual evoked potentials
(E) auditory evoked potentials

115. Which of the following is true about MS?

(A) Males are affected twice as often as females.
(B) Typical age of onset is in the fifth or sixth decade of life.
(C) Eighty percent of patients have the relapsing-remitting type MS.
(D) Fifty percent of patients have primary progressive MS.
(E) Optic neuritis typically is bilateral.

116. Which of the following medications is useful to hasten clinical recovery with an acute relapse of MS?

(A) interferon beta-1b
(B) cyclosporin
(C) methotrexate
(D) corticosteroids
(E) penicillins

117. A 40-year-old man last used IV drugs more than 10 years ago. Since that time he has been a moderate drinker of beer and wine. In the American population at large, what is the prevalence of the viral illness that is most likely to cause him to need a liver transplant?

(A) 0.1%
(B) 1%
(C) 2%
(D) 3%
(E) 4%

Questions 118 through 120

A 41-year-old man reports that he washes his hands 50 times a day. In the evening, he will check the doors, windows, and stove at least a dozen times before retiring for the night. He is fearful of the number 3; for example, he will not write out a check with a 3 in the number, and he will not stop his car if the odometer number ends in 3.

118. Which of the following is the most likely diagnosis?

(A) paranoid disorder
(B) paranoid schizophrenia
(C) schizotypal personality disorder
(D) obsessive-compulsive disorder (OCD)
(E) presenile dementia

119. Of the following drugs, which is recommended as a first choice to control this man's symptoms?

(A) fluvoxamine
(B) alprazolam
(C) buspirone
(D) risperidone
(E) lithium

120. The man wants to know if he can be treated nonpharmacologically. Successful therapeutic intervention would most likely be accomplished by which of the following?

(A) ECT
(B) behavioral therapy
(C) hypnosis
(D) short-term dynamic psychotherapy
(E) transcranial magnetic stimulation (TMS)

Questions 121 and 122

A 3-day-old term infant presents with progressive vomiting and abdominal distention. On questioning the nursery staff, they report that the child passed meconium at 48 h, but only after receiving a glycerin suppository. He has not tolerated oral feeds, and urine output has decreased over the preceding 12 h.

121. Which of the following diagnostic and/or therapeutic interventions is essential prior to transporting the child to a regional pediatric hospital?

(A) nasogastric tube decompression and IV fluid resuscitation
(B) sweat chloride determination
(C) plain abdominal radiographs
(D) blood and urine cultures, followed by initiation of broad-spectrum antibiotics
(E) barium enema

122. On arrival at the receiving pediatric hospital, which of the following is the most appropriate approach to establishing the diagnosis?

(A) anorectal manometry
(B) plain radiographs, followed by a barium enema, and subsequent rectal biopsy
(C) abdominal ultrasound
(D) sweat chloride
(E) laparotomy

123. A patient smokes two packs of cigarettes per day, and is an alcoholic. You tell him that he should stop smoking and that he should stop drinking alcohol. You explain that smokers have an average reduction in life expectancy of 6.6 years. What is the average change in life expectancy for alcoholics?

(A) 0.3 years
(B) no change
(C) 1 year
(D) –5 years
(E) –20 years

124. You apply a purified protein derivative (PPD) skin test to a 60-year-old healthy male from a rural area in the United States who is applying for a job in a hospital. Between 48 and 72 h later, you measure induration to be 6 mm and tell him the result was negative. Three weeks later, the test is repeated and induration measures 13 mm. Which of the following is the most appropriate next step in management?

(A) Repeat again in 2 months.
(B) Treat the new infection.
(C) Consider this to probably be a booster effect.
(D) Obtain sputum for culture.
(E) Check again immediately.

125. What is the current recommended strategy for lung cancer screening?

(A) chest x-ray every other year in a patient with greater than 50 pack-years of smoking
(B) chest x-ray every other year for everyone over 50 years old
(C) chest x-ray every year in a patient with greater than 50 pack-years of smoking
(D) chest x-ray every year for everyone over 50 years old
(E) screening is not recommended

126. Which of the following is a side effect of methotrexate?

(A) congestive heart failure
(B) peripheral neuropathy
(C) bone marrow depression
(D) hemorrhagic cystitis
(E) conduction hearing loss

127. A worker is returning to more active duty after having recovered from a difficult episode of radicular low back pain. She wants to avoid a recurrence. Her job will be to walk around on a concrete shop floor delivering parcels that weigh 15 lbs. Which of the following recommendations is most likely to help her avoid a recurrence?

(A) Seek transfer to a sit-down job on the light assembly line.
(B) Wear a back belt when lifting and carrying parcels.
(C) Use both hands to hold the parcel when holding a parcel out in an extended reach.
(D) Do light stretching, including back extensions, several times per day.
(E) Take ibuprofen 400 mg PO tid with food.

128. A 36-year-old alcoholic patient has cirrhosis and pancreatic insufficiency due to recurrent pancreatitis. He complains of night blindness, decreased ability to taste food, and dry skin with hyperpigmentation. These complaints suggest deficiency of which of the following?

(A) copper
(B) zinc
(C) selenium
(D) chromium
(E) manganese

129. Which of the following classes of medications causes chronic cough?

(A) angiotensin-converting enzyme (ACE) inhibitors
(B) calcium channel blockers
(C) fluoroquinolones
(D) HMG coreductase inhibitors
(E) cephalosporins

Questions 130 and 131

An investigator studies breast cancer. She enrolls 300 disease-free women to take part in a 10-year randomized prospective investigation designed to determine whether specific risk factors are responsible for disease.

130. Which of the following issues are inherent disadvantages of this type of study?

(A) It has a large potential for loss to follow-up.
(B) It is difficult to choose an appropriate control group.
(C) It is not good for studying more than one outcome.
(D) It not good for studying rates.
(E) It is not good for studying rare risk factors.

131. At the conclusion of the study, the investigator calculates the relative risk of developing breast cancer for a particular risk factor. Which of the following calculations will she do to calculate relative risk?

(A) (incidence in exposed persons + incidence in unexposed persons) – (incidence in unexposed persons)
(B) (incidence in exposed persons) – (incidence in unexposed persons)
(C) (incidence in exposed persons – incidence in unexposed persons)/ incidence in exposed persons
(D) (incidence in exposed persons)/ (incidence in unexposed persons)
(E) (incidence in exposed persons × incidence in unexposed persons)/100

Questions 132 and 133

A 52-year-old patient is seen in a walk-in medical clinic complaining of a headache. On examination, his BP is noted to be 210/140 mmHg. His retina shows hemorrhages and papilledema. Electrocardiogram shows left ventricular hypertrophy (LVH). BUN and creatinine are both elevated at 56 and 28.

132. On what basis can the diagnosis of malignant hypertension be made?

(A) the level of systolic BP
(B) the level of diastolic BP
(C) headache
(D) funduscopic changes
(E) heart size

133. Which of the following provides the best information regarding the prognosis of the malignant hypertension?

(A) the level of systolic BP
(B) the level of diastolic BP
(C) abnormalities of renal function
(D) future compliance
(E) heart size

134. A 64-year-old woman is brought to your office by her husband for evaluation of forgetfulness. She also has some word-finding problems and some paranoid delusions about the next-door neighbor. Which of the following is most specific for Alzheimer disease?

(A) normal score on the Beck Depression Inventory
(B) poor score on the Folstein mini-mental status examination
(C) mild cerebral atrophy on a brain CT scan
(D) rapid, resting tremor
(E) decreased bilateral parietal lobe activity on positron emission tomography (PET) scan

135. After a motor vehicle accident, your 49-year-old male patient presents complaining of pain in his left lower leg. On examination, you note bruising over his left calf and 1+ edema in his lower left leg. Compression ultrasonography immediately is ordered and is negative for DVT. Which of the following is the best next step in management?

(A) no follow-up needed
(B) venography
(C) CT scan of left leg
(D) referral to orthopedics
(E) repeat ultrasonography in 1 week

Answers and Explanations

1. **(C)**

2. **(D)**

Explanations 1 and 2

Antibiotic-associated colitis often occurs in elderly persons, after exposure to antibiotics, and is caused by enterotoxins produced by *C. difficile*. Whereas abdominal x-rays and CT scanning can demonstrate abnormal findings, detection of toxin in the stool will yield a definitive diagnosis. The appropriate treatment of patients with dehydration and abdominal symptoms would be IV fluids and admittance to the hospital for monitoring of their disease, discontinuation of the antibiotics that precipitated the disease, and institution of metronidazole. Barium enema should be avoided because it may precipitate complications. Whereas proctoscopy may be helpful, colonoscopy may precipitate perforation and should be avoided. *(Townsend et al., pp. 1428–1429; Greenfield et al., p. 196)*

3. **(E)** The single most effective intervention a physician can make in smoking cessation is delivering an unambiguous, nonjudgmental, informative statement on the need to quit smoking. It is especially helpful to deliver this message consistently over successive visits, and if effective and adapted, assistance and follow-up are provided. Physicians can help establish a "quit date," prepare the patient for withdrawal symptoms, and supply positive reinforcement on successive visits. Nicotine products may be useful for many smokers withdrawing from tobacco products. It is surprising how often clinicians fail to counsel smoking patients to stop using tobacco products. As per the year 2000 Public Health Service Guideline, the five "As" of tobacco cessation are: ask (whether smokes), advise (not to use tobacco), assess (readiness to quit), assist (in quit attempt), and arrange (for follow-up). *(U.S. Preventive Services Task Force p. 602; Wallace and Doebbeling, p. 812; U.S. Public Health Service, www.surgeongeneral.gov.; Lang and Hensrud, 2004)*

4. **(C)** Duodenal atresia presents with vomiting on the first day of life. The diagnosis is suspected when the abdominal film shows the "double bubble" sign shown in Fig. 7-1. Surgical repair is usually successful, and prognosis is excellent. Pyloric stenosis typically manifests after the second to third week of life, and the vomiting grows progressively worse as the pyloric muscle hypertrophies. The obstruction is rarely present at birth. Adrenogenital syndrome presents with vomiting at birth or shortly thereafter. Electrolyte abnormalities are a major issue. Esophageal atresia is excluded by passing a nasogastric tube into the stomach. Cystic fibrosis does not present with vomiting unless meconium ileus is present at birth. *(Townsend et al., pp. 2104–2108, 2111–2112)*

5. **(E)** This young man has psychotic symptoms. Of the medications listed, quetiapine is the only antipsychotic. This is a benzothiazepine with high affinity for serotonin types 2 and 6 (5-HT_2 and 5-HT_6), moderate affinity for dopamine type 2 (D_2) receptors, and lower for dopamine type 1 (D_1) and lower still for dopamine type 4 (D_4). It has been found effective for various psychotic disorders and is fairly new among the antipsychotic agents. Buspirone is a nonbenzodiazepine anxiolytic agent. Bupropion is an antidepressant drug recently experiencing renewed use in smoking cessation programs. Fluvoxamine, an antidepressant (selective serotonin reuptake inhibitor [SSRI]), and clomipramine, an antidepressant, have been of particular value in the treatment of OCD. *(Kaplan and Sadock, pp. 497–498, 1029–1032, 1127)*

doxycycline or a single dose of azithromycin would be effective treatment. For a pregnant woman, one would, for example, prescribe a course of amoxicillin, 500 mg by mouth three times per day for 7 days, or erythromycin, 500 mg by mouth four times per day for 7 days, or azithromycin, 1 g by mouth as a single dose, and maintain abstinence for 7 days. Repeat testing 3 weeks after treatment. *(USPSTF, pp. 1–80)*

22. (B)

23. (A)

Explanations 22 and 23

The presentation of a painful swelling involving the nipple areolar complex associated with erythema and subareolar fluid in a young woman are the typical findings of periductal mastitis and abscess. The organisms responsible for the disease are staphylococcal species and anaerobes. The diagnosis can be confused with inflammatory carcinoma, whose presentation includes peau d'orange, a solid mass, and other findings that usually involve larger areas of skin of the breast rather than localized to the nipple areolar complex. Paget's disease of the nipple is characterized by an eczematoid lesion; Mondor's disease usually affects the peripheral breast and represents superficial thrombophlebitis; and intraductal papilloma is usually nonpalpable and presents with a nipple discharge without inflammatory changes. An abscess can be treated with aspiration and antibiotics that cover both aerobic and anaerobic bacteria. Antibiotics alone would not be sufficient for an abscess, but can be used in patients with periareolar inflammation without abscess formation. Incision and drainage can be used, particularly if the abscess does not respond to nonoperative measures, but the patient must care for an open wound that may require weeks for healing. Lumpectomy and excisional biopsy are not appropriate therapies. *(Greenfield et al., p. 1349)*

24. (E) Levonorgestrel 0.75 mg every 12 h for two doses will prevent 75% of pregnancies when taken within 72 h of unprotected intercourse. This is sold as plan B. Effective postcoital contraception requires inhibition of the preovulatory luteinizing hormone (LH) surgery and subsequent ovulation. A triphasic oral contraceptive taken daily for 21 days will not prevent ovulation when begun on cycle day 16. Metho-trexate causes necrosis of actively dividing cells (e.g., trophoblasts) and will not suppress ovulation. Moreover, there is no clinical trial to demonstrate its effectiveness as a postcoital contraceptive. DES may be an effective postcoital contraceptive, but it has not been evaluated for this and will cause significant nausea and vomiting. Likewise, danazol has never been tested as a postcoital contraceptive. *(Scott et al., p. 555)*

25. (B) The Women's Health Initiative (WHI) is a National Institute of Health (NIH) funded randomized, prospective, controlled, double blind clinical trial of combination estrogen + progestin, estrogen only (in women who had a prior hysterectomy), and no HRT. After 5.5 years the investigators stopped the combination HRT arm of the study because of a 26% increase in breast cancer (38/10,000 vs. 30/10,000 women). About 1 year later, the estrogen only arm was stopped because of an increase in breast cancer in the treated group. Though the increase in both arms was not statistically significant, the treatment arms were stopped because the frequency exceeded the predicted acceptable risk established by the study's Data Safety Monitoring Board before the study began. Primarily as a consequence of the WHI results, the Food and Drug Administration (FDA) has established recommendations for the use of HRT: (1) indicated for relief of menopausal symptoms (hot flashes, vaginal dryness), (2) the lowest effective dose, (3) the shortest possible duration of treatment, (4) use of alternatives if the indication is other than symptomatic relief, such as osteoporosis prevention. The addition of a progestin does not seem to reduce this risk, and may actually increase the risk further. Despite serious concerns about methodologic problems in these studies (small number of women with breast cancer, selection bias, ascertainment bias, and so forth), women should be informed of this potential risk, but also informed of the benefits of HRT.

Although estrogen given alone increases the risk of endometrial adenocarcinoma three-to eight-fold, estrogen replacement given with adequate progesterone supplementation actually decreases the likelihood of developing endometrial carcinoma. At least 70 mg of medroxyprogesterone acetate (Provera, Cycrin) monthly is necessary to prevent an increased risk of endometrial cancer. Culture and attitude, plus the availability of a suitable sexual partner, is more responsible than estrogen deficiency for the decline in sexual activity and response after menopause. Estrogen replacement will stabilize bone mineral density but will not increase it. Evidence is increasing that estrogen replacement decreases the risk of colon cancer. *(Speroff and Fritz, pp. 689–777)*

26. (C) Roseola infantum (also known as exanthema subitum) is a common disease of childhood. It is seen predominantly in infants between the ages of 6 and 24 months and typically causes temperatures as high as 38.9–40.5°C (102–105°F) for 3–5 days without accompanying symptoms. Physical examination is frequently normal but may reveal mild pharyngeal injection, suboccipital lymphadenopathy, or a bulging anterior fontanel. Defervescence then occurs, followed closely by the development of a truncal maculopapular rash, which fades after 2–3 days. It is most often caused by human herpes virus-6. It is the appearance of a rash after the cessation of fever that differentiates roseola infantum from other infectious exanthems. Measles is characterized by a generalized red, blotchy rash in a febrile individual with cough, coryza, conjunctivitis, and photophobia. The typical fine red papular rash of scarlet fever usually appears at the height of fever. Kawasaki disease is characterized by conjunctivitis, oral lesions, cervical adenitis, fever for 5 days, palmar or plantar erythema, and desquamation from the fingers or toes. The accompanying red rash is nonspecific. The rash in erythema infectiosum is a bright red rash on the cheeks (slapped cheek), followed by a reticular rash on the extremities. *(Rudolph et al., pp. 1029, 1031, 1222–1223)*

27. (D) Patients with terminal illnesses have specific needs and present particular problems for in-hospital and outpatient management. Families are often fearful, confused, and unclear as to how to relate to these patients. House officers are not immune to this problem. Analgesics for pain relief are generally more efficacious when administered on a regular schedule, allowing the patient to refuse. The inappropriate use of prn regimens stems from a prevalent but unsubstantiated fear that patients will become addicted to the medication. In fact, studies have shown that fewer than 1% of patients treated with pain medication become addicted. Patients confronting death are acutely socially sensitive, and miscommunications or evasive discussions are interpreted with the most negative outlook. Patients generally prefer honest information, especially if they have to make decisions about subjecting themselves to often painful procedures and treatments. Checking with the patient on how much information he or she would like about the illness helps clarify the direction the physician will follow to effectively address the patient's information needs. Studies of groups of terminally ill patients with metastatic carcinoma described group therapy as an exceptionally effective mode of treatment. It offers a close support system based on a common bond and allows the patients to learn from each other how to cope and how to help their loved ones cope with the stresses of terminal illness. *(Kaplan and Sadock, pp. 1338–1347)*

28. (A) Congenital adrenal hyperplasia may be caused by many different defects of steroidogenesis. The most common defect, 21-hydroxylase deficiency, accounts for about 95% of these disorders and is transmitted as an autosomal-recessive trait. These patients have aldosterone deficiency, which results in hyponatremia, hyperkalemia, hypotension, and shock. They also have glucocorticoid deficiency and, therefore, have hypoglycemia. The electrolyte abnormalities are the key to the diagnosis. None of the other diseases listed would cause this degree of electrolyte abnormality. *(Rudolph et al., p. 2030)*

29. (A) The leading cause of massive bleeding per rectum in the older population is angiodysplasia and diverticulosis of the colon. The absence of abdominal findings suggests these possibilities rather than an inflammatory process. *(Way and Doherty, pp. 736–738)*

30. **(E)** A sentinel, or herald, bleed is common in patients with an aortoenteric fistula. The key point in the history is prior aneurysm repair with a graft. The location of the fistula is the third or fourth portion of the duodenum, so UGI endoscopy to the duodenal bulb would miss the lesion. Immediate operation is indicated because these patients will suffer a subsequent life-threatening bleed. *(Townsend et al., p. 1255)*

31. **(G)** Colon carcinoma may be the source of chronic blood loss that often presents with fatigue and orthostasis, particularly from a right-sided lesion. Abdominal fullness and tenderness is suggestive of a large, right-sided colon cancer. *(Townsend et al., pp. 1457–1458; Way and Doherty, pp. 718–719)*

32. **(I)** Bleeding from acute gastric ulcer may occur and become life threatening, especially in the elderly taking nonsteroidal anti-inflammatory drugs (NSAIDs). Immediate operation is indicated following resuscitation. *(Greenfield et al., pp. 762–763, 1048–1049)*

33. **(H)** Varices account for 10% of UGI bleeding and are suggested in patients with an alcohol history and examination findings suggestive of cirrhosis. *(Way and Doherty, p. 580)*

34. **(F)** Peptic ulcer disease is the most common cause of acute UGI hemorrhage. Duodenal ulcers occur slightly more frequently than gastric ulcers. Brisk hemorrhage occurs from the gastroduodenal artery from a posterior penetrating ulcer in the duodenal bulb. *(Greenfield et al., pp. 760–761, 1048–1049)*

35. **(B)** The features of ulcerative colitis include age of onset usually between 15 and 40 years, bloody diarrhea, abdominal pain, and fever. Bloody diarrhea is the major symptom in 25% of patients. *(Greenfield et al., pp. 1073–1074; Townsend et al., p. 1428)*

36. **(C)** The most common cause of secondary amenorrhea in reproductive-age women is pregnancy. Therefore, a pregnancy test should be the first step in the evaluation of secondary amenorrhea. Her complaint of hot flashes and vaginal dryness suggest estrogen deficiency as a cause of her amenorrhea. Estrogen deficiency may occur as a result of hypothalamic-pituitary failure and the loss of FSH and LH secretion leading to a diminished ovarian estrogen secretion. The presence of hot flashes suggests that the loss of estrogen is the result of ovarian failure, because hot flashes typically occur as a result of (a) presence of estrogen, followed by loss of estrogen and (b) increased FSH and LH concentrations. Hypothyroidism and hyperprolactinemia can also cause secondary amenorrhea. Serum estradiol concentrations are less useful in assessing the cause of amenorrhea than measurement of FSH. A decreased estradiol concentration occurs with either hypothalamic-pituitary failure or ovarian failure. A decreased serum FSH concentration indicates hypothalamic-pituitary failure, whereas, an elevated FSH concentration indicates ovarian failure. A serum testosterone concentration is appropriate only if the amenorrhea is accompanied by signs of androgen excess (e.g., hirsutism, deepening of the voice, clitoral enlargement, and so forth). *(Speroff and Fritz, pp. 404–409)*

37. **(A)** Oral contraceptives are absolutely contraindicated in women over 35 who smoke because there is an additive risk of smoking and estrogen for heart attack and stroke. The other choices are all relative contraindications that require clinical judgment, thorough discussion with the patient about contraceptive options, and informed consent. The discussion and consent must be documented in the medical record. In this author's opinion, the patient should be counseled to choose a nonhormonal contraceptive method or at least a hormonal contraceptive that does not contain estrogen (e.g., a progestin-only oral contraceptive or Depot medroxyprogesterone acetate). Transdermal and transvaginal contraception likely have the same heart attack and stroke risk as a combination oral contraceptive. *(Speroff and Fritz, p. 906)*

38. **(B)** DDH, formerly called congenital dislocation of the hip, is a relatively common problem, with a frequency of 1.5–10 per 1000 live births. Genetic factors seem to have a major role, with the disorder being especially prevalent among certain ethnic groups. It is common in Northern Italy and Japan and among Navajo Native Americans, but rare in Blacks and Chinese. Girls are affected six to eight times more often than are boys. However, nongenetic factors also play a part. Uterine crowding and mechanical problems in the uterus appear to predispose to DDH. For example, DDH is more common with breech presentation and more common in firstborn children. Type of delivery is not related to the incidence of DDH. *(Rudolph et al., pp. 2434–2436)*

39. **(E)** NMS is a rare, potentially fatal complication of the use of antipsychotic medication. Symptoms typically include high fever, delirium, and rigidity, and they usually develop within a week of starting a new drug or raising the dosage of the currently prescribed drug. Once NMS is suspected, the antipsychotic drug should be stopped and emergency supportive measures begun. Mortality from NMS has been reported to be as high as 20%. *(Kaplan and Sadock, pp. 993–994)*

40. **(A)** To determine the likelihood that a person with a positive test truly has the disease (to determine the positive predictive value of the test), you must know the sensitivity of the test and also must know the prevalence. If no one has the disease, no one testing positive will have the disease. If everyone has the disease, everyone testing positive will have the disease. Positive predictive value = true positives divided by true positives plus false positives. *(Greenberg et al., p. 79)*

41. **(C)**

42. **(E)**

43. **(E)**

Explanations 41 through 43

This patient has carbon monoxide poisoning, first requiring oxygen. Initial fluid resuscitation in burn injury is isotonic crystalloid. Colloid is not recommended in the first 24 h because of the profound capillary leak associated with the early injury phase. The most common formula for fluid resuscitation in burn injury is the Parkland formula. This is based on body weight and percentage of body surface area (BSA) burned; that is, 4 mL × body weight (kg) × %BSA = mL resuscitation fluid/first 24 h. One-half of this amount is given in the first 8 h after the burn, with the remainder over the next 16 h. This fluid is given in addition to the patient's maintenance fluid requirements. Patients with circumferential burn injury are at risk of developing compartment syndrome. Burn wound edema increases the enclosed compartment pressure above systemic perfusion pressures, resulting in tissue ischemia. The patient will have pain in the affected extremity, especially with passive stretch. The limb will demonstrate signs of decreased distal perfusion, including pallor, decreased sensation, and motor weakness. Compartment pressure is relieved with emergency escharotomy. Elevation of the extremity is not appropriate as it will further diminish distal perfusion. Supplemental oxygen by mask is an ineffective means of increasing oxygen delivery because of diminished perfusion to the affected limb. *(Townsend et al., pp. 576–578; Greenfield et al., pp. 433–436, 439–440)*

44. **(A)** Raloxifene is a SERM that acts as an estrogen in some systems and as an antiestrogen in others. Currently, it is approved by the FDA only for prevention and treatment of osteoporosis. Bone mineral density is increased approximately 3% after 24 months. Raloxifene exerts no effect on HDL cholesterol concentrations but does lower total cholesterol and LDL cholesterol concentrations. Evidence that there is a cardioprotective effect in humans is currently mixed. It acts as an antiestrogen in the hypothalamus; as a result, approximately 25% of women who take raloxifene experience hot flashes (vs. approximately 18% receiving a placebo). It also acts as an antiestrogen in the reproductive tract. Endometrial stripe thickness does not increase in response to raloxifene, and there is no change from an atrophic endometrium with its use. Preliminary data support the conclusion that raloxifene reduces the risk of breast cancer by

about 60% after 4 years of continuous use. *(Speroff and Fritz, p. 700)*

45. **(D)** Aspirin is well absorbed from both the stomach and small intestine. Removal from the body involves both hepatic and renal pathways. Treatment is indicated when the ingested dose exceeds 100 mg/kg, and intensity of therapy is guided by the severity of the ingestion as estimated by serum salicylate levels in relationship to time since ingestion. Therapeutic intervention is aimed at limiting absorption of aspirin from the gastrointestinal tract (effectively accomplished by gastric lavage and administration of activated charcoal) and enhancing renal excretion of the drug. Maintenance of high urine flow aids rapid clearance and alkalinization of the urine results in an ionized form of the drug that is poorly reabsorbed from the renal tubule, thus increasing excretion. *N*-acetylcysteine has no place in the treatment of aspirin poisoning. It is, however, quite effective in preventing the hepatotoxicity associated with severe acetaminophen overdose. Induced emesis is rarely used in the emergency department because it tends to delay the administration of activated charcoal. Several studies have not shown any benefit from the addition of cathartics to charcoal in the management of acute aspirin ingestions. *(Ellenhorn, pp. 210–221)*

46. **(A)** The third U.S. Preventive Services Task Force (USPSTF) strongly recommends that clinicians routinely screen all sexually active women aged 25 and younger, and other asymptomatic women at increased risk, for chlamydia. *(USPSTF, pp. 1–80)*

47. **(C)** Carpal tunnel syndrome is secondary to compression of the median nerve at the wrist. This compression neuropathy affects women more often than men. The patient may experience weakness of the hand, which is typically worse at night and relieved by shaking the hand on awakening. There is hypesthesia in the median nerve distribution, and when long-standing, there may be atrophy of the thenar muscles. Management includes wrist splinting, anti-inflammatory agents, steroid injection, and avoiding repetitive movement of the hand and wrist. Surgical decompression may be required if nonoperative measures do not relieve symptoms. Compression of the digital nerve of the thumb produces paresthesias limited to the affected digit. The motor branch of the median nerve may be compressed in the palm secondary to direct trauma. Median nerve compression by the pronator teres is usually associated with forearm pain in addition to paresthesias in the nerve distribution. *(Townsend et al., p. 2221; Way and Doherty, p. 1280; Greenfield et al., pp. 2123–2124)*

48. **(E)** Postpartum amenorrhea in a woman with postpartum hemorrhage, especially if the pregnancy was complicated by hypertension, is most likely the result of Sheehan syndrome. This is a disorder caused by pituitary necrosis and resulting in gonadotropin deficiency. More severe forms will include deficiency of other pituitary trophic hormones, including TSH and ACTH. The clinical clue that reinforces this diagnosis is the inability to lactate. This is presumed to be the result of necrosis of pituitary lactotropes and severely decreased pituitary prolactin secretion. Endometrial sclerosis or cervical stenosis would be more likely if the history included a postpartum dilation and curettage (D&C) to control the hemorrhage. Although there is no clinical information to exclude polycystic ovary syndrome or premature ovarian failure, these are unlikely and, for premature ovarian failure, would be coincidental, not causally related to the obstetric hemorrhage. *(Cunningham et al., p. 638)*

49. **(C)** Dislocation of the radial head, also known as "nursemaid's elbow," is a very common condition of young children between the ages of 1 and 4 years. It is caused by sudden traction on the forearm, resulting in dislocation of the radial head from the capitulum of the humerus. The child holds the affected arm in flexion at the elbow with the forearm pronated. X-rays reveal no abnormalities. Treatment is by swift supination of the forearm; further treatment is usually not necessary with the first occurrence. *(McMillan et al., p. 1037)*

50. (E) Acne is a skin disorder with its onset in puberty, when testosterone derived from the gonads and adrenal glands stimulates sebaceous gland activity. This results in the formation of sebum, which contains triglycerides, squalene, wax esters, sterol esters, and phospholipids. Propionibacterium acnes, an anaerobic pleomorphic skin organism, produces a lipase that releases free fatty acids from the sebum mixture, including highly irritating medium-chain triglycerides. Individuals prone to acne seem to have an increased turnover of abnormally cohesive keratinized cells in the sebaceous duct; these accumulate, plug the duct, and inhibit the release of sebum to the skin surface. Acne tends to persist until the late teens or early twenties. Too frequent or too vigorous face washing can be irritating to the skin and actually worsen the acne. Diet seems to be of little importance in the etiology of acne. The treatment goals are to decrease the risk of scarring and to alleviate the psychologic stress during these critical years of social and sexual development. Adolescents with mild to moderate acne usually respond to topical treatment. Therapy should be individualized, but benzoyl peroxide and tretinoin is a reasonable combination for initial therapy. *(Rudolph et al., pp. 1208–1210)*

51. (C) Neurally mediated syncope (also called vasovagal or neurocardiogenic) is most common as a cause of syncope. Studies from the 1980s showed that approximately 24% of syncope is neurally mediated and 34% had an unknown cause. More recently, through increased use of tilt table testing, about 50–66% of the cases previously classified as unknown are now thought to be neurally mediated. Medications cause approximately 3%, psychiatric disorders 2%, and arrhythmias 14%. *(Kapoor, pp. 1856–1862)*

52. (B) In a historical cohort study, the cohort is formed in the past, classified by exposure status, and followed forward in time to determine the development of disease. This study is not ecologic in design, because information on individual subjects was collected. It was not a cross-sectional design, because new occurrences of bronchitis since employment were used to calculate risk. It was not a randomized, controlled trial, because the investigator did not have anything to do with who works inside or outside of the post office. It was not a prospective cohort design, because the cohort was defined in the past. *(Wallace and Doebbeling, pp. 18, 19; Greenberg et al., pp. 116, 117)*

53. (C) A mass immunization program is indicated. Preventive treatment with rifampin is usually limited to close contacts such as household members, day care center contacts, and people exposed to the patient's oral secretions. Sending students home 2 months early will only redistribute exposed persons. A case-control study will be difficult, since there are so many exposure variables and it will take time to do. An education campaign can help with early detection, not with prevention. Immunizations will be more effective. Most of the sporadic outbreaks in this country are due to serotype C meningococcus, which is covered by the vaccine. Rates of asymptomatic carriage are high, and it may be impractical to eliminate all carriage in a population. It is not clear why a general population with many carriers may suddenly erupt with several cases of disease. Preventing disease through vaccination remains the best method in the face of an outbreak. Note that immunization is not protective for the serotype that generally affects children of less than 1 year of age. *(Wallace and Doebbeling, p. 206; Lang and Hensrud, 2004)*

54. (B)

55. (C)

Explanations 54 through 55

Cardiac tamponade results from rapid accumulation of fluid in the pericardial sac, compromising cardiac filling and resulting in decreased cardiac output. The clinical findings of tachycardia, hypotension, and distant heart sounds in the presence of penetrating chest trauma should alert the physician to this diagnosis. Patients may also demonstrate jugular venous distention from decreased venous return to the right heart, and a diminished pulse pressure. Penetrating trauma with an entry wound in this location (fifth intercostal space midclavicular line) would be unlikely to injure the descending aorta. From anatomic landmarks, the left atrium and left ventricle are directly in the path of penetration. A massive hemothorax or tension pneumothorax would be associated with respiratory compromise, decreased breath sounds on the side of injury, and tracheal shift to the contralateral side. Phrenic nerve paralysis would affect diaphragmatic function and lead to altered ventilatory mechanics secondary to paradoxical movement of the hemidiaphragm. Pericardiocentesis is both diagnostic and therapeutic and should be the first step in management. Aspiration of as little as 10–20 mL may improve the patient's hemodynamic status. Once stabilized, the patient should be transferred to the operating room for definitive management of the underlying penetrating cardiac injury. This patient does not have respiratory compromise and would, therefore, not require assisted ventilation or chest tube insertion. The patient's hypotension may not respond to IV fluid bolus, but requires urgent pericardial decompression to improve venous return and cardiac output. Emergency department thoracotomy is reserved for patients with penetrating chest trauma who arrive in the emergency department with measurable vital signs and subsequently suffer cardiopulmonary arrest. The thoracotomy permits open cardiac massage, and attempt at manual control of blood loss from the site of injury, in preparation for rapid transfer to the operating room. *(Townsend et al., pp. 506, 508–510)*

56. **(C)** Reported rates of stillbirth in mothers with syphilis were 14–34%, a dramatic increase as compared to the 0.7% in the general population. Mean birth weights are decreased significantly in infected mothers. This is the result of both preterm labor and intrauterine growth restriction. Women with primary or secondary syphilis are more likely to transmit infection to their fetus than are those with late or latent syphilis. Most infants with early congenital syphilis do not develop evidence of active disease for 10–14 days after birth. Despite the possibility of immune suppression in HIV-infected women, serologic tests for syphilis are accurate in mother and infant. *(Sweet and Gibbs, pp. 150–161)*

57. **(B)** Septic pelvic thrombophlebitis should be suspected in women with postpartum fever that fails to respond to broad-spectrum antibiotics, and whose physical examination is normal. CT scan or MRI of the pelvis may disclose pelvic vein phlebitis. The clinical impression that anticoagulant doses of heparin result in a rapid defervescence is not supported by convincing clinical data. Infectious causes of postpartum fever usually respond to broad-spectrum antibiotics within 48–72 h. A pelvic abscess is usually easy to palpate on bimanual examination and may be anterior or posterior to the uterus. Subinvolution of the uterus, increased uterine tenderness, and increased postpartum bleeding with a foul lochia are the signs of postpartum endometritis. Pyelonephritis should also have responded to antibiotics within 48–72 h. Breast engorgement may cause a fever within 24–48 h postpartum, but the fever resolves without antibiotics. *(Cunningham et al., pp. 681–682)*

58. **(C)** The most likely illness is staphylococcal food poisoning, resulting from contamination by a food handler. Often, the handler has evidence of an infection. The victims exhibit classic symptoms of abrupt, often violent nausea, vomiting, abdominal cramps, and prostration. They frequently feel feverish and perspire, but they are not febrile. Diarrhea is frequent, but not the dominant complaint. The illness is caused by a heat-stable enterotoxin produced from *S. aureus*. Regarding the food handler, *S. aureus* is a common organism found in mucocutaneous infections. In outbreaks like this, infected lesions on food handlers can sometimes be found. Transmission is usually from an infected food handler to foodstuffs that are prepared ahead of time and then held at suboptimal temperatures, which allows the organism time to replicate and produce enterotoxin. Because the toxin is heat stable, rewarming the food and keeping it hot on a serving table will not neutralize it. The toxin is preformed when ingested, so there is no incubation time required in the victim. Therefore, onset is usually rapid. *(Wallace and Doebbeling, pp. 724, 727)*

59. **(B)** The clinical symptoms of iron toxicity are divided into stages. In a significant ingestion, the first stage begins immediately after the ingestion and lasts 6–24 h. Vomiting, diarrhea, abdominal pain, pallor, lethargy, and hypotension can be seen. These result from the direct toxicity to the GI tract and GI hemorrhage can occur. Liver failure and an associated coagulopathy can occur but not typically until 12–24 h after the ingestion. Arrhythmias and respiratory symptoms are not seen with iron ingestions. If a patient does not develop symptoms within 6 h of ingestion, it is unlikely that iron toxicity will develop. *(Ellenhorn, pp. 1558–1562)*

60. **(C)** Numerous complications of Epstein-Barr virus-associated mononucleosis have been described, such as hematologic complications, hemolytic anemia, and thrombocytopenia. Neuro-logic complications include aseptic meningitis, encephalitis, optic neuritis, Guillain–Barré syndrome, transverse myelitis, and Bell's palsy. Splenic rupture is rare but potentially fatal. Often, it follows mild trauma. Although liver involvement is not uncommon acutely, chronic active hepatitis has not been described. Pancreatitis and azotemia have not been described. *(Rudolph et al., pp. 1035–1038)*

61. **(C)** Interviewing the patient is critical to determining her needs. Ideally, this would be with her alone. Patients frequently will provide important information about themselves. They may not if a family member is present. All other options listed are premature. Prescribing sertraline, lorazepam, or ECT require a thorough evaluation of the patient's history, symptoms, psychosocial situation, and so forth before determining a course of action. A family conference may be of real value, but should follow interview of the patient. *(Kaplan and Sadock, pp. 229–233)*

62. **(D)** If you observe a pattern consistent with poisoning by a chemical weapon of mass destruction, leave the scene and call 911 immediately. Do not become the next helpless victim. Rapidly developing (over the course of minutes) twitching, vomiting, difficulty breathing, pinpoint pupils, coma, and death are typical of poisoning with the potent organophosphate nerve gas sarin. *(Wallace and Doebbeling, pp. 1169– 1173)*

63. **(A)** Dose-related and cumulative renal insufficiency is the major dose-limiting toxicity of cisplatin. The main route of excretion of cisplatin is through the kidneys, and good hydration may help minimize potential tubular damage. Other toxic reactions include myelosuppression and neurotoxicity. Dermatitis, cystitis, and decreased visual acuity are not toxic effects of cisplatin. Cisplatin is commonly used to treat ovarian cancer. *(Frank, pp. 48–58; Kasper et al., pp. 475, 555)*

64. **(C)** When the prevalence of the screened-for-disease increases in a population, the positive predictive value of the screening test also increases. (If no persons in the population have the disease, the PPV will be 0%. If all persons in the population have the disease, the PPV will be 100%.) The sensitivity and specificity of the test are not affected by the prevalence of the disease. Accuracy refers to the specificity and sensitivity of the test, which are characteristics of the test itself, and thus is not affected by prevalence. A reliable test reproduces the same results when it is repeated. (Just as a very reliable gun will always hit a target in exactly the same place, although it may not be hitting the bull's eye.) *(Wallace and Doebbeling, pp. 907–908)*

65. **(B)** The triad of hypertension, hyperreflexia, and proteinuria in pregnancy establishes the diagnosis of preeclampsia. The etiology is still unknown, and the only accepted treatment at term pregnancy is delivery of the infant. The risk of eclampsia is not proportional to the increase in systolic or diastolic pressure and has been reported to occur at the time of normal BP readings. Beta blockers are not contraindicated in pregnancy, although ACE inhibitors are contraindicated. Beta-blocking drugs effectively lower BP, and are most effectively used when the pregnant woman is early in the third trimester and prolongation of pregnancy is desired. The risk of abruptio placenta, not the risk of placenta previa, is increased in hypertensive pregnant women. Perinatal mortality is significantly increased in pregnant women with hypertension and proteinuria. In one study, it was increased threefold in women whose diastolic BPs were 105 torr or higher. *(Cunningham et al., pp. 569–608)*

66. (B) Classically, there are three stages of labor. The first stage begins with the onset of regular uterine contractions that cause cervical dilation and ends with complete dilatation of the cervix. The first stage can be divided into a latent phase and an active phase. In a primigravida, the length of the latent and active phases average 8.6 and 4.9 h, respectively. Both times are shorter in women who have had a child. The second stage begins with complete dilatation of the cervix and ends with delivery of the infant. The third stage begins after delivery of the infant and ends with delivery of the placenta. Subsequent events such as myometrial contractions, inspection of the cervix and vagina, and repair of an episiotomy or laceration are not recognized as a stage of labor. *(Cunningham et al., pp. 252–262)*

67. (B) Taxol is frequently used in the treatment of advanced epithelial ovarian cancers. Originally, it was derived from the bark of the western yew tree, but can now be chemically synthesized. It is a mitotic spindle inhibitor, but acts in a manner different from other such inhibitors. Taxol promotes assembly of microtubules and stabilizes them, thus preventing depolymerization and cell duplication. Myelosuppression is the major toxic effect that limits the utility of taxol, and other typical side effects of chemotherapy, such as alopecia, nausea, vomiting, and peripheral neuropathies, are also seen. *(Snow et al., pp. 57–64)*

68. (B) According to the transtheoretical model of behavior change, a patient in the contemplation stage of behavior change is a person who has some motivation to change and has made a commitment to do so within the next 6 months. The precontemplation stage represents a stage at which an individual has no consideration of change and this may be because he/she is not aware of the behavior or its consequences. The action stage occurs when individuals modify their activities, experiences, or environment in order to change behavior. It represents the first 6 months of actual behavior change. The maintenance stage represents the period during which the individual works toward preventing relapse. It usually represents the period after the first 6 months of behavior change. A preparation stage is sometimes added to refer to those planning definitive change within 1 month and having already initiated some changes in behavior. Relapse also is sometimes referred to as a stage. *(Lang and Hensrud, pp. 61–63; Wallace and Doebbeling, p. 812)*

69. (E) Hypertension before the third trimester, uterine size greater than dates, and the absence of a fetus with a detectable heartbeat after 6 postmenstrual weeks strongly suggests a diagnosis of gestational trophoblastic disease, most likely a hydatidiform mole. A multiple pregnancy is not a consideration because gestational sacs, each containing a fetus, with cardiac activity in each sac, would be seen by transvaginal ultrasonography after 6 postmenstrual weeks. Although the absence of an intrauterine pregnancy is ultrasonic evidence of a tubal pregnancy, the ectopic gestational sac is usually seen when the hCG concentration is 10,000 mIU/mL or higher. The presence of a significantly enlarged uterus does not favor a diagnosis of tubal pregnancy. Serum hCG concentrations are lower than expected with a blighted ovum, and the uterus tends to be smaller than the gestational age. The elevated hCG concentration, the hypertension, and the absence of a fetus with a heartbeat is against the diagnosis of a normal intrauterine pregnancy in a woman with a myomatous uterus. Management of this patient is evacuation of the uterus by suction curettage and serial hCG measurements for 1 year to be certain that this woman does not subsequently develop choriocarcinoma. *(Scott et al., pp. 1019–1030)*

70. (B) Any condition that causes narrowing of the upper airway may result in inspiratory stridor. This includes acute laryngotracheobronchitis or croup. This patient has the typical history and examination seen in patients with croup. Laryngomalacia is a condition of unusual softness of the larynx, resulting in inspiratory collapse and stridor. The condition is present early in infancy and usually resolves by 3–5 years. Patients with laryngomalacia have chronic stridor. Conditions that cause narrowing of the conducting system of the lower respiratory tract, such as bronchiolitis, result in wheezing. Foreign bodies are more common in children between the ages of 1 and 4 years, when they tend to put things in their mouths. Peritonsillar abscess is seen in older children and adolescents. *(Kliegman, pp. 83–84)*

71. **(D)** Down syndrome, fragile X syndrome, fetal alcohol syndrome, and cri-du-chat syndrome all are associated with mental retardation. Persons with Turner syndrome (XO) have a female habitus, but because of the lack of the second X chromosome, there is an agenesis or dysgenesis of the gonads. No secondary sexual characteristics develop without treatment. Short stature, webbed neck, and low posterior hairline are common. Later medical management is necessary to assist them with their infertility and absence of secondary sexual characteristics. *(Kaplan and Sadock, pp. 733, 1161–1178)*

72. **(A)** Down syndrome results from trisomy 21 and occurs in 1/1000 live births. Clinical features include hypotonia, upward slanted palpebral fissures, midface depression, flat, wide nasal bridge, simian creases, short stature, and frequent congenital heart problems. Fragile X syndrome is a recessive syndrome that results from a mutation of the X chromosome, and occurs in 1/1000 male births and 1/3000 female births. It is the second most common cause for mental retardation. The traditional phenotype includes a long head and ears, short stature, hyperextensible joints and postpubertal macroorchidism. Fetal alcohol syndrome results in mental retardation and a typical phenotype of hypertelorism, microcephaly, short palpebral fissures, inner epicanthal folds, and a short turned up nose. Cri-du-chat (cat's cry) syndrome results from a lack of chromosome #5. These children are severely retarded and often have microcephaly, low set ears, micrognathia, and hypertelorism and make a characteristic cat-like cry caused by laryngeal abnormalities. *(Kaplan and Sadock, pp. 1161–1178)*

73. **(C)** Psychologic assessment techniques are, like most tools, useful for a diversity of purposes. Their worth partially depends on the training, competence, and ethical values of the tester. In the hands of a competent clinician, the results of an IQ examination, when correlated with other information from the person's history or present status, are valuable data. In 1896, the French clinician Binet began a project to develop an objective measure by which to quantify individual differences in mental abilities (intelligence). From 1905 to 1908, Binet and Simon introduced a series of standardized IQ tests in which correct responses to items that differed progressively in level of difficulty were correlated with a child's chronologic age. In 1916, Terman, at Stanford University, revised the Binet–Simon Intelligence Scale. The Stanford–Binet Test was quickly adopted in the United States for assessing the intelligence of children. Wechsler, as chief psychologist at Bellevue Hospital in New York, introduced the next major development in the history of intelligence testing. Before Wechsler, IQ testing was primarily used with children 15 years old or younger. Wechsler developed scales that compared the performance of a child with the performance of his or her own agemates on the same test items. The Bellevue–Wechsler Scale was introduced in 1939. In 1949, this scale was used as the model for a revised test specifically for children (ages 6–16 years), the WISC. Restandardization of the Bellevue–Wechsler Scale led to the introduction of the Wechsler Adult Intelligence Scale (WAIS) in 1958, with norms for ages 16–75 years. The WISC and WAIS are currently the most widely accepted tests of intelligence in use today. The Metropolitan Achievement Test and the Vineland Social Maturity Scale are contemporary standardized tests of school readiness and grade-level achievement and acquisition of culture-based social skills, respectively. *(Kaplan and Sadock, pp. 1156–1160)*

74. **(D)** Candida vaginitis is the only local infection in which the vaginal pH is less than 4.5. Figure 7-2 shows the branching hyphae diagnostic of candidal infection. The absence of clue cells and no amine odor excludes bacterial vaginosis due to *G. vaginalis*. Trichomonas vaginitis is due to a unicellular, flagellated organism that would demonstrate flagellar motion on a saline

wet smear. Chlamydia and syphilis present with no diagnostic vaginal discharge. *(MMWR, pp. 45–48)*

75. **(B)** Either oral or vaginal antifungal agents are usually effective in eradication of *Candida* species from the vagina. Metronidazole is used to treat trichomoniasis or bacterial vaginosis. Ceftriaxone is the current treatment of choice for gonorrhea. Oral azithromycin is recommended as cotherapy with ceftriaxone to eradicate concurrent *Chlamydia* infection, present in up to 50% of women with a positive gonococcal culture (even if the LCR is negative for chlamydia). Oral or vaginal clindamycin is effective therapy for bacterial vaginosis, giving cure rates comparable to metronidazole (about 95%). *(MMWR, pp. 45–48)*

76. **(A)** Anorexia nervosa is a disorder of unknown cause that primarily affects young women. Its onset most frequently occurs during adolescence and its highest incidence is among White females of Western countries. The clinical picture is predominated by signs of starvation, and obsessive-compulsive traits are often present. Affected individuals are frequently good students who have been characterized as achievers. A loss of 25% or more of total body weight is almost always included in the diagnostic criteria. Hypothermia and bradycardia are seen with severe weight loss. Patients with bulimia tend to binge and then purge. They are often of normal weight. Hyperthyroidism is not common in adolescents but can occur. It can cause weight loss, but this patient does not have other signs of hyperthyroidism, such as tachycardia. Diabetes in adolescents typically is of abrupt onset, with the classic symptoms of polyphagia, polydipsia, and polyuria. Depression can cause weight loss, but patients tend to withdraw from their activities, and mood changes are the dominant symptom. *(Rudolph et al., pp. 232–233, 2074–2077, 231, 2112–2119)*

77. **(C)** The following factors contribute to a favorable prognosis for children with ALL: age between 3 and 7 years, absence of lymphadenopathy, female gender, initial WBC of 10,000, hemoglobin of 7 g/100 mL, and platelet count of at least 100,000. All of these factors except gender lose their prognostic significance after 2 years of complete and continuous remission. Unfavorable prognostic factors include the presence of a mediastinal mass, Ph1 chromosome, decreased immunoglobulins, T- or B-cell surface markers on lymphoblasts, more than 25% blast cells in the bone marrow 14 days after treatment, and L2 or L3 lymphoblasts. *(McMillan et al., pp. 1493–1501)*

78. **(A)** This patient seems to be suffering from a full-blown manic episode, coming after a previous depressive episode. Bipolar I disorder is characterized by at least one full-blown manic episode. Bipolar II disorder is characterized by periods of major depression which alternate with hypomanic periods which do not reach the level of psychosis seen in this patient. This patient's prominent mood-related symptoms make the diagnosis of paranoid schizophrenia unlikely as an explanation for his psychotic symptoms. Although both hypothyroidism and hyperthyroidism can cause mood disorders, and should be ruled out in patients presenting with mood disorders, particularly when accompanied by other symptoms of thyroid disease (such as weight gain, fatigue, and cold intolerance in hypothyroidism, and tachycardia and heat intolerance in hyperthyroidism), they are less frequent as a cause of manic symptoms than is bipolar I disorder. *(Kaplan and Sadock, pp. 542–544)*

79. **(A)** The anticonvulsant valproic acid is well established as an effective treatment for the manic phase of bipolar I disorder, and is used about as frequently as lithium carbonate for that purpose. Fluoxetine, bupropion, and venlafaxine are antidepressants that can be effective in the treatment of the depressed phase of individuals with bipolar I disorder, but one runs the risk of exacerbating a manic episode by using antidepressants in such patients. Clonazepam, a benzodiazepine, is a useful adjunctive medication in the treatment of bipolar I disorder, but is not well established as a first-line treatment of mania, as are medications such as valproic acid and lithium. *(Kaplan and Sadock, pp. 570–572)*

80. **(E)** A karyotype of peripheral lymphocytes is the most appropriate option of the listed choices. It will be 46,XX in this patient. The normal height, normal breast, and pubic hair development, absent cervix and uterus, and a negative family history point to a diagnosis of vaginal and Müllerian agenesis. In general, a karyotype is a useful early step in the evaluation of primary amenorrhea because 45,X gonadal dysgenesis is the most common cause of primary amenorrhea, and because several causes of primary amenorrhea are associated with the presence of a Y chromosome. Approximately 30% of women with a Y chromosome will develop a gonadal malignancy by the age of 30 years. A pelvic ultrasound is unnecessary if the pelvic examination is reliable in revealing the absence of a cervix and uterus, but should be done if there is any doubt about the pelvic findings. Breast development signifies the presence of estrogen, which means that the hypothalamic-pituitary-gonadal axis is intact. A serum estradiol or CT scan of the pituitary are, therefore, unnecessary. A laparoscopy is a reasonable procedure to remove the testes in a 46,XY female with testicular feminization, but is an inappropriate and unnecessary diagnostic tool for this patient. *(Speroff and Fritz, pp. 419–423)*

81. **(C)** The absence of a uterus can only be due to Müllerian agenesis or testicular feminization (androgen insensitivity syndrome). The presence of mature breasts indicates estrogen secretion (unless there is a history of long-standing estrogen therapy); normal breast development is present in both disorders. The presence of an adult pubic hair pattern excludes testicular feminization because the deficiency or absence of androgen receptors in the pubis will result in sparse or absent pubic hair. Thus, the most likely diagnosis is Müllerian agenesis. Because these women have normally functioning ovaries, a test to detect ovulation also establishes the diagnosis of Müllerian agenesis: a biphasic basal temperature graph or a serum progesterone concentration over 5 ng/mL. Women with anorexia nervosa have deficient hypothalamic secretion of gonadotropin-releasing hormone (GnRH) and secondarily decreased secretion of FSH, LH, and ovarian estradiol and progesterone. The presence of breast growth indicates that this woman was exposed to estrogen at some time. The exposure may have been in the past and may have been from exogenous sources. However, anorectic women have a cervix and uterus. The normal height and the presence of breasts excludes gonadal dysgenesis (e.g., Turner syndrome), as these women are never taller than 157.5 cm (62 in.), and the streak gonads are incapable of estrogen production. There is one exception to this height limit: women with 46,XX or 46,XY gonadal dysgenesis will have a normal height. However, women with any form of gonadal dysgenesis (streak gonads) will have a uterus and cervix, even those with 46,XY gonadal dysgenesis. This is so because the gonads are so dysgenetic (literally translated: *malformed*) that the streak gonads of a woman with 46,XY gonadal dysgenesis are so malformed that they never produce Müllerian duct regression factor. Women with 17α-hydroxylase deficiency have hypertension and are sexually infantile, because this steroid enzyme deficiency does not permit normal cortisol, androgen, or estrogen biosynthesis. Deficient cortisol biosynthesis results in increased ACTH secretion, which stimulates an increased adrenal secretion of mineralocorticoids and results in hypertension. *(Speroff and Fritz , pp. 419–423)*

82. **(E)** Creation of the vagina will enable this woman to have satisfactory coitus, including orgasm. Daily use of vaginal dilators of increasing length and diameter is a nonoperative means of creating a vagina. This usually requires daily use of the dilators for 6–12 months to achieve adequate vaginal depth. The most common operative method to create a vagina is to sew a split-thickness skin graft taken from the buttocks over a mold. The mold with covering skin graft is then placed into a space created between the bladder and rectum. This is called the McIndoe procedure. Removal of the gonads is inappropriate, because they are normally functioning ovaries. Any form of HRT is inappropriate for the same reason. Glucocorticoid therapy is indicated only in women with certain forms of congenital adrenal hyperplasia (21-hydroxylase deficiency, 11-hydroxylase deficiency, 17α-hydroxylase deficiency). *(Speroff and Fritz, pp. 420–421)*

83. **(C)** Of all the patients with dementia, 50–60% have the most common type of dementia—Alzheimer's dementia. The second most common type is vascular dementia. Dementia is differentiated from delirium in that it involves a more chronic and insidious cognitive decline, and the patient is usually alert and the cognitive changes are more stable over time. Pick disease is another form of dementia which involves a preponderance of frontotemporal atrophy and involves personality changes more frequently along with cognitive decline.

A dementia workup is initiated to make sure the appropriate treatments are initiated for the form of dementia which presents. Some forms of dementia rarely can be resolved (e.g., B_{12} deficiency leading to cognitive decline), and one does not want to miss such an opportunity to correct this. RPR (test for syphilis), liver enzymes, TSH, CBC, UA, renal function, blood and urine drug screens, erythrocyte sedimentation rate, HIV screening, neuroimaging, EEG, and physical examination (looking for neurologic findings characteristic of vascular dementias) with mini-mental status examination are parts of a routine dementia workup. *(Kaplan and Sadock, pp. 322, 329–344)*

84. **(A)** Tuberculous meningitis is characterized pathologically by a thick, gelatinous exudate in the subarachnoid space. The predilection of this material for the base of the brain explains the frequency of cranial nerve findings in afflicted children. Although the concentration of protein in the CSF usually is elevated, levels of 1 g/100 mL or greater generally indicate obstruction of the ventricular system. The tuberculin test is negative in about 10% of patients, especially those with advanced disease. Although the onset may occasionally be acute, signs and symptoms generally begin gradually or insidiously. The prognosis is guarded, and for those who present with advanced neurologic findings such as coma, the prognosis is poor, even with appropriate therapy. *(Rudolph et al., pp. 618)*

85. **(C)**

86. **(C)**

87. **(D)**

Explanations 85 and 87

A common response to frightening news and a possible life-threatening illness is regression—a return to an earlier form of behavior that is more childlike. It is an attempt to flee overwhelming anxiety and fear. It is a seeking to be cared for and protected. Borderline personality disorder and PMS, though possible, require further investigation, and from the information given are not well-supported diagnoses. Sometimes clinicians, in their own angry countertransference to such patients, may "act out" by labeling the patient with these, since both terms can have a negative connotation. The nurses' anger in this case is an example of countertransference, which are feelings and attitudes of the therapist (medical personnel) toward the patient that may arise from the past or be a reaction to the patient's transference feelings or attitudes toward the therapist. In this case, for example, if the countertransference anger led to angry demands to medicate or to restrain this patient, we would also have an example of "acting out." Although the consulting psychiatrist must be cognizant of the reason for referral "to medicate," he or she must quickly determine what the real and most therapeutic goal is. Given the case scenario, the psychiatrist needs to first determine why this woman is acting the way she is. One would presume that once this woman is encouraged to talk about her angry feelings, she will be able to get to the underlying fears, which might include fear of mutilation, fear for her children, fear of losing her job or her husband's love, and fear of losing life itself. Appropriate medications may be indicated to help this woman deal with her fears and anxieties. *(Stoudemire [1998b], pp. 3–35, 70–77)*

88. **(B)** The initial evaluation of hirsutism should include measurement of serum 17-hydroxyprogesterone, testosterone, and perhaps dehydroepiandrosterone sulfate (DHEAS). Appropriate tests to evaluate her anovulatory menstrual cycles

include serum prolactin and thyroid function. A pelvic ultrasound is appropriate if the bimanual part of the pelvic examination is unsatisfactory: obesity or voluntary guarding. An ACTH stimulation test is appropriate only in those women who may have congenital adrenal hyperplasia, suggested by a positive family history of hirsutism and oligomenorrhea, and significantly increased DHEAS levels. One milligram of dexamethasone at 11:00 p.m. should suppress the next morning's cortisol concentration to less than 5 g/dL. Failure to do so suggests the possibility of an adrenal tumor, and CT scan of the adrenal glands should be done. Measurement of FSH should be done only if the woman has any climacteric symptoms. *(Speroff and Fritz, pp. 504–513)*

89. **(A)** Polycystic ovary syndrome was first described in 1935 by Stein and Leventhal. It is important to understand the features of the disorder as a syndrome that likely has multiple causes. There is growing sentiment to discard the terms polycystic ovary syndrome and Stein–Leventhal syndrome in favor of a more descriptive term, such as chronic estrogenic anovulation. In this way, the disorder can more easily be recognized as one with a spectrum of causes and clinical manifestations. At least 75% of women with chronic estrogenic anovulation will have what has been called polycystic ovary syndrome. The normal 17-hydroxyprogesterone concentration effectively excludes attenuated 21-hydroxylase deficiency and an adrenal adenoma. The normal prolactin concentration tends to exclude a pituitary adenoma, although some pituitary tumors do not appear to secrete any hormones. The history of oligomenorrhea and hirsutism since puberty, plus the normal bimanual examination, makes a Sertoli–Leydig cell tumor unlikely. Abrupt cessation of menses, followed by the onset of hirsutism plus unilateral ovarian enlargement, is the usual presentation of a virilizing ovarian tumor. *(Speroff and Fritz, pp. 470–476)*

90. **(C)** DVT is variable in its presentation. A patient may have pain, discoloration, and a palpable cord, but these classic findings are low in sensitivity and specificity. Unilateral leg edema may be the only finding and is the most sensitive indicator of DVT. Duplex scanning is the most sensitive and specific of methods, especially for DVT above the knee, with a sensitivity of 95%, but is less sensitive for clots below the knee. Impedance plethysmography is also an option, but has a high rate of false positives. Venography is the most definitive technique for detection, but is uncomfortable, costly, technically difficult, and may even induce thrombophlebitis. Although she is at risk for pulmonary embolus (PE), her respiratory rate is normal, and there is nothing to suggest PE, so VQ scan, pulmonary angiography, and pulse oximetry are not crucial. *(Kasper et al., pp. 1491–1492)*

91. **(B)**

92. **(C)**

Explanations 91 and 92

Heparin-induced thrombocytopenia (HIT) has been increasing in incidence and is an important immunologic drug reaction because of its potential complications. Evidence suggests that its risk is dose-dependent. The highest risk occurs when heparin is given at full doses, and risk is lower with intermediate-dose heparin (7500 U twice daily). It usually occurs 5–15 days into therapy, and thrombocytopenia is moderate (counts range from 25,000 to 100,000). Typically, an IgG antibody (very rarely IgM, but not IgA) binds to heparin. Risk of HIT is higher with bovine rather than porcine heparin. Serious thrombotic complications can occur, both arterial and venous, with venous four times as common. Bleeding is not a common complication. Stroke and skin necrosis can occur, but less commonly. *(Kasper et al., pp. 675, 689, 692)*

93. **(A)** Acrodermatitis enteropathica is an autosomal-recessive disorder characterized clinically by dermatitis, alopecia, malabsorption, infections, growth retardation, and, rarely, hypogonadism. Children with this disorder manifest the clinical findings soon after being weaned from breast feeding because of the decreased bioavailability

of zinc in cow's milk. Malabsorption is characterized by severe steatorrhea, lactose intolerance, and malnutrition. Some patients are known to develop cutaneous candidiasis, bacterial infections, and eye manifestations, including blepharitis and photophobia. Chronic zinc deficiency is the cause of the disorder. The treatment of choice is the administration of 10–45 mg/day of elemental zinc. *(Rudolph et al., pp. 1176, 1177)*

94. **(C)** Intussusception, a telescoping of one portion of the gut into another, is the most common cause of intestinal obstruction between the ages of 2 months and 6 years. Typically, there is the onset of severe paroxysmal pain in a previously healthy child. Stools containing both blood and mucus, known as currant jelly stools, are characteristic of this disorder and are passed by 60% of these patients. Constipation can cause abdominal pain and can be palpated in the abdomen if severe enough. It does not cause bloody stools. Patients with infectious gastroenteritis can have blood in their stools, but this patient does not have diarrhea. Meckel's diverticulum causes painless rectal bleeding. *(Kliegman, pp. 258–259; Townsend et al., pp. 2112–2113; Way and Doherty, pp. 1323–1324)*

95. **(D)** Hirschsprung's disease, or congenital aganglionic megacolon, is associated with an absence of ganglion cells in part of the colon. It is the most common cause of intestinal obstruction of the colon and accounts for 33% of all neonatal obstructions. Patients present with constipation as neonates. Duodenal stenosis and esophageal atresia would cause vomiting. Breast-feeding failure can also cause constipation, but this baby has regained her birth weight, so it is obvious that her intake is adequate. Functional constipation does not occur in the first few days of life. *(Kliegman, pp. 258–259; Townsend et al., pp. 2113–2114; Way and Doherty, pp. 1321–1322)*

96. **(C)** Meckel's diverticulum is present in 2–3% of the population. Symptoms and signs can occur at any age but usually are manifested in the first 2 years of life. The most common sign is painless rectal bleeding. Anal fissures commonly cause rectal bleeding in infants, but it is a small amount of blood that typically coats the stool. Intussusception can cause bloody stools but usually also causes intermittent abdominal pain. Milk allergy would not occur this acutely. If the patient had a bloody stool with a volvulus, he would be ill-appearing and have abdominal pain. *(Kliegman, pp. 323–331; Townsend et al., pp. 1366–1368)*

97. **(B)** von Willebrand disease is an autosomal-dominant disorder. von Willebrand disease is characterized by a prolonged bleeding time, various abnormalities of the factor VIII complex, and a prolonged PTT. In contrast, the bleeding time is normal in hemophilia and factor IX deficiency, and the PTT is normal in idiopathic thrombocytopenic purpura. Factors II, VII, IX, and X are vitamin K–dependent and may be deficient in a variety of disorders, including liver disease, malabsorption, and altered bowel flora. *(Behrman et al., pp. 1513–1515)*

98. **(E)** Infants with fever, especially those less than 1 month of age, are at high risk for serious bacterial infection. Approximately 9% of these infants who look well on examination will have a serious bacterial infection. History and physical examination alone are not sensitive in detecting these infections. Laboratory evaluation is essential. Bacteremia, urinary tract infection, and meningitis are all possibilities in this age group, and so all of these tests must be done. *(Kliegman, pp. 1066–1067)*

99. **(B)** Group B *Streptococcus* is the most common cause of neonatal sepsis and meningitis in many medical centers. Gram-negative organisms, *L. monocytogenes*, and *Salmonella* are also possible, but less common. *H. influenzae*, type b, causes invasive disease, but the incidence has decreased dramatically since universal immunization was instituted. *S. aureus* would be an unusual organism unless the infant had some type of break in the skin. *(Kliegman, pp. 1066–1067)*

100. **(A)** Group A *Streptococcus* is the most likely organism. The next most common would be *Staphylococcus aureus*. *H. influenzae* and

Streptococcus pneumoniae do not cause adenitis. *P. multocida* is an organism found in the mouths of cats, which can cause a wound infection after a cat bite. *(Kliegman, pp. 973, 974)*

101. **(D)** From a case-control study, the incidence (risk) of colon cancer cannot be calculated directly, because the cases and controls have been selected based on their disease status. Thus, choices (A), (C), and (E) should be excluded as possible correct answers. Choice (B) gives the odds of ionizing radiation exposure in those with colon cancer (rather than without colon cancer), and so cannot be selected as an answer. Thus, the only correct answer is (D), in which the relative risk of colon cancer associated with exposure to ionizing radiation is approximated by an odds ratio. The odds ratio is the odds that a case was exposed divided by the odds that a control was exposed. Here the odds ratio is 1.3. *(Gordis, p. 33)*

102. **(E)** This patient is in severe distress and needs immediate therapy. Inhaled albuterol is the initial treatment of choice. Cromolyn sodium is a drug with efficacy in the prevention of acute exacerbations of allergen- and exercise-induced asthma. It has no bronchodilatory activity and should not be used in the treatment of acute asthma. Aminophylline is rarely used in the acute treatment of asthma, because studies have shown that it does not add to the efficacy of inhaled albuterol. Diagnostic studies may need to be done later when the patient's respiratory distress has been relieved. *(Rudolph et al., pp. 1959–1961)*

103. **(C)** Wounds resulting from animal bites may become infected with the typical skin and soft-tissue infectious agents, *Staphylococcus aureus* and *Streptococcus pyogenes*. Occasionally, they are infected with normal flora of the animal's mouth. Cat bite wounds may become infected with *P. multocida*. These infections can be quite severe and may require surgical drainage because the long slender teeth of cats enable deep inoculation of the organism. Dog bite wounds may become infected with *E. corrodens*. Rat bite wounds may result in rat bite fever, of which *S. minus* is one causative agent. *R. henselae* causes cat scratch disease. *F. tularensis* is the etiologic agent for tularemia. *(McMillan et al., pp. 1208–1209)*

104. **(A)** The Institute of Medicine Committee on Nutritional Status during Pregnancy and Lactation indicates that women who are overweight or obese at the onset of pregnancy should be advised to gain less total weight during the pregnancy. The appropriate weight gain for a woman with a prepregnancy BMI over 29 is roughly 13–18 lbs. The fetus, expanded blood volume, uterine enlargement, breast tissue growth, and other products of conception generate an estimated 13–17 lbs. Because weight gain during pregnancy is not based solely on these tissues, acceptable weight gain in women with normal BMIs may be greater. *(Institute of Medicine, p. 10)*

105. **(A)** Generalized seizures frequently occur starting 12–24 h after a patient with alcohol dependence stops drinking. Although patients in alcohol withdrawal can have periods of lethargy, they generally alternate with periods of hyperexcitability in patients with delirium tremens. Patients with long-term severe alcohol abuse are more likely to suffer from hypoglycemia, hyponatremia, and hypomagnesemia, all of which can result in seizures, than from hyperglycemia, hypernatremia, or hypermagnesemia. *(Kaplan and Sadock, pp. 403–405)*

106. **(B)** Wernicke's encephalopathy, which, if left untreated, can result in a chronic amnestic condition known as Korsakoff syndrome, is caused by thiamine deficiency in patients with alcohol dependence. If a patient with alcohol dependence who is at risk for the syndrome is to be given IV glucose, the IV glucose should include 100 mg of thiamine to each liter of the glucose solution, or the condition may be worsened. Oral thiamine should be given after IV thiamine is started. Lorazepam, diazepam, and haloperidol will not prevent the progression of Wernicke–Korsakoff syndrome. *(Kaplan and Sadock, p. 406)*

107. (E) *S. pneumoniae* is the most common bacterial pathogen in community acquired pneumonia. This is the case no matter if the patient is young or old or immunocompromised. If the pneumonia goes undiagnosed and the patient does not improve, you certainly would consider *C. psittaci* given the birds in her home, but this is a rare cause of pneumonia. Also, *H. influenzae* is more common in patients with COPD but still not as common as *S. pneumoniae* *(Bartlett et al. [1998], pp. 811–838)*

108. (C) Dose response and biological plausibility are helpful in determination of causation, but the clearest criterion for causation is temporality. The cause must precede the effect. The other proposed answers are also relevant. *(Rom, p. 173; LaDou, pp. 232–233)*

109. (A) Primary prevention aims to preserve health by preventing disease before it has occurred. Pasteurization removes the risk of illness before a population is exposed to potential disease. Secondary prevention aims to detect disease at an early stage in order to minimize morbidity. Most screening programs are considered secondary prevention. Tertiary prevention involves the care of established disease, with attempts made to minimize the negative effects of disease, and prevent disease-related complications. The terms "quaternary prevention" and "prophylactic prevention" were added as distractors. *(Lang and Hensrud, pp. 3–4)*

110. (A) The highest incidence of primary hyperparathyroidism occurs in women over the age of 60. Most patients are asymptomatic and found on screening tests. Those patients with symptoms most often manifest emotional disorders (e.g., depression) and hypercalciuria. Five to 10% of patients with first-time renal colic have primary hyperparathyroidism. Most patients with primary hyperparathyroidism have disease limited to one gland rather than multigland disease. MEN syndromes I and IIa manifest parathyroid disease, but are rare and are associated with other endocrinopathies. Carcinoma is rare. *(Greenfield et al., pp. 1293–1297)*

111. (E) Inhalational anthrax occurs very rarely in persons working with animals. It potentially can result from inhalation of weaponized spores, which can be made readily respirable. One to six days of incubation are followed by about 3 days of mild symptoms such as low-grade fever, malaise, myalgia, fatigue, nonproductive cough, and sometimes precordial oppression. This is followed by sudden onset of dyspnea, profuse sweating, and cyanosis, which generally proceeds to death unless treated early in its course. Widening of the mediastinum and pleural effusions are seen on chest x-ray. Doxycycline or ciprofloxacin or amoxicillin are approved for treatment of anthrax. Recovered persons develop immunity, but the generalizability and durability of this are uncertain. Inhalational anthrax is not contagious as an inhalational disease. Cattle do tend to get an intestinal form of anthrax, but this results in catastrophic illness for the animal. *(Wallace and Doebbeling, p. 357; Bell D, et al., pp. 222–225)*

112. (D) Occult bacteremia refers to the finding of a positive blood culture in a child who appears well enough to be treated as an outpatient. The response to antipyretics or lack of response does not change the risk for bacteremia. The risk of occult bacteremia correlates statistically with an elevated WBC (15,000) and fever (39°C [102.2°F]). Occult pneumococcal bacteremia is most common between 6 months and 2 years of age, and the incidence declines after the second birthday. Occult bacteremia occurs with essentially the same frequency in all socioeconomic groups. The most common organism found is *Streptococcus pneumoniae* followed by *Salmonella* and *N. meningitidis*. The treatment of children with occult bacteremia is dependent on lab findings and clinical status *(Kliegman, pp. 1063–1066)*

113. (C)

114. (B)

115. (C)

116. (D)

Explanations 113 through 116

Bilateral internuclear ophthalmoplegia is very characteristic of MS. Careful physical examination reveals evidence of multiple lesions, such as afferent pupillary defect and bilateral upgoing toes. Memory loss may occur later in the course of illness. Autonomic injury may produce constipation, but this is not specific for MS. Intention tremor is a manifestation of cerebellar involvement, but again not specific for MS. Periventricular plaques on brain MRI are characteristic and found in over 90% of patients with known MS. MRI is much more sensitive than brain CT scan and should be the first step. CSF is abnormal in 95% of MS patients. Increases in IgG and oligoclonal IgG bands are specific and suggest increased risk of disseminated disease and should also be done. Visual and auditory evoked potentials are abnormal in demyelinated tracts and serve as additional supporting evidence of MS. EEG is not helpful. Relapsing-remitting MS is the type present in 80% of patients; primary progressive MS affects approximately 20%. Symptoms typically begin in the second or third decade of life. MS affects females approximately twice as often as males. Optic neuritis typically is unilateral. Corticosteroids often hasten clinical recovery during acute relapses of MS. Interferons and immune globulin are medications useful to reduce the rate of clinical relapse. There is no clear evidence that cyclosporin or methotrexate are effective. *(Noseworthy et al., pp. 938–952)*

117. (B) About 1% (2.7 million persons) of Americans have chronic active hepatitis C. No vaccine is available for hepatitis C, the results of medical treatment of hepatitis C are mediocre after it has become chronic, and chronic active hepatitis C is the leading cause of need for liver transplants. Persons with chronic active hepatitis C should absolutely avoid consumption of alcoholic beverages, as alcohol accelerates progression to liver failure. *(Wallace and Doebbeling, pp. 182–185; www.cdc.gov/ncidod/diseases/hepatitis/resources/dz_burden02.htm)*

118. (D)

119. (A)

120. (B)

Explanations 118 through 120

Persons who have significantly disabling obsessions (persistent, intrusive thoughts or impulses) or exhibit disruptive compulsive behavior (stereotyped, purposeful, repetitive behavior that is felt as no longer controllable by the individual) are suffering from OCD. Obsessive thoughts can be distinguished from psychotic thoughts by the affected person's recognition that these thoughts are their own and have not emanated from an external source. Affected persons typically display few cognitive deficits except those imposed by the concentration and attention demands of the OCD. Treatment of OCD can be multifaceted. Effective pharmacotherapeutic agents include the tricyclic antidepressants, especially clomipramine, and the SSRIs, which include fluoxetine, sertraline, paroxetine, citalopram, and fluvoxamine. These are the drugs of first choice. If these are partially effective, other medications may be added. An anxiolytic (e.g., buspirone) or a benzodiazepine (e.g., alprazolam or clonazepam) may be tried, especially if anxiety is prominent. Lithium may be added for prominent affective symptoms such as depression. Antipsychotics (e.g., risperidone) may also be used in the event of psychotic symptoms. Behavioral therapy, designed to reduce anxiety, also can be effective. The technique of progressively delaying compulsive responses to anxiety or obsessional thoughts has been helpful in many cases. Group therapy can be useful in providing support, sharing successful intervention techniques, and reducing the fear in persons with OCD that they are crazy. TMS is a noninvasive technique for stimulating the cerebral cortex with an electrical magnetic field without inducing seizures. TMS is currently being studied for the treatment of depression. *(Kaplan and Sadock, pp. 616–623, 1144)*

121. (A)

122. (B)

Explanations 121 and 122

This infant presents with the clinical picture of a bowel obstruction. Initial management should include IV fluid resuscitation and nasogastric decompression. These interventions are essential before safe transport of the child to another center for further diagnostic studies. A septic workup, with initiation of antibiotic therapy, would be indicated only if there were perinatal risk factors for sepsis. Progressive abdominal distention, vomiting, and delayed passage of meconium are suggestive of Hirschsprung disease. Plain abdominal radiographs will demonstrate multiple dilated bowel loops. A contrast enema is important to exclude other causes of distal bowel obstruction in the neonate. Hirschsprung disease is then confirmed with rectal biopsy. Anorectal manometry is a useful diagnostic tool in older children because it requires the subject's cooperation and communication skills. *(Townsend et al., pp. 2113–2114; Way and Doherty, pp. 1321–1322; Greenfield et al., pp. 1998–2000)*

123. (E) Mortality associated with alcoholism often occurs relatively early in life, whether due to liver failure or suicide or motor vehicular accidents. Injuries precipitated by alcoholics may also result in the deaths of others. Alcoholism results in large loss of productive life years. The average change in life expectancy for alcoholics is –20 years. This reinforces the need for prevention and for treatment of alcoholism. *(Wallace and Doebbeling, pp. 818–849)*

124. (C) If a person has not had a skin test for tuberculosis within the past year, and is getting a baseline PPD, it is wise that it be done as a "two step." In the standard Mantoux skin test, 5 tuberculin units of PPD is injected intradermally, and the diameter of induration is read 48–72 h later. Induration of up to 15 mm can be considered negative in low risk persons, up to 10 mm in persons from areas where tuberculosis is endemic, and up to 5 mm in persons likely to be infected or with a compromised immune response. A person who was exposed to tuberculosis in the past, but who does not have active infection, may have a small response to the initial PPD, but has a stronger response after that response has been boosted by exposure to PPD. A positive response to PPD 6 months after an initial negative may, therefore, be misconstrued to be due to a new infection. A "two step" better establishes a baseline by repeating the PPD to see whether the immune response was strengthened by the initial PPD. This is particularly indicated if the response to the initial PPD was equivocal and if it has been years since the person last had a skin test for tuberculosis. *(Wallace and Doebbeling, p. 211)*

125. (E) Screening trials using chest x-ray and cytologic sputum evaluation have failed to show a decrease in lung cancer mortality. Screened groups had the same number of deaths from lung cancer as control groups. Studies are underway to investigate the benefit of using CT scanning for lung cancer screening. *(Patz et al., pp. 1627–1633)*

126. (C) Bone marrow depression is the most serious toxic effect of methotrexate. Other toxic effects include megaloblastic anemia, diarrhea, stomatitis, vomiting, vasculitis, and pulmonary fibrosis. Myocardial damage leading to heart failure, peripheral neuropathy, hemorrhagic cystitis, and hearing loss are not side effects of methotrexate, but may occur with other chemotherapeutic agents. *(Kasper et al., pp. 471, 2013)*

127. (D) Sitting actually increases the pressure on lumbar disks relative to standing. National Institute for Occupational Safety and Health (NIOSH) has not found backbelts to be helpful in prevention of low back pain. Holding weight out away from the body greatly increases pressure on the lumber disks and should be avoided. Weight should be kept close to the body. Being active, including light stretching (generally back extension exercises such as

McKenzie exercises, if this does not produce radicular pain), and maintenance of good posture may help control symptoms. *(Wallace and Doebbeling, pp. 656–657; McCunney, p. 324; LaDou, pp. 56–57)*

128. (B) Several disease states predispose to zinc deficiency, including cirrhosis, alcoholism, poor nutrition, and pancreatic insufficiency. Zinc deficiency can cause growth retardation, hypogonadism, anorexia, impaired sense of taste and smell, diarrhea, alopecia, dermatitis, hyperpigmentation, and poor wound healing. Night blindness due to combined zinc and vitamin A deficiencies improves only if both substances are replenished. Zinc deficiency in cirrhosis is associated with hepatic coma. Adult copper deficiency is also rare and is associated with Keshan disease, a fatal cardiomyopathy occurring in children. Chromium deficiency causes impaired growth and abnormal lipid, glucose, and protein metabolism. Hypomagnesemia is associated with weight loss, dermatitis, change in hair color, and hypocholesterolemia. *(Kasper et al., pp. 409–412)*

129. (A) Postnasal drip syndromes (such as allergic rhinitis and chronic sinusitis), asthma, gastroesophageal reflux, and chronic bronchitis (usually in patient with a long smoking history) are common causes of chronic cough. ACE inhibitors may cause chronic coughing. With discontinuation of the drug, coughing should improve or resolve within 4 weeks. *(Irwin and Madison, 2000)*

130. (A) Disadvantages seen commonly with cohort studies are that they often use large sample sizes, they often require lengthy follow-ups, and loss of follow-up can bias results. Cohort studies have the advantage of being able to evaluate multiple outcomes. Choice of control is more of an issue when using a case-control method of study. Ethical and legal issues are more commonly a concern in randomized controlled trials. *(Wallace and Doebbeling, pp. 18–19)*

131. (D) Relative risk is calculated by dividing the incidence in exposed persons by the incidence in unexposed persons. Total incidence—incidence in unexposed is the calculation used for determining population attributable risk. Incidence in exposed—incidence in unexposed persons is the calculation for attributable risk and (incidence in exposed—incidence in unexposed)/incidence in exposed is used to identify attributable risk percent. *(Lang and Hensrud, pp. 16–17)*

132. (D)

133. (C)

Explanations 132 and 133

Malignant hypertension is defined by the presence of papilledema and endorgan changes rather than the absolute BP level. Headache may not be the result of his elevated BP, and heart size can be related to factors other than hypertension, such as heart failure and cardiomyopathy. Impairment of renal function provides the best index to prognosis in malignant hypertension. The level of systolic or diastolic BP and size of the heart are features that are readily reversible and do not relate quantitatively to prognosis. A larger heart and more florid retinopathy do not necessarily portend a poorer prognosis, but numerous studies have documented that the worse the renal impairment, the poorer the prognosis. Compliance may play a role in BP control, but is not reliable for predicting prognosis. *(Kasper et al., pp. 1478, 1480)*

134. (E) Patients with Alzheimer disease often have symptoms that may mimic depression (lack of enthusiasm, moodiness) along with their intellectual decline and, therefore, may score poorly on a depression screening inventory. In early stages, they may be able to perform well on formal mental status testing. CT and MRI scans are not specific for Alzheimer's and may be normal early in the course of the disease. The earliest metabolic changes in Alzheimer's occur in the parietal cortex and can be seen with PET scanning. Tremor is uncommon with Alzheimer's, but is seen with Parkinson's. Pathologic features include brain atrophy, neurofibrillary tangles, and granulovacuolar neuronal degeneration. Initial symptoms generally begin after the age of 45 years, with progressive memory loss leading to global dementia. Some familial clustering is reported, but most cases are sporadic.

Choline acetyltransferase activity is reduced, not increased, and hallucinations and delusions are common. EEG may be normal or show nonspecific slowing. *(Kasper et al., pp. 2393–2400)*

135. **(E)** Compression ultrasonography is the diagnostic test of choice for assessment of DVT. Sensitivity and specificity are more than 95% for proximal deep-venous thrombosis but sensitivity falls to around 70% for isolated DVT in the calf. Imaging of calf veins often is not routinely performed. Given the clinical suspicion, follow-up ultrasonography in 1 week is advisable to detect possible extension from the calf into proximal veins. If the test is negative at 1 week, proximal extension then is highly unlikely. *(Bates and Ginsberg, pp. 268–277)*

REFERENCES

American Diabetes Association. Standards of medical care for patients with diabetes mellitus. *Diabetes Care* 2001;24(1):S33–S43.

Bartlett JG, Breiman RF, Mandell LA, et al. Community-acquired pneumonia in adults: guidelines for management. *Clin Infect Dis* 1998; 26:811–838.

Bates SM, Ginsberg JS. Treatment of deep-vein thrombosis. *N Engl J Med* 2004;351:268–277.

Behrman RE, Kliegman RM, Arvin AM. *Nelson Textbook of Pediatrics*, 16th ed. Philadelphia, PA: W.B. Saunders, 2000.

Bell D, Kozarsky P, Stephens D. Clinical issuses in the prophylaxis, diagnosis, and treatment of anthrax. *Emerg Infect Dis* 2002;8(2):222–225.

Copeland LJ. *Textbook of Gynecology*. Philadelphia, PA: W.B. Saunders, 2000.

Cunningham FG, Gant NF, Leveno KL, et al. *Williams Obstetrics*, 21st ed. New York, NY: McGraw-Hill, 2001.

Ellenhorn MJ. *Ellenhorn's Medical Toxicology: Diagnosis and Treatment of Human Poisoning*, 2nd ed. Baltimore, MD: Williams & Wilkins, 1997.

Frank RN. Diabetic retinopathy. *N Engl J Med* 2004;350:48–58.

Gordis L. *Epidemiology*, 3rd ed. Philadelphia, PA: W.B. Saunders, 2004.

Greenberg RS, Daniels SR, et al. *Medical Epidemiology*, 3rd ed. New York, NY: McGraw-Hill, 2001.

Greenfield LJ, Mulholland M, Oldham KT, et al. (eds.). *Surgery: Scientific Principles and Practice*. Philadelphia, PA: Lippincott-Raven, 2001.

Institute of Medicine. Committee on Nutritional Status During Pregnancy and Lactation. *Nutrition During Pregnancy: Part I, Weight Gain: Part II Nutrient Supplements*.

Iwin RS, Madison JM. The diagnosis and treatment of cough. *N Engl J Med* 2000;343(23):1715–1721.

Kaplan HI, Sadock BJ. *Synopsis of Psychiatry: Behavioral Sciences Clinical Psychiatry*, 8th ed. Baltimore, MD: Williams & Wilkins, 2003.

Kapoor WN. Syncope. *N Engl J Med* 2000;343(25): 1856–1862.

Kasper DL, Braunwald E, Fauci A, et al. *Harrison's Principles of Internal Medicine*, 16th ed. New York, NY: McGraw-Hill, 2005.

Kliegman RM. *Practical Strategies in Pediatric Diagnosis and Therapy*. Philadelphia, PA: W.B. Saunders, 1996.

LaDou J. *Current Occupational & Environmental Medicine*, 3rd ed. New York, NY: McGraw-Hill, 2003.

Lang, RS, Hensrud, DD. *Clinical Preventive Medicine*, 2nd ed. Chicago, IL: AMA Press, 2004.

McCunney RJ. *A Practical Approach to Occupational and Environmental Medicine*, 3rd ed. Philadelphia, PA: Lippincott Williams & Wilkins, 2003.

McMillan JA, DeAngelis CD, Feigin RD, et al. *Oski's Pediatrics: Principles and Practice*, 3rd ed. Philadelphia, PA: JB Lippincott, 1999.

Noseworthy JH, Lucchinetti C, Rodriquez M, et al. Multiple sclerosis. *N Engl J Med* 2000;343(13): 938–952.

Olin JW. Thromboangiitis obliterans (Buerger's disease). *N Engl J Med* 2000;343(12):864–869.

Patz EF, Goodman PC, Bepler G. Screening for lung cancer. *N Engl J Med* 2000;343(22):1627–1633.

Rom WN (ed.). *Environmental and Occupational Medicine*, 3rd ed. Philadelphia, PA: Lippincott-Raven, 1998.

Rudolph AM, Hoffman JIE, Rudolph CD. *Pediatrics*, 20th ed. Stamford, CT: Appleton & Lange, 1996.

Scott JR, Gibbs RS, Karlan BY, et al. (eds.). *Danforth's Obstetrics and Gynecology*, 9th ed. Philadelphia, PA: Lippincott Williams & Williams, 2003.

Snow V, Barry P, Fihn S, et al. Evaluation of primary care patients with chronic stable angina: guidelines from the American College of Physicians. *Ann Intern Med* 2004;141:57–64.

Speroff L, Fritz MA. *Clinical Gynecologic Endocrinology and Infertility*, 7th ed. Baltimore, MD: Lippincott Williams & Wilkins, 2005.

Stoudemire A (ed.). *Human Behavior: An Introduction for Medical Students*, 2nd ed. Philadelphia, PA: JB Lippincott, 1998b.

Sweet RL, Gibbs RS. *Infectious Diseases of the Female Genital Tract*, 3rd ed. Baltimore, MD: Williams & Wilkins, 1995.

Townsend CM Jr, Beauchamp RD, Evers BM, et al. (eds.). *Sabiston Textbook of Surgery: The Biologic Basis of Modern Surgical Practice*, 17th ed. Philadelphia, PA: Elsevier, 2004.

U.S. Preventive Services Task Force. *Guide to Clinical Preventive Services, 3rd ed.* Agency for Healthcare Research and Quality. http://www.ahrq.gov. (Note that this is now a rolling document, frequently updated, and incorporates recommendations from the 2nd ed. LM, October 2004.)

U.S. Public Health Service. *Treating Tobacco Use and Dependence.* www.surgeongeneral.gov. Summary, June 2000.

Wallace RB, Doebbeling BN (eds.). *Maxcy-Rosenau-Last Public Health & Preventive Medicine*, 14th ed. Stamford, CT: Appleton & Lange, 1998.

Way LW, Doherty GM (eds.). *Current Surgical Diagnosis and Treatment*, 11th ed. New York, NY: McGraw-Hill, 2003.

SUGGESTED READINGS

ACOG Technical Bulletin. *Immunization During Pregnancy*, no. 160, October 1991.

Adrogue HJ, Madias NE. Management of life-threatening acid–base disorders. *N Engl J Med* 1998;338:26–34.

Ameli S, Shah PK. Cardiac tamponade. *Cardiovasc Clin* 1991;9:665–673.

American Academy of Pediatrics. *Report of the Committee on Infectious Diseases*, 24th ed. Evanston, IL: American Academy of Pediatrics, 1997.

American Psychiatric Association (APA). *Diagnostic and Statistical Manual of Mental Disorders*, 4th ed. Text Revision. Washington, DC: American Psychiatric Association, 2000.

Andreason NC, Black DW. *Introductory Textbook of Psychiatry*, 2nd ed. Washington, DC: American Psychiatric Association, 1995.

Bar-Or O. *Pediatric Sports Medicine for the Practitioner.* New York, NY: Springer-Verlag, 1983.

Bartlett JG, Mundy LM. Community-acquired pneumonia. *N Engl J Med* 1995;333:1618–1624.

Berkowitz CD. *Pediatrics: A Primary Care Approach.* Philadelphia, PA: W.B. Saunders, 1996.

Byrne TN. Spinal cord compression from epidural metastases. *N Engl J Med* 1992;327:614–619.

Centers for Disease Control and Prevention. National Center for Infectious Diseases. *Viral Hepatitis Surveillance*, 2005. Available at: www.cdc.gov/ncidod/diseases/hepatitis/resource/d2_burden-02.htm

Champion LAA, Schwartz AD, Luddy RE, et al. The effects of four commonly used drugs on platelet function. *J Pediatr* 1976;89:653–656.

Coffey RL, Zile MR, Luskin AT. Immunologic tests of value in diagnosis. I. Acute phase reactants and autoantibodies. *Postgrad Med* 1981;70:163–178.

Committee on Drugs. Treatment guidelines for lead exposure in children. *Pediatrics* 1995;96:155–160.

Creasy RK, Resnik R. *Maternal–Fetal Medicine: Principles and Practice*, 3rd ed. Philadelphia, PA: W.B. Saunders, 1994.

Dajani AS, Taubert KA, Wilson W, et al. Prevention of bacterial endocarditis: recommendations by the American Heart Association. *JAMA* 1997;277:1794–1801.

DeArce MA, Kearns A. The fragile X syndrome: the patients and their chromosomes. *J Med Genet* 1984;21:84–91.

Diabetes Control and Complications Trial Research Group. The effect of intensive treatment of diabetes on the development and progression of long-term complications in insulin-dependent diabetes mellitus. *N Engl J Med* 1993;329:977–986.

DiSaia PJ, Creasman WT. *Clinical Gynecologic Oncology.* St. Louis, MO: Mosby, 1997.

Dixon AC, Parrillo JE. Managing the cardiovascular effects of sepsis and shock. *J Crit Illness* 1991;6: 1197–1214.

Feigin RD, Cherry JD. *Textbook of Pediatric Infectious Diseases*, 3rd ed. Philadelphia, PA: W.B. Saunders, 1992.

Feinstein AR. *Principles of Medical Statistics*. Boca Raton, FL: Chapman & Hall, 2002.

Fink JN, Fauci A. Immunological aspects of cardiovascular disease. *JAMA* 1982;248:2716–2721.

Fitzpatrick TB, Johnson RA, Polano MK, et al. *Color Atlas and Synopsis of Clinical Dermatology*, 2nd ed. New York, NY: McGraw-Hill, 1994.

Gartner LM. Neonatal jaundice. *Pediatr Rev* 1994;15:422–432.

Giammarco R, Edmeads J, Dodick D. *Critical Decisions in Headache Management*. Hamilton, BC Decker, Malden, MA: Blackwell Science, 1998.

Goroll AH, Lawrence AM, Mulley AG. *Primary Care Medicine*, 3rd ed. Philadelphia, PA: JB Lippincott, 1995.

Guyer B, Martin J, MacDorman M, et al. Annual summary of vital statistics—1996. *Pediatrics* 1997;100:905–918.

Hales RE, Frances AJ (eds.). *Psychiatry Update: American Psychiatric Association Annual Review*, vol. 6. Washington, DC: American Psychiatry Press, 1987.

Hogan DE. The emergency department approach to diarrhea. *Emerg Clin North Am* 1996;14:673–692.

Hoskins WJ, Perez CA, Young RC. *Principles and practice of Gynecologic Oncology*, 3rd. ed. Philadelphia, PA: Lippincott Williams & Wilkins, 2000.

Hurst JW. *Medicine for the Practicing Physician*. Stamford, CT: Appleton & Lange, 1996.

Hurwitz S. *Clinical Pediatric Dermatology: A Textbook of Skin Disorders of Childhood and Adolescence*. Philadelphia, PA: W.B. Saunders, 1981.

Joint National Committee on Prevention, Detection, Evaluation and Treatment of High Blood Pressure. Seventh Report of the Joint National Committee on the Prevention, Detection, Evaluation and Treatment of High Blood Pressure. N/H Pub. No. 04–5230. Bethesda, MD: National Heart, Lung, and Blood Institute, 2004.

Koehler JE. Bartonella infections. *Adv Pediatr Infect Dis* 1996;11:1–27.

Laine L, Suchower L, Connors A, et al. Twice-daily, 10-day triple therapy with omeprazole, amoxicillin, and clarithromycin for *Helicobacter pylori* eradication in duodenal ulcer disease: results of three multicenter, double-blind, United States trials. *Am J Gastroenterol* 1998;93:2106–2112.

Last JM (ed.). *Maxcy–Rosenau-Last Public Health & Preventive Medicine*, 13th ed. East Norwalk, CT: Appleton & Lange, 1992.

Light RW. Parapneumonic effusions and empyema: current management strategies. *J Crit Illness* 1995;10:832–842.

McAnarney ER, Kreipe RE, Orr DP, et al. *Textbook of Adolescent Medicine*. Philadelphia, PA: W.B. Saunders, 1992.

The Medical Letter on Drugs and Therapeutics: Drugs for Treatment of Acute Otitis Media in Children, vol. 36. New Rochelle: Medical Letter, 1994, pp. 19–21.

Norman ME. Vitamin D in bone disease. *Pediatr Clin North Am* 1982;29:947–971.

Oski FA, DeAngelis CD, Feigin RD, et al. *Principles and Practice of Pediatrics*, 2nd ed. Philadelphia, PA: JB Lippincott, 1994.

Paulson WD. Identifying acid-base disorders: a systematic approach. *J Crit Illness* 1999;14(2):103–109.

Rankin AC, Brooks R, Ruskin JN, et al. Adenosine and the treatment of supraventricular tachycardia. *Am J Med* 1992;92:655–664.

Relman DA, Schmidt TM, MacDermott RP, et al. Identification of the uncultured bacillus of Whipple's disease. *N Engl J Med* 1992;327:293–301.

Rock JA, Thompson JD. *TeLinde's Operative Gynecology*, 8th ed. Philadelphia, PA: Lippincott-Raven, 1997.

Schumacher HR (ed.). *Primer on the Rheumatic Diseases*, 10th ed. Atlanta, GA: Arthritis Foundation, 1993.

Stenchever MA, Droegemueller W, Herbst AL, et al. *Comprehensive Gynecology*, 4th ed. St. Louis, MO: Mosby, 2001.

Stoudemire A (ed.). *Clinical Psychiatry for Medical Students*, 3rd ed. Philadelphia, PA: JB Lippincott, 1998a.

Tancredi LR. Emergency psychiatry and crisis intervention: some legal and ethical issues. *Psychiatr Ann* 1982;12:799–806.

Tecklenburg FW, Wright MS. Minor head trauma in the pediatric patient. *Pediatr Emerg Care* 1991;7: 40–47.

Tomb DA. *Psychiatry*, 5th ed. Baltimore, MD: Williams & Wilkins, 1995.

Traugott L, Alpers A. In their own hands. *Arch Pediatr Adolesc Med* 1997;151:922–927.

Wedding D. *Behavior and Medicine*, 2nd ed. St. Louis, MO: Mosby, 1995.

Workowski K, Levine W. Sexually transmitted diseases treatment guidelines. *Morbidity and Mortality Weekly Report* 2002;*51(RR06): 1–80.*

Yamada T, Alpers D, Owyang C, et al. *Textbook of Gastroenterology*. Philadelphia, PA: JB Lippincott, 1991.

Yen SSC, Jaffe RB. *Reproductive Endocrinology: Physiology, Pathophysiology and Clinical Management*, 3rd ed. Philadelphia, PA: W.B. Saunders, 1991.

Zinner MJ. *Maingot's Abdominal Operations*, 10th ed., vols. 1 and 2. Stamford, CT: Appleton & Lange, 1997.

Subject List: Practice Test 1

Question Number and Subject

PREVENTIVE MEDICINE

3. Disease control
8. Toxicology
18. Clinical prevention
40. Biostatistics
46. Clinical prevention
52. Biostatistics
53. Disease control
58. Disease control
62. Disaster response, toxicology
64. Biostatistics
68. Clinical prevention
101. Biostatistics
108. Causation, epidemiology
109. Clinical prevention
111. Disaster response
117. Epidemiology, infectious disease
123. Epidemiology
124. Secondary prevention, infectious disease
125. Clinical prevention
127. Occupational medicine
130. Biostatistics
131. Biostatistics

OBSTETRICS AND GYNECOLOGY

9. Oncology
19. Management of delivery
20. Dysmenorrhea
21. Infectious Diseases
24. Birth control
25. Endocrinology
36. Dysmenorrhea
37. Birth control
44. Endocrinology
48. Management of delivery/dysmenorrhea
56. Management of delivery
57. Management of delivery
65. Pregnancy
66. Delivery
69. Endocrine
74. Infectious diseases
75. Infectious diseases
80. Genetics/endocrine
81. Genetics/endocrine
82. Genetics/endocrine
88. Endocrine
89. Endocrine
104. Pregnancy

PSYCHIATRY

5. Assessment/psychopharmacology
6. Psychopathology
7. Psychopathology
17. Psychopathology/assessment
27. Consultation psychiatry
39. Psychopharmacology
61. Assessment/consultation psychiatry
71. Child psychiatry
72. Child psychiatry
73. Child psychiatry
78. Assessment/psychopathology
79. Intervention/psychopharmacology
83. Psychopathology
85. Assessment
86. Assessment
87. Assessment
105. Psychopathology
106. Psychopharmacology
118. Assessment/psychopathology
119. Intervention/psychopharmacology
120. Intervention/psychotherapy

INTERNAL MEDICINE

15. Endocrine
16. Endocrine
51. Neurology
63. Toxicology
67. Pharmacology
90. Cardiovascular
91. Cardiovascular
92. Cardiovascular
107. Infectious diseases
113. Nervous system diseases
114. Nervous system diseases
115. Nervous system diseases
116. Nervous system diseases
126. Pharmacology
128. Nutrition
129. Pharmacology
132. Cardiovascular
133. Cardiovascular
134. Neurology
135. Cardiovascular

PEDIATRICS

14. Genetics/respiratory
26. Infectious diseases
28. Endocrine/metabolic
38. Structural
45. Toxicology
49. Trauma
50. Dermatologic
59. Toxicology
60. Infectious diseases
70. Infectious diseases
76. Psychopathology
77. Neoplastic
84. Infectious diseases
93. Nutrition
94. Structural
95. Structural
96. Structural
97. Hematology
98. Infectious diseases
99. Infectious diseases
100. Infectious diseases
102. Allergy
103. Infectious diseases
112. Infectious diseases

SURGERY

1. Infectious diseases
2. Infectious diseases
4. Structural
10. Oncology/endocrine
11. Oncology/endocrine
12. Oncology/endocrine
13. Oncology/genetics
22. Infectious diseases/breast
23. Infectious diseases/breast
29. Digestive system diseases
30. Digestive system diseases
31. Digestive system diseases
32. Digestive system diseases
33. Digestive system diseases
34. Digestive system diseases
35. Digestive system diseases
41. Trauma
42. Trauma
43. Trauma
47. Nervous system diseases
54. Trauma
55. Trauma
110. Endocrine diseases
121. Pediatrics/GI
122. Pediatrics/GI

CHAPTER 8

Practice Test 2

Questions

DIRECTIONS (Questions 1 through 36): Each of the numbered items in this section is followed by five or more answer options. Select the ONE lettered answer or completion that is BEST in each case.

Questions 1 and 2

A 55-year-old man presents to the physician's office complaining of persistent heartburn of 10 years' duration. He also complains of a chronic cough and regurgitation at night for 3 years despite raising the head of his bed 30 degrees. He self-medicated intermittently for 7 years, initially with antacids and then H_2 blockers, but the severity of his symptoms increased and he was placed on a proton-pump inhibitor 3 years ago. His heartburn is partially improved, and he still complains of nighttime regurgitation and cough. His physical examination is normal, and he is referred for upper endoscopy that reveals superficial linear ulcerations of his distal esophagus with 3 cm of epithelial changes consistent with Barrett's esophagus (Fig. 8-1, see color plate 1). Biopsies reveal esophagitis and high-grade dysplasia of the Barrett's epithelium.

1. Early treatment with which of the following would most likely have prevented this condition?

    (A) H_2 blockers
    (B) diet modification
    (C) Nissen fundoplication
    (D) proton-pump inhibitor
    (E) regular schedule of antacids

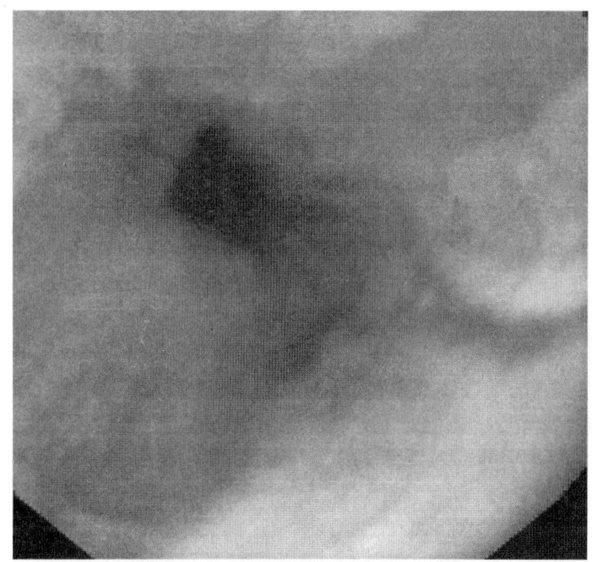

FIG. 8-1 Also see Color Plate 1. *(Reprinted with permission from Zinner MJ.* Maingot's Abdominal Operations, *10th ed., vol. 1. Stamford, CT: Appleton & Lange, 1997.)*

2. Which of the following should be recommended for this patient?

    (A) double dose proton-pump inhibitor and repeat endoscopy in 3 months
    (B) proton-pump inhibitor and H_2 blocker, followed by repeat endoscopy in 3 months
    (C) antibiotic treatment for *Helicobacter pylori* with proton-pump inhibitor
    (D) Nissen fundoplication
    (E) esophagectomy

3. A 7-year-old girl is brought to the clinic with a 2-day history of right ear pain. She has not had fever, congestion, or other symptoms. On physical examination, she is afebrile. She has pain when you move the pinna. There is drainage in the right ear canal that obscures the tympanic membrane. Which of the following is the most likely diagnosis?

   (A) acute otitis media with perforation
   (B) contact dermatitis
   (C) foreign body in the ear canal
   (D) mastoiditis
   (E) external otitis

4. In 2000, the Public Health Advisory Committee on Immunization Practices changed its recommendation for immunizing children under 4 years old against polio. The old recommendation included use of oral polio vaccine. The new recommendation is for a series of four doses of injectable polio vaccine. This recommendation reflected the fact that

   (A) injectable vaccine was less expensive than oral vaccine due to cost of preparation
   (B) the risk of contracting vaccine-associated paralytic polio from oral vaccine is now higher than the risk of contracting wild-strain polio
   (C) no cases of wild-strain paralytic polio had been reported in 15 years
   (D) injectable vaccine is more protective than oral vaccine
   (E) injectable polio vaccine is available worldwide

5. In the ER, you see a 25-year-old female, with no history of human immunodeficiency virus (HIV) infection, who was just sexually assaulted. She wants an HIV test immediately, which you provide. You propose follow-up testing with an enzyme-linked immunosorbent assay (ELISA) test based on the delay between infection and appearance of detectable antibodies.

   In general, ELISA detectable antibodies appear how long after infection with HIV?

   (A) 2–10 days
   (B) 5–21 days
   (C) 10 days to 1 month
   (D) 2–9 weeks
   (E) 4 weeks to 3 months

6. A worker from a company that uses and ships a lot of organic solvents sees you because he feels very fatigued. He appears to be anemic, and a complete blood count (CBC) reveals anemia, leukopenia, and thrombocytopenia. Which of the following is most likely to cause this profile?

   (A) acetone
   (B) mushroom toxin
   (C) toluene
   (D) benzene
   (E) diesel exhaust

7. You refer a 45-year-old male with type I diabetes to an ophthalmologist because he is complaining of blurred vision. The visit to the ophthalmologist office is considered which of the following types of preventive measures?

   (A) primary prevention
   (B) secondary prevention
   (C) tertiary prevention
   (D) quaternary prevention
   (E) predisease prevention

8. Based on evidence-based practices you are asked to prioritize who will be receiving Papanicolaou (Pap) tests. For which one of the following women would you be most likely to perform a Pap test?

   (A) a 78-year-old female who has three grown children, a history of normal Pap tests, and no Pap test in the past 5 years
   (B) a 27-year-old female who had a total hysterectomy 1 year ago, and who had a history of noninvasive cancer of the cervix
   (C) a 38-year-old female who has never been sexually active, and who has not had a Pap test in the past 10 years

(D) a 37-year-old female who is sexually active, has had normal Pap tests every 3 years since age 20, and had a normal Pap test 1 year ago
(E) a 30-year-old female who is sexually active, has a history of normal Pap tests, had a total hysterectomy for uterine fibroids, and has not had a Pap test in 10 years

9. A 35-year-old granite quarry worker presents to his primary care physician with the complaint of a persistent productive cough. A chest x-ray reveals nodules in the middle and upper lung fields. A tuberculin skin test is done and is read as positive. In addition to this patient's tuberculosis, what comorbid condition is highly likely in this patient?

(A) asbestosis
(B) silicosis
(C) coal worker's pneumoconiosis
(D) berylliosis
(E) siderosis

10. A fox bites a man camping in a rural area of Texas. The fox escapes after the incident and the man is unable to capture or track him. Which of the following is the most appropriate follow-up therapy for this individual?

(A) postexposure therapy with both rabies vaccine and immunoglobulin
(B) postexposure therapy for tetanus based on immunization status only, fox rabies is uncommon in North America
(C) postexposure therapy with rabies vaccine and tetanus toxoid regardless of immunization status
(D) postexposure therapy with rabies vaccine, rabies immunoglobulin, and tetanus prophylaxis based on the individual's immunization status
(E) postexposure therapy with rabies immunoglobulin and tetanus toxoid

11. You are reviewing data in order to determine whether there is an association between measured systolic and diastolic blood pressures in the general population, and what is the magnitude of the trend. Which of the following statistical analysis techniques would be most appropriate?

(A) Wilcoxon Two-Group Rank Sum test
(B) Mann–Whitney U-test
(C) Wilcoxon Signed-Ranks test
(D) linear model of regression
(E) odds ratio

12. A 34-year-old male is admitted with fever and shortness of breath to a Chicago hospital. Chest x-ray reveals pneumonia and blood cultures grow *Streptococcus pneumoniae*. Which of the following antibiotics is best empiric choice for treatment?

(A) ceftriaxone
(B) penicillin
(C) vancomycin
(D) amoxicillin
(E) azithromycin

13. During a daytime church picnic, a wild fox suddenly appears from the woods and attacks a young woman, biting her several times on the leg. The fox then proceeds to wander around the picnic, attacking brightly colored coolers. A man attempts to catch the fox and is bitten several times on his hands and head in the process. Animal control officers arrive and safely trap the fox. Which of the following is the best course of action?

(A) Observe the fox for 10 days.
(B) Submit the fox head for rabies testing and treat victims based on results.
(C) Begin treatment with tetanus antitoxin.
(D) Begin treatment of bite victims with rabies vaccine.
(E) Begin treatment of bite victims with rabies immune globulin and rabies vaccine.

14. A 31-year-old White woman is pregnant at 31 weeks' gestation. She and her husband just read an article in Good Housekeeping magazine about cystic fibrosis (CF) and ask you what their chances are of having a child with CF. Neither have been tested for the CF gene. You know that the gene frequency in a White population is approximately 1 in 25. You tell them that the probability of having a child with CF is approximately

(A) 0, because neither of the couple has symptoms of CF
(B) 1 in 50
(C) 1 in 625
(D) 1 in 1350
(E) 1 in 2500

15. A 17-year-old girl has moderate dysmenorrhea that began about 1 year after menarche. Physical examination, including the pelvic examination, is normal. Which of the following medications most often provides effective relief for her primary dysmenorrhea?

(A) fluoxetine
(B) acetaminophen
(C) bromocriptine
(D) ibuprofen
(E) hydrocortisone

16. A 15-year-old boy comes to the emergency department with sudden onset of respiratory distress. He states that he was studying 1 h ago, when he developed chest pain and dyspnea. He has no history of any previous respiratory problems. On physical examination, he is tachypneic, has moderate retractions, and has decreased breath sounds over the left lung fields. Which of the following is the most likely diagnosis?

(A) aspiration of a foreign body
(B) exacerbation of asthma
(C) empyema
(D) pneumonia
(E) pneumothorax

Questions 17 and 18

A 2-week-old boy is brought to your office for a checkup. He has been doing well at home. The results of his newborn screen indicate that he has sickle cell disease (hemoglobin SS disease).

17. Which of the following is the most important next step in his management?

(A) avoiding heat exposure
(B) immunizing with pneumococcal vaccine
(C) prescribing folic acid supplements
(D) prescribing iron supplements
(E) prescribing prophylactic penicillin

18. Six months later, this same patient returns to your office with a 3-day history of lethargy and fever. He has also had rhinorrhea and a cough. On physical examination, he is pale, tachycardic, and has a left upper quadrant mass. His hemoglobin is 4 g/dL, platelet count is 100,000, and white blood cell (WBC) is 15,000 with 50% segmented neutrophils. His reticulocyte count is 15%. Which of the following is the most likely diagnosis?

(A) acute chest syndrome
(B) acute splenic sequestration
(C) aplastic crisis
(D) intussusception
(E) vasoocclusive crisis

19. A 2-year-old boy is diagnosed with severe mental retardation after a referral for lack of any language development. Which of the following epidemiologic characteristics is seen in severe mental retardation?

(A) female predominance
(B) about 80% correlation with advanced maternal age
(C) prevalence nearly evenly distributed across social classes
(D) life expectancy equal to the general population
(E) less than half of cases are genetic in origin

Questions 20 through 22

A 55-year-old man presents to the emergency department with an acute onset of excruciating substernal chest and epigastric pain following a prolonged episode of vomiting. His past history is significant for hypertension, diabetes, and a 30 pack-year smoking history. Vital signs show a blood pressure (BP) of 90/60 mmHg, pulse rate 100/min, respiratory rate 18/min, and temperature of 100°F. Examination reveals an ill-appearing man with subcutaneous emphysema and distant breath sounds on the left. A chest x-ray reveals pneumomediastinum and a left hydropneumothorax. A left chest tube is placed, and IV fluids are administered with resolution of his hypotension.

20. Which of the following is the most likely diagnosis?

(A) bronchopleural fistula
(B) esophageal perforation
(C) Mallory–Weiss tear
(D) spontaneous pneumothorax
(E) gastric perforation

21. Which of the following is the most appropriate diagnostic test?

(A) computed tomography (CT) scan
(B) esophagogram
(C) analysis of the pleural fluid
(D) esophagoscopy
(E) tracheobronchogram

22. Which of the following factors has the most influence on outcome?

(A) choice of antibiotics
(B) time to definitive treatment
(C) intensive care management
(D) early intubation and mechanical ventilation
(E) history of smoking

23. A researcher is conducting a study to determine whether a new medication causes insomnia. He surveys a group of study individuals taking the medication. The survey tool asks individuals to score their responses on a scale, rating the quality of their sleep as being poor, fair, good, or excellent. The data that is being collected by the researcher can be categorized as which of the following?

(A) dimensional
(B) ordinal
(C) binary
(D) nominal
(E) categorical

24. An individual is studying length of survival associated with chemotherapy for a particular cancer. He has looked at 25 individuals who have survival times ranging from 2 months to 2 years. Three of his study participants are still alive so their true survival time is still unknown. Which of the following measures of central tendency can be used at this point to analyze the data?

(A) mean
(B) mode
(C) median
(D) midrange
(E) midmode

25. A 26-year-old man presents to the emergency room with complaints of seeing and feeling bugs crawling on him (there are none per your thorough examination). He is tremulous, diaphoretic, disoriented, and his pulse rate is 120/min with a BP of 200/100 mmHg. Which of the following psychotropic drugs is he most likely withdrawing from?

(A) amitriptyline
(B) alprazolam
(C) chlorpromazine
(D) benztropine
(E) lithium carbonate

26. A young couple is going on their honeymoon to Mexico and wish to avoid travelers' diarrhea. You advise them to avoid water, ice, salads, and raw vegetables. What organism is the usual culprit?

(A) *Shigella*
(B) *Salmonella*
(C) *Vibrio parahaemolyticus*
(D) *Escherichia coli*
(E) *Campylobacter jejuni*

Questions 27 and 28

A healthy 23-year-old woman has her first prenatal visit. She has regular menses at 28- to 30-day intervals. Her last menstrual period (LMP) began December 1, 2001.

27. Which of the following is her estimated due date (EDD)?

(A) August 24, 2002
(B) September 1, 2002
(C) September 8, 2002
(D) September 15, 2002
(E) September 22, 2002

28. This woman has a pelvic examination at this prenatal visit. Her uterus is palpated midway between her symphysis and umbilicus. By physical examination, which of the following is her gestation age?

(A) 6 weeks
(B) 12 weeks
(C) 16 weeks
(D) 20 weeks
(E) 28 weeks

29. A 73-year-old man has been experiencing increasing drowsiness and incoherence. He has a history of arrhythmias and has fallen twice in the past 2 weeks. There are no focal deficits on neurologic examination. A contrast CT scan of the head is shown in Fig. 8-2. Which of the following is the treatment of choice?

(A) give parenteral antibiotics
(B) give antifungal therapy

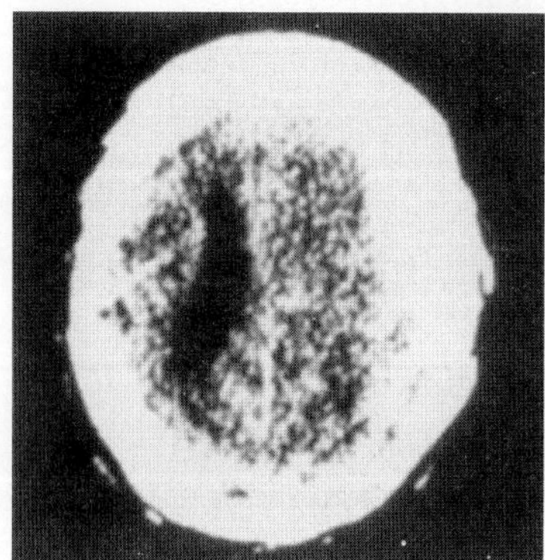

FIG. 8-2

(C) drill burr holes
(D) observe the patient and repeat the CT scan in 1 month
(E) give fibrinolytic therapy

30. A 21-year-old female comes to you for information about HIV and condom use. She has intermittently had sexual intercourse with several different men over the past 3 years. She consistently assures you that condoms are used. She wants to know whether condoms will protect her from HIV transmission from an HIV positive partner. Which of the following about condoms and HIV is true?

(A) If a woman has frequent sexual intercourse with an HIV positive man for a period of years, the risk of transmission of HIV with consistent condom use becomes similar to the risk of transmission without condoms.
(B) Latex condoms are less effective than natural membrane condoms in prevention of HIV transmission.
(C) Condoms treated with nonoxynol-9 are more than twice as effective at preventing transmission of HIV when compared with condoms not treated with this spermicide.
(D) Abstinence is the only way to prevent HIV transmission.
(E) Lubrication with petroleum jelly increases the likelihood that latex condoms fail.

31. The concerned mother of a 13-year-old girl states that her daughter has been sleeping late, easily becomes irritated with her younger brother, and insists on locking her bedroom door. She is doing well in school and is on the middle school soccer team. On physical examination, she is Tanner stage 4 and the rest of her physical findings are normal. Which of the following is the most appropriate next step in her management?

(A) checking her thyroid function
(B) obtaining a urine drug screen
(C) ordering a pregnancy test
(D) questioning the patient about possible abuse
(E) reassuring the mother

32. A 12-month-old boy is brought to the emergency department after having a generalized seizure at home. He has also vomited three times and been very irritable. He has never had a seizure previously and in general is in good health. On examination, he has a temperature of 40°C. He is irritable and does not seem to recognize his mother. A cerebrospinal fluid (CSF) sample obtained shows the following: 2000 WBCs (98% segmented neutrophils), protein of 155, and glucose of 20. Which of the following organisms is the most likely cause of his infection?

(A) enterovirus
(B) group A *Streptococcus*
(C) group B *Streptococcus* (GBS)
(D) *Streptococcus pneumoniae*
(E) *Mycobacterium tuberculosis*

Questions 33 and 34

A 55-year-old woman presents to the emergency department with malaise, fever, chills, anorexia, and nausea of 2 weeks' duration. Her past history is pertinent for a cholecystectomy 5 years ago and chronic diverticulitis of the sigmoid colon, manifesting as recurrent episodes over the last 2 years, for which she has been treated nonoperatively, the last episode occurring 6 weeks ago. On examination, she weighs 198 lbs and is febrile to 101°F, with a BP of 120/80 mmHg and pulse rate of 85/min, and has mild right upper quadrant abdominal tenderness. Laboratory data reveal a WBC of 18,000 and mildly elevated alkaline phosphatase and bilirubin.

33. Which of the following is the most appropriate diagnostic imaging procedure for this patient?

(A) radionuclide gallium scan
(B) abdominal ultrasound
(C) CT scan
(D) radionuclide technetium-99m sulfur colloid liver scan
(E) magnetic resonance imaging (MRI)

34. An imaging procedure (Fig. 8-3) demonstrates multifocal hepatic abscesses of different sizes. Which of the following is the most appropriate course of initial management?

(A) broad-spectrum antibiotics alone
(B) percutaneous drainage alone
(C) surgical drainage alone
(D) broad-spectrum antibiotics and percutaneous drainage
(E) broad-spectrum antibiotics and surgical drainage

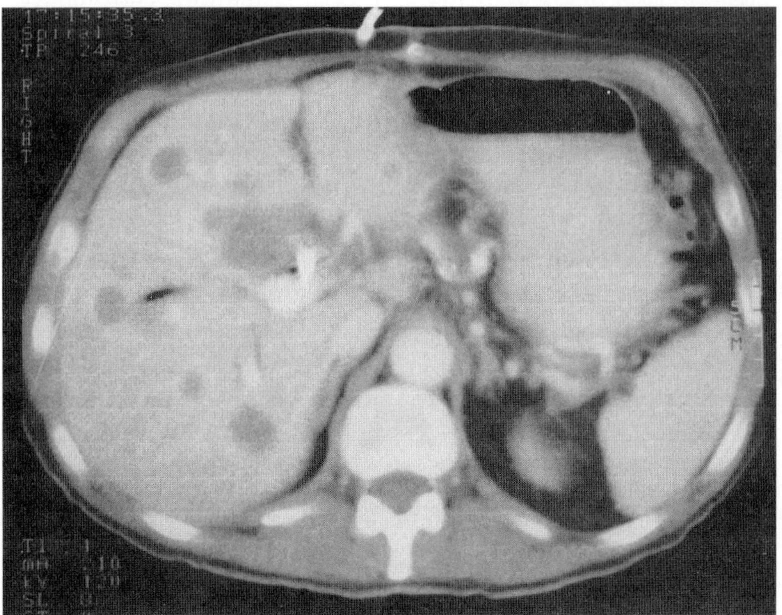

FIG. 8-3 *(Reprinted with permission from Zinner MJ.* Maingot's Abdominal Operations, *10th ed., vol. 2. Stamford, CT: Appleton & Lange, 1997.)*

Questions 35 and 36

A 10-year-old boy is brought to your office with a 3-year history of behavioral problems. Last week, he was suspended from school for bullying kids at the bus stop. Last year, he killed his family's cat by putting it in the dryer. His mother reports he ran away from home twice last year, each time for more than 2 days. He was previously arrested for burning down a warehouse. His mother says having him born was a mistake. The boy reports his mood is "good."

35. Which of the following is the most likely diagnosis?

(A) antisocial personality disorder
(B) oppositional defiant disorder
(C) no axis I disorder
(D) Tay-Sachs disorder
(E) conduct disorder

36. Which of the following statements is correct regarding this disorder?

(A) An estimated 15–20% of boys and 2–9% of girls under age 18 have the disorder.
(B) Low levels of plasma dopamine beta-hydroxylase have been implicated in some children with this disorder.
(C) There is no correlation between parental alcoholism and the emergence of this disorder.
(D) Attention deficit disorder cannot, by definition, coexist with this disorder.
(E) The average age of boys is the same as that of girls at the onset of this disorder.

DIRECTIONS (Questions 37 through 46): For each numbered item, select the ONE best lettered option that is most closely associated with it. Each lettered option may be selected once, more than once, or not at all.

For each patient with amenorrhea, select the most likely diagnosis.

(A) anorexia nervosa
(B) endometrial sclerosis
(C) polycystic ovary syndrome
(D) postpill amenorrhea
(E) pregnancy
(F) premature ovarian failure
(G) prolactin-secreting pituitary tumor
(H) Sertoli–Leydig cell tumor
(I) 17α-hydroxylase deficiency
(J) Sheehan syndrome
(K) testicular feminization syndrome
(L) Turner syndrome
(M) 21-hydroxylase deficiency
(N) true hermaphroditism
(O) Müllerian agenesis

37. A 24-year-old nulligravida last menstruated 3 years ago. One month ago, she took medroxyprogesterone acetate for 10 days but failed to bleed vaginally. Her medical history is unremarkable except for chronic schizophrenia, for which she takes an antipsychotic medication. Her BP is normal. She is 165 cm (5 ft 6 in.) tall and weighs 59 kg (130 lb). Nipple secretion is present bilaterally. Her vagina is dry, and there is no mucus within the cervical canal. Her pelvic examination and the remainder of her examination are normal.

38. A 19-year-old woman has never menstruated. She has never developed breasts or pubic hair. Physical examination confirms that she has Tanner stage 1 breast development and pubic hair. Her BP is 142/94 mmHg. Her pelvic examination is normal for a prepubertal female.

39. A 22-year-old woman began to menstruate at the age of 13 years, but has menstruated irregularly at $1^1/_2$- to 5-month intervals since. For the past 6 years, she has noted increasing hair growth on her face, chest, and abdomen. She now shaves every other day. She has no family history of irregular menses or hirsutism. Her BP is normal. She has no galactorrhea. The examination confirms the hirsutism. Her pelvic examination is normal except for a male escutcheon. Her serum dehydroepiandrosterone sulfate (DHEAS) concentration is normal.

40. A 38-year-old woman is now 6 months postpartum, but has not resumed menstruation. She did not breast feed; in fact, she was unable to do so because she did not form milk. Preeclampsia and uterine atony causing an estimated blood loss of 1200 mL within 3 h after the birth of her child complicated her pregnancy. The uterine atony responded to uterine massage and intramuscular ergot injections.

41. A 16-year-old girl has never menstruated, nor has she developed breasts. She has Tanner stage 2 pubic hair. A trial of oral medroxyprogesterone acetate failed to induce menstruation. She is 150 cm tall and weighs 46 kg (101 lb). Examination confirms the absence of breasts and scant development of pubic hair. A small cervix is seen on speculum examination, and a small uterus is palpated on bimanual examination. She has a webbed neck, cubitus valgus, and widely spaced nipples. Her serum follicle-stimulating hormone (FSH) level is 86 mIU/mL.

42. A 20-year-old woman has never menstruated, but developed breasts to Tanner stage 5 beginning at age 12 years. She has a maternal cousin who has never menstruated. Her BP is normal. Pubic hair is sparse. Her vagina is short, and there is no cervix seen on speculum examination. There is no palpable uterus on bimanual examination.

43. A 31-year-old woman has not menstruated since she had a dilation and curettage (D&C) 6 months ago for an incomplete spontaneous abortion complicated by endometritis.

44. A 35-year-old woman last menstruated 3 months ago. Until then, her menses were monthly and associated with premenstrual symptoms and mild dysmenorrhea. She discontinued oral contraceptives 3 months ago, and her last menses was a withdrawal from the contraceptive. She has noted some breast soreness, fatigue, and increased urinary frequency. Her vaginal epithelium appears slightly cyanotic.

45. A 32-year-old woman ceased to menstruate 1 year ago and has noticed a slight decrease in breast size. Before she stopped menstruating altogether, she recalls that her menses began to occur at irregular intervals at age 26. In the past year, she has noticed short episodes of flushing and perspiration 8–10 times daily, which have awakened her at night. She also complains of being tired all the time. Three years ago, a 5-day course of medroxyprogesterone acetate induced a menstrual period; 6 months ago, it did not. Her vaginal epithelium is dry, and there is no mucus within the cervical canal. Her FSH concentration is 53 mIU/mL.

46. A 25-year-old woman had monthly menses until they stopped abruptly 9 months ago. Since that time, she has noted progressive facial hair growth and deepening of her voice. Noteworthy on her physical examination is a prominent male escutcheon and slight enlargement of her clitoris. On bimanual examination, her right ovary has a diameter of approximately 7 cm, while the left ovary is about 4 cm. Her serum DHEAS concentration is normal. Her serum testosterone concentration is elevated at 183 ng/dL.

DIRECTIONS (Questions 47 through 58): Each of the numbered items or incomplete statements in this section is followed by answers or by completions of the statement. Select the ONE lettered answer or completion that is BEST in each case.

47. A muscular 25-year-old man presents to the emergency room with pressured speech, decreased need for sleep, grandiosity, hypersexuality, and racing thoughts worsening over 2 weeks. He has no family history of mental illness, but you find out he has been taking a medication he obtained illegally for the past month. Which one of the following medications is the most likely cause of this patient's symptoms?

(A) morphine
(B) cannabis
(C) alprazolam
(D) anabolic steroid
(E) lithium carbonate

48. A 25-year-old male develops low-grade fever, loss of appetite, dark urine, and then jaundice 3 weeks after a 2-week long humanitarian relief tour requiring extensive back country travel in an underdeveloped country. During the relief effort, he had close contact with young children and lived in the homes of area residents. He relied on locally prepared food and water sources. A laboratory test shows a high titer of immunoglobulin M (IgM) antihepatitis A virus (HAV). Which of the following would have been the best method to prevent this from happening?

(A) administration of a dose of immunoglobulin 1 week before leaving
(B) ingesting only foods cooked to high temperature and bottled water
(C) daily doses of bismuth subsalicylate (Pepto-Bismol) and ciprofloxacin
(D) administration of a dose of immunoglobulin immediately after returning
(E) vaccination with hepatitis A vaccine 10 years earlier

49. A 2-month-old infant is brought to the clinic with a diaper rash. Her mother states that it started as a red rash in the diaper area 1 week ago. She treated it with over-the-counter diaper cream, but it continued to spread and then began to peel 2 days ago. On physical examination, she is afebrile, has a diaper rash (Fig. 8-4, see color plate 2), and otherwise has a normal physical examination. Which of the following is the most likely diagnosis?

(A) allergic dermatitis
(B) bullous impetigo
(C) *Candida* dermatitis
(D) irritant dermatitis
(E) seborrheic dermatitis

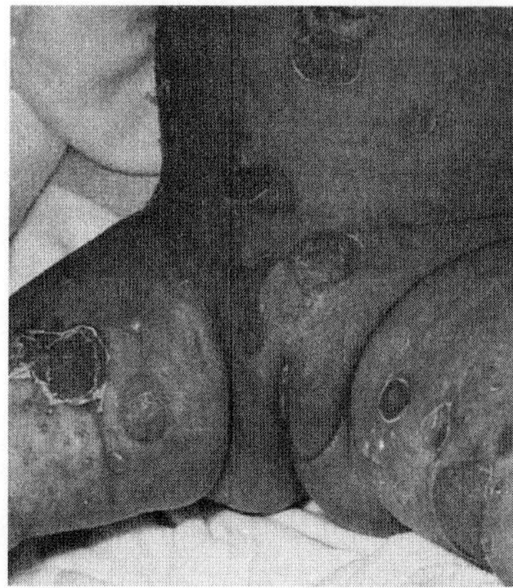

FIG. 8-4 Also see Color Plate 2. *(Courtesy of M. L. Williams. Reprinted with permission of Yearbook Medical Publishers.)*

50. Your next patient is a 4-month-old infant who is returning to have her ear checked. You diagnosed her with otitis media 2 weeks ago, and she has taken amoxicillin for 10 days. She is feeling well, and her mother's only concern is that she has developed a diaper rash over the last 3 days. She has been using emollient creams on it, which have not helped. On physical examination, there are no abnormal findings except for the rash (Fig. 8-5, see color plate 3). Which of the following is the most likely diagnosis?

(A) allergic dermatitis
(B) bullous impetigo
(C) *Candida* dermatitis
(D) irritant dermatitis
(E) seborrheic dermatitis

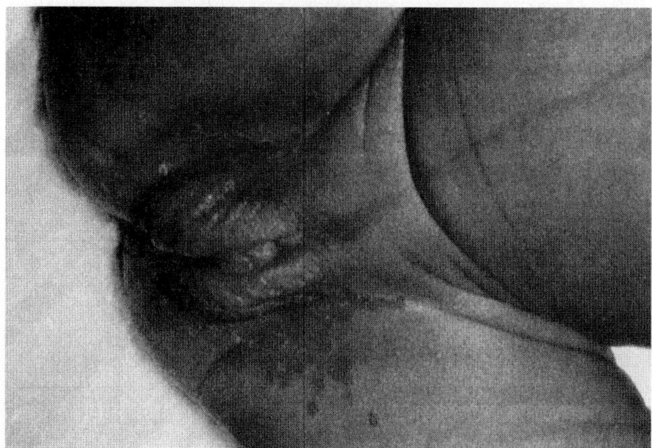

FIG. 8-5 Also see Color Plate 3. *(Courtesy of Neil S. Prose)*

Questions 51 and 52

A 33-year-old woman presents to the physician's office with a 2-month history of a left breast mass. The mass is nontender, and there is no associated nipple discharge or skin dimpling. Her past history is unremarkable. Her LMP started 2 weeks ago. Current medications include birth control pills. Family history is positive for breast cancer in a maternal grandmother. Physical examination reveals a 2-cm, firm, well-defined, very mobile, oval mass in the upper outer quadrant of the left breast without regional adenopathy. Mammography shows dense breasts. Ultrasonography demonstrates a well-marginated solid mass (Fig. 8-6).

51. Which of the following is the most likely diagnosis?

(A) invasive ductal carcinoma
(B) ductal carcinoma *in situ*
(C) fibrocystic changes
(D) fibroadenoma
(E) intraductal papilloma

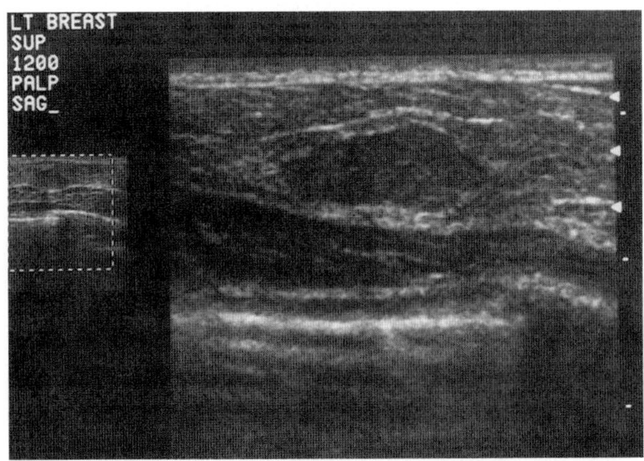

FIG. 8-6

52. Which of the following should be recommended as part of management of the mass?

(A) discontinuation of birth control pills
(B) reexamination after the next menstrual cycle
(C) needle biopsy
(D) excisional biopsy
(E) repeat ultrasound in 6 months

53. A 23-year-old female presents to your office with a rash. She reports that she is experiencing low-grade fevers and headache, in addition to the rash. She also relates having noticed a small ulcer in her genital area approximately 6 weeks earlier that has now healed. On physical examination, diffuse lymphadenopathy is noted along with the rash pictured in Fig. 8-7 (see color plate 4). Of the following disorders, which is most likely to be the correct diagnosis?

(A) leprosy
(B) secondary syphilis
(C) chancroid
(D) acquired immune deficiency syndrome (AIDS)
(E) tinea

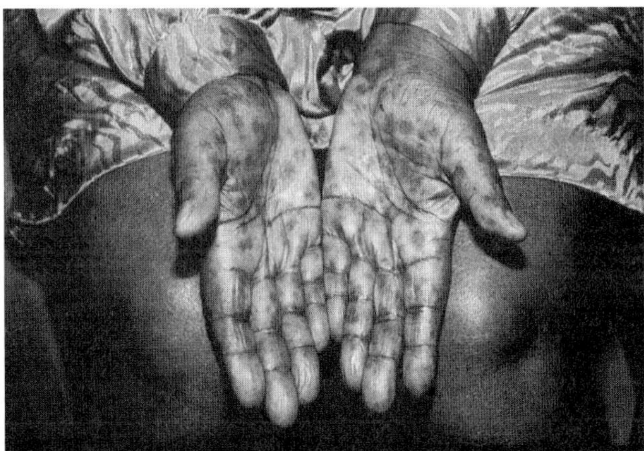

FIG. 8-7 Also see Color Plate 4. *(Courtesy of Neil S. Prose)*

54. A 7-year-old girl is brought to the clinic with a rash. His mother states that the rash has developed over the last several days. It began as a small red bump and has continued to grow (Fig. 8-8, see color plate 5). He has also had fever, headache, and malaise over the last several days. On physical examination, he has the rash and otherwise has a normal examination. Which of the following is the most likely diagnosis?

(A) contact dermatitis
(B) erythema marginata
(C) erythema migrans
(D) erythema multiforme
(E) tinea corporis

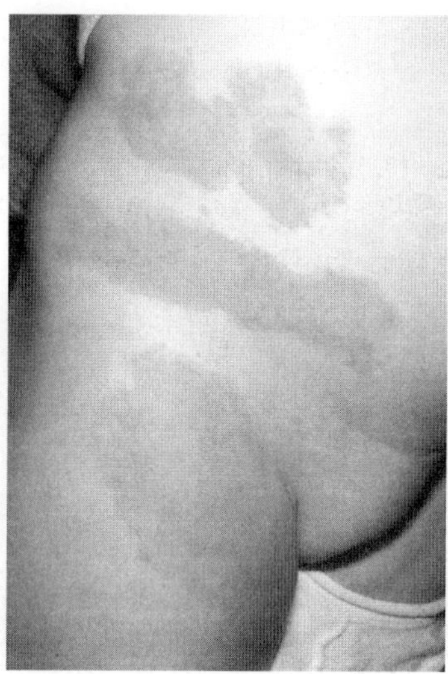

FIG. 8-8 Also see Color Plate 5. *(Courtesy of M. L. Williams)*

55. A 7-day-old infant is brought to the clinic with a rash. He was born at term and is the first child in the family. He had no problems at birth and has been doing well at home. On examination, he is afebrile. Other than the rash (Fig. 8-9, see color plate 6), which is found only on the top of his scalp, his examination is normal. Which of the following organisms is most likely the cause of his rash?

(A) enterovirus
(B) GBS
(C) herpes simplex virus
(D) *Staphylococcus aureus*
(E) varicella-zoster virus

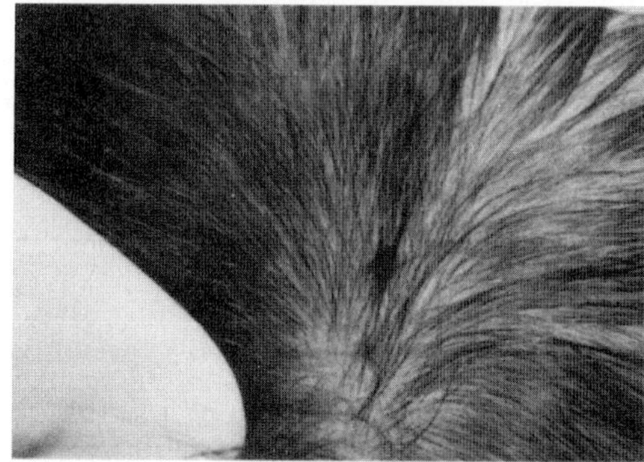

FIG. 8-9 Also see Color Plate 6. *(Courtesy of Neil S. Prose)*

56. A 6-year-old girl is brought to the office with a rash. Her mother states that 1 week ago she had a fever, headache, and malaise, which lasted for 3 days and then resolved. Now she feels well except for some pruritus with the rash. Her mother has also noted that the rash becomes more prominent when she is outside in the sun. On examination, she has no abnormal findings, except for the rash. Her cheeks are intensely red, and on her extremities she has the rash shown in Fig. 8-10 (see color plate 7). Which of the following is the most likely diagnosis?

(A) erythema infectiosum
(B) Kawasaki disease
(C) measles
(D) roseola
(E) scarlet fever

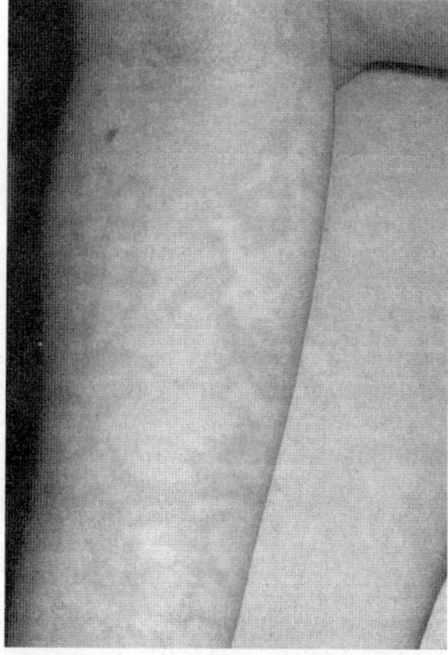

FIG. 8-10 Also see Color Plate 7. *(Courtesy of I. Frieden)*

57. A healthy 28-year-old woman begins prenatal care at 8 weeks' gestation. Her hemoglobin concentration is 13.5 g/dL. She began to take an over-the-counter multivitamin about 3 months before conception. Which of the following statements about folic acid is correct?

(A) 0.4–1.0 mg daily reduces the risk of a neural tube defect (NTD).
(B) It prevents a microcytic anemia.
(C) The amount should be increased to 1–2 mg/day in a woman who previously had a child with spina bifida.
(D) Prenatal vitamins should be started when pregnancy is recognized.
(E) Prescription prenatal vitamins have 0.4 mg of folic acid.

58. A 17-year-old adolescent comes to the clinic for a sports physical. He has no concerns about his health. He is a senior and is looking forward to playing baseball. He states that he is sexually active and has had three partners in the last 6 months. They usually use condoms for birth control. His physical examination is normal except for the lesion shown in Fig. 8-11 (see color plate 8). On further questioning, he first noted it 2 weeks ago. It has not been bothering him at all, so he did not mention it. Which of the following is the most likely cause of this lesion?

(A) condylomata acuminata infection
(B) herpes simplex infection
(C) staphylococcal infection
(D) trauma
(E) primary syphilis infection

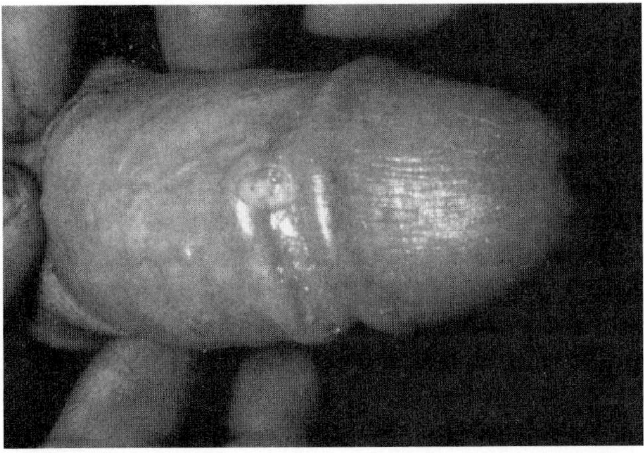

FIG. 8-11 Also see Color Plate 8. *(Courtesy of Neil S. Prose)*

DIRECTIONS (Questions 59 and 60): For each numbered item, select the ONE best lettered option that is most closely associated with it. Each lettered option may be selected once, more than once, or not at all.

For each of the following children with birth defects, select the most likely diagnosis.

(A) Beckwith–Wiedemann syndrome
(B) Cornelia de Lange syndrome
(C) defects associated with maternal use of coumadin derivatives
(D) fetal alcohol syndrome
(E) fetal hydantoin syndrome
(F) Noonan syndrome
(G) Prader–Willi syndrome
(H) Williams syndrome

59. A 3-year-old boy was hypotonic at birth. He also has moderate short stature and the physical features shown in Fig. 8-12.

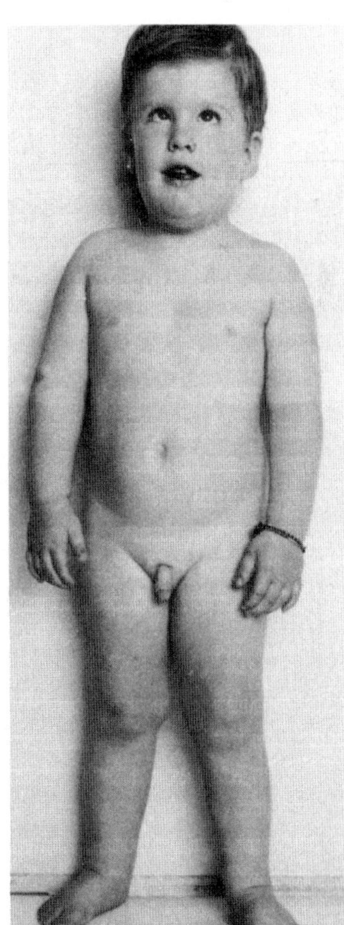

FIG. 8-12 *(Reprinted with permission from Rudolph AM.* Rudolph's Pediatrics, *20th ed. Stamford, CT: Appleton & Lange, 1995)*

60. A 12-month-old boy has a history of failure to thrive and developmental delay. He also has a cleft palate, a ventricular septal defect, and hearing loss. He has the facial features shown in Fig. 8-13.

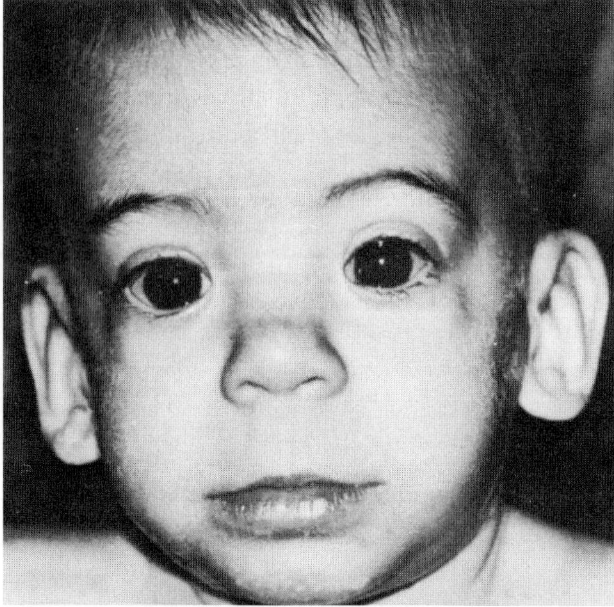

FIG. 8-13 *(Reprinted with permission from Rudolph AM.* Rudolph's Pediatrics, *20th ed. Stamford, CT: Appleton & Lange, 1995.)*

DIRECTIONS (Questions 61 through 64): Each of the numbered items or incomplete statements in this section is followed by answers or by completions of the statement. Select the ONE lettered answer or completion that is BEST in each case.

61. A 42-year-old man has the fingernails shown in Fig. 8-14. He also has arthritis involving the fingers. Which of the following is the most likely associated skin condition?

(A) pityriasis rosea
(B) erythema nodosum
(C) erythema multiforme
(D) psoriasis
(E) bullous pemphigoid

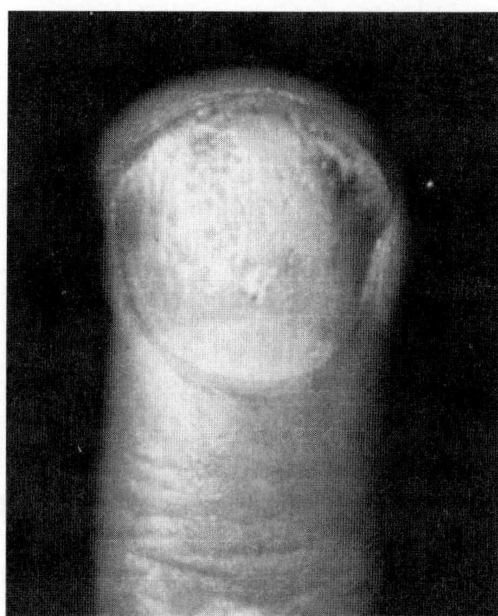

FIG. 8-14 *(Reprinted with permission from Zais N.* The Nail in Health and Disease, *2nd ed. East Norwalk, CT: Appleton & Lange, 1990.)*

62. An 18-year-old college student presents with sudden onset of severe pain in both legs. Her hematocrit is 26. Her peripheral blood smear is shown in Fig. 8-15 (see color plate 9). Which of the following is the most likely diagnosis?

(A) sickle cell anemia
(B) iron-deficiency anemia
(C) alpha-thalassemia major
(D) beta-thalassemia minor
(E) anemia of chronic disease

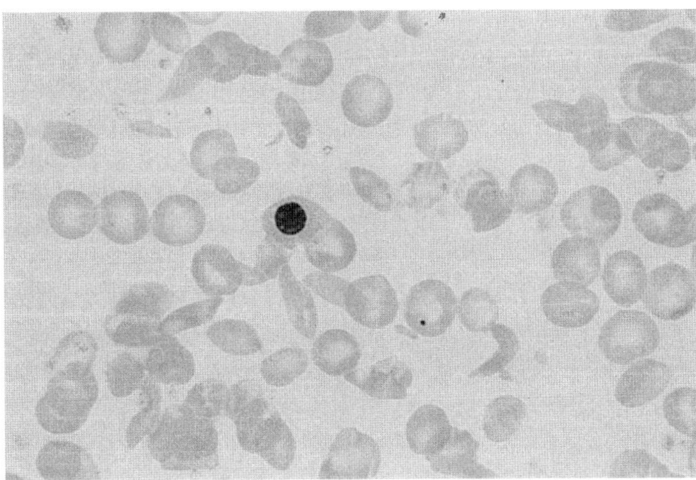

FIG. 8-15 Also see Color Plate 9. *(Reprinted with permission from Hurst JW.* Medicine for the Practicing Physician, *4th ed. Stamford, CT: Appleton & Lange, 1996.)*

63. A 30-year-old, previously healthy woman slips on the ice while crossing the street and strikes her head on the pavement. Bystanders report that she has loss of consciousness for 2 min, following which she is lucid but complaining of a headache. She is taken to a nearby emergency department. Over the next few hours, the patient develops a decreased level of consciousness, a dilated right pupil, and left hemiparesis. Which of the following is the most likely diagnosis?

(A) right occipital intracranial hematoma
(B) right subdural hematoma
(C) right epidural hematoma
(D) left epidural hematoma
(E) subarachnoid hemorrhage

64. A scientist working with ionizing radiation experiences a malfunction with his personal protective equipment and is exposed to about three Sieverts of radiation. What is the most likely form of acute radiation syndrome that he will experience?

(A) cerebral form
(B) gastrointestinal form
(C) hematopoietic form
(D) pulmonary form
(E) renal form

DIRECTIONS (Questions 65 through 68): For each numbered item, select the ONE best lettered option that is most closely associated with it. Each lettered option may be selected once, more than once, or not at all.

For each patient with rectal bleeding, select the most likely diagnosis.

(A) ischemic colitis
(B) peptic ulcer
(C) Meckel's diverticulum
(D) diverticulosis of the colon
(E) colonic polyp
(F) ulcerative colitis
(G) carcinoma of colon

65. A 70-year-old woman presents with vague abdominal pain and bloody diarrhea 3 days after an abdominal aortic aneurysm repair.

66. A 50-year-old alcoholic man with epigastric pain and tarry black, foul-smelling stools.

67. A 60-year-old previously healthy man presents with massive rectal bleeding.

68. A 75-year-old woman with recent onset of constipation, small-caliber stools, and intermittent dark red blood per rectum.

DIRECTIONS (Questions 69 through 96): Each of the numbered items or incomplete statements in this section is followed by answers or by completions of the statement. Select the ONE lettered answer or completion that is BEST in each case.

Questions 69 and 70

A 16-year-old boy comes to the clinic for a sports physical. You have followed him for many years and he has always been healthy. He continues to be healthy and has no concerns. On physical examination, the only abnormality that you discover is an irregular heart rhythm. You order a rhythm strip which is shown in Fig. 8-16.

69. Which of the following is the most likely diagnosis?

(A) atrial premature beats
(B) sick sinus syndrome
(C) sinoatrial block
(D) sinus arrhythmia
(E) supraventricular tachycardia

70. After identifying the particular rhythm, you arrange for further testing. Which of the following diagnostic tests would be the most appropriate initial step in caring for this patient?

(A) chest x-ray
(B) echocardiogram
(C) electrocardiogram (ECG)
(D) repeat rhythm strip in 1 week
(E) no further diagnostic tests are necessary

Questions 71 and 72

A 17-year-old previously healthy teenager suffers a direct blow to the upper abdomen during a hockey game. He complains of moderate epigastric pain at the time of the injury. Forty-eight hours later, the boy develops progressively increasing bilious emesis. On arrival in the emergency department, his abdomen is nondistended, with mild tenderness on palpation in the epigastrium and right upper quadrant. Laboratory investigations demonstrate a hematocrit of 36, WBC of 11,000, and an amylase of 235 IU.

71. Which of the following is the most likely diagnosis?

(A) pancreatitis
(B) gastritis
(C) acute cholecystitis
(D) duodenal hematoma
(E) small bowel perforation

72. Which of the following is the treatment of choice?

(A) immediate exploration
(B) nasogastric decompression and parenteral alimentation
(C) retrocolic gastrojejunostomy
(D) antacids and H_2 blockers
(E) cholecystectomy

Questions 73 and 74

A 26-year-old man complains to his family physician that he finds it difficult to perform adequately in his job as an accountant at a law firm because he feels the need to wash his hands at least once every half-hour, both at home and at work. He washes his hands for at least 5 min at a time, and he finds that his hands are beginning to get raw and red. The man reports that he has been engaging in this behavior for the past 2 months. He washes his hands in response to fears that they may have been contaminated by his touching telephones and other objects that other people have used.

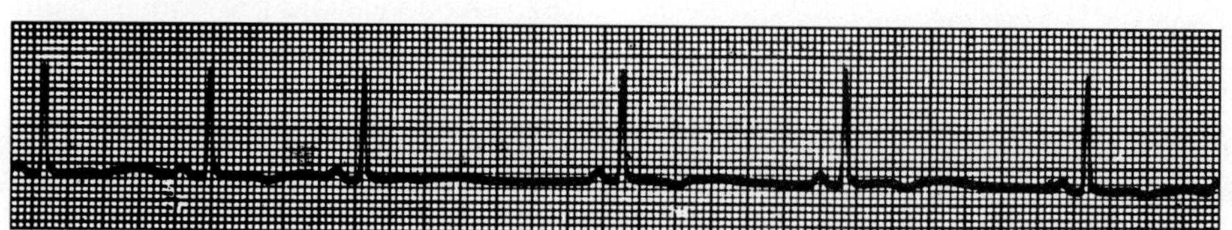

FIG. 8-16 *(Reprinted with permission from Rudolph C et al.* Rudolph's Pediatrics, *21st ed. New York: McGraw-Hill, 2003.)*

73. Which of the following is the most likely diagnosis?

(A) generalized anxiety disorder
(B) panic disorder without agoraphobia
(C) panic disorder with agoraphobia
(D) specific phobia
(E) obsessive-compulsive disorder

74. Which of the following medications is most likely to be effective in the treatment of the individual's disorder?

(A) lorazepam
(B) fluoxetine
(C) clonazepam
(D) haloperidol
(E) risperidone

Questions 75 and 76

75. A healthy, 28-year-old, primigravid woman at 40 weeks' gestation has had regular uterine contractions for 7 h. Her cervix is 7-cm dilated and 70% effaced. The vertex is at a +1 station. Which one of the following statements is correct?

(A) She is having false labor pains.
(B) She is in the latent phase of the first stage of labor.
(C) She is in the active phase of the first stage of labor.
(D) She is in the second stage of labor.
(E) She is in the third stage of labor.

76. At a +1 station, which one of the following statements best describes the location of the fetal vertex?

(A) It is floating above the pelvic inlet.
(B) It is below the pelvic inlet and above the ischial spines.
(C) It is at the level of the ischial spines.
(D) It is below the ischial spines and above the perineum
(E) It is visible at the perineum during a contraction.

77. A 53-year-old male just received notice from the blood bank that his most recent blood donation tested positive for HIV. He is from South Dakota, is well known by you, is believed to be trustworthy, and gives blood annually. He reports that for the past 20 years he has been in a mutually monogamous relationship with his wife, and that they have never used intravenous drugs or transfusions. The blood bank uses an ELISA to test for HIV.

Which of the following would be the most correct about this patient?

(A) He is at very low risk of having HIV. He should abstain from sex or practice safe sex while awaiting the results of a repeat ELISA.
(B) He is at very low risk of having HIV. He should abstain from sex or practice safe sex while awaiting the results of a confirmatory test such as a Western Blot test.
(C) Based on the specificity of the ELISA test, he has approximately a 13% chance of being infected with HIV. He should abstain from sex or practice safe sex while awaiting the results of a repeat ELISA.
(D) Based on the specificity of the ELISA test, he has approximately a 13% chance of being infected with HIV. He should abstain from sex or practice safe sex while awaiting the results of a confirmatory test such as a Western Blot test.
(E) He should immediately be offered post exposure prophylaxis, which would be initiated while awaiting results from confirmatory testing.

Questions 78 and 79

A 53-year-old male with a prior history of a sigmoid colon resection for diverticular disease presents to the emergency department with a 2-day history of crampy abdominal pain and progressive abdominal distention. He has had several episodes of bile-stained vomiting. His last bowel movement was 24 h before presentation. On examination, the patient has moderate abdominal distention, with intermittent high-pitched bowel sounds.

78. Initial management and evaluation of this patient should include which of the following?

(A) IV fluids and nasogastric decompression, followed by plain abdominal radiographs
(B) IV fluids and analgesics
(C) plain abdominal radiographs
(D) a barium enema
(E) a Fleet's enema and stool softeners

79. Over the next 6 h, the patient does not improve. A plain abdominal radiograph is shown in Fig. 8-17. Which of the following is the most appropriate next step in management?

(A) to continue serial examinations and repeat abdominal radiographs in the morning
(B) insertion of a rectal tube for colonic decompression
(C) insertion of a Cantor tube for small bowel decompression
(D) colonoscopy
(E) urgent exploratory laparotomy

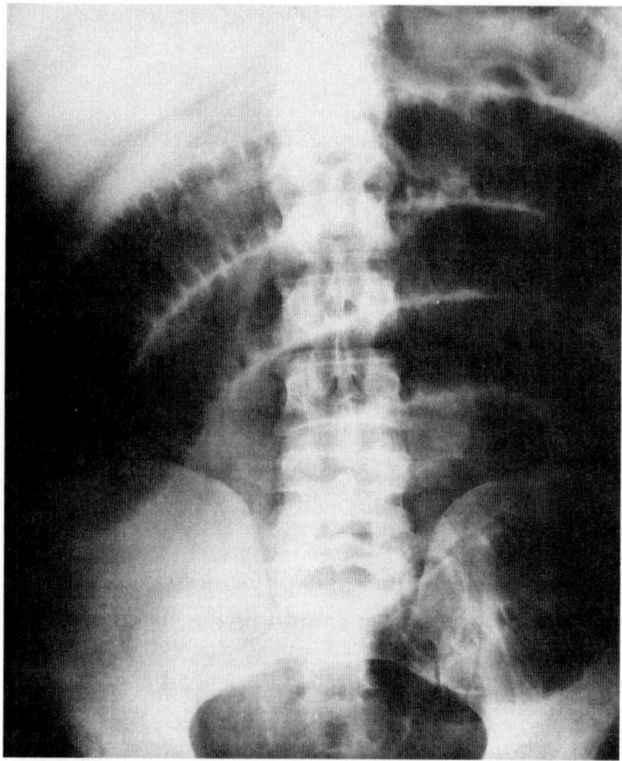

FIG. 8-17 *(Reprinted with permission from Zinner MJ.* Maingot's Abdominal Operations, *10th ed., vol. 2. Stamford, CT: Appleton & Lange, 1997.)*

80. A child is able to use a pincer grasp (thumb–first digit) to pick up a raisin. He can stand with support. He says "mama" and "dada." He is shy around strangers. You correctly note that he is developing normally. How old is he?

(A) 6 months
(B) 9 months
(C) 12 months
(D) 15 months
(E) 18 months

81. A 2-month-old infant is brought to the emergency department after having a seizure at home. The baby has not been ill, and there is no history of trauma. On examination, the baby is afebrile and is very lethargic. You are concerned about the possibility of child abuse. What physical finding would suggest that the child had injuries from violent shaking?

(A) Kernig's sign
(B) neck tenderness

(C) overlapping cranial sutures
(D) positive rooting reflex
(E) retinal hemorrhages

82. A 9-week-old infant has a hemoglobin of 9.2 g/dL. The rest of his CBC is normal. He has not had any health problems and was born at term without complications. Which of the following statements is true about anemia in infants at this age?

(A) Breast-fed infants commonly develop iron deficiency at this age.
(B) A congenital hemoglobinopathy is likely.
(C) Lead toxicity is a common cause of anemia at this age.
(D) This is likely his physiologic nadir.
(E) Transfusion should be considered for any hemoglobin less than 10 g/dL.

83. Your hospital is about to launch a new breast cancer awareness program. In preparation for determining the effectiveness of the initiative, you are asked to determine the current rate of mammographies among women admitted to your hospital. What type of study would be most appropriate for this purpose?

(A) a case-control study
(B) a cohort study
(C) a cross-sectional study
(D) a randomized trial
(E) a clinical trial

84. You have been treating an otherwise healthy 35-year-old male assembly line worker for sciatica, secondary to lumbar disk herniation at L4–L5. He is improving, several modified duty jobs are available. Which of the following would be least hazardous for him?

(A) assembly of 20 5-lb parts per hour while standing at a table and repeatedly leaning across the table to tighten bolts with a wrench
(B) inspection of dense 15-lb metal parts while standing or sitting at a table, and 10 times per hour carrying the part 10 ft at waist level to another table
(C) assembly of three 1-lb parts per minute while continuously seated at the assembly line, and doing job rotation to other similar positions two times per shift
(D) picking up 10-lb boxes of parts from the floor without squatting and transferring them to a waist-level conveyor once per minute
(E) keeping him off work until he can work without restrictions

Questions 85 and 86

85. A 27-year-old woman presents with cauliflower-like lesions of the external genitalia, vagina, and cervix. They vary in size and are discrete and nontender (see Fig. 8-18). Which of the following is the most likely cause of the lesions?

(A) herpes simplex
(B) gonorrhea
(C) *Hemophilus ducreyi*
(D) human papillomavirus (HPV)
(E) *Chlamydia trachomatis*

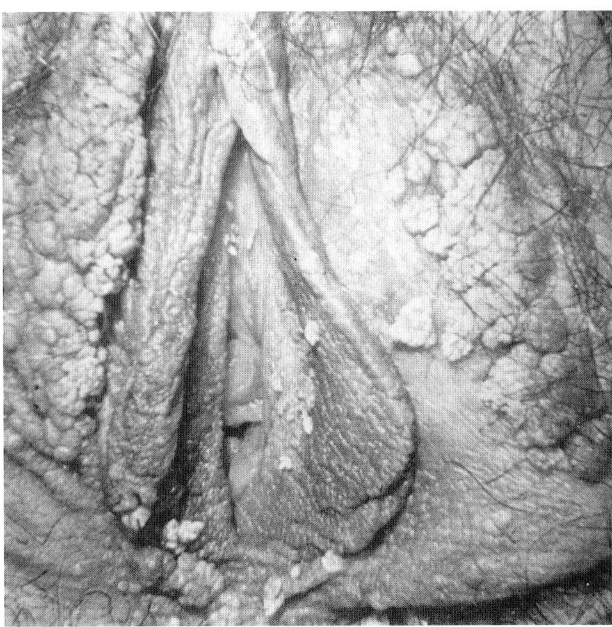

FIG. 8-18

86. A 33-year-old woman presents to your office with the vulvar lesions shown in Fig. 8-18. Which one of the following statements is correct?

(A) A biopsy or excision of the lesions should be done to establish the diagnosis.
(B) Type-specific human papilloma virus (HPV) nucleic acid testing should be done to confirm the diagnosis.
(C) The presence of these lesions increases the risk of cervical cancer.
(D) Successful medical or surgical therapy reduces the risk of future transmission.
(E) The lesions most commonly occur as a result of sexual transmission.

87. A 41-year-old women requests information about cervical cytology (Pap smear). In your counseling you tell her each of the following statements. Which one of the following statements is correct?

(A) The first Pap smear should be done at age 18 or when the woman becomes sexually active, whichever is first.
(B) A Pap smear should be done annually in all women.
(C) A CIN I (cervical intraepithelial neoplasia, mild dysplasia) Pap result will progress to cervical cancer in more than 50% of women.
(D) Cigarette smoking reduces the risk of cervical cancer.
(E) Liquid-based cervical cytology (Thin-Prep, Autocyte) yield have a higher true-positive rate than cytology interpreted from a microscopic slide.

Questions 88 through 90

A 55-year-old homeless woman with a long history of schizophrenia is seen for monitoring of her medications. As she talks, she frequently protrudes her tongue and grimaces. Her arms and hands jerk and bizarrely gesticulate as she talks. She is constantly squirming as she sits. She has been on fluphenazine 20 mg po bid for many years.

88. The abnormal movements strongly suggest which of the following?

(A) an exacerbation of catatonic schizophrenia
(B) tardive dyskinesia
(C) akathisia
(D) pseudoparkinsonism
(E) Huntington disorder

89. Which of the following is a risk factor for the above condition?

(A) young age
(B) being male
(C) low dose of medication
(D) being homeless
(E) having a mood disorder

90. Which of the following is a primary initial treatment strategy in this case?

(A) increasing the dose of fluphenazine
(B) add clonazepam to the regimen
(C) switch from fluphenazine to quetiapine
(D) add benztropine
(E) add propranolol

91. A 50-year-old professor was traveling across the country to attend a conference where he was to present. He took a medicine to help him get some sleep on the flight. The day following his presentation (which witnesses report he did give), he has no memory of giving the presentation. Which of the following medications most likely caused his memory loss?

(A) fluoxetine
(B) triazolam
(C) clonazepam
(D) diazepam
(E) tamazepam

Questions 92 and 93

A 20-year-old college student seems very uneasy as you walk in the examination room at the student health office. He tells you he has painful sores on his penis and admits that he has had intercourse with several different coeds in the past several months. The lesions are shown in Fig. 8-19.

92. Which of the following is the most likely diagnosis?

(A) herpes zoster
(B) syphilis
(C) herpes simplex
(D) condyloma acuminatum
(E) lymphogranuloma venereum

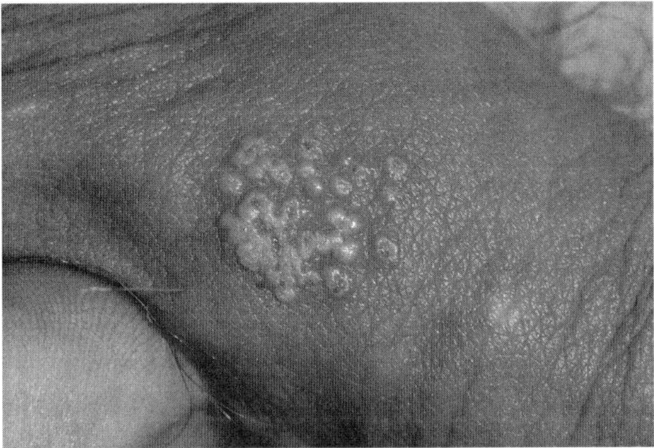

FIG. 8-19 *(Reprinted with permission from Fitzpatrick TB.* Color Atlas and Synopsis of Clinical Dermatology. *New York: McGraw-Hill, 1997.)*

93. The student has lots of questions about this infection. Which of the following is important for him to know about this condition?

(A) He can continue sexual activity with the lesions present as long as he uses a condom.
(B) Shedding of the organism will cease when the lesions are gone.
(C) Doxycycline is an effective treatment.
(D) He is at very low risk of having a recurrent episode if he uses condoms.
(E) Infection can be transmitted even when he is asymptomatic.

94. A 6-year-old boy has a purpuric and petechial rash over the buttocks and lower extremities. He appears to be well and is afebrile, but has swelling of the right knee. His CBC is normal. Which of the following is the most likely diagnosis?

(A) idiopathic thrombocytopenic purpura (ITP)
(B) systemic lupus erythematosus (SLE)
(C) meningococcemia
(D) Henoch–Schönlein (anaphylactoid) purpura
(E) juvenile rheumatoid arthritis

95. A 6-week-old male infant presents with a 5-day history of progressively worsening vomiting. He has not had a stool in 2 days. On physical examination, he is dehydrated. Serum electrolytes are:

Na^+	K^+	Cl^-	HCO_3^{-1}
136	3.0	88	36

Which of the following is the most likely diagnosis?

(A) congenital adrenal hyperplasia
(B) gastroesophageal reflux
(C) pyloric stenosis
(D) renal tubular acidosis
(E) gastroenteritis

96. A 27-year-old man is psychiatrically evaluated in jail for making threats to kill himself. He has been arrested for violation of parole, operating a drug house, and selling cocaine. He is enraged with the police for doing this, his fifteenth or "maybe twentieth" arrest since age 15. He feels they are out to get him. He admits to using alcohol and "crack" since age 12; they were easy to obtain because both parents used them. The highest grade achieved was 10th, during which he quit because "both the teachers and principal had it in for him." He was truant most of the time, anyway. Currently, he operates his own "chop shop" and talks with pleasure about the "kids" who provide him with cars for the shop and about his dealers who buy parts. "We take care of each other." He admits to hearing voices "occasionally" but denies ever being depressed or manic, except while on crack.

Which of the following personality disorders best describes this man?

(A) histrionic personality disorder
(B) narcissistic personality disorder
(C) avoidant personality disorder
(D) borderline personality disorder
(E) antisocial personality disorder

DIRECTIONS (Questions 97 through 100): For each numbered item, select the ONE best lettered option that is most closely associated with it. Each lettered option may be selected once, more than once, or not at all.

For each clinical setting described below, select the diagnosis that fits.

(A) migraine headache
(B) muscle contraction headache
(C) subarachnoid hemorrhage
(D) subdural hematoma
(E) brain tumor
(F) cluster headache
(G) sinus headache

97. a 42-year-old secretary with pain in her forehead that is worse when she bends over

98. a 32-year-old football coach with the worst headache of his life on the top of his head

99. a 50-year-old alcoholic man with pain around his right eye and excessive tearing

100. a 16-year-old girl with unilateral pain in the frontotemporal area associated with nausea

DIRECTIONS (Questions 101 through 116): Each of the numbered items or incomplete statements in this section is followed by answers or by completions of the statement. Select the ONE lettered answer or completion that is BEST in each case.

101. A 44-year-old man undergoes evaluation for worsening headaches. His posteroanterior and lateral arteriograms are shown in Fig. 8-20. What is the most likely complication?

(A) hypopituitarism
(B) subarachnoid hemorrhage
(C) hypercalcemia
(D) tentorial herniation
(E) chronic meningitis

Questions 102 through 105

A 60-year-old previously healthy woman is scheduled for an elective colon resection for a nonobstructing sigmoid colon carcinoma. The patient began a clear liquid diet 2 days preoperatively. Oral antibiotics were started the day before surgery, in addition to magnesium citrate. The patient vomited after the first dose of magnesium citrate and was not able to tolerate a second oral dose. At surgery, the patient received a third-generation cephalosporin intravenously on

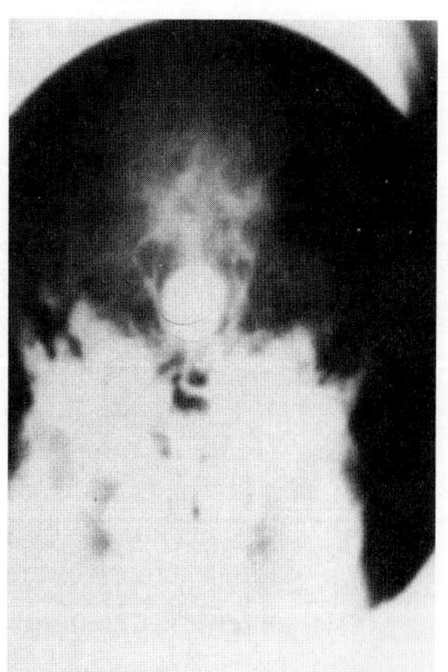

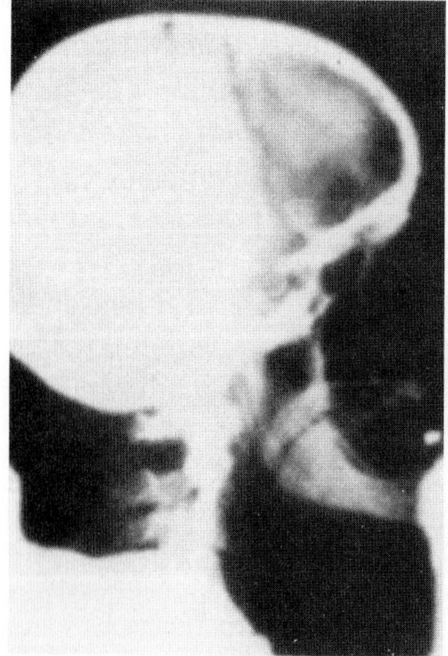

FIG. 8-20

induction of anesthesia. During the colonic anastomosis, there was gastrointestinal spillage.

102. This operative procedure would be classified as

(A) class I clean
(B) class II clean-contaminated
(C) class II clean-contaminated with inadequate bowel preparation and gastrointestinal spillage
(D) class III contaminated
(E) class IV dirty

103. Thirty-six hours after surgery, the patient has a persistent low-grade fever and mild tachypnea. On examination of the chest, there is decreased air entry at the lung bases. The abdominal dressing is clean and dry, and urine output via catheter is clear and adequate in volume. Which of the following is the most likely cause of the patient's fever?

(A) a wound infection
(B) a urinary tract infection
(C) pneumonia
(D) atelectasis
(E) a pelvic abscess

104. Appropriate evaluation and management should include which of the following?

(A) empiric antibiotic therapy
(B) blood, urine, and sputum cultures, followed by empiric antibiotic therapy
(C) pulmonary toilet with incentive spirometry and chest physiotherapy
(D) removal of the urinary catheter
(E) CT scan of the abdomen, with percutaneous abscess drainage

105. By the 6th postoperative day, the patient has normal bowel function and is tolerating a full oral diet. However, she develops a spiking fever pattern and complains of increasing incisional discomfort. On examination, there is a small amount of drainage on the wound dressing, and the incision is erythematous and tender. Appropriate evaluation and management at this point should include which of the following?

(A) blood, urine, and sputum cultures; chest x-ray and abdominal CT scan
(B) discharging the patient on oral antibiotics
(C) culture of the wound drainage, and initiation of IV antibiotics
(D) opening the incision, culture of the wound drainage, and initiating local wound care
(E) opening the incision, culture of the wound drainage, and initiating IV antibiotics

106. At her first prenatal visit at 8 weeks' gestation, a woman who is pregnant for the second time has a culture of her cervix that is positive for GBS. Her first child was delivered at 35 weeks after spontaneous rupture of the amniotic membranes and spontaneous onset of labor. During her first labor, she had several recorded temperatures of 101.6°F. Which of the following is the most appropriate next step in management?

(A) Prescribe oral amoxicillin for 1 week and repeat the cervical culture in 4 weeks.
(B) Repeat the cervical culture at 36 weeks' gestation and administer amoxicillin if it is positive.
(C) Administer IV penicillin when she goes into labor.
(D) Perform a cesarean section to prevent neonatal infection.
(E) Do nothing, because the attack rate to the infant is very low.

107. A 33-year-old woman with two children requests your advice about contraceptive choices. She and her partner desire no more children. Both are healthy, nonsmoking adults. She is especially interested in the method with the lowest failure rate. Which one of the following has the lowest failure rate as used?

(A) oral contraceptives
(B) intrauterine device (IUD)
(C) condoms
(D) tubal ligation
(E) vasectomy

108. A study finds that the incidence of asthma in your community is higher than what is reported for the state, and that 40% of the homes in your community are heated with forced air. The study design described here is best described as which of the following?

(A) an ecologic study
(B) a cross-sectional study
(C) a cohort study
(D) a case-control study
(E) a randomized clinical study

109. The mother of a 2-year-old boy asks you how tall you think he will be. His father is an NBA player and his mother is wondering if the child might follow in his footsteps. Currently his height is 37.5 in. You tell the mother that her son will most likely be how tall?

(A) about 5 ft tall
(B) about 7 ft tall
(C) about 6 ft tall
(D) 5 ft 3 in. tall
(E) there is no way to tell

110. During a routine yearly checkup, an 8-year-old boy is found to have 2+ proteinuria on urinalysis. Which of the following is the most appropriate diagnostic test to order?

(A) blood urea nitrogen (BUN) and serum creatinine
(B) urine culture
(C) intravenous pyelogram (IVP)
(D) a repeat urinalysis
(E) renal sonogram

111. A 42-year-old alcoholic woman is admitted to the hospital after suffering a seizure. She is febrile, cachectic, ill-kempt, and has poor oral hygiene. A chest examination is normal; her chest x-ray is shown in Fig. 8-21. Which of the following is true regarding this lesion?

(A) often found as multiple lesions
(B) often associated with periodontal disease
(C) often due to aerobes
(D) often due to gram-negative bacilli
(E) second-generation cephalosporin is the drug of choice

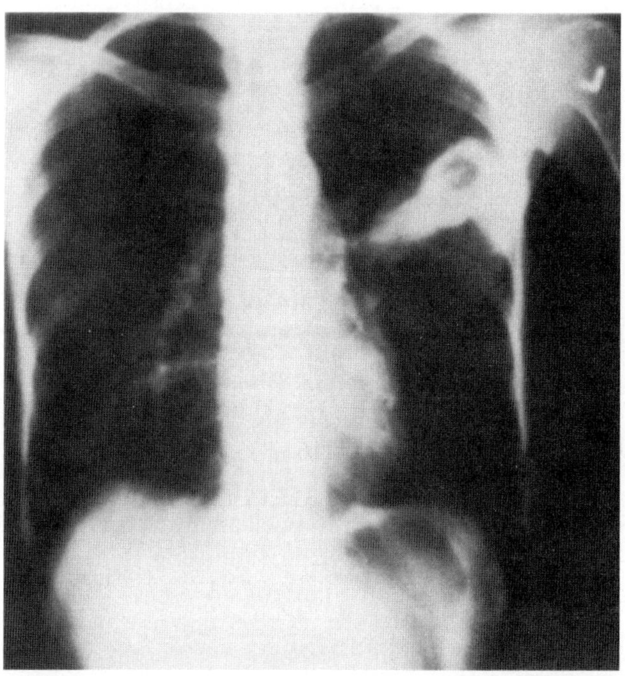

FIG. 8-21

112. In reviewing your clinical practice, you notice that almost one quarter of the hospital inpatients you have seen in the past 3 months have carried the diagnosis of congestive heart failure. Which of the following best describes about how common this disorder is among patients currently in the hospital?

(A) incidence
(B) prevalence
(C) positive predictive value
(D) negative predictive value
(E) relative risk

113. A 61-year-old man is admitted to the cardiac care unit (CCU) with crushing chest pain and the ECG shown in Fig. 8-22. He is agitated, pale, and diaphoretic. Peripheral pulses are weak, and systolic BP is 90 mmHg. Neck veins are distended, Kussmaul's sign is present, but lungs are clear. There is an S_3 gallop but no murmur. Which of the following is the most likely cause of the hypotension?

(A) acute mitral regurgitation
(B) aortic dissection
(C) bacterial endocarditis
(D) right ventricular infarct
(E) pericardial tamponade

Questions 114 through 116

An 8-month-old girl is brought to the clinic with a 3-day history of fever, vomiting, and irritability. She has never had a similar problem. On physical examination, her temperature is 40.0°C. She appears moderately dehydrated. She vomits twice during the visit. Her initial workup shows a WBC of 20,000 with 70% neutrophils. Her catheterized urinalysis shows a specific gravity of 1.030, 1+ protein, and trace blood. The microscopic examination reveals 0–5 red blood cells per high-power field, numerous WBCs per high-power field, and moderate bacteria. A urine culture is sent.

114. Which of the following is the most appropriate next step in her management?

(A) Prescribe trimethoprim-sulfamethoxazole and see her tomorrow in the office.
(B) Give IM ceftriaxone and see her tomorrow in the office.
(C) Admit her to the hospital for IV hydration and IV antibiotics.
(D) Wait for the urine culture and treat her if it is positive.
(E) Start oral rehydration in the office and prescribe amoxicillin.

115. Her urine culture is positive the next day. Which of the following organisms is the most likely cause of her infection?

(A) *Escherichia coli*
(B) *Klebsiella*
(C) nontypeable *Haemophilus influenzae*
(D) *Pseudomonas aeruginosa*
(E) *Staphylococcus aureus*

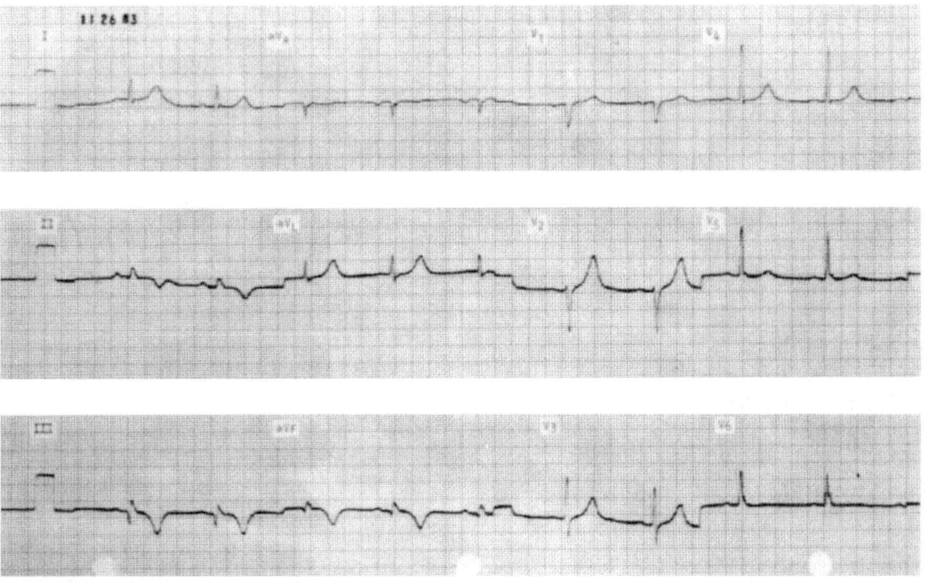

FIG. 8-22

116. You see her in the office 3 weeks later after the infection has been treated. All of her symptoms have resolved, and she has a normal physical examination. Which of the following is the most appropriate next step in her management?

(A) Order a renal ultrasound.
(B) Order a voiding cystourethrogram.
(C) Order a renal ultrasound and a voiding cystourethrogram.
(D) Order a nuclear medicine renal scan.
(E) No tests are necessary.

DIRECTIONS (Questions 117 through 126): Each set of matching Questions in this section consists of a list of lettered options followed by several numbered items. For each item, select the ONE best lettered option that is most closely associated with it. Each lettered option may be selected once, more than once, or not at all.

Questions 117 through 122

Certain side effects are typically caused by psychiatric medication. In the case reports below, identify the medication that is most likely the cause of the side effect described.

(A) clozapine
(B) fluvoxamine
(C) haloperidol
(D) imipramine
(E) lithium carbonate
(F) lorazepam
(G) thioridazine
(H) trazodone

117. A routine blood test showed a WBC of 1.9 K/mm^3 in a man with chronic schizophrenia. Because of this, he was directed to discontinue the medication that had significantly controlled his hallucinations better than any of the many medications he had tried in the past.

118. A young man was successfully medically treated for feelings of discouragement, an early morning awakening sleep disturbance, poor appetite, and sense of hopelessness. Several months after starting this medication, he sought help in the emergency department because of a penile erection that would not subside.

119. A 35-year-old woman with a history of major depression with psychosis appeared in the emergency department. Her eyes were, as she said, "locked up in my head." She had started a drug approximately 2 weeks before this episode.

120. A 45-year-old woman with a history of erratic, hostile behavior, pressured speech, flight of ideas, and impulsiveness has had her symptoms controlled with medication. She is seen by her psychiatrist for a routine visit and complains that she might be getting "the flu." She describes symptoms of nausea and diarrhea. As she speaks, the psychiatrist notes that she slurs her words and is tremulous and ataxic.

121. A young man with a history of psychotic symptoms has responded well to a low-potency, high-anticholinergic drug. He complains to his psychiatrist that he is embarrassed that his semen seems to go "in" rather than "out." He wonders if he is going crazy again.

Questions 122 through 126

For each of the following patients with a respiratory illness, select the most likely pathogen.

(A) adenovirus
(B) *Bordetella pertussis*
(C) *Chlamydia trachomatis*
(D) coxsackievirus
(E) Epstein-Barr virus
(F) *Haemophilus influenzae*
(G) herpes simplex 1
(H) *Moraxella catarrhalis*
(I) *Mycoplasma pneumoniae*
(J) parainfluenza virus
(K) respiratory syncytial virus (RSV)
(L) rotavirus
(M) *Staphylococcus aureus*
(N) *Streptococcus agalactiae* (group B)
(O) *Streptococcus pneumoniae*
(P) *Streptococcus pyogenes* (group A)

122. a 3-month-old infant with wheezing and history of 3 days of cough, congestion, and rhinorrhea

123. a 9-year-old with gradual onset of fever, malaise, and worsening cough over 5 days and rales in the area of the right upper lobe

124. a 3-month-old infant with history of eye drainage at 2 weeks of age who now has insidious onset of staccato cough and is afebrile, with bilateral rales on examination

125. a 6-month-old with history of 2 weeks of congestion and rhinorrhea, who now has worsening paroxysms of coughing

126. a 2-year-old with 2 days of rhinorrhea and cough, now with hoarseness and a barky cough

DIRECTIONS (Questions 127 through 133): Each of the numbered items or incomplete statements in this section is followed by answers or by completions of the statement. Select the ONE lettered answer or completion that is BEST in each case.

Questions 127 and 128

A young man develops wheezing after eating lobster and presents to the emergency department 15 min later with persistent breathing difficulty.

127. Which of the following is the most important initial treatment?

(A) oral beta-blocker
(B) topical steroid
(C) IV steroid
(D) subcutaneous epinephrine
(E) intramuscular diphenhydramine

128. Which of the following is associated with this type of immediate hypersensitivity?

(A) immunoglobulin A (IgA) binding to mast cells or basophil membranes
(B) delayed skin rash
(C) immediate appearance of symptoms, with self-limited resolution within one-half hour
(D) intrinsic asthma
(E) symptoms including laryngeal edema and bronchospasm

129. A 30-year-old employee has had audiometric testing done as a part of the company's Hearing Conservation Program. You notice that on the right there is a 10 dB hearing loss at both 3000 Hz and 4000 Hz. On the left, there is a 5 dB loss at 3000 Hz and a 10 dB loss at 4000 Hz. Which of the following is the most appropriate course of action?

(A) Return this person to work with ear plugs.
(B) Wash out an accumulation of cerumen.
(C) Refer to an ear, nose, and throat specialist to rule out acoustic neuroma.
(D) Assume a recent middle ear infection and recheck in 2 weeks.
(E) Alert the primary care physician to the possibility that an ototoxic is inducing hearing loss.

Questions 130 and 131

A 33-year-old man presents to the emergency room complaining of left-sided chest pressure and shortness of breath that began about an hour ago. He is otherwise healthy with no significant past history and a recent normal physical examination. His cholesterol was 168 with an HDL of 75. He has no family history of coronary artery disease. His ECG is shown in Fig. 8-23.

130. What is the abnormality on the ECG?

(A) acute pericarditis
(B) acute anteriolateral wall myocardial infarction (MI)
(C) acute inferior wall MI
(D) congestive heart failure
(E) atrial fibrillation

131. Which of the following is the most likely cause of these findings?

(A) cocaine use
(B) coronary artery disease
(C) viral pericarditis
(D) pulmonary embolism
(E) congestive heart failure

132. A young farm worker who was working with pesticides is brought to the emergency room with headache, vomiting, salivation, diarrhea, muscle fasciculations, difficulty walking and difficulty speaking. His clothing has been removed, he has been washed, and he has been given activated charcoal. What is the most effective remaining treatment for this case of pesticide poisoning?

(A) epinephrine
(B) chelation
(C) a spironolactone
(D) atropine
(E) supportive therapy

133. A 72-year-old patient presents at your office uncertain if he can afford your services. He does have a Medicare card. Which of the following is the most applicable to Medicare Part B?

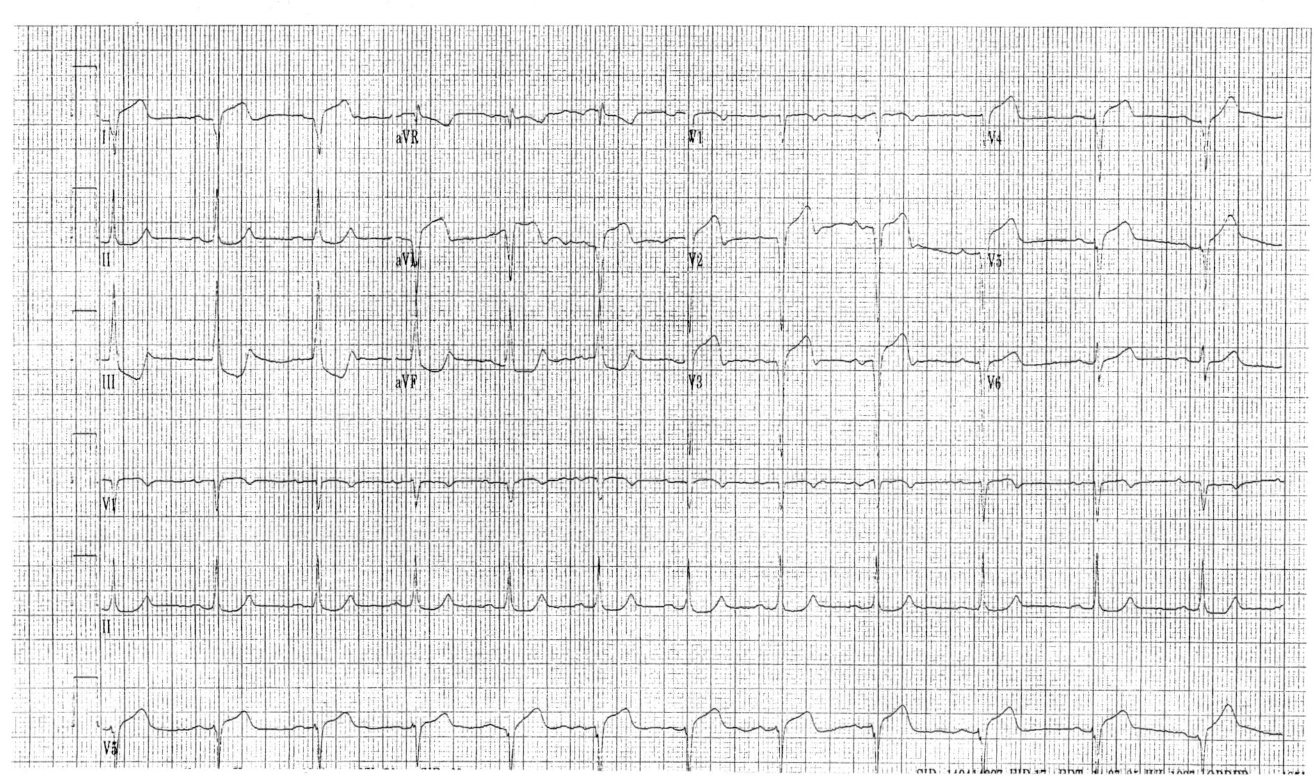

FIG. 8-23

(A) It is a joint federal state program.
(B) It categorizes diagnoses and conditions into Diagnosis Related Groups (DRGs).
(C) It reimburses based on the Resource Based Relative Value Scales (RBRVSs).
(D) It corresponds to Title 19 of the Social Security Act.
(E) It provides a minimum set of services to the needy.

DIRECTIONS (Questions 134 through 140): For each numbered item, select the ONE best lettered option that is most closely associated with it. Each lettered option may be selected once, more than once, or not at all.

Question 134 through 140

A 24-year-old man is brought to a general hospital emergency room by local police. They explain that the man is well known to them as a "troublemaker." The police report that he suffers from mild mental retardation, and that he has been very upset for the past month because of the recent death of his mother, who he had visited every week while he lived in a group home. They report that the young man is also mentally ill and that his behavior has recently deteriorated, resulting in his eviction from the group home 1 day earlier. The physician on call obtains the patient's past medical record from the file room, and learns that the patient has a history of asthma and type II diabetes mellitus, for both of which he is seen in a hospital clinic. The records also indicate that the patient has a history of impulsive and self-destructive behavior, and that he was diagnosed at age 18 as having borderline personality disorder. At age 21, the records indicate, the patient began to experience auditory hallucinations and to believe that the FBI was out to get him. Since then, he has carried the diagnosis of chronic paranoid schizophrenia.

In the Diagnostic and Statistical Manual of Mental Disorder, 4th Edition, Text Revision (DSM-IV-TR), a multiaxial diagnostic system is used. Using the above case, match the axis below to the diagnostic features listed.

(A) axis I
(B) axis II
(C) axis III
(D) axis IV
(E) axis V

134. mild mental retardation

135. ejection from group home

136. chronic paranoid schizophrenia

137. borderline personality disorder

138. asthma

139. type II diabetes mellitus

140. recent death of mother

Answers and Explanations

1. **(C)**

2. **(E)**

Explanations 1 and 2

The complications of gastroesophageal reflux disease (GERD) include esophagitis, esophageal ulceration, stricture, and Barrett's esophagus, among others. Although some patients with GERD respond well to medical therapy, such as a proton-pump inhibitor, regurgitation, and coughing attacks, some may not improve with medical treatment alone. The results of treatment by antireflux surgery, such as Nissen fundoplication, are generally good under these circumstances and may prevent the progression of the Barrett's. Once present, Barrett's rarely regresses following surgery. Once high-grade dysplasia is found within Barrett's epithelium, up to half of esophagi removed for such a condition demonstrate foci of invasive cancer. Therefore, the recommended treatment for high-grade dysplasia within Barrett's is esophagectomy. There is no evidence to suggest that *H. pylori* is involved in GERD or esophagitis. *(Greenfield et al., pp. 666–676; Townsend et al., pp. 1142–1144, 1163)*

3. **(E)** External otitis is an infection of the external auditory canal. The primary symptom is ear pain, which is worsened when the pinna is moved. This distinguishes it from otitis media. A foreign body is easily seen in the canal, unless there is secondary infection and drainage. Mastoiditis is a complication of otitis media. Patients have fever, and as the process progresses, displacement of the pinna. Contact dermatitis in the ear is usually due to an earring and would occur on the pinna. *(Rudolph et al., pp. 1255–1256)*

4. **(B)** Disease from wild poliovirus was eliminated from the United States. However, approximately eight cases of paralytic polio associated with oral vaccine were occurring every year. Since this complication does not arise with injectable inactivated poliovirus vaccine (IPV), the recommendation was made to change the schedule to four doses of IPV. (When polio was still endemic, oral vaccine had been preferable, since oral vaccines were more efficient at preventing intestinal infection without disease, and therefore transmission of polio that can occur in vaccinated persons.) *(CDC website: www.cdc.gov; Wallace and Doebbeling, p. 124)*

5. **(E)** ELISA detectable antibodies to HIV generally appear within 4–12 weeks after infection with HIV. They are detectable within 6 months in more than 95% of cases. Note that since 2002, rapid HIV tests are available, which require blood or an oral swab. Positive results require confirmatory testing with Western Blot of immunofluorescent assay. *(USPSTF, 2nd ed., Screening: HIV, pp. 304–305; CDC website: www.cdc.gov; MMWR, 2004)*

6. **(D)** Chronic exposure to benzene, which is used in many industrial processes, is a very well documented cause of bone morrow depression. Benzene-induced aplastic anemia can be fatal. Chronic exposure also is known to cause an increased risk of leukemia. Acute exposure to high concentrations will cause CNS depression. *(Wallace and Doebbeling, p. 514; LaDou, p. 224)*

7. **(C)** Tertiary prevention activities involve the care of established disease, with attempts made to restore to highest function, minimize the negative effects of disease, and prevent disease-related complications. In this scenario, the patient has established disease or diabetes, and referral to the ophthalmologist's office is an attempt to minimize the negative effects of his diabetes-induced retinopathy. Primary prevention is used to prevent disease before it has

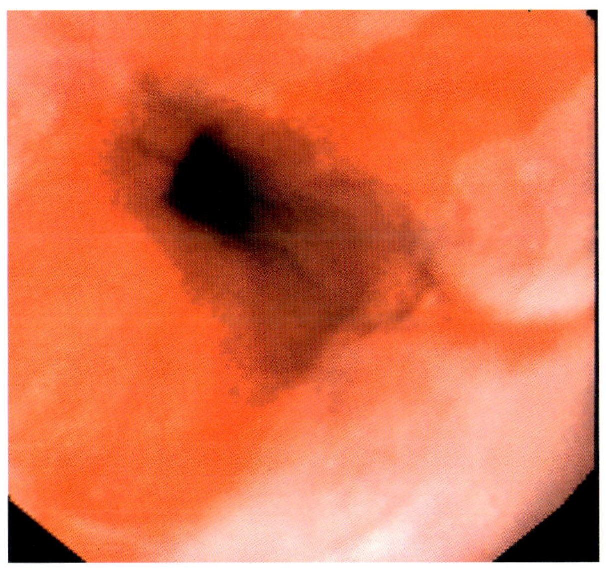

Color Plate 1 (Figure 8–1)

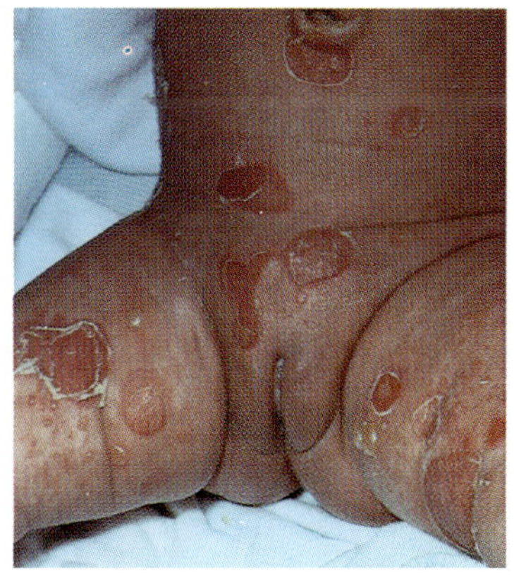

Color Plate 2 (Figure 8–4)

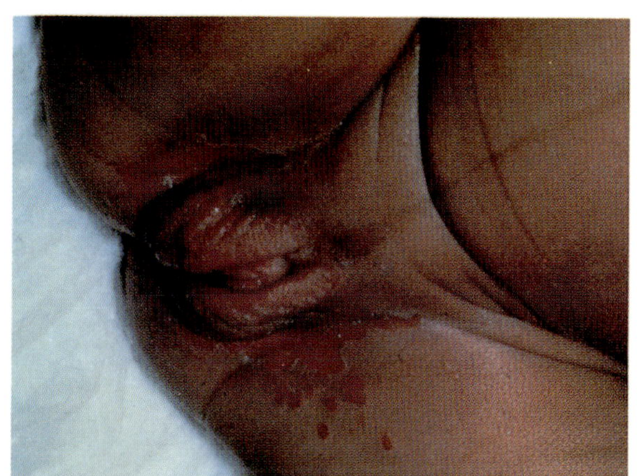

Color Plate 3 (Figure 8–5)

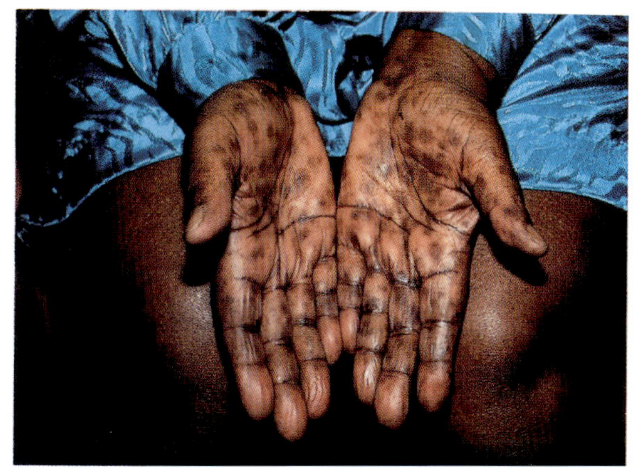

Color Plate 4 (Figure 8–7)

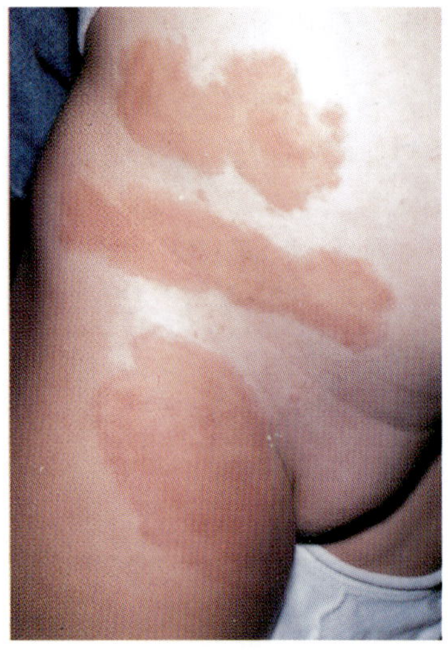

Color Plate 5 (Figure 8–8)

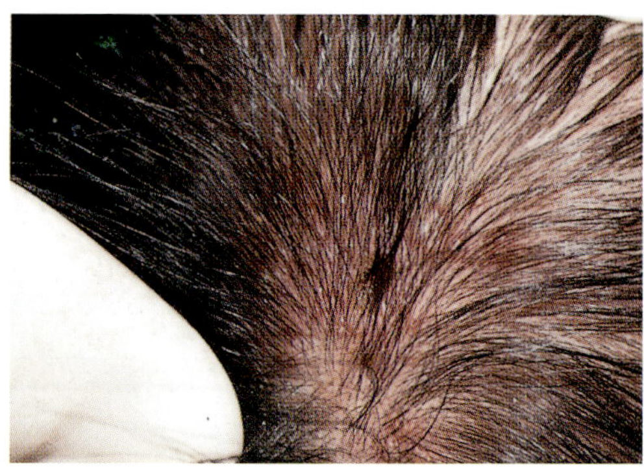

Color Plate 6 (Figure 8–9)

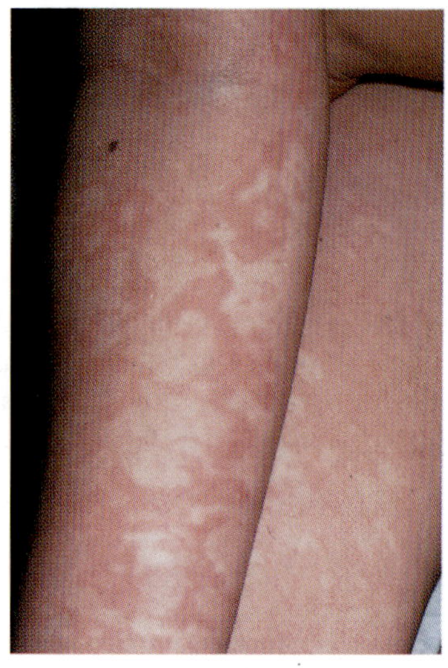

Color Plate 7 (Figure 8–10)

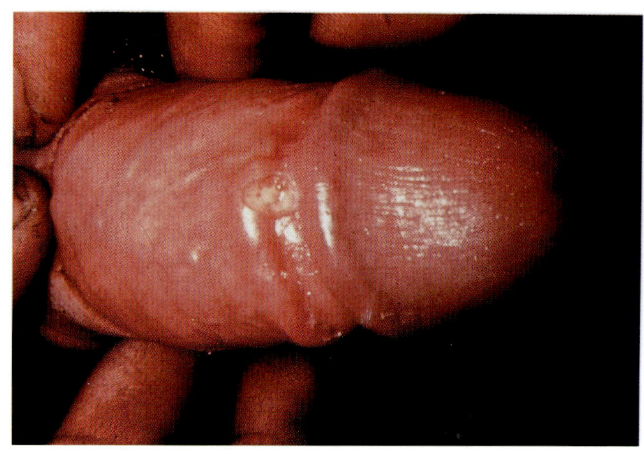

Color Plate 8 (Figure 8–11)

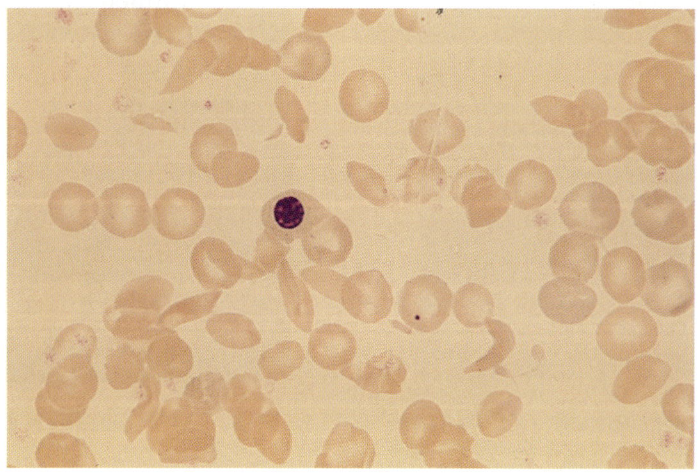

Color Plate 9 (Figure 8–15)

occurred, i.e., immunization programs. Secondary prevention aims to detect presymptomatic disease at an early stage in order to prevent or minimize morbidity. Quaternary and predisease prevention are not terms used to refer to the three main types of prevention. *(Lang and Hensrud, pp. 3–4)*

8. **(C)** Pap testing should be done for all women who have been sexually active and who have a cervix. It should be started when sexual activity is initiated, be repeated at least every 3 years, and probably can be stopped at age 65 if all previous Pap tests have been normal. If a woman has had a hysterectomy for invasive cancer of the cervix or has a history of diethylstilbestrol (DES) exposure, Pap tests (cell cytology) should be continued despite absence of the cervix (evidence for this practice is not strong, but it is the current recommendation). Cancer of the cervix seems to occur almost exclusively or exclusively in association with active infection with a pathogenic strain of HPV. *(USPSTF, 3rd.: Periodic Updates. Screening: Cervical Cancer, 2003)*

9. **(B)** Silicosis is often seen in quarry workers working with compounds with high free crystalline silica such as quartz, sandstone, granite, and slate. Involvement of the lungs by silicosis increases susceptibility to tuberculosis infection. There is no added risk of tuberculosis after exposure to asbestos or other nonsilica dust. Coal worker's pneumoconiosis, as the name implies, is more commonly seen in coal workers. Asbestosis is more commonly seen in those who have a history of exposure to asbestos containing compounds or materials, or the mining or milling of asbestos. Siderosis refers to the lung disease caused by inhalation of iron dust. Siderosis is not considered to increase susceptibility to tuberculosis. *(Wallace and Doebbeling, p. 487; LaDou, p. 337)*

10. **(D)** Fox rabies is still a serious problem in North America. Furthermore, foxes act as a common reservoir of rabies in parts of Texas. The appropriate management of this patient would include postexposure prophylaxis with both rabies vaccine and immune globulin. The patient's tetanus immunization status should also be reviewed and postexposure prophylaxis administered if the immunization status is incomplete or unknown. *(Wallace and Doebbeling, pp. 349–352)*

11. **(D)** Linear regression with calculation of the regression coefficient is commonly used to assess whether there is a relationship between two variables and to assess the magnitude of that trend. The regression coefficient is the slope of the line. If the line is essentially horizontal, the slope is close to zero, and the variables have little relationship to each other. It must be remembered that a high level of correlation indicates strong association, but does not necessarily mean that there is a causal relationship between the two variables. The odds ratio is used to contrast two proportions. The Wilcoxon Two-Group Rank Sum test, Mann–Whitney U-test, and Wilcoxon Signed-Ranks test are nonparametric rank tests that use ranks of observed data rather than original values. *(Feinstein, pp. 372, 381)*

12. **(A)** Resistance to penicillin has increased significantly in the last decade and approaches 20–30% in some areas. Third-generation cephalosporins (ceftriaxone) are a preferred antibiotic for initial treatment. After streptococcus culture sensitivities return, antibiotic therapy can be tailored depending on antibiotic susceptibilities. *(Bartlett et al., 1998, pp. 811–838)*

13. **(E)** Although testing of an animal specimen can give a diagnosis in less than 24 h, immediate treatment is indicated because the fox's behavior is clearly abnormal and highly suggestive of rabies. It is appropriate after such an attack to begin preventive treatment immediately for presumptive rabies exposure. In 1999, the Immunization Practices Advisory Committee (ACIP) confirmed that recommended postexposure prophylaxis is a five-shot series of immunizations given over 28 days. A dose of rabies-specific immunoglobulin, calculated by weight, is given with the first immunization. One-half of the dose is administered in the area of the bite(s), the remainder in the gluteus. In the United States, no cases of rabies have occurred after prompt and complete postexposure

prophylaxis. Observation of wildlife for rabies is never indicated because the period in which rabies may be communicable is unknown. *(CDC website: www.cdc.gov; Wallace and Doebbeling, pp. 351–352)*

14. **(E)** CF is an autosomal-recessive disorder. The CF gene has been mapped to chromosome 7q3.1. To date, more than 150 gene mutations causing CF have been identified, although the mutation designated delta F508 accounts for approximately 70% of the gene mutations in a White population. Most laboratories analyze 38–31 mutations for diagnosis or carrier screening. This is sufficient to identify 90–95% of mutations in a White population. The frequency of mutations in a Black population is approximately 1 in 65, and is rare in an Asian population. Each of this couple has a 1 in 25 chance of carrying a CF gene. The probability that both carry a CF gene is $(1/25)^2$, or 1 in 625. As an autosomal-recessive disorder, 1 in 4 children will have CF if both parents carry a CF gene. Thus, the empiric probability that this couple will have an affected child is the product of the probability that both carry a CF gene and the 25% probability that the child will inherit the CF gene from both parents: 1/625 times 1/4 or 1 in 2500. As carrier screening becomes more available, routine testing for CF carrier status is becoming the standard of care for all pregnant women. *(Creasy and Resnick, pp. 927–928)*

15. **(D)** Prostaglandin inhibition is the key to control of primary dysmenorrhea. Even the dysmenorrhea associated with endometriosis is thought to be secondary to excess prostaglandin formation. Nonsteroidal anti-inflammatory drugs (NSAIDs) such as ibuprofen and others are usually effective in controlling the pain of primary dysmenorrhea (pain with menstruation in the absence of pelvic pathology). Inhibition of ovulation with oral contraceptives, depot medroxyprogesterone acetate, or a gonadotropin-releasing hormone agonist is also effective. Oral contraceptives decrease prostaglandin synthesis by causing atrophy and decidualization of the endometrium. Relief of dysmenorrhea may be enhanced by the combined use of oral contraceptives and an NSAID taken on a scheduled basis, i.e., the woman is instructed to begin the NSAID with the onset of premenstrual symptoms and continue on a scheduled (not prn) basis until she is far enough into her menstrual cycle that the dysmenorrhea usually disappears. Bromocriptine and corticosteroids have no discernible effect on ovulation or the production of prostaglandins and are ineffective in relieving primary dysmenorrhea. Although fluoxetine or other selective serotonin reuptake inhibitors (SSRI) are useful to treat the premenstrual syndrome (PMS) or the premenstrual dysphoric disorder (PMDD), these are ineffective in relieving dysmenorrhea. The presence of pelvic pathology, such as a pelvic mass or nodularity of the uterosacral ligaments suggesting endometriosis, should be evaluated before prescribing medication. The preferred method of evaluation of suspected pelvic pathology is a diagnostic laparoscopy. *(Speroff and Fritz, pp. 539–540)*

16. **(E)** Spontaneous pneumothorax can be seen in otherwise healthy adolescents. It presents very suddenly with chest pain and dyspnea. You would expect to hear wheezing or decreased breath sounds bilaterally if this were an exacerbation of asthma resulting in this much respiratory distress. Pneumonia and empyema would not present over such a short time. He would also be febrile. A foreign body aspiration is unlikely in this age group. *(Kliegman et al., p. 65)*

17. **(E)** Patients with sickle cell disease are at risk for overwhelming infection, especially with encapsulated organisms. This is especially true in infants and young children. The use of prophylactic penicillin has dramatically decreased this risk. It is started as soon as the diagnosis is made. He will need a pneumococcal vaccine, but it is not effective in neonates. It is usually given at age 2 years. Neonates with sickle cell disease are not at any greater risk for iron deficiency than normal infants. These patients are at higher risk for folate deficiency. However, controlled studies have not documented the need for routine folic acid supplementation, so some centers have elected to stop routine supplementation. The only caution in avoiding heat for these patients is that dehydration can exacerbate sickling. When exposed to heat, patients need to be diligent about adequate fluid intake. *(Rudolph et al., pp. 1531–1534, 2233–2234)*

18. **(B)** This is the classic presentation of splenic sequestration, which occurs in these patients in the first few years of life, before the spleen autoinfarcts. Acute chest syndrome, intussusception, and vasoocclusive crisis are not associated with severe anemia. If this were an aplastic crisis, a very low reticulocyte count would be expected. *(Rudolph et al., pp. 1532–1532)*

19. **(C)** The prevalence of severe mental retardation is spread about equally across all social classes. Mild mental retardation is seen more predominantly in children of lower social classes. Severe mental retardation has also been found to have a male excess with a male to female ratio of 1.1 to 1.4. About 30% of severe mental retardation is attributed to trisomies, and thus, although advanced maternal age is a strong predictor of trisomy, the correlation is much less than 80%. The life expectancy of persons with severe mental retardation is considerably shorter than that of the general population. *(Wallace and Doebbeling, pp. 1049–1051)*

20. **(B)**

21. **(B)**

22. **(B)**

Explanations 20 through 22

Clinical features of spontaneous esophageal perforation (Boerhaave syndrome) include acute onset of excruciating pain after straining, such as in the case of vomiting. Associated clinical findings may include subcutaneous emphysema, fever, hypotension, tachycardia, and dyspnea. Initial treatment includes resuscitative efforts to stabilize the patient. The diagnostic test of choice is a contrast study of the esophagus. A CT scan is helpful in atypical presentations or to demonstrate related complications. Esophagoscopy is rarely needed to diagnose a perforation. Analysis of the pleural fluid may be suggestive of a perforation, but radiologic studies would be required to make a definitive diagnosis. Time to definitive treatment is the factor that most influences outcome. Poorer survival has been noted in patients in whom a delay in treatment of more than 24–48 h has occurred. *(Townsend et al., pp. 1110–1115)*

23. **(B)** The main characteristic of the ordinal scale is that the categories have a logical or ordered relationship to each other. This type of scale permits the measurement of degrees of difference, but not the specific amount of difference. The intervals between dimensional scales have distinct measurable differences between them that look at specific quantifiable amounts of difference, i.e., 1, 2, 3, 4 h. A binary scale has only two categories, i.e., male, female, yes, no, and so forth. In a nominal scale the categories have no rankings or relationship to each other, i.e., blue, black, brown, categories for eye color. Categorical is similar to nominal. *(Feinstein, pp. 10–13)*

24. **(C)** The median is useful when looking at longitudinal data when the data set is still incomplete. The median survival time is the length of survival that is met or exceeded by 50% of the study population. The median does not incorporate the values at the extremes and therefore will not be affected by the remaining values that are still not recorded. The mean takes into account all values and therefore cannot be calculated at this time. There is not enough information provided to determine whether a mode can be calculated on this example. If there are more than three study participants with a particular survival time, the lengths of the remaining study participants will be irrelevant, but if the maximum number of participants with a particular survival time is less than 3, we will have to wait and find out what the remaining survival times are. The midrange is calculated by dividing the sum of the minimum and maximum items by two. The maximum value is still unknown, therefore the midrange cannot be calculated yet. Midmode is not a statistical measure of central tendency. *(Feinstein, p. 31)*

25. **(B)** Short-acting benzodiazepines especially, such as alprazolam, can produce significant

symptoms when abruptly discontinued, a sign of physiologic dependence. Mild symptoms can include anxiety, irritability, sleep disruption, tremor, and nausea; the development of paranoia, depression, delirium, and seizures are serious complications of sudden drug withdrawal. The likelihood of significant withdrawal symptoms increases with dosage, length of treatment, and shorter half-life. *(Kaplan and Sadock, pp. 1027–1028)*

26. **(D)** Most cases of travelers' diarrhea are due to *E. coli*. *Shigella* and *Salmonella* infections occur in the United States as well. *Vibrio* is obtained from eating undercooked seafood. *Campylobacter* is a common cause of diarrhea in many areas, and is particularly common in children under 5 years and in college-aged people. *(Braunwald et al., p. 836)*

27. **(C)** The EDD is calculated according to Naegele's rule by adding 7 days to the first day of the LMP, then subtracting 3 months. For this to be accurate, the woman must have reasonably regular menstrual intervals of 28–32 days. The mean duration of pregnancy is 266 days from conception or 280 days from the first day of the last menses if menstrual intervals are about 28 days. An ultrasound should be done between 14 and 20 gestational weeks (estimated from uterine size) in women with an uncertain LMP or irregular menstrual intervals. *(Scott et al., p. 5)*

28. **(C)** The uterine fundus in pregnancy does not grow beyond the pelvis until after 12 postmenstrual weeks. Subsequently, gestational age can be estimated from fundal height in two ways. At 14, 16, and 18 weeks, the uterus is palpable one-fourth, one-half, and three-fourths the distance from the symphysis pubis to the umbilicus. The fundus is palpable at the level of the umbilicus at 20 gestational weeks. Between 16 and 36 weeks, the distance from the symphysis pubis to the uterine fundus (in cm) approximates the weeks' gestation. *(Scott et al., p. 8)*

29. **(C)** The CT scan shown in Fig. 8-2 demonstrates a smooth, biconvex lens-shaped mass in the periphery of the right temporoparietal region. This picture is characteristic of a subdural hematoma that is a result of laceration of veins bridging the subdural space. Unlike an epidural hematoma, which expands quickly and progresses rapidly to coma, a subdural hematoma is initially limited in size by increased intracranial pressure and expands slowly. Symptoms may follow the inciting trauma by several weeks. Altered mental status is often more prominent than focal signs and may progress from confusion to stupor to coma. Treatment consists of evacuation of the clot via burr holes. Antibiotics and antifungal agents have no role, and fibrinolytic therapy or delay in treatment could be harmful. *(Braunwald et al., pp. 2436–2438)*

30. **(E)** The most effective strategies for preventing heterosexual transmission of HIV are abstinence or having sex with an uninfected partner in a mutually monogamous relationship. Studies have also shown that consistent and correct use of latex condoms is highly effective in preventing the sexual transmission of HIV infection. The strongest evidence for this comes from studies of couples in which one member is known to be infected with HIV and the other is known to be initially uninfected. In a 2-year study, 124 couples of this sort reported consistent condom use during about 15,000 episodes of intercourse. None of the seronegative partners became infected with HIV. In contrast, in couples who used condoms inconsistently, 10% of the initially uninfected partners acquired HIV infection over the same time period. That rate is similar to the rate of HIV transmission in nonusers of condoms. Condoms made from natural membrane (lamb cecum) are more porous to viral particles than are latex condoms. Condoms treated with nonoxynol-9, contrary to expectations, have not been demonstrated to decrease likelihood of HIV transmission. Exposure of latex to petroleum products causes it to deteriorate and to tear more easily. *(Wallace and Doebbeling, pp. 1196–1197)*

31. **(E)** One of the major developmental tasks of adolescence is the acquisition of independence from the parents. Spending time in their own personal space is a part of this. Although prevalent adolescent problems, such as abuse, pregnancy, and drug abuse, can also result in withdrawal from the family, some change in their functioning at school would be expected. If she were hypothyroid, you would expect to see some changes in her physical examination. *(Rudolph et al., pp. 224–226)*

32. **(D)** The patient has the typical CSF findings of bacterial meningitis, with elevated WBCs and a predominance of neutrophils, elevated protein, and decreased glucose. These values would not be expected in patients with tuberculosis or enteroviral meningitis. Typical bacteria that cause meningitis in this age group are *S. pneumoniae* and *Neisseria meningitidis*. Group B *Streptococcus* is the most common bacterial cause of meningitis in neonates. Group A *Streptococcus* does not commonly cause meningitis. *(Kliegman et al., pp. 955–965)*

33. **(C)**

34. **(D)**

Explanations 33 and 34

Pyogenic hepatic abscesses may occur following intraabdominal sepsis, such as diverticulitis. A typical presentation may include fever, abdominal pain, anorexia, and nausea of relatively short duration, along with an elevated WBC and elevation in liver function tests. The most sensitive imaging procedure is the CT scan. An ultrasound is a very useful screening test, especially for suspected biliary tree abnormalities, but may be limited in obese patients or those with nonhomogeneous livers. Radionuclide imaging studies are not as useful as CT or ultrasound. The treatment of pyogenic abscesses includes both antibiotics and drainage. Percutaneous drainage of most hepatic abscesses is safe and effective. Surgical drainage is advised for patients exhibiting signs of continued sepsis despite percutaneous drainage and appropriate antibiotics. *(Greenfield et al., pp. 958–959; Townsend et al., pp. 1534–1539)*

35. **(E)** Symptoms of conduct disorder must begin before the age of 13 for the diagnosis to be made, and 3 of 15 behaviors must have been present including: bullying, truancy, cruelty to or hurting animals, threatening or intimidating others, often initiating fights, cruelty to people, stealing or raping, purposeful firesetting, lies to or cons others, staying out at night despite parents prohibiting, and running away from home. Differential diagnoses include mood disorders, psychotic disorders, and oppositional defiant disorder. Children with oppositional defiant disorder do not typically violate the rights of others where those with conduct disorder do. Children with conduct disorder are more likely to develop antisocial personality disorder, but this disorder cannot be diagnosed till adulthood. Tay-Sachs disease is a disorder which is caused by a defect of the enzyme hexosaminidase A and leads to seizures and spasticity. *(Kaplan and Sadock, pp. 1167, 1232–1238)*

36. **(B)** Almost 10% of boys 18 years of age or younger meet the diagnostic criteria for conduct disorder. Although this prevalence rate is significantly higher than in girls, the incidence of the disorder actually is higher in postpubertal girls than in postpubertal boys. Parental alcoholism, sociopathy, neglect, or absence can predispose to the development of conduct disorder in their children. In some children, hyperactivity precedes the emergence of conduct disorder. Various etiologic factors contributing to the development of conduct disorders have been explored. These include attempts to define specific neurologic factors. One such theory states that there is decreased noradrenergic functioning in conduct disorder. The enzyme dopamine beta-hydroxylase, which converts dopamine to norepinephrine, has been found to be in low levels in the plasma of some children with conduct disorder. In addition, it has been found that attention deficit disorder and conduct disorder often coexist in some children. Other studies indicate the probability of psychosocial etiologic factors, including having parents with serious psychopathology, substance abuse, and alcohol abuse disorders. The number of boys with the disorder is higher, and the age of onset is younger (for boys, 10–12 years vs. 14–16 years for girls). *(APA, pp. 93–99; Kaplan and Sadock, pp. 1234–1238)*

37. (G) Amenorrhea and galactorrhea are usually concurrent findings in women with significantly increased prolactin concentrations. The differential diagnosis of hyperprolactinemia is: thyroid dysfunction resulting in increased hypothalamic thyrotropin-releasing hormone secretion, certain psychotropic and antihypertensive medications, a pituitary tumor, and idiopathic. Although it is uncertain that this patient has a pituitary adenoma, this is the most likely diagnosis in her situation of anestrogenic amenorrhea and galactorrhea. A serum prolactin concentration exceeding 100 ng/mL (normal is usually less than 20) is associated with a pituitary adenoma in at least 80% of these women. This woman should have a serum prolactin concentration measured, and then a CT scan or MRI of her pituitary if the prolactin concentration is this high. Tumors develop as a result of chronic lactotrope stimulation (or chronic suppression of dopamine secretion from the hypothalamus). First-line treatment is oral bromocriptine (Parlodel) or cabergoline (Dostinex). *(Speroff and Fritz, pp. 429–436)*

38. (I) Hypertension in a sexually infantile woman with primary amenorrhea is 17α-hydroxylase deficiency until proven otherwise. This is an autosomal-recessive disorder in which cortisol, androgen, and estrogen secretion is deficient. The gene for 17α-hydroxylase is on chromosome 10q24, and a variety of mutations result in the clinical picture seen in this woman. The mineralocorticoid pathway is the only steroid biosynthetic pathway that is not impaired. Mineralocorticoid (11-desoxycorticosterone, corticosterone, and aldosterone) secretion is increased because the decreased cortisol causes an increased, adrenocorticotropic (ACTH) hormone secretion. Serum pregnenolone and progesterone concentrations will be elevated, while 17-hydroxypregnenolone and 17-hydroxyprogesterone concentrations will be low. Treatment is glucocorticoid replacement to suppress high levels of ACTH. *(Speroff and Fritz, p. 352)*

39. (C) Irregular menstrual intervals in women with signs of androgen excess (hirsutism, temporal balding, voice changes, clitoral enlargement, and so forth) suggest a functional rather than a neoplastic disorder if the problem is chronic and dates from the time of puberty. The absence of a family history, normal BP, and a normal DHEAS level eliminate 21-hydroxylase deficiency. Deficiency of 17α-hydroxylase causes sexual infantilism, not hirsutism. Moderate increases in serum prolactin levels may cause irregular menses, but not hirsutism. Sertoli–Leydig cell tumor is the only other hyperandrogenic disorder listed. Clinical presentation of women with this tumor is usually abrupt onset of amenorrhea and unilateral ovarian enlargement. *(Speroff and Fritz, pp. 470–475)*

40. (J) Postpartum amenorrhea in a woman with a history of hypertension and hemorrhage is most likely the result of pituitary necrosis and inability to secrete gonadotropins (FSH and luteinizing hormone). Prolactin secretion is also impaired, and lactation is not possible in these women. ACTH and thyroid-stimulating hormone (TSH) secretion may also be impaired, and this woman should be evaluated with an AM serum cortisol and TSH concentration. *(Speroff and Fritz, p. 438; Yen and Jaffe, pp. 521–522)*

41. (L) Key to making the diagnosis of Turner syndrome (gonadal dysgenesis) is the recognition that 150 cm (4 ft, 11 in.) is short. Streak gonads (i.e., gonadal dysgenesis) should be the first consideration in any woman with primary amenorrhea who is under 5 ft tall. Other signs of gonadal dysgenesis in this young woman are the webbed neck, cubitus valgus, shield chest and wide spaced nipples, heart murmur, and others. A karyotype should be obtained to confirm the diagnosis and ensure that there is no Y chromosome. The presence of a Y chromosome requires removal of the gonads because these women have about a 30% chance of developing a gonadal tumor, such as gonadoblastoma. The increased FSH concentration confirms that this woman's amenorrhea is the result of gonadal failure, not hypothalamic-pituitary failure. *(Speroff and Fritz, p. 445; Yen and Jaffe, pp. 367–371)*

42. (K) Testicular feminization is a disorder in which 46,XY individuals lack androgen receptors or have androgen receptors that do not respond normally to adult male levels of testosterone secretion. This disorder is also known as complete androgen insensitivity. The gonads are testes and are located intraabdominally or in hernia sacs in the inguinal canals. A cervix and uterus are absent because the testes secreted Müllerian duct inhibiting factor during early embryonic life. Because of the risk of a testicular tumor, they should be removed. Orchiectomy can safely be delayed until puberty is complete in subjects with the complete form of testicular feminization. The testes should be removed soon after the diagnosis is made in those with partial forms of androgen insensitivity, because variable degrees of masculinization will occur beginning at the time of puberty. These women require estrogen replacement after removal of the gonads to maintain breast development and prevent osteoporosis. Sparse pubic hair indicates that this is not Müllerian agenesis. In Müllerian agenesis, the karyotype would be 46,XX. *(Speroff and Fritz, pp. 338–342, 349)*

43. (B) The triad of a pregnancy, endometrial trauma, and endometrial infection in a woman who subsequently becomes amenorrheic is almost pathognomonic of endometrial sclerosis (Asherman syndrome). No treatment is necessary unless the woman wants to conceive. Treatment consists of lysing the intrauterine adhesions by hysteroscopy, insertion of an IUD or pediatric foley catheter into the uterus and high-dose estrogen therapy (e.g., conjugated estrogens 2.5 mg daily) for 4–8 weeks. The IUD prevents uterine adhesions from reforming by keeping the opposing walls of the endometrium apart. The estrogen stimulates growth and proliferation of any endometrium still present. *(Speroff and Fritz, p. 419)*

44. (E) The most common cause of amenorrhea in women of reproductive age is pregnancy. Breast soreness, fatigue, and increased urinary frequency are symptoms of pregnancy. A sensitive pregnancy test should be done on all amenorrheic women of reproductive age, even if the possibility of pregnancy is denied. The cyanosis of the vaginal epithelium is Chadwick sign, a sign of pregnancy that appears at about 6 postmenstrual weeks. It is doubtful that postpill amenorrhea is a frequent disorder. Available evidence demonstrates that conception rates after stopping oral contraceptives are similar to those of women who did not use a contraceptive. If amenorrhea persists for 3–6 months or longer after stopping oral contraceptives, it should be evaluated, just as it would under any circumstance. *(Cunningham et al., pp. 22–29)*

45. (F) Premature ovarian failure is suggested by the presence of hot flashes, failure to menstruate after medroxyprogesterone acetate, physical evidence of estrogen deficiency (dry vaginal epithelium and no cervical mucus), and increased FSH concentrations. This disorder affects approximately 1% of all women under 40 years of age. Ten percent of women with secondary amenorrhea and as many as 28% of women with primary amenorrhea will have some form of premature ovarian failure. Most have premature menopause secondary to depletion of oocytes. However, approximately 20% of women with premature ovarian failure will have either the gonadotropin-resistant ovary syndrome or autoimmune ovarian failure. In these women, there are a normal number of oocytes for their age, and pregnancy is theoretically possible, although extremely unlikely. Chemotherapy, radiation therapy, galactosemia, and overwhelming ovarian infection are other causes of premature ovarian failure. Treatment is hormone replacement with estrogen and progestin. *(Speroff and Fritz, pp. 412–414)*

46. (H) Abrupt cessation of menses coincident with or followed shortly by signs of masculinization suggest the possibility of a virilizing ovarian tumor, especially if one ovary is enlarged significantly more than the other. The most common virilizing tumor in women of reproductive age is a Sertoli–Leydig cell tumor. The degree of masculinization is variable and seems to depend on the number of testosterone-producing interstitial cells present in the tumor. A pure Sertoli cell tumor will not cause signs of masculinization. It is commonly stated that testosterone concentrations less than 200 ng/dL suggest a functional process, whereas concentrations greater than 200 ng/dL suggest a tumor. This is a reasonable clinical guide, but with many exceptions. *(Speroff and Fritz, pp. 983–984; Hoskins et al., pp. 1082–1085; Copeland, pp. 1397–1398)*

47. **(D)** Abuse of anabolic steroids is most likely to be associated with the development of such manic-like symptoms as euphoria, irritability, and reckless behavior. Depression can result from drug withdrawal, and suicides have occurred. Abuse of anabolic steroids can produce drug dependence. *(Stoudemire [1998a], p. 414; Kaplan and Sadock, pp. 466–468)*

48. **(E)** Although prior administration of human immunoglobulin containing anti-HAV before or within 2 weeks after exposure is 75–85% effective, prior immunization against hepatitis A is even more effective. A two-dose vaccination schedule is 95% effective in preventing disease in adolescents and adults. Immunity is believed to last at least 10 years, and perhaps 20 or 30 years. Consuming untreated water and uncooked food in endemic areas is a risk factor; therefore, relying on bottled water and cooked food is reasonable. However, this will not protect against contact with younger children who often have subclinical infections and remain significant sources of disease transmission. Pepto-Bismol and ciprofloxacin are preventive treatments for travelers' diarrhea. *(Wallace and Doebbeling, pp. 76–77, 175–178)*

49. **(B)** Diaper dermatitis is a very common problem in infants. This infant's rash is due to bullous impetigo. The classic presentation of this illness is erythema of the skin, followed by the development of bullae that rupture. Allergic dermatitis and irritant dermatitis are most prominent on the convex areas and are intensely red. *Candida* dermatitis is red without bullae and has satellite lesions at the margins. In seborrheic dermatitis, children tend to have the rash on the scalp, neck, and face also. It is scaly and more prominent in the intertriginous areas. *(Hurwitz, pp. 34–38)*

50. **(C)** Diaper dermatitis is a very common problem in infants. This infant's rash is due to *Candida*. *Candida* dermatitis is red without bullae and has satellite lesions at the margins. It is common in infants, especially when they have been on antibiotics. In bullous impetigo, the skin is initially erythematous and then bullae develop. Allergic dermatitis and irritant dermatitis are most prominent on the convex areas and are intensely red. In seborrheic dermatitis, children tend to have the rash on the scalp, neck, and face also. It is scaly and more prominent in the intertriginous areas. *(Hurwitz, pp. 27–29)*

51. **(D)**

52. **(C)**

Explanations 51 and 52

Fibroadenoma represents the most common breast tumor in young women. They are usually well defined, mobile, and firm on examination. Invasive ductal carcinoma is much less frequent in this age group. Ductal carcinoma *in situ* is usually nonpalpable, but may on occasion present as a mass. Fibrocystic changes can present as a mass, but a well-defined mass identified by sonography is more suggestive of fibroadenoma. Intraductal papillomas have an average size of 3–4 mm and are rarely palpable. Excisional biopsy is not necessary for all fibroadenomas, and the patient should be given the option of observation if the physical examination, imaging studies, and needle biopsy (triple test) are all benign. *(Greenfield et al., pp. 1345–1346; Donegan and Spratt, pp. 71–73, 329–330)*

53. **(B)** Syphilis is a sexually transmitted infection caused by the bacterium *Treponema pallidum*. After an average incubation period of 21 days, a painless papule forms and gradually forms a clean ulcer (chancre). The secondary stage begins about 4–8 weeks after the appearance of the primary chancre. Malaise, sore throat, fever, and headache are common. The diagnosis can be made by dark-field examination and serologic testing (serologic test for syphilis [STS], Venereal Disease Research Laboratory [VDRL], fluorescent treponemal antibody-absorption test for syphilis [FTA-ABS]). Leprosy may present with hypopigmented macules, plaques, or papules, but fever and headache are not typical symptoms. Chancroid presents with an inflammatory macule that forms a pustule and then ulcerates. Adenopathy may be noted with chancroid, but fevers and headaches are not typical. The gram-negative organism responsible for chancroid (*H. ducreyi*) may be obtained by culture. The history of a genital ulcer followed by the rash pictured should raise the suspicion of syphilis as the most likely cause. *(MMWR, pp. 18–25)*

54. **(C)** Erythema migrans is the exanthem seen in Lyme disease. It starts as a red macule or papule and then expands to an annular plaque with a raised border. It is seen 3–5 weeks after the tick bite at the site of the bite. Patients often have systemic symptoms at the same time. Erythema marginatum is the exanthem in acute rheumatic fever. It is also an annular lesion that usually occurs on the trunk. This patient does not have the other symptoms consistent with rheumatic fever. Contact dermatitis is not annular but intensely erythematous and shaped according to the offending article, such as in a necklace shape if the patient is allergic to a metal necklace. Erythema multiforme classically has target lesions. Tinea corporis is also annular, but has central clearing and is typically not as large as erythema migrans. *(American Academy of Pediatrics, pp. 329–330; Hurwitz, pp. 306–310)*

55. **(C)** Neonates are exposed to herpes at birth if the mother has a genital infection. Transmission of the infection to the infant is much more likely if the infection is primary. The characteristic lesions are grouped vesicles on an erythematous base. They are likely to occur at a traumatized location such as the scalp if a monitor has been used during delivery. Varicella also is vesicular, but one would expect to see numerous lesions, which usually start on the trunk. GBS and *Staphylococcus* can cause cellulitis in the newborn, but the rash would not be vesicular. Exanthems are common with enterovirus but are macular and are present all over the body. *(American Academy of Pediatrics, pp. 309–318)*

56. **(A)** Erythema infectiosum (fifth disease) is caused by parvovirus. This patient has the typical presentation with a prodromal illness, followed by the characteristic "slapped-cheek" rash on the face and the reticular rash on the extremities. Kawasaki disease is diagnosed clinically. Patients have fever, conjunctivitis, adenopathy, oral changes, and rash and are usually ill. Measles presents with the classic triad of the three Cs—conjunctivitis, coryza, and cough—followed by the rash. Roseola usually occurs in infants. Patients have several days of high fever, followed by a rash on the trunk, which is macular or maculopapular. The rash in scarlet fever is a fine papular rash (sandpaper-like). *(Rudolph et al., pp. 1058–1059, 1221–1224)*

57. **(A)** Folic acid in doses of 0.4–1 mg daily reduce the risk of a NTD, such as spina bifida, from approximately 1 in 1000 to 1 in 2000 when begun 1–3 months before conception and continued through the first 3 months of pregnancy. Over-the-counter multivitamins typically contain 0.4 mg folic acid, whereas prescription prenatal vitamins typically contain 1 mg. Folic acid prevents or corrects a macrocytic, megaloblastic anemia. Women who previously delivered an infant with a NTD should begin 4 mg/day folic acid at least 1 month before conception and continue this dose until 12 weeks' gestation to reduce the risk of a recurrent NTD. The dose may then be reduced to 1 mg daily because closure of the embryonic neural tube is complete by this time. The primary reason to prescribe a prenatal vitamin is to provide 60–65 mg elemental iron daily, rather than the 25–30 mg in most over-the-counter multivitamins. *(Creasy and Resnick, p. 938)*

58. **(E)** The primary syphilitic lesion or chancre starts as a papule and over several weeks develops into a small plaque with an erosive surface. It occurs at the site of penetration of the treponemes and is most commonly found on the genitalia. It is not painful. Herpes infection lesions are typically grouped vesicles on an erythematous base. Lesions from trauma and staphylococcal infections would be painful. Lesions from condylomata acuminata are soft, flesh-colored, and nodular. *(Hurwitz, pp. 302–305)*

59. **(G)** These are the classic history and physical findings seen in Prader–Willi syndrome. Typical features are obesity, almond-shaped eyes, and narrow bifrontal diameter. Patients also have severe neonatal hypotonia, hypoplastic genitalia, small hands and feet, polyphagia, and mental retardation. It is inherited sporadically, and many affected individuals have an abnormality of chromosome 15. *(Rudolph et al., pp. 2022, 2303)*

60. **(D)** This child has fetal alcohol syndrome. The facial features shown include narrow palpebral fissures; a short nose with a broad, low bridge; midfacial hypoplasia; and a long philtrum with a narrow vermilion border. Associated anomalies are cleft palate; cardiac malformations (especially atrial and ventricular defects); hearing loss; and joint, skin, and skeletal abnormalities. There are also varying degrees of growth failure and developmental delay. The severity of the defects seems to be proportional to the amount of alcohol consumed during the pregnancy. *(Rudolph et al., pp. 775–778)*

61. **(D)** Psoriasis is a chronic skin disease characterized by well-demarcated, erythematous papules and plaques covered by flakes or scales. Common sites of involvement are the scalp, back, extensor surfaces of the knees and elbows, perianal region, and genitalia. Psoriasis is associated with nail dystrophy (pits, grooves, or crumbling), arthritis (usually monarthric, involving the digits), and acute anterior uveitis (common to the human lymphocyte antigen [HLA]-B27–related diseases). The other skin findings do not have any association with nail pitting. *(Freedberg et al., pp. 407–415)*

62. **(A)** This smear demonstrates sickling of red blood cells. Sickle cell anemia is caused by the homozygous state for the abnormal beta-globin chain gene, resulting in the production of hemoglobin S (Hb S) rather than normal Hb A. During deoxygenation, polymerization of Hb S occurs, resulting in sickled red cells. These cells lead to hemolysis, splenic and hepatic red cell sequestration, and occlusion of microvasculature, the latter being responsible for the pain symptoms. *(Braunwald et al., pp. 669–671)*

63. **(C)** An epidural hematoma most commonly occurs in the temporoparietal region as a result of hemorrhage from the middle meningeal artery. There may be an initial brief loss of consciousness secondary to a concussive event, followed by a variable lucid interval. As the hematoma expands and exerts a mass effect, there is a deteriorating level of consciousness, with tentorial herniation and eventual midbrain compression. The patient develops an ipsilateral dilated fixed pupil and contralateral hemiparesis. Therefore, this patient with a dilated right pupil and left hemiparesis has a right epidural hematoma. An occipital intracranial hematoma will present with visual defects. A subdural hematoma develops from injury to the dural venous sinuses, with an acute subdural hematoma presenting with signs of rapidly increasing intracranial pressure and herniation. Subarachnoid hemorrhage is associated with a severe headache and photophobia, without a significant alteration in level of consciousness. *(Greenfield et al., p. 2144)*

64. **(C)** The hematopoietic form is most commonly seen at radiation levels of 2–10 Sieverts. The main phase of the illness is seen about 3–6 weeks after exposure and can consist of weakness leukopenia and thrombocytopenia. If bone marrow suppression is significant, then resulting death from infection and/or hemorrhage may occur. The cerebral form of acute radiation syndrome occurs at exposures of greater than 50 Sieverts. This form usually presents with nausea, vomiting, diarrhea, and headache. Coma, convulsions, and death may also occur on the first day. The gastrointestinal form is seen at exposure rates of 10–20 Sieverts and can have effects that present up to 2 weeks after exposure. The pulmonary form occurs at exposures of greater than 6 Sieverts of irradiation to the lung tissue. Effects are most commonly seen about 30–90 days after exposure. If significantly extensive, it can result in respiratory failure, pulmonary fibrosis, or cor pulmonale. Renal forms are not commonly recognized as one of the main forms of acute radiation syndrome. *(Wallace and Doebbeling, pp. 621–624)*

65. **(A)**

66. **(B)**

67. **(D)**

68. **(G)**

Explanations 65 through 68

Ischemic colitis after aortic aneurysm repair is a result of ligation of the inferior mesenteric artery, with compromise to the perfusion of the distal colon. It is associated with crampy lower abdominal pain, and bloody stools from mucosal sloughing. Bleeding from a gastrointestinal source above the ligament of Treitz (such as a peptic ulcer) will result in melena, which is characterized by tarry, foul-smelling stools. Meckel's diverticulum presents with painless rectal bleeding in children. Diverticulosis is the most common cause of massive rectal bleeding, which is usually bright red and painless. Colonic polyps may be singular or multiple, and usually bleed at the time of stooling, or when the polyp sloughs spontaneously. Patients with ulcerative colitis may have diarrhea, abdominal cramps, and weight loss, with a clinical course that may be associated with a severe exacerbation. With severe colitis, there is increased frequency of bloody stools, and signs of systemic toxicity (fever and leukocytosis). Carcinoma of the colon should be suspected in a patient presenting with rectal bleeding and a history of a change in bowel habits. *(Greenfield et al., pp. 1144–1158; Way and Doherty pp. 736–737)*

69. **(D)** Sinus arrhythmia is a normal variant that is common in pediatric patients. It usually varies with the respiratory cycle, slowing with expiration. On the strip, each normal QRS wave is preceded by a normal P wave. This excludes the diagnosis of atrial premature beats that would have premature P waves that were shaped differently. Patients with sick sinus syndrome usually have episodes of tachycardia and episodes of sinus arrest. In sinoatrial block, the sinoatrial pacemaker is discharging, but occasionally the impulse does not depolarize the atria. The strip shows pauses that approximate the normal P-P interval. This patient does not have a tachycardic rhythm, and patients with supraventricular tachycardia usually have symptoms of palpitations or a sensation of their heart racing. *(Rudolph et al., pp. 1853–1854)*

70. **(E)** Because this is a normal variant, no further diagnostic testing is necessary. *(Rudolph et al., p. 1853)*

71. **(D)**

72. **(B)**

Explanations 71 and 72

A direct blow to the epigastrium compresses the duodenum against the vertebral column, with a shearing injury resulting in an intramural hematoma. With the breakdown of hemoglobin in the hematoma, there is an increase in the oncotic pressure and imbibement of fluid into the hematoma, leading to progressive obstruction. This can contribute to the delay in presentation, which is commonly several days after the initial injury. Bilious vomiting is secondary to obstruction at the junction of the second and third parts of the duodenum. There may be mild hyperamylasemia, related either to the duodenal wall injury or to an associated pancreatic injury. Pancreatitis from blunt abdominal trauma usually presents at the outset with progressive abdominal tenderness and significant elevation of serum amylase. There is often a delay in the diagnosis of small bowel perforation, with the development of tachycardia, fever, and peritonitis on abdominal examination. Gastritis is usually secondary to an acute infectious agent, and cholecystitis occurs in the presence of cholelithiasis. Patients with obstruction from intramural duodenal hematoma are managed with nasogastric decompression and parenteral nutrition. In the majority of cases, the obstruction will resolve in 7–10 days. Operative intervention is not usually required. *(Townsend et al., pp. 515–517; Way and Doherty, pp. 253–254; Greenfield et al., pp. 347–348)*

73. **(E)** Obsessive-compulsive disorder is characterized by obsessions, which are recurrent and persistent intrusive thoughts which often lead to compulsions, repetitive behaviors, such as hand washing, that the person feels driven to perform in response to the obsession. Generalized anxiety disorder is characterized by chronic, excessive, and uncontrollable worry about multiple life circumstances, often accompanied by concentration problems and muscle tension, but unrelated to obsessions. Panic disorder is characterized by discrete episodes of intense anxiety, often coupled with a fear of dying, which may occur out of the blue. They are sometimes accompanied by agoraphobia (a fear of going into areas, such as shopping malls, where the panic attacks have occurred). A specific phobia is an unreasonable fear of a particular item, such as fear of spiders. *(Kaplan and Sadock, pp. 616–623)*

74. **(B)** Fluoxetine and other SSRIs are effective in the treatment of obsessive-compulsive disorder, as is the highly serotonergic tricyclic antidepressant clomipramine. Benzodiazepines such as lorazepam and clonazepam may reduce anxiety in patients with obsessive-compulsive disorder, but do not alleviate the core symptoms of the disorder. Such antipsychotic medications as haloperidol and risperidone are not effective alone in the treatment of obsessive-compulsive disorder, but in selected patients with tics, schizotypal features, or delusions in addition to their obsessive-compulsive symptoms, the addition of an antipsychotic to an SSRI may be useful. *(Kaplan and Sadock, pp. 622–623)*

75. **(C)** False labor or Braxton Hicks contractions occur at irregular intervals and usually last 30 s or less. Although they may cause slight cervical dilation and effacement, only true labor will cause the amount of cervical dilation and effacement present in this woman. The first stage of labor is defined as the interval from onset of regular uterine contractions sufficient to cause cervical dilation to complete cervical dilation, 10 cm. The first stage is subdivided into a latent phase and active phase. The latent phase is characterized by slow cervical dilation of 1 cm/h or less. When the rate of cervical dilation increases to 1.5 cm/h or greater, the woman is in the active phase of the first stage of labor. The second stage of labor is the interval from complete cervical dilation to delivery of the infant. The third stage is the interval from delivery of the infant to delivery of the placenta. *(Cunningham et al., pp. 252, 310)*

76. **(D)** Station of the presenting part is divided between –3 and +3. At –5, the presenting part is above the pelvic inlet. At 0 station, the presenting part is at the level of the ischial spines. Stations –4 to –1 are between the pelvic inlet and ischial spines. At +5 station, the presenting part is visible at the perineum, eventually even between contractions. Stations +1 to +4 are between the ischial spines and perineum. Descent of the presenting part progresses from –5 to +5 station. *(Cunningham et al., pp. 311–312)*

77. **(A)** The diagnosis of HIV infection depends on the demonstration of antibodies to HIV and/or the direct detection of HIV or one of its components. The standard screening test for HIV is an ELISA, which detects antibodies to HIV. Antibodies to HIV generally become detectable in the circulation 4–12 weeks after infection. The sensitivity of the ELISA test approaches 100% in persons with clinical AIDS. The specificity of the ELISA test is generally above 99.5%. This means that among 1000 normal persons, up to 5 may be expected to be falsely identified as being seropositive for HIV. In a study of a group of volunteer blood donors, for example, only 13% of ELISA-positive individuals truly had HIV infection. (The positive predictive value of the test was 13%.) The individual described in this question is from an even lower risk group, for which the positive predictive value of the ELISA test would be even lower, meaning that an even larger proportion of positives would be false-positives. Factors associated with false-positive ELISA tests include large exposure to many antigens, as in receiving multiple transfusions, and having autoantibodies, hepatic disease, or recent influenza vaccination. Positive results thus must be confirmed. A person initially testing positive with an ELISA test should first have the ELISA test repeated. If it is still positive, confirmatory testing should be done with a test such as a Western Blot. A negative Western Blot allows one to conclude with certainty that the ELISA reactivity was a false-positive. Clinicians should have these tests performed only at qualified laboratories. *(Wallace and Doebbeling, p. 157; USPSTF, 2nd ed., Screening: HIV, pp. 303–317)*

78. (A)

79. (E)

Explanations 78 and 79

This patient presents with symptoms and signs of a small-bowel obstruction, most probably from intraabdominal adhesions related to previous abdominal surgery. The diagnosis is strongly suspected on the basis of the clinical presentation. Appropriate initial management should, therefore, include nasogastric decompression to prevent further distention from swallowed air, and initiation of IV fluid resuscitation before obtaining abdominal radiographs. Analgesics may mask physical signs of impending bowel ischemia. A barium enema may be helpful in patients with suspected colonic obstruction, but should not be obtained before resuscitation and plain radiographs. This patient does not have a history of constipation, and, therefore, enemas and stool softeners are not indicated. This patient has clinical and radiographic signs of a complete small-bowel obstruction. Because of the risk of intestinal ischemia, surgery is indicated after initial resuscitative maneuvers to correct fluid and electrolyte abnormalities. Continued nonoperative management is appropriate only in patients with partial obstruction who show continued clinical improvement when reexamined. A rectal tube or colonoscopy is not indicated for a small-bowel obstruction, and a "long tube" (Cantor tube) has no additional advantage over standard nasogastric decompression. *(Townsend et al., pp. 1334–1340; Way and Doherty, pp. 683–687)*

80. (B) The pincer grasp is attained in the second 6 months of life. Ninety percent of children can do this by age 10 months. The milestone of object constancy (the understanding that an object continues to exist even if the child does not see it) occurs around 9 months. The infant then recognizes the difference between people he knows well and strangers, which leads to the development of stranger anxiety. Ninety percent of infants can stand with support by 10 months. Between 8 and 10 months, babbling becomes more complex, with "mama" and "dada" used nonspecifically. *(Behrman et al., pp. 43–44)*

81. (E) Retinal hemorrhages in young children, when seen with other evidence of trauma, especially when the history is not consistent with the physical examination, are pathognomonic of child abuse. Kernig's sign is a sign of meningeal irritation and is seen with meningitis. The rooting reflex is normal in infants. Overlapping cranial sutures can be a normal finding shortly after a vaginal birth. They also can occur when the infant has microcephaly. Neck tenderness could be due to abuse or accidental trauma and of itself does not suggest abuse. *(Rudolph et al., pp. 2176, 2238)*

82. (D) At birth, the average hemoglobin is 17 g/L because of the relatively hypoxic intrauterine environment. After birth, the PaO_2 rises, and erythropoiesis decreases. Red cell life span is shorter at this time as well. These two processes lead to the physiologic nadir in hemoglobin that occurs around 2 months of age. Iron deficiency is the most common anemia in childhood but is not typically seen until after 6–12 months. Lead toxicity is not seen until children can put objects in their mouths. The patient could have a congenital hemolytic anemia with a normal hemoglobin, but this is much less likely. Transfusion is not indicated in this patient unless there are symptoms or signs of cardiac failure. *(Kliegman et al., pp. 803–817)*

83. (C) A cross-sectional study is a survey, and is appropriate to answer this question. Cross-sectional studies often produce biased results. Subjects selected for survey may not be representative of the desired population, or only an unrepresentative subset of those selected may actually respond to the survey (selection bias). Subjects, interviewers, or test instruments may systematically record information in an unrepresentative manner (information bias). The effect of an extraneous variable may be mixed with the effect of the studied exposure on the studied disease (confounding). Trials and cohort studies generally refer to prospective studies. A case-control study generally identifies a group of individuals with an uncommon disease and compares the historical profiles of those "cases" with those of disease-free individuals who otherwise are generally comparable. *(Gordis, pp. 173–174; Greenberg and Daniels, pp. 144–150)*

84. **(B)** Early return to appropriate work is associated with improved functional outcome. Opportunities to change posture frequently improve tolerance and outcome in low back pain. Carrying weight close to the waist and without bending moderately increases pressure on intervertebral disks. Extended forward reach, bending at the waist, and sitting do markedly increase pressure on the lumbar intervertebral disks. *(Wallace and Doebbeling, pp. 652–657)*

85. **(D)** This is a classic case of condyloma (venereal warts). Condyloma acuminatum is caused by the HPV. Because this is a sexually transmitted disease (STD), women with condyloma should be screened for other STDs, such as gonorrhea, *Chlamydia*, syphilis, and possibly hepatitis B and C. Annual Pap smears are crucial, because several strains of HPV are associated with a high risk of developing cervical dysplasia or neoplasia (HPV types 16/18, 45, and 46). Venereal warts are usually caused by strains of HPV yielding a low to intermediate risk of cervical dysplasia or neoplasia, but women can be infected with more than one strain of HPV. *(MMWR, pp. 53–59)*

86. **(E)** The woman has a classic picture of condyloma acuminata. There is no persuasive evidence that transmission occurs in any manner other than sexual. This is caused by one or more strains of HPV. A biopsy or excision is not necessary to establish the diagnosis. However, there are several circumstances when a biopsy should be done: the diagnosis is uncertain (e.g., similar lesions in older women may be verrucous carcinoma), the lesions do not respond or worsen with standard therapy, the patient is immunocompromised, or the warts are pigmented, indurated, fixed, and ulcerated. No data support the use of type-specific HPV nucleic acid testing. There is no evidence that the presence of vulvar condylomata is associated with an increased risk of cervical cancer. However, certain strains of HPV are associated with cervical dysplasia or carcinoma (types 16, 18, 31, 33, and 35). It is uncertain if medical or surgical therapy to reduce the viral DNA load affects future transmission. *(MMWR, pp. 53–55)*

87. **(E)** Liquid-based cytology diagnosed 36% to more than 200% more cases of low-grade squamous intraepithelial lesion (LSIL) than the conventional slide technique of Pap smears. However, the degree of improved sensitivity with liquid-based Pap smears and the difference in specificity from slide-based cytology is uncertain. With liquid-based cytology the remaining liquid (commonly retained 2–4 weeks) can be assayed for HPV serotypes in women with an atypical squamous cells of undetermined significance (ASCUS) to ascertain the presence of high-risk serotypes for cervical dysplasia and cancer. Women with LSIL or high-grade squamous intraepithelial lesion (HSIL) Pap smears are presumed to have exposure to high-risk strains of HPV. In a review of the literature since 1950, 57% of patients with CIN I underwent spontaneous regression whereas only 1% of women with CIN I progressed to invasive cervical cancer. In programs with organized and systematic screening for cervical cancer, there was little advantage of annual Pap smears over a Pap smear every 2–3 years. The American College of Obstetricians and Gynecologists currently recommend annual Pap smears until age 30. Women over 30 who have had three consecutive negative Pap smears may then be screened every 2–3 years. More frequent screening should be continued for women with certain risk factors for cervical dysplasia or cancer: women with HIV, immunosuppressed women, and women exposed to DES *in utero*. While cigarette smoking appears to decrease the risk of endometrial cancer, the risk of cervical cancer is increased in these women. *(Creasy and Resnick, pp. 11–17; Stenchever et al., pp. 869–872)*

88. **(B)** Tardive dyskinesia is a frequent side effect of long-term administration of typical antipsychotics and presents with involuntary, irregular choreoathetoid movements of the tongue, mouth, and sometimes limbs and the trunk. *(Kaplan and Sadock, p. 995)*

89. **(E)** Being homeless is not a known risk factor for tardive dyskinesia, but length of treatment and increased dose of dopamine receptor antagonist medication, increasing age, female sex, and the presence of mood disorder all are risk factors for development of tardive dyskinesia. *(Kaplan and Sadock, p. 995)*

90. **(C)** Vitamin E, propranolol, diazepam, and others all have varied effects on the disordered movements of tardive dyskinesia, but none have been entirely effective. Benztropine is not effective for tardive dyskinesia but is used quite effectively for other extrapyramidal effects of the neuroleptics, such as tremors, pseudoparkinsonism, and the dystonias. Switching from a dopamine receptor antagonist to a serotonin-dopamine antagonist (quetiapine) would be the best treatment option of those given. Newer antipsychotics, such as olanzapine, risperidone, ziprasidone, aripiprazole, and quetiapine, seem to have little extrapyramidal effects and may offer successful treatment of psychosis without risk of tardive dyskinesia. Ideally, a discontinuation of all antipsychotics would prevent the worsening of the movement disorder. The dire effects of this on the psychotic disorder, however, make it a rare option. *(Kaplan and Sadock, pp. 995, 1051–1066; Stoudemire [1998a], pp. 178–179, 645–647)*

91. **(B)** Triazolam is a high potency benzodiazepine and short acting benzodiazepine that has been associated with anterograde amnesia. *(Kaplan and Sadock, p. 1027)*

92. **(C)**

93. **(E)**

Explanations 92 and 93

In Figs. 8-2, a group of vesicles with early central crusting on a red base can be seen on the shaft of the penis. This is characteristic of genital herpes simplex. Syphilis is usually a painless chancre that develops into an ulcer. Lymphogranuloma venereum is an organism that belongs to the *Chlamydia* group of parasites. The primary genital lesion is a small painless papule that heals spontaneously. Condyloma acuminatum is a wart caused by HPV that may be pinpoint or cauliflower-like. Herpes zoster represents reactivation of the varicella-zoster virus and is not sexually transmitted. Patients with genital herpes need to be warned that infection can be transmitted even when asymptomatic. Shedding of the organism does not stop when the lesions are gone. Patients should refrain from sexual activity while the lesions are present because condoms are not reliably protective. Patients also need to be told about the risk of having a recurrent episode. Acyclovir is the antiviral used to treat herpes. Doxycycline is the treatment of choice for lymphogranuloma venereum. *(Freedberg et al., Chap. 214)*

94. **(D)** Henoch–Schönlein purpura (HSP), the most common vasculitis of childhood, is characterized by petechiae or purpura of the buttocks and lower extremities and occasionally arthritis, nephritis, abdominal pain due to gastrointestinal bleeding, or other fasculitic complications. Remember, HSP is characterized by nonthrombocytopenic purpura. A normal platelet count rules out ITP. SLE, more commonly afflicting females, is not often encountered in children. Children with meningococcemia are acutely ill and febrile. Petechiae are not a feature of juvenile rheumatoid arthritis. *(Behrman et al., pp. 677–678)*

95. **(C)** Children with one of the salt-losing forms of congenital adrenal hyperplasia have aldosterone deficiency. In the absence of this hormone, the kidney does not retain sodium normally, and there is inappropriate retention of potassium and hydrogen ions, resulting in hyponatremia, hyperkalemia, and metabolic acidosis. The characteristic serum electrolyte aberrations observed

in patients with hypertrophic pyloric stenosis include hypokalemia, hypochloremia, and metabolic alkalosis. Children with renal tubular acidosis often present with hyperchloremic metabolic acidosis and hypokalemia. Patients with gastroesophageal reflux usually present with vomiting over several weeks. Patients with gastroenteritis usually have vomiting and diarrhea. *(Kliegman et al., pp. 301–317)*

96. **(E)** Antisocial personality disorder is characterized by an ongoing disregard for and violation of the rights of others. Patterns of these behaviors and attitudes begin in early childhood or adolescence. Persons with such a disorder fail to conform to social norms and are frequently deceitful and manipulative to achieve their aims. They are impulsive and fail to plan ahead. They also tend to be irritable and may get into physical fights as well as assaultive behaviors. *(APA, pp. 701–706; Stoudemire [1998a], pp. 218–221)*

97. **(G)**

98. **(C)**

99. **(F)**

100. **(A)**

Explanations 97 through 100

Sinus headache is usually acute in onset, worse on awakening, better on standing, and can worsen on bending over. Often, there is a purulent nasal discharge and pain over the involved sinus. Subarachnoid hemorrhage is often described as "the worst headache of my life" and is very abrupt in onset. Cluster headache predominantly occurs in middle-aged men, and its typical presentation involves intense unilateral headache that is searing, stabbing, and accompanied by ipsilateral lacrimation, nasal stuffiness, and facial flushing. Alcohol is believed to be a precipitant, although alcohol is well tolerated between attacks. Migraine headache is more common in women, and usually begins in childhood or young adult life. Migraine may or may not have an aura, but is unilateral, of pulsating quality, and accompanied by nausea or vomiting, photophobia, or phonophobia. Subdural hematoma is also a subtle condition with earlier head trauma that may be forgotten until the patient displays mental status changes or focal neurologic deficits. A patient with a brain tumor may be asymptomatic other than headache initially, but usually neurologic deficits will be found as the time progresses. Muscle contraction headache is typically worse as the day goes on, bilateral in the frontotemporal area, and described as a tight band around the head. *(Rowland, pp. 36–38)*

101. **(B)** The arteriograms in Fig. 8-20 demonstrate a large aneurysm arising from the basilar artery. Intracranial aneurysms occasionally present with new onset or worsening of headaches or may be asymptomatic and found coincidentally during evaluation of an unrelated disorder. Frequently, they leak or rupture, resulting in a subarachnoid hemorrhage with sudden onset of severe headache and meningeal symptoms and signs (e.g., nuchal rigidity, photophobia). Rapid progression to stroke, coma, or death may follow. Intracranial aneurysms are not associated with hypercalcemia, hypopituitarism, or chronic meningitis and rarely cause tentorial herniation without rupturing. Surgical approaches to intracranial aneurysms include excision and ligation. *(Giammarco et al., pp. 131–138)*

102. **(D)** Surgical procedures are classified into four categories, based on the risk of wound infection. Elective colon surgery with an adequate bowel preparation, and no spillage of gastrointestinal contents, is classified as a clean-contaminated (class II) procedure. In this patient, there was an incomplete, and hence, inadequate bowel prep, with resultant soilage at surgery, converting this to a class III contaminated procedure. *(Townsend et al., pp. 258–259, 301–303)*

103. **(D)**

104. **(C)**

105. **(D)**

Explanations 103 through 105

Evaluation of postoperative fever should begin with a thorough clinical history and examination of the patient. Empiric cultures and antibiotic therapy are not indicated and are not cost-effective. Therapy should be targeted at clearly identified foci. Atelectasis is the most common cause of postoperative fever in the first 24–48 h. It is managed with aggressive pulmonary toilet, chest physiotherapy, ambulation, and adequate pain control. Postoperative wound infection usually presents between the 5th and 10th postoperative days, with fever, increased incisional discomfort, wound erythema, and purulent drainage. Management is directed at opening the wound for adequate drainage and local wound care. Therapy with antibiotics is not usually required if adequate drainage is achieved. A urinary tract infection may develop postoperatively, but usually does not present before the third to fifth postoperative day. There is an increased risk in patients with indwelling urinary catheters for greater than 5 days.

Nosocomial pneumonia is a significant problem in the surgical patient but does not usually present in the first few days after elective surgery. Patients with inadequate pain control, poor pulmonary toilet, and prolonged preoperative hospitalization are at greater risk. Intraabdominal abscess may develop as a complication after colonic surgery, either as a consequence of intraoperative fecal contamination, or as a result of an anastomotic leak. Established pelvic infection does not usually present before the fifth to seventh postoperative day. Management options include percutaneous CT-guided drainage. *(Townsend et al., pp. 267–268, 299–303, 305–307; Way and Doherty, pp. 25–26, 36)*

106. **(C)** As many as 15–40% of women have GBS in their lower genital tract. The overall attack rate for early onset neonatal sepsis is 1–2 per 1000 births. In women whose lower genital tracts are known to be colonized, the attack rate is 1–2%. Because of the low attack rate and the high rate of recolonization after antibiotic treatment, antibiotic therapy of the initial positive culture is neither beneficial nor cost-effective. For the same reason, a repeat culture and treatment of a positive culture at 36 weeks is not justified. There is no evidence that a cesarean section reduces the probability of neonatal GBS sepsis. The woman who is likely to benefit the most from intrapartum antibiotic prophylaxis is one who has a known positive culture and one or more of the following risk factors *(Creasy and Resnick, pp. 674–677)*:

- preterm labor (37 weeks)
- preterm, premature rupture of the membranes (37 weeks)
- prolonged rupture of the membranes (18 h)
- sibling affected by symptomatic GBS infection
- maternal fever during labor

107. **(E)** Two statistics are given to express failure rates of a contraceptive method: the failure rate with perfect use and the failure rate with typical use (both rates after 1 year of use). The latter is the most relevant because nonsterilization methods are not always used, or are used incorrectly. Reported failure rates with typical use are:

- oral contraceptives 3%
- IUD 0.1–2.0%
- condoms 14%
- female sterilization 0.05–1.0%
- male sterilization 0.15%

The best answer is male sterilization because of the widely reported failure rates with female sterilization. This variation depends on such factors as experience of the surgeon, type of tubal sterilization procedure, age of the woman (fertility declines with age), frequency of coitus and others. The Mirena (levonorgestrel impregnated) IUD has a lower failure rate than the Copper T-380 (ParaGard), as reflected in the figures given above. *(Speroff and Fritz, p. 829; Stenchever et al., p. 542)*

108. **(A)** Ecologic studies compare groups not individuals. The unit of observation in the above study was a community not individuals. A cross-sectional study design would have looked at the incidence of asthma in those who also owned a particular home heating system at a particular point in time. A cohort study would have taken disease-free individuals in the community who also owned the home heating system and followed them over time to see who developed disease. A case-control approach would have taken individuals with and without asthma and identified how many from each group also had the particular home heating system. A randomized clinical trial would have randomly selected certain families to live in homes with the two different heating systems and would have monitored outcomes after a set period of time. *(Wallace and Doebbeling, pp. 18-19; Gordis, pp. 204–205)*

109. (C) Children usually reach 50% of their expected adult height by the age of 2 years. Additionally, at 2 years of age, children reach approximately 20% of their expected adult weight and 85% of their expected adult head circumference. *(Behrman et al., p. 43)*

110. (D) Many healthy children have intermittent proteinuria that can be quite substantial and can be exaggerated by vigorous exercise. In those in whom it is intermittent and not accompanied by hematuria, chronic renal disease is unusual. A child who has proteinuria on a single specimen, thus, will need repeated urinalyses to establish the intermittent nature of the finding. Careful examination of the sediment to look for red blood cells and casts should also be performed. BP should be determined at each visit. Some clinicians also suggest protein determinations on 12-h specimens, collected while these children are active and again while they have been resting for 12 h, thus establishing the link to exercise. If proteinuria remains intermittent, most physicians do not perform invasive procedures such as a biopsy. Proteinuria alone is unlikely to be an indicator of urinary tract infection or structural kidney disease; thus, an IVP and urine culture are unlikely to be helpful. Likewise, with isolated and intermittent proteinuria as the only abnormality, BUN and creatinine levels are highly unlikely to be abnormal. *(Rudolph et al., pp. 413–420)*

111. (B) Lung abscesses are localized cavities with pus. They are usually a result of aspiration of infected material from the upper airway and often associated with periodontal disease or poor oral hygiene. The most common pathogens are anaerobes. Penicillin is the drug of choice for most of these anaerobic infections. *(Kasper et al., pp. 942–945, 1536–1537)*

112. (B) Prevalence is the number of affected persons in a population divided by the total number of persons in the population at that time. Incidence is the number of new cases of a disease that occur during a specified period of time within a population at risk. Both require knowledge of population numbers. Calculation of prevalence requires knowledge of the total number of individuals in the population from which the cases arose. Calculation of incidence requires knowledge of the total number of individuals in the population at risk at the beginning of the study. *(Gordis, pp. 35–37)*

113. (D) The ECG demonstrates T-wave inversions in II, III, and AVF, inferior wall leads. About one-third of patients with inferoposterior wall left ventricular infarction have some degree of right ventricular necrosis, and an occasional patient has extensive right ventricular MI. The predominant clinical feature of right ventricular MI is severe right ventricular failure with jugular venous distention but no pulmonary vascular congestion, Kussmaul's sign (increased jugular venous distention with inspiration), and often hypotension. The mainstay of treatment is volume expansion. Pressor agents, preload and afterload reducing drugs, and intraaortic balloon counterpulsation may also be required. *(Kasper et al., pp. 1416, 1456)*

114. (C)

115. (A)

116. (C)

Explanations 114 through 116

The patient seems to have pyelonephritis. Treatment is directed toward treating the most commonly acquired community organism, *E. coli*, and ensuring good hydration. Many pediatric textbooks also recommend initial treatment in the hospital for all patients less than 1 year of age. In this patient, because she is vomiting and has signs of dehydration, initial management with IV fluids and antibiotics is indicated. Aggressive therapy for pyelonephritis is especially critical for younger patients because their risk for renal scarring is the greatest. Pediatric patients with pyelonephritis are relatively likely to have an anatomic abnormality or vesicoureteral reflux. A renal ultrasound and voiding cystourethrogram are done to check for these. A renal scan could also be used to detect anatomic abnormalities but is more expensive and exposes the patient to radiation, which ultrasound does not. *(Kliegman et al., pp. 403–411)*

117. **(A)** Clozapine is a relatively new antipsychotic used in treatment-resistant schizophrenia, as well as in patients who experience severe extrapyramidal side effects of tardive dyskinesia with the standard antipsychotic drugs. Unfortunately, agranulocytosis occurs in 1–2% of patients treated with clozapine. Immediate discontinuation of the drug is required because this condition can be fatal. Monitoring of the WBC, starting off weekly, has been required since clozapine has been available. Because most cases occur within the first 6 months of clozapine treatment, there is hope that in the future this requirement will be eased. *(Kaplan and Sadock, pp. 1070–1074)*

118. **(H)** Trazodone, an antidepressant drug, is used not only for depression, but also for sleep because of its sedating properties. It is associated with the rare occurrence of priapism, a prolonged erection in the absence of sexual stimulation. If not treated early, the condition may develop into an emergent situation. *(Kaplan and Sadock, pp. 1123–1125)*

119. **(C)** Haloperidol is a butyrophenone antipsychotic drug with a high degree of extrapyramidal effects. The oculogyric syndrome is an example of an extrapyramidal effect called a dystonia. Thioridazine, a piperidine phenothiazine, has some potential to cause extrapyramidal symptoms, but this is significantly less than that seen with haloperidol. *(Kaplan and Sadock, pp. 497, 1053)*

120. **(E)** Lithium carbonate is a naturally occurring salt used as a mood stabilizer in the treatment of bipolar disorders. Because of the potential for toxicity, periodic monitoring of blood level is required. In addition, monitoring is required to confirm a blood level within the therapeutic range, usually 0.6–1.2 meq/L. As serum levels rise above 1.5 meq/L, symptoms of toxicity emerge in a somewhat predictable manner from early signs such as nausea, vomiting, and diarrhea to more severe signs of coarse tremor, ataxia, lethargy, and coma. Sensitivity to the significance of observable clinical signs provides a means for the clinician to identify toxicity, even though a blood level is not immediately available. *(Kaplan and Sadock, pp. 1067–1074)*

121. **(G)** Thioridazine causes retrograde ejaculation in men. This is harmless, but nevertheless a cause of embarrassment. *(Kaplan and Sadock, p. 1057)*

122. **(K)**

123. **(I)**

124. **(C)**

125. **(B)**

126. **(J)**

Explanations 122 through 126

The most common cause of lower respiratory infections in infants is RSV. It commonly presents during the winter months with rhinorrhea and wheezing. Infants typically are afebrile. Adenovirus can present with wheezing but more typically also includes conjunctivitis and pharyngitis. *Mycoplasma pneumoniae* is the most common cause of pneumonia in school-aged children. The typical course is a gradual onset of fever, cough, and malaise. *S. pneumoniae* can cause pneumonia in this age group but typically presents more acutely. *C. trachomatis* is the most common cause for conjunctivitis in the first few months of life. Infants acquire it at birth from their mothers. In some infants, it progresses to pneumonitis with the classic "staccato" cough.

Adenovirus can cause a respiratory infection as well as conjunctivitis, but the two symptoms occur concurrently. Pertussis presents with an insidious prodrome over several weeks, which is difficult to differentiate from other upper respiratory infections, except that it lasts longer. The second phase is the paroxysmal phase, with the episodic cough that can be quite severe. Although pertussis vaccine is in widespread use, the disease is relatively common. The reservoir of infection is typically adults whose immunity has waned. Many pathogens cause respiratory infections in children. In this patient, the course is too long for a typical viral infection and not acute enough for bacterial pneumonia, such as that caused by GBS. Croup is a common respiratory infection that occurs in the autumn. The typical course is a few days of cough, rhinorrhea, and low-grade fever, followed by the onset of paroxysms of barky or seal-like cough. It is typically worse at night and resolves in 2 days. The most common cause is parainfluenza virus. *(Kleigman et al., pp. 43–69)*

127. (D)

128. (E)

Explanations 127 through 128

Treatment must to be prompt, because death can occur within minutes with a severe anaphylactic reaction. Administration of subcutaneous or IV epinephrine should be given as soon as possible to control symptoms. Beta blockers are relatively contraindicated. Topical steroids are of no benefit, and IV steroids are not effective for the acute event, but may help later recurrence of bronchospasm. Diphenhydramine is appropriate for urticaria, but is second to epinephrine. Type 1 immediate hypersensitivity reactions are characterized by early symptoms such as urticaria, laryngeal edema, bronchospasm, and vasomotor collapse. They result from mast cell or basophil binding by IgE (not IgA) or activated complement fragments C3a or C5a (so-called anaphylatoxins). A persistent delayed rash is not seen with type 1 reactions. The early cutaneous hypersensitivity response of wheal and flare is seen within 15 min and resolves in about 90 min. Foods, bee stings, drugs, and pollens are examples of inciting agents. Extrinsic (but not intrinsic) asthma is an example of a type 1 allergic reaction. *(Kasper et al., pp. 1949–1952)*

129. (A) This pattern of loss is typical for very mild noise-induced hearing loss. The employee would, if exposed to loud noise on the job and in the OSHA-mandated Hearing Conservation Program, be fitted with and provided with hearing protection, trained in hearing conservation, and returned to work. Obstruction with cerumen would decrease hearing more profoundly and at all frequencies. An acoustic neuroma generally produces a rapidly progressive (and soon more profound) hearing loss that is unilateral and may be associated with new onset of tinnitus. Middle ear infection may cause some temporary loss at all frequencies, and generally can be revealed by history and otoscopic examination. Ototoxins generally cause loss in a pattern similar to that of presbycusis, in which most loss occurs at the highest frequencies. *(Rom, pp. 1345–1355; McCunney, pp. 381–393; LaDou, pp. 112–118)*

130. (B) The ST-T segment elevation in the anterior and lateral leads (V_2–V_6, I, AVL) in this ECG is indicative of an acute anterolateral wall MI. Acute pericarditis causing ST segment elevation would cause ST-T elevation in all of the leads. An acute inferior wall MI would show changes in the inferior leads (II, III, AVF) and not ST-T elevation in the anterolateral leads. Pulmonary embolism and congestive heart failure would not typically cause focal ST-T elevation. *(Kasper et al., pp. 1316–1318)*

131. (A) This patient is young and has no risk factors for coronary artery disease. Specifically, his cholesterol profile is excellent, and he has no family history of coronary disease. Cocaine would be most likely in this patient as the cause of the infarct. *(Kasper et al., p. 1410)*

132. (D) This man has been poisoned with an organophosphate insecticide such as parathion. Organophosphates are the most common cause of insecticide poisonings. Symptoms may develop during or up to about 12 h after exposure. Respiratory, dermal, and gastrointestinal absorption routes are all possible. Organophosphates lead to nicotinic, muscarinic, and central nervous system overstimulation. DUMBELS (diarrhea, urination, miosis, bronchospasm, emesis, lacrimation, and salivation) is a mnemonic for the muscarinic (cholinergic) signs seen with organophosphate poisoning. Atropine is an anticholinergic agent. *(Rom, pp. 1157–1163; LaDou, pp. 186–187)*

133. **(C)** Medicare (Title 18 of the Social Security Act) covers people aged 65 and older, and the permanently and totally disabled persons, and people with end-stage renal disease. It is a federal program divided into part A (paying for hospital services according to DRGs) and part B (paying physician services according to RBRVSs). Medicaid (Title 19 of the Social Security Act), covers people who are needy by providing a minimum set of services. It is a federal-state program with benefits that vary from state to state. *(Wallace and Doebbeling, p. 1128)*

134. **(B)**

135. **(D)**

136. **(A)**

137. **(B)**

138. **(C)**

139. **(C)**

140. **(D)**

Explanations 134 through 140

The multiaxial diagnostic system of DSM-IV-TR is used to code information about several facets of a patient's condition. Clinical psychiatric disorders, other than personality disorders and mental retardation, are coded on axis I. Chronic paranoid schizophrenia is an example of such a clinical disorder. Personality disorders (such as borderline personality disorder) and mental retardation are coded on axis II. General medical conditions, such as asthma and type II diabetes mellitus, that are potentially relevant to the understanding or management of an individual's mental disorder are coded on axis III. Psychosocial and environmental problems, such as the recent death of this patient's mother and his ejection from his group home, are coded on axis IV, and a global assessment of an individual functioning on a scale from 1 to 100 is coded on axis V. *(APA, pp. 27–35)*

Guyer B, Martin J, MacDorman M, et al. Annual summary of vital statistics—1996. *Pediatrics* 1997;100:905–918.

Hales RE, Frances AJ (eds.). *Psychiatry Update: American Psychiatric Association Annual Review*, vol. 6. Washington, DC: American Psychiatry Press, 1987.

Hatcher RA, Trussell J, Stewart F, et al. *Contraceptive Technology*, 16th ed. New York, NY: Irvington Publishers, 1994.

Hogan DE. The emergency department approach to diarrhea. *Emerg Clin North Am* 1996;14:673–692.

Hurst JW. *Medicine for the Practicing Physician*. Stamford, CT: Appleton & Lange, 1996.

Joint National Committee on Prevention, Detection, Evaluation and Treatment of High Blood Pressure. The sixth report. *Arch Intern Med* 1997;157:2413–2446.

Kasper DL, Braunwald E, Fauci A, et al. *Harrison's Principles of Internal Medicine*, 16th ed., New York, NY: McGraw-Hill, 2005.

Kelley WN. *Textbook of Internal Medicine*, 2nd ed. New York, NY: JB Lippincott, 1992.

Koehler JE. Bartonella infections. *Adv Pediatr Infect Dis* 1996;11:1–27.

Laine L, Suchower L, Connors A, et al. Twice-daily, 10-day triple therapy with omeprazole, amoxicillin, and clarithromycin for *Helicobacter pylori* eradication in duodenal ulcer disease: results of three multicenter, double-blind, United States trials. *Am J Gastroenterol* 1998;93:2106–2112.

Last JM. *Public Health and Human Ecology*, 2nd ed. Stamford, CT: Appleton & Lange, 1997.

Light RW. Parapneumonic effusions and empyema: current management strategies. *J Crit Illness* 1995;10:832–842.

McAnarney ER, Kreipe RE, Orr DP, et al. *Textbook of Adolescent Medicine*. Philadelphia, PA: W.B. Saunders, 1992.

The Medical Letter on Drugs and Therapeutics: Drugs for Treatment of Acute Otitis Media in Children, vol. 36. New Rochelle, NY: Medical Letter, 1994, pp. 19–21.

Oski FA, DeAngelis CD, Feigin RD, et al. *Principles and Practice of Pediatrics*, 2nd ed. Philadelphia, PA: JB Lippincott, 1994.

Rankin AC, Brooks R, Ruskin JN, et al. Adenosine and the treatment of supraventricular tachycardia. *Am J Med* 1992;92:655–664.

Relman DA, Schmidt TM, MacDermott RP, et al. Identification of the uncultured bacillus of Whipple's disease. *N Engl J Med* 1992;327:293–301.

Rock JA, Thompson JD. *TeLinde's Operative Gynecology*, 8th ed. Philadelphia, PA: Lippincott-Raven, 1997.

Schuchat A, Whitney C, Zangwill K. Prevention of perinatal group B streptococcal disease: a public health perspective. *Morb Mortal Wkly Rep* 1996; 45(RR-7):1–24.

Schumacher HR (ed.). *Primer on the Rheumatic Diseases*, 10th ed. Atlanta, GA: Arthritis Foundation, 1993.

National Cholesterol Education Program. Second Report of the Expert Panel on Detection, Evaluation and Treatment of High Blood Cholesterol in Adults. *Circulation* 1994;87(3):1333–1445.

Stoudemire A (ed.). *Human Behavior: An Introduction for Medical Students*, 2nd ed. Philadelphia, PA: Lippincott-Raven, 1998b.

Sweet RL, Gibbs RS. *Infectious Diseases of the Female Genital Tract*, 3rd ed. Baltimore, MD: Williams & Wilkins, 1995.

Tancredi LR. Emergency psychiatry and crisis intervention: some legal and ethical issues. *Psychiatr Ann* 1982;12:799–806.

Tecklenburg FW, Wright MS. Minor head trauma in the pediatric patient. *Pediatr Emerg Care* 1991;7: 40–47.

Tomb DA. *Psychiatry*, 5th ed. Baltimore, MD: Williams & Wilkins, 1995.

Traugott L, Alpers A. In their own hands. *Arch Pediatr Adolesc Med* 1997;151:922–927.

Wedding D. *Behavior and Medicine*, 2nd ed. St. Louis, MO: Mosby, 1995.

World Health Organization. Available at: www.who.int/en/

Yamada T, Alpers D, Owyang C, et al. *Textbook of Gastroenterology*. Philadelphia, PA: JB Lippincott, 1991.

Zais N. *The Nail in Health and Disease*, 2nd ed. East Norwalk, CT: Appleton & Lange, 1990.

Zenz C. In: Dickerson BO, Horvath EP (eds.), *Occupational Medicine*, 3rd ed. St. Louis, MO: Mosby, 1994.

Zinner MJ. *Maingot's Abdominal Operations*, 10th ed., vols. 1 and 2. Stamford, CT: Appleton & Lange, 1997.

Subject List: Practice Test 2

Question Number and Subject

OBSTETRICS AND GYNECOLOGY

14. Genetics
15. Dysmenorrhea
27. Prenatal care
28. Prenatal care
37. Amenorrhea
38. Amenorrhea
39. Amenorrhea
40. Amenorrhea
41. Amenorrhea
42. Amenorrhea
43. Amenorrhea
44. Amenorrhea
45. Amenorrhea
46. Amenorrhea
53. Infectious diseases
57. Physiology of pregnancy
75. Physiology of pregnancy
76. Physiology of pregnancy
85. Infectious diseases
86. Infectious diseases
87. Oncology
106. Perinatal infections
107. Birth control

PSYCHIATRY

25. Psychopharmacology
35. Child psychiatry/epidemiology
36. Child psychiatry
47. Psychopathology
73. Geriatric psychiatry
74. Psychopathology
88. Psychopharmacology
89. Psychopharmacology
90. Psychopharmacology
91. Psychopharmacology
96. Assessment/psychopathology
117. Psychopharmacology
118. Psychopharmacology
119. Psychopharmacology
120. Psychopharmacology
121. Psychopharmacology
134. Psychopathology
135. Psychopathology
136. Psychopathology
137. Psychopathology
138. Psychopathology
149. Psychopathology
140. Psychopathology

INTERNAL MEDICINE

12. Pharmacology
26. Gastroenterology
29. Neurology
61. Dermatology
62. Hematology
92. Infectious diseases
93. Infectious diseases
97. Neurology
98. Neurology
99. Neurology
100. Neurology
101. Neurology
111. Infectious diseases
113. Cardiovascular
127. Allergy
128. Allergy
130. Cardiovascular
131. Cardiovascular

PEDIATRICS

3. Infectious diseases
16. Structural
17. Infectious diseases
18. Circulatory

31. Child development
32. Infectious diseases
49. Infectious diseases
50. Infectious diseases
54. Infectious diseases
55. Infectious diseases
56. Infectious diseases
58. Infectious diseases
59. Genetic/structural
60. Toxic
69. Cardiac
70. Cardiac
80. Growth and development
81. Trauma
82. Hematology
94. Hematology
95. Structural
109. Growth and development
110. Metabolic
114. Infectious diseases
115. Infectious diseases
116. Infectious diseases
122. Infectious diseases
123. Infectious diseases
124. Infectious diseases
125. Infectious diseases
126. Infectious diseases

PREVENTIVE MEDICINE

4. Disease control
5. Public health/sexually transmitted disease
6. Toxicology
7. Epidemiology
8. Clinical preventive services
9. Occupational medicine
10. Clinical prevention
11. Biostatistics
13. Disease control
19. Epidemiology
23. Biostatistics
24. Epidemiology
30. Public health/sexually transmitted disease
48. Assessment
64. Occupational medicine
77. Public health/bloodborne pathogens
83. Epidemiology
84. Occupational medicine
108. Epidemiology
112. Biostatistics
129. Occupational medicine
132. Occupational medicine
133. Health services administration

SURGERY

1. Digestive system diseases
2. Digestive system diseases
20. Digestive system diseases
21. Digestive system diseases
22. Digestive system diseases
33. Infectious diseases
34. Infectious diseases
51. Oncology/breast
52. Oncology/breast
63. Trauma
65. Digestive system diseases
66. Digestive system diseases
67. Digestive system diseases
68. Digestive system diseases
71. Trauma
72. Trauma
78. Digestive system diseases
79. Digestive system diseases
102. Digestive system diseases
103. Digestive system diseases
104. Digestive system diseases
105. Digestive system diseases/infectious diseases

Index

Page numbers followed by italic *f* denote figures.